WHEATER'S
FUNCTIONAL
HISTOLOGY

For my parents, John and Isabel Young, without
whom none of this would have been possible.
B.Y.

For my parents, Frank and Vi Heath, and my brother
Graham, for their guidance and encouragement of
the pursuit of excellence.
J.W.H.

Dedicated to the memory of

Paul Richard Wheater
1951–1989

Commissioning Editor: Timothy Horne
Project Development Manager: Jim Killgore
Project Manager: Nancy Arnott
Designer: Erik Bigland
Page make-up: Kate Walshaw

WHEATER'S FUNCTIONAL HISTOLOGY

A TEXT AND COLOUR ATLAS

FOURTH EDITION BY

BARBARA YOUNG
BSc Med Sci Hons (St. Andrews), PhD (Cambridge), MB BChir (Cambridge), MRCP(UK), FRCPA

Senior Staff Specialist in Anatomical Pathology, Royal North Shore Hospital, Sydney, Australia and Clinical Senior Lecturer in Pathology, University of Sydney.

JOHN W. HEATH
BSc Hons(Melbourne), PhD (Melbourne)

Associate Professor in Anatomy, The University of Newcastle, New South Wales, Australia

WITH CONTRIBUTIONS BY

ALAN STEVENS
MBBS, FRCPath

Senior Lecturer in Histopathology, University of Nottingham Medical School, Nottingham, UK

JAMES S. LOWE
BMedSci, BMBS, DM, FRCPath

Professor of Neuropathology, University of Nottingham Medical School, Nottingham, UK

DRAWINGS BY

PHILIP J. DEAKIN
BSc Hons (Sheffield), MB ChB (Sheffield)

General medical practitioner, Sheffield, UK

THIRD EDITION BY

H. GEORGE BURKITT
BARBARA YOUNG
JOHN W. HEATH

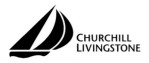
CHURCHILL LIVINGSTONE

EDINBURGH LONDON NEW YORK OXFORD PHILADELPHIA ST LOUIS SYDNEY TORONTO 2000

CHURCHILL LIVINGSTONE
An imprint of Elsevier Science Limited

First edition 1979
Second edition 1987
Third edition 1993
Fourth edition 2000
Reprinted 2000, 2001 (twice), 2002, 2003 (twice)

ISBN 0443 05612 9

International Student Edition ISBN   0443 05618 8
Reprinted 2000, 2001, 2002

British Library Cataloguing in Publication Data
A catalogue record for this book is available from the British
Library

Library of Congress Cataloguing in Publication Data
A catalogue record for this book is available from the Library
of Congress

Medical knowledge is constantly changing. As new
information becomes available, changes in treatment,
procedures, equipment and the use of drugs become
necessary. The authors and contributors and the publishers
have, as far as it is possible, taken care to ensure that the
information given in this text is accurate and up-to-date.
However, readers are strongly advised to confirm that the
information, especially with regard to drug usage, complies
with the latest legislation and standards of practice.

 your source for books,
journals and multimedia
in the health sciences
www.elsevierhealth.com

The
publisher's
policy is to use
**paper manufactured
from sustainable forests**

Printed in Spain by Grafos, S.A. Arte sobre papel

Preface to the Fourth Edition

In writing the fourth edition of Functional Histology, we have maintained the general format and approach of the previous three editions, which have proved enormously popular with both students and teachers of histology. The aim of this fourth edition is to keep the subject matter up to date and as relevant as possible to modern histology courses. Scientific and medical knowledge are constantly changing and expanding, and in particular huge advances have been made in molecular and cellular biology since the third edition. We have incorporated these into the 'functional' component of the book. We have retained the organisation of the subject matter into three sections: The Cell, Basic Tissue Types and Organ Systems, which we feel is the logical way to tackle the subject, the first two sections laying the groundwork for the third. The enlargement of the book to A4 size has been made largely to allow for larger illustrations and font size, which we feel will add to the 'user friendliness' of the book This does not signal a major increase in the text.

The retirement of George Burkitt from the authorship team has been a great loss. His abilities as a writer and his grasp of all the details in production of the book have been sorely missed in the preparation of this new edition.

In this edition we have added many new colour photomicrographs to expand and improve on the quality of the illustrations. The emphasis remains on human tissues, with animal tissues being used only where suitably fixed specimens of normal human tissue were not available. All the new light micrographs are of human tissue. Many of the superb illustrations from the first two editions have however been retained. These were photographed by the late Paul Wheater and are of such high quality that we see no need to attempt to replace them. Likewise new electron micrographs have been included, some to improve existing illustrations. The line diagrams in this edition have been extensively updated and converted to full colour format to improve clarity. New diagrams have been added to illustrate or summarise the material in the text, particularly in the area of cell biology. Another new feature of this Edition is the insertion of an 'approach to microscopy' at the beginning of Chapter 1, which we hope will be useful to students in their interpretation of images throughout the book. Several new tables have been introduced to highlight structural and functional differences in similar structures. Chapter 1 has been totally restructured to bring together light and electron micrographs demonstrating cellular components. Again the aim here is to make the book as easy to use as possible for the student. The entire text has been reviewed and updated. We have however endeavoured, as in previous editions, to avoid the inclusion of superfluous detail. In today's medical courses, far less time is devoted to the study of histology than previously and we have aimed to include all the information required for medical undergraduates and most other science students. The book is also designed so that the information is accessible for students in integrated Problem Based Learning medical courses who may need to dip into different sections of the book rather than reading from beginning to end.

We hope that the reader finds this new edition of Functional Histology a useful resource and an enjoyable read.

Sydney, Australia   B. Young
2000   J.W. Heath

Preface to the First Edition

Histology has bored generations of students. This is almost certainly because it has been regarded as the study of structure in isolation from function; yet few would dispute that structure and function are intimately related. Thus, the aim of this book is to present histology in relation to the principles of physiology, biochemistry and molecular biology.

Within the limits imposed by any book format, we have attempted to create the environment of the lecture room and microscope laboratory by basing the discussion of histology upon appropriate micrographs and diagrams. Consequently, colour photography has been used since it reproduces the actual images seen in light microscopy and allows a variety of common staining methods to be employed in highlighting different aspects of tissue structure. In addition, some less common techniques such as immunohistochemistry have been introduced where such methods best illustrate a particular point.

Since electron microscopy is a relative new technique, a myth has arisen amongst many students that light and electron microscopy are poles apart. We have tried to show that electron microscopy is merely an extension of light microscopy. In order to demonstrate this continuity, we have included resin-embedded thin sections photographed around the limit of resolution of the light microscope; this technique is being applied increasingly in routine histological and histopathological practice. Where such less conventional techniques have been adopted, their rationale has been outlined at the appropriate place rather than in a formal chapter devoted to techniques.

The content and pictorial design of the book have been chosen to make it easy to use both as a textbook and as a laboratory guide. Wherever possible, the subject matter has been condensed into units of illustration plus relevant text; each unit is designed to have a degree of autonomy whilst at the same time remaining integrated into the subject as a whole. Short sections of non-illustrated text have been used by way of introduction, to outline general principles and to consider the subject matter in broader perspective.

Human tissues were mainly selected in order to maintain consistency, but when suitable human specimens were not available, primate tissues were generally substituted. Since this book stresses the understanding of principles rather than extensive detail, some tissues have been omitted deliberately, for example the regional variations of the central nervous system and the vestibulo-auditory apparatus.

This book should adequately encompass the requirements of undergraduate courses in medicine, dentistry, veterinary science, pharmacy, mammalian biology and allied fields. Further, it offers a pictorial reference for use in histology and histopathology laboratories. Finally, we envisage that the book will also find application as a teaching manual in schools and colleges of further education.

Nottingham
1979

Paul R. Wheater
H. George Burkitt
Victor G. Daniels

Acknowledgements

Our thanks are due to many individuals who contributed material to the first two editions of this book. In particular, thanks to Paul Beck of the Department of Human Morphology for producing a large number of valuable specimens. Many of the original electron micrographs were prepared by his colleagues John Kugler and Annette Tomlinson, to whom we are deeply indebted. From the Department of Biology, University of York, Peter Crosby provided most of the scanning electon micrographs, Brian Norman provided several light microscopic sections and Dr Robert Lang produced the freeze-etched preparation used in Figure 1.5(b). The otolith specimen used in Figure 21.27(c) was lent by Mr Roger Gray FRCS, Addenbrookes Hospital, Cambridge and Professor N. Dilly, St. George's Hospital, Tooting. Donald Canwell of the Physiological Laboratory, University of Cambridge, contributed many sections from his personal collection, several of which enhanced the second edition. Dr Graham Robinson and Stan Terras of the Department of Pathology, University of Nottingham, each provided several electron micrographs, and with their colleague Linda Burns provided the thin resin sections used for light microscopy. Dr Terry Bennett of the Department of Physiology, University of Nottingham contributed figure 7.11. Dr Pat Cooke of the Department of Genetics, City Hospital, Nottingham lent the chromosome preparation used in Figure 2.2. Pathologists Dr David Ansell of City Hospital, Nottingham, Drs Hugh Rice and Peter James of Nottingham General Hospital and Dr Pauline Cooper of Addenbrooke's Hospital, Cambridge, made available various tissue specimens and slides. Peter Squires and Hugh Pulsford of Huntingdon Research Centre, Cambridgeshire, were a great help in providing the primate tissues used when suitable human tissues were unavailable. Bill Brackenbury of the Department of Pathology, University of Nottingham, performed much of the macrophotography, and Leonard Beard of the Department of Medical Illustration, Hinchingbrooke Hospital, Huntingdon, photographed the two thin sections in black and white. The remaining colour photomicrographs in the first two editions were the work of the late Paul Wheater. Special thanks also to Dr Grahame Kidd who photographed five of the new electron micrographs in the third edition.

In relation to this new edition, our profound thanks to Alan Stevens and Jim Lowe who helped with revisions in several chapters as well as supplying superb quality illustrations. Their help was vital in getting the manuscript finished on time and has added immeasurably to the quality of this new edition.

We gratefully acknowledge the help of the medical and scientific staff of the Department of Anatomical Pathology, Royal North Shore Hospital Sydney, Australia, for their tireless work in cutting and staining sections for photography. Thank you also to pathologists and trainees at Royal North Shore Hospital, who generously provided material for photography. A JEOL 1200EX electron microscope was used for all of the new electron micrographs; we are most grateful to Gary Weber for his careful maintenance of this instrument. Dr. Gerald Little kindly provided the scanning electron micrograph for Figure 12.7.

Finally, we thank our families and friends for their forbearance and support throughout this challenging project, which consumed much time.

Contents

PART ONE
THE CELL

1. Cell structure and function   2
2. Cell cycle and replication   33

PART TWO
BASIC TISSUE TYPES

3. Blood   46
4. Supporting/connective tissues   65
5. Epithelial tissues   80
6. Muscle   97
7. Nervous tissues   116

PART THREE
ORGAN SYSTEMS

8. Circulatory system   144
9. Skin   157
10. Skeletal tissues   172
11. Immune system   193
12. Respiratory system   222
13. Oral tissues   237
14. Gastrointestinal tract   249
15. Liver and pancreas   274
16. Urinary system   286
17. The endocrine glands   310
18. Male reproductive system   328
19. Female reproductive system   341
20. Central nervous system   372
21. Special sense organs   380

Notes on staining methods   406

Index   408

THE CELL

1. Cell structure and function 2
2. Cell cycle and replication   33

1. Cell structure and function

Introduction to microscopy

The study of histology, the subject of this text and atlas, is carried out using microscopes of various types in order to visualise the structure of body tissues. Structure is closely related to function and much can be deduced about the function of cells and tissues by careful examination of their component parts. Taken together with information gathered from biochemistry, physiology and other basic sciences, this study can provide a powerful tool to understand the normal functioning of the body. In addition, acquiring this knowledge is a necessary first step for the understanding of disease. Histology is about looking at structure, and in this introductory section we aim to provide some guidelines to assist the absolute beginner in examining and interpreting the images in this book.

This book mainly uses photomicrographs taken with the *light microscope (LM)* (almost all coloured images) and the *electron microscope (EM)* (black and white images). Simply put, the LM and EM differ in *optical resolution* and *available magnification.* In practical terms 'resolution' refers to the capacity of an optical system to reveal detail in a specimen. The resolution available from a conventional LM is only about 0.2 µm. Thus at distances of less than 0.2 µm, objects that are actually separate from one another will appear to merge. In contrast, EM resolution for biological specimens is as little as 1 nm so that the resolving power is about 200-fold better than LM. In addition, maximum 'available magnification' is limited to about × 1000 in most student LMs, whereas an EM readily achieves 100-fold greater magnification, or about × 100 000. EM images are therefore said to display cell and tissue *ultrastructure.*

EM images may be two- or three-dimensional

There are two types of electron microscope: *scanning EM* and *transmission EM*. Scanning EM produces three-dimensional (3-D) images, but these are restricted to the surface of the object with the internal structure concealed from view. Transmission EM is so-named because the electron beam must pass through the specimen to form an image. To achieve this, ultrathin sections (50–100 nm) must be cut. Transmission of the electron beam through the tissue results in a 2-D image of the plane of the section. In practice, transmission EM is more informative of biological ultrastructure and these images predominate in this book. We have supplemented these with scanning EM images where it helps with 3-D conceptualisation (cf. Figs 16.13 and 16.14). As a matter of convention the abbreviation EM can be assumed to be a transmission EM, while we have identified scanning EMs as SEM.

Light and electron microscopy are complementary

The strengths of LM and EM differ yet complement one another very effectively. With LM one can observe large areas of a specimen (usually several cm²). A wide range of staining methods, some empirical, some specific, are available for LM, permitting identification of cell and tissue features; many of these stains are polychromatic, i.e. they produce multiple colours in the specimen which, besides looking pretty, help to identify different components. For certain specimens, sections slightly thicker than usual may be used to demonstrate 3-D features. Thus from LM, students can expect to gain an understanding of overall cell and tissue architecture.

The superior resolution and magnification of EM permit visualisation of many features which simply cannot be seen by LM. Yet in some respects EM is less flexible than LM. For example, the available area in EM specimens is generally less than 1 mm² and this may make it difficult to obtain representative fields. Few staining methods are available for EM and these produce only monochromatic (black and white) images. EM is also costly and time-consuming and usually not available to the average student.

Hints for interpreting EMs

Interpretation of EMs can be quite challenging due to the wide range of magnifications available (× 500 – × 190 000 in this book). In other words an EM image is not necessarily of very high magnification. In fact, there is an overlap in the magnification ranges of EM and LM. It is a good idea consciously to note the magnification and/or scale bar on each image in the book.

The terms *electron-dense* and *electron-lucent* are used to describe the relative darkness and lightness, respectively, as they appear in transmission EM images. Sections examined by EM are almost featureless unless stained with heavy metals (e.g. uranium and lead salts) that bind to cell and tissue components to varying degrees. Significant binding of metal stain to a particular structure will impede transmission of the electron beam through the specimen at that point; the structure will apear dark grey or black and is said to be electron-dense (really too dense to allow passage of electrons). Other structures with little or no affinity for the stain will appear lighter grey or white and are termed electron-lucent because they permit greater transmission of the electron beam.

A useful starting point in interpreting EMs is to select several commonly found structures that you can confidently identify and memorise their dimensions. These can then be used as 'internal rulers' to gauge the dimensions of numerous other features in the field. For example, plasma membrane and organelle membranes will be visible at medium magnifications as thin electron-dense lines that measure about 10 nm wide. Thus, structures such as intermediate filaments (10 nm in diameter and solid) and microtubules (20–25 nm in diameter but hollow) can be identified. Similarly, individual ribosomes and glycogen particles are 20–30 nm in diameter. Being alert to major size differences between organelle types will instil further confidence. For example, nuclear diameter (5–10 μm in most cells) is up to 10 times greater than the diameter of lysosomes and mitochondria (0.2–1.0 μm) and up to 100 times greater than individual Golgi transport vesicles (50–100 nm). The next step is to actively look for the unique set of features that characterises and distinguishes each organelle and inclusion. For example, only mitochondria and the nucleus possess a double membrane, and in mitochondria the inner of these two membranes is thrown into highly characteristic folds.

High magnification electron micrographs are often required to demonstrate particular features but usually display only a tiny region of the cell. Therefore, do not be surprised if many of the common organelles are not seen in the field. A reliable indicator of high magnification is if an individual membrane appears trilaminar rather than as a single electron-dense line. At low magnification, EM interpretation can actually be more difficult because membranes and the smallest organelles are no longer clearly visible. Get orientated by looking first for the biggest objects, i.e. nuclei and boundaries of the cells themselves, and next for the mid-sized organelles such as mitochondria. Regions of interface between cells and extracellular tissue can give clues about tissue heterogeneity.

Specific localisation methods for LM and EM

The traditional staining techniques of histology, developed in the last century from dyes used in the textile industry, remain valuable and widely used as empirical methods for LM. Subsequently, a range of specific methods were developed, enabling LM visualisation of defined intracellular and extracellular constituents. More recently, technical refinements have allowed conceptually similar specific localisations to be achieved at EM level.

One major group of specific methods, known as *histochemical techniques*, employs reagents known to react with defined cellular constituents (e.g. lipids, glycogen and DNA) thereby producing selective colouration recognisable by LM. In a subset known as *enzyme histochemistry* the activity of enzymes can similarly be demonstrated by staining for their specific substrates or end products; these methods are often applicable for both EM and LM. A further subset, termed *immunohistochemistry*, has gained rapid acceptance. Immunologically based, this newer method offers high specificity and sensitivity of localisation. In essence, antibodies are raised against specific cellular components (in this context, the antigen) and then conjugated with a visual marker appropriate for LM or EM (e.g. dyes, enzymes, tiny particles of colloidal gold). When the antibody is then applied to the tissue under study, it binds to the antigen. Hence, the site of antibody–antigen binding becomes flagged by the chosen visual marker (e.g. Fig. 1.9; Notes on staining techniques, p. 406).

Constraints in LM and EM: aspects of tissue preparation

A problem common both to light and electron microscopy is the need to prevent autolytic degeneration and to preserve cellular ultrastructure. Fixatives such as *formaldehyde* and *glutaraldehyde* are used for this purpose. *Fixation* causes cross-linking of macromolecules, which reduces and often arrests biological activity, at the same time rendering the cells more amenable to staining. Most tissues are too thick to be examined directly in the microscope and must therefore be cut into very thin slices (*sections*). To facilitate the cutting of thin sections, the tissue is usually *embedded* in a hard medium such as paraffin wax (LM) or a plastic resin (EM); fixed tissues generally require dehydration with organic solvents before the embedding step. Each stage in the fixation, dehydration, embedding, sectioning and final staining sequence may induce *artefacts* (distortions in cell and tissue architecture, e.g. shrinkage). In situations where preservation of biological activity of cell constituents (e.g. enzymes) is the major objective, thin sections for histochemistry can be obtained from minimally fixed or unfixed frozen tissue; such *frozen sections* have their own peculiar artefactual distortions. As noted above, unstained sections are quite lacking in contrast when viewed by conventional LM or EM. However, special types of LM (*phase contrast, interference contrast*) have been developed to address this limitation and are frequently used, for example, to monitor living tissue cultures.

Introduction to the cell

The cell is the functional unit of all living organisms. The simplest organisms such as bacteria and algae consist of a single cell. More complex organisms consist of many cells held together by connections between cells, and between cells and *extracellular matrix* (e.g. the matrix of bone). The cells of multicellular organisms, such as humans, show a great variety of functional and morphological specialisations which have developed during the process of evolution by amplification of one or other of the basic functions common to all living cells. Despite this extraordinary range of morphological forms, all *eukaryotic* cells conform to a basic structural model, which is the subject of this chapter. Students will be well aware that the term *eukaryote* refers to the group of organisms whose cells have a defined nucleus surrounded by a nuclear membrane. This group includes most living organisms other than bacteria. *Prokaryotes* (mainly bacteria) have some major structural differences and are not discussed here. The process by which cells assume specialised structure and function is known as *differentiation.*

Even with early light microscopy, it was evident that cells are divided into at least two components: the *nucleus* and the *cytoplasm.* As microscopical techniques advanced it became increasingly obvious that both the cytoplasm and nucleus contain a number of subcellular elements, called *organelles.*

Fig. 1.1 **The cell** *(illustration opposite)* EM × 15 000

The basic structural features common to all cells are illustrated in this electron micrograph of a hormone-secreting cell from the pituitary gland. All cells are bounded by an external limiting membrane called the *plasma membrane* or *plasmalemma* **PM** which serves as a dynamic interface between the internal environment of the cell and the external environments. In this particular example, the cell interacts with two types of external environment: adjacent cells **C** and intercellular spaces **IS**. The functions of the plasma membrane include transfer of nutrients and metabolites, attachment of the cell to adjacent cells and other structures, and cell–cell communications. These functions depend to some extent on the specialised nature of the cell.

The nucleus **N** is the largest organelle and its substance, often referred to as the *nucleoplasm*, is bounded by a membrane system called the *nuclear envelope* **NE**. The cytoplasm contains a variety of organelles, most of which are also bounded by membranes. An extensive system of flattened membrane-bound tubules, saccules and flattened cisterns, collectively known as the *endoplasmic reticulum* **ER**, is widely distributed throughout the cytoplasm. A second discrete system of membrane-bound saccules, the *Golgi apparatus* **G**, is typically located close to the

nucleus. Scattered free in the cytoplasm are a number of relatively large, elongated organelles called *mitochondria* **M** which have a smooth outer membrane and a convoluted inner membrane system. In addition to these major organelles, the cell contains a variety of other membrane-bound structures, an example of which are the numerous, electron-dense *secretory vesicles* **V** (in this case containing hormone) seen in this micrograph.

Thus the cell is divided into a number of membrane-bound compartments, each of which has its own particular biochemical environment. Membranes therefore serve to separate incompatible processes. In addition, enzyme systems are found embedded in membranes so that membranes are themselves the site of many specific biochemical reactions.

The cytoplasmic organelles are suspended in a fluid medium called the *cytosol* in which many metabolic reactions take place. Within the cytosol, there is a network of minute tubules and filaments, collectively known as the *cytoskeleton*, which provides structural support for the cell and its organelles, as well as providing a mechanism for transfer of materials within the cell and movement of the cell itself.

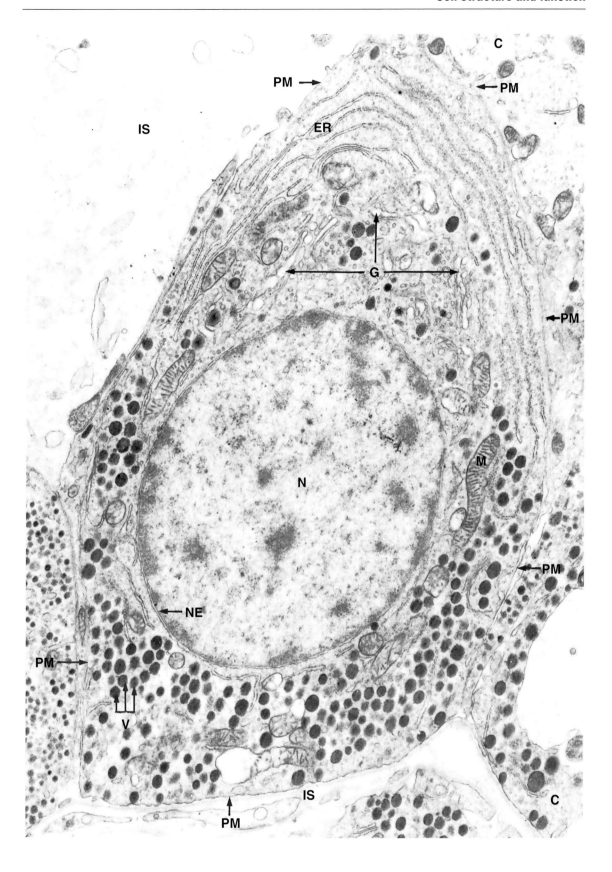

Functional Histology

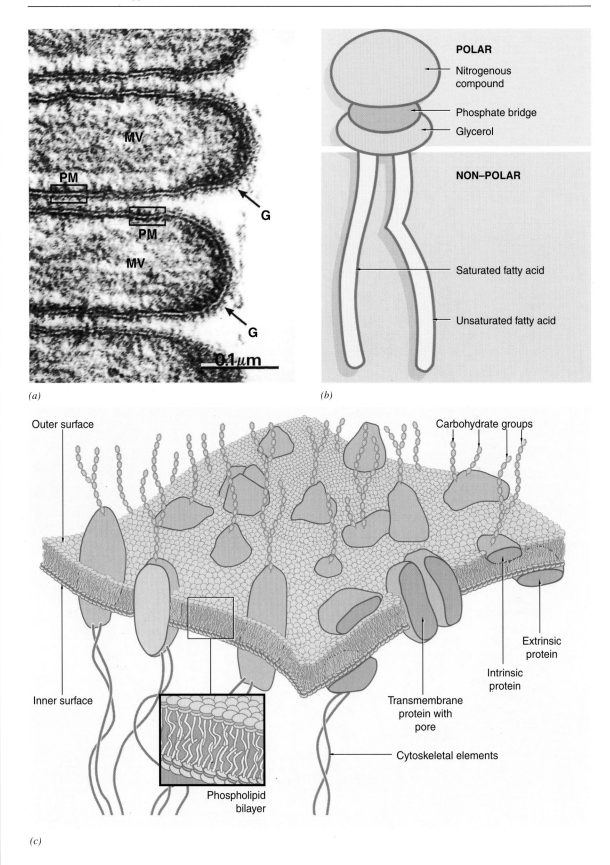

(a)

(b)

POLAR

Nitrogenous compound

Phosphate bridge

Glycerol

NON–POLAR

Saturated fatty acid

Unsaturated fatty acid

Outer surface

Carbohydrate groups

Inner surface

Phospholipid bilayer

Transmembrane protein with pore

Cytoskeletal elements

Intrinsic protein

Extrinsic protein

(c)

Membrane structure

Our current knowledge of membrane structure is the result of many years of study. The permeability of membranes to lipids gave the first indication that cell membranes were composed of lipid as well as protein. Later it was calculated that there was sufficient lipid in the cell membrane to form a bilayer, and an early model was developed of a lipid bilayer sandwiched between two layers of protein. This model, however, failed to explain selective membrane permeability to non-lipid-soluble molecules. Singer and Nicholson, in the early 1970s, proposed the *fluid mosaic model* of membrane structure which has been confirmed by many independent researchers and is now generally accepted.

Fig. 1.2 **Membrane structure** *(illustrations opposite)*

(a) EM × 210 000 (b) Phospholipid structure (c) Fluid mosaic model of membrane structure

Cell membranes consist of a bilayer of phospholipid molecules which are *amphipathic,* i.e. they consist of a polar, *hydrophilic* (water-loving) head and a non-polar, *hydrophobic* (water-hating) tail. The polar heads are mainly derived from glycerol conjugated to a nitrogenous compound such as choline, ethanolamine or serine via a phosphate bridge as shown in diagram (b). The phosphate group is negatively charged, whereas the nitrogenous group is positively charged. The non-polar tail of the phospholipid molecule consists of two long-chain fatty acids, each covalently linked to the glycerol component of the polar head. In most mammalian cell membranes, one of the fatty acids is a straight-chain saturated fatty acid, whilst the other is an unsaturated fatty acid which is 'kinked' at the position of the unsaturated bond. Because of their amphipathic nature, phospholipids in aqueous solution will spontaneously form a bilayer with the hydrophilic (polar) heads directed outwards and the hydrophobic tails forced together inwards. The weak intermolecular forces which hold the bilayer together allow individual phospholipid molecules to move relatively freely within each layer and sometimes to 'flip' between layers.

The fluidity and flexibility of the membrane is increased by the presence of unsaturated fatty acids which prevent close packing of the hydrophobic tails. Cholesterol molecules are also present in the bilayer in an almost 1:1 ratio with phospholipids. Cholesterol molecules themselves are amphipathic and have a kinked conformation, thus preventing overly dense packing of the phospholipid fatty acid tails whilst at the same time filling the gaps between the 'kinks' of the unsaturated fatty acid tails. Cholesterol molecules thus stabilise and regulate the fluidity of the phospholipid bilayer.

Protein molecules make up almost half of the total mass of the membrane. Some protein molecules are incorporated within the membrane (*intrinsic* or *integral proteins*) whereas others are held to the inner or outer surface by weaker electrostatic forces (*extrinsic* or *peripheral proteins*). Some intrinsic proteins span the entire thickness of the membrane (*transmembrane proteins*) to be exposed to each surface. Transmembrane proteins are held within the membrane by a hydrophobic central zone which allows the protein to float freely in the plane of the membrane (somewhat akin to the pudding known as 'floating islands'). The parts of these proteins protruding beyond the lipid bilayer are hydrophilic. Some membrane proteins are anchored to cytoplasmic structures by the cytoskeleton.

On the external surface of the plasma membranes of animal cells, many of the membrane proteins and some of the membrane lipids are conjugated with short chains of polysaccharide; these *glycoproteins* and *glycolipids,* respectively, project from the surface of the bilayer forming an outer coating which may be analogous to the cell walls of plants, bacteria and fungi. This polysaccharide layer has been termed the *glycocalyx* and appears to vary in thickness in different cell types; a similar layer is often also present on membrane surfaces within the cell that are not exposed to the cytosol (e.g. luminal aspects of membrane systems). The glycocalyx appears to be involved in cell-recognition phenomena, in the formation of intercellular adhesions and in the adsorption of molecules to the cell surface; in some situations the glycocalyx also provides mechanical and chemical protection for the plasma membrane.

The electron micrograph in (a) provides a high magnification view of the plasma membrane **PM** of the minute surface projections (*microvilli*) **MV** of a lining cell from the small intestine. The characteristic trilaminate appearance is made up of two outer electron-dense layers separated by an electron-lucent layer. The outer dense layers are thought to correspond to the hydrophilic 'heads' of phospholipid molecules, whilst the electron-lucent layer is thought to represent the intermediate hydrophobic layer mainly consisting of fatty acids and cholesterol. On the external surface of the plasma membrane is a fibrillary coat, called the 'fuzzy coat', representing the glycocalyx **G.** This is an unusually prominent feature of small intestinal lining cells where it incorporates a variety of digestive enzymes.

Transport across plasma membranes

Plasma membranes mediate the exchange of materials and information between the internal and external environments of the cell, enabling the cell to control the quality of its internal environment. Transport of materials across the plasma membrane occurs by four principal mechanisms.

- **Passive diffusion.** This type of transport is entirely dependent on the presence of a concentration gradient across the plasma membrane. Lipids and lipid-soluble molecules such as ethanol pass freely through plasma membranes which also offer little barrier to the diffusion of gases such as oxygen and carbon dioxide. The plasma membrane is, in general, impermeable to hydrophilic molecules. Nevertheless, some small molecules, including water and urea, and inorganic ions such as bicarbonate, are able to pass down osmotic and electrochemical gradients through the membrane via hydrophilic regions, the nature of which remains obscure.

- **Facilitated diffusion.** This type of transport is also concentration-dependent and involves the movement of larger hydrophilic molecules, such as glucose and amino acids, which may occur in either direction. This process is strictly passive but requires the presence of protein carrier molecules (known as **gated pores**) to which the molecules bind specifically but reversibly. When glucose, for example, is bound to its carrier protein, the transmembrane protein undergoes a change in shape which moves the glucose molecule to the interior of the cell, where it is able to dissociate from the carrier which then returns to its original shape.

- **Active transport.** This mode of transport is not only independent of concentration gradients, but also often operates against extreme concentration gradients. The classic example of this form of transport is the continuous movement of sodium out of the cell by the '**sodium pump**', a transmembrane protein complex (**Na^+-K^+ ATPase**) which exchanges a sodium for a potassium ion across the membrane. ATP is converted to ADP in the process to generate the energy required.

- **Bulk transport.** Transport of large molecules or small particles into the cell occurs by a range of mechanisms collectively known as **endocytosis**. The various types of endocytosis, including **phagocytosis** and **receptor-mediated endocytosis,** are discussed in some detail later in this chapter. **Exocytosis** uses similar mechasims in reverse to secrete cell products into the external enviroment. **Pinocytosis** involves the uptake of small volumes of extracellular fluid in a non-specific manner. Materials taken up by pinocytosis may be transported across the cell and excreted at another face of the cell; this is described as **transcytosis**.

Both active and passive transport processes are enhanced if the area of the plasma membrane is increased by folds or projections of the cell surface as exemplified by the absorptive cells lining the small intestine (see Fig. 1.2). Histologically, these transport processes can only be observed indirectly; for example, cells suspended in hypotonic solutions swell due to passive uptake of water, whereas cells placed in hypertonic solutions tend to shrink due to outflow of water. Radioisotope labelling techniques can be used to follow active transport processes. Bulk transport, however, is readily observable by microscopy (see Fig. 1.12).

Information must also be transported from the external environment to the interior of the cell, informing the cell that it is time to divide, produce more or less of a particular product, contract, respond to a foreign substance and so on. Messages may be transported across the plasma membrane by three main methods.

- The messenger molecule may be lipid-soluble and pass directly through the cell membrane to deliver its message by binding directly to an intracellular receptor, as is the case with the steroid hormone cortisol. One disadvantage of this method of delivery is that the information is delivered to all cells.

- More commonly, the messenger molecule is a protein which binds to a specific receptor on the cell surface. An enormous range of cell surface receptors is now known to exist and these share many structural similarities with transmembrane transport proteins. When the receptor is bound to its specific messenger protein, e.g. the hormone insulin, a change in the shape of the receptor allows it to modify cytoplasmic components known as the **second messenger,** thus passing on the information. Many of these membrane receptors are enzymes which become activated on binding to their specific messenger molecule or **ligand**. These activated enzymes then modify a component of the second messenger system, e.g. by adding or taking away a phosphate residue and altering the activity of that enzyme.

- A third method of information tranfer occurs between nerve cells, or between a nerve cell and a muscle cell. A chemical **neurotransmitter** is released from a nerve cell and binds to a receptor on the adjacent nerve or muscle cell, opening an ion channel and thus depolarising the membrane. In this case, a specific chemical interaction is converted to an electrical signal at the cell membrane.

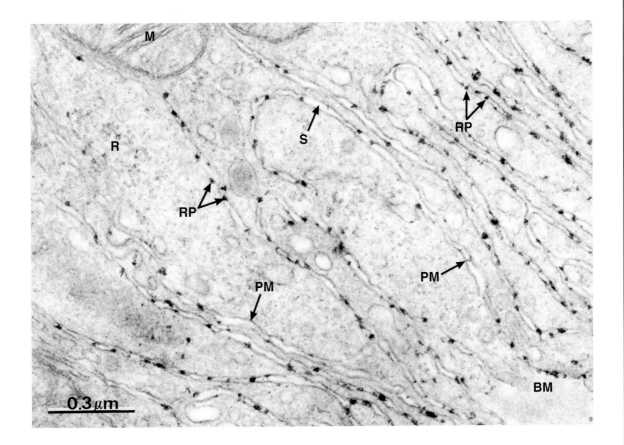

Fig. 1.3 **Active transport across membranes** EM × 80 000

This electron micrograph applies the technique of enzyme histochemistry to electron microscopy. The tissue shown is the proximal convoluted tubule of the kidney (see Ch. 16). At their bases, these cells have multiple finger-like processes that interdigitate with each other so that the interface between each cell and the extracellular space is very large. This space is known as the basolateral space **S.** The plasma membranes of the two cells **PM** can be seen outlining the individual cell processes, which contain the usual cytoplasmic organelles such as mitochondria **M** and ribosomes **R**. A small amount of basement membrane **BM** can be seen at the bottom right of the micrograph.

Proximal convoluted tubule cells are very active in the transport of ions across the plasma membrane into the basolateral space and this is facilitated by the very extensive basolateral space. Embedded within the plasma membrane is the enzyme *Na$^+$-K$^+$ATPase* (*Na$^+$-K$^+$ activated ATPase*) which exchanges one Na$^+$ for one K$^+$ ion across the plasma membrane. In this micrograph the tissue has been manipulated so as to produce an electron-dense reaction product **RP** which can be seen at intervals in the intercellular space, thus identifying the position of the Na$^+$-K$^+$ ATPase. Note that in order to see this reaction product, the rest of the specimen has been very lightly stained and thus the cytoplasmic details are faint.

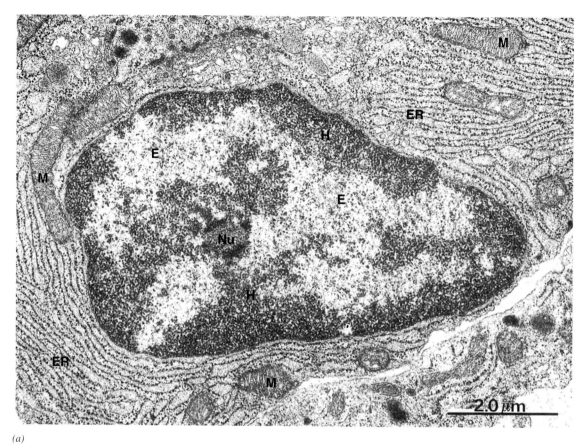

(a)

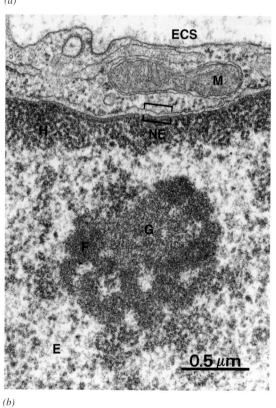

(b)

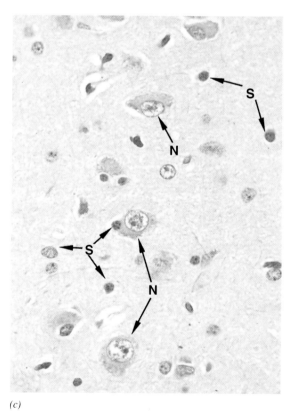

(c)

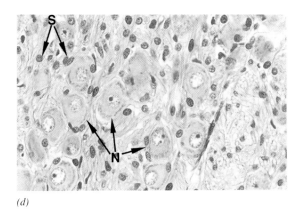

(d)

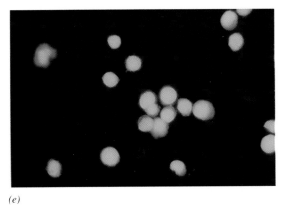

(e)

Fig. 1.4 **Nucleus** *(illustrations (a), (b) and (c) opposite)*
(a) EM × 15 000 (b) EM × 37 000 (c) H & E × 480 (d) Azan × 320 (e) Acridine orange × 320

Micrograph (a) illustrates the nucleus of a *plasma cell* which secretes large amounts of a protein called *antibody.* Typical of protein-secreting cells, the cytoplasm contains plentiful ribosome-studded or rough *endoplasmic reticulum* **ER** and many *mitochondria* **M,** which produce the energy required for such a metabolically active cell.

The nucleus contains DNA (making up less than 20% of its mass), protein called *nucleoprotein* and some RNA. Nucleoprotein is of two major types: low molecular weight, positively charged *histone proteins* which bind tightly to DNA and control the coiling of the DNA strand, and *non-histone proteins,* including enzymes for the synthesis of DNA and RNA and regulatory proteins. All nucleoproteins are synthesised in the cytoplasm and imported into the nucleus. Nuclear RNA includes newly synthesised messenger, transfer and ribosomal RNA which has not yet passed into the cytoplasm.

Except during cell division, the *chromosomes*, each a discrete length of DNA with bound histone proteins, exist as tangled strands which cannot be visualised individually. Nuclei are heterogeneous structures with electron-dense and electron-lucent areas. The dense areas, called *heterochromatin* **H**, consist of tightly coiled inactive chromatin found in irregular clumps often around the periphery of the nucleus. In females, the inactivated X-chromosome forms a small discrete mass, the *Barr body.* Barr bodies are sometimes seen at the edge of the nucleus in female cells when cut in a favourable plane of section. The electron-lucent nuclear material, called *euchromatin* **E,** represents that part of the DNA which is active in RNA synthesis. Collectively, heterochromatin and euchromatin are known as *chromatin,* a name derived from the strong colour of nuclei when stained for light microscopy.

Many nuclei, especially those of cells highly active in protein synthesis, contain one or more dense structures called *nucleoli* **Nu** which are the sites of ribosomal RNA synthesis and ribosome assembly. Ribosomal RNA and proteins, which are imported from the cytoplasm, are assembled into subunits which then pass back to the cytoplasm to aggregate into complete ribosomes. Micrograph (b) shows a typical nucleolus. Ultrastructurally, nucleoli are quite variable in appearance. In this example the nucleolus consists of reticular *nucleolonema* with dense *filamentous components* **F** and paler *granular*

components **G**. The filamentous components are thought to be the sites of ribosomal RNA synthesis, while ribosome assembly takes place in the granular components. Note also euchromatin **E** and heterochromatin **H** within the nucleus which is bounded by the nuclear envelope **NE**. A thin rim of cytoplasm containing a mitochondrion **M** separates the nucleus from the extracellular space **ECS**.

In general, the degree of activity of any cell may be judged by the appearance of its nucleus. Inactive cells have small nuclei with condensed chromatin and small or absent nucleoli. In highly active cells, the nuclear material is dispersed (euchromatin) with prominent nucleoli.

The specimen shown in micrograph (c) is of brain tissue which has been stained with *haematoxylin and eosin* (H & E), the 'standard' histological staining method. Haematoxylin is blue in colour and eosin is pink. Haematoxylin, a basic dye which binds to negatively charged DNA and RNA, is principally employed to demonstrate nuclear form. Eosin, an acidic dye, has affinity for positively charged structures such as mitochondria and many other cytoplasmic constituents. *Acidophilic* (positively charged) structures are therefore *eosinophilic* when stained by the H & E method. The highly active nerve cells **N** seen in micrograph (c) have huge nuclei with relatively pale-stained, dispersed nuclear chromatin and prominent nucleoli. In contrast, the surrounding relatively inactive support cells **S** have small nuclei with intensely stained heterochromatin and no visible nucleoli.

Micrograph (d) also shows nerve tissue, but stained by the Azan method which contains a basophilic dye giving the nucleus a red colour, and a blue green acidophilic dye. Note how the nuclear form of the neurones **N** and support cells **S** corresponds to that in micrograph (c) despite the difference in colour.

In micrograph (e), the specimen has been stained with a dye that combines with DNA and RNA. When viewed using a *fluorescence microscope,* the DNA is seen as yellow-green fluorescence and the RNA as orange-red fluorescence, thereby highlighting the nuclei and cytoplasm, respectively. The micrograph shows plasma cells and lymphocytes in a smear of bone marrow aspirate; the plasma cells, which are very active in protein synthesis, have plentiful cytoplasmic RNA, whereas the quiescent lymphocytes have almost none.

THE CELL

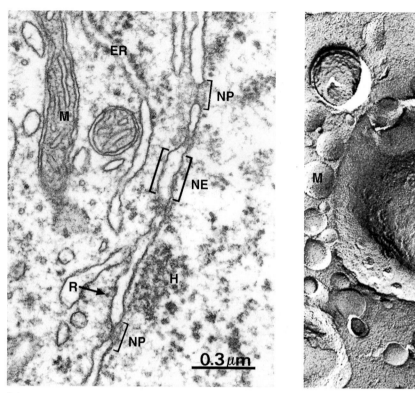
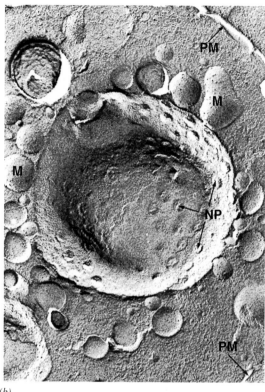

(a)   *(b)*

Fig. 1.5 Nuclear envelope (a) EM × 59 000 (b) Freeze-etched preparation SEM × 34 000

The *nuclear envelope* **NE**, which encloses the nucleus, consists of two layers of membrane (each layer of standard phospholipid bilayer structure) with the *intermembranous space* between. The outer lipid bilayer is continuous with the endoplasmic reticulum **ER** and has ribosomes **R** on its cytoplasmic face. On the inner aspect of the nuclear envelope, there is an electron-dense fibrillar layer, the *nuclear lamina,* consisting of polypeptides called *lamins* which link membrane proteins and heterochromatin **H.**

The nuclear envelope contains numerous *nuclear pores* **NP** at the margins of which the inner and outer membranes become continuous. Each pore contains a *nuclear pore complex,* an elaborate cylindrical structure consisting of proteins which form a central channel. Nuclear pores permit and regulate the exchange of metabolites, macromolecules and ribosomal subunits between nucleus and cytoplasm. The mechanism of transport through a nuclear pore is unknown but requires energy derived from ATP. The nuclear pore complex may also hold together

the two lipid bilayers of the nuclear envelope. Note that mitochondria **M** are also identifiable in the cytoplasm.

Micrograph (b) shows an example of a technique called *freeze-etching.* Briefly, this method involves the rapid cooling of cells to subzero temperatures; the frozen cells are then fractured. Internal surfaces of the cell are thus exposed (in a somewhat random manner), the fracture lines tending to follow natural planes of weakness. Surface detail is obtained by 'etching' or subliming excess water molecules from the specimen at low temperature. A thin carbon impression is then made of the surface and this mirror image is viewed by conventional electron microscopy. Freeze-etching provides a valuable tool for studying internal cell surfaces at high resolution. In this preparation, the plane of cleavage has included part of the nuclear envelope in which nuclear pores **NP** are clearly demonstrated. Note also the outline of the plasma membrane **PM** and mitochrondria **M.**

Protein synthesis

Proteins are not only a major structural component of cells but, in the form of enzymes, transport proteins and regulatory proteins, mediate many metabolic processes. Thus the nature and quantity of proteins within any individual cell determine the activity of that cell. All cellular proteins are subject to wear and tear and are replaced continuously. Many cells also synthesise proteins for export; such proteins include glandular secretions and the extracellular structural components of tissues. Protein synthesis is, therefore, an essential and continuous activity of all cells and the major function of some cells.

The principal organelles involved in protein synthesis are the nucleus and *ribosomes.* The nucleus of every cell contains within its DNA the code for every protein that could be produced by that individual. Production or *expression* of selected proteins is characteristic of differentiated cells. The presence of a particular protein within a cell is one possible method of identifying different cell types, e.g. the presence of actin and myosin in muscle cells.

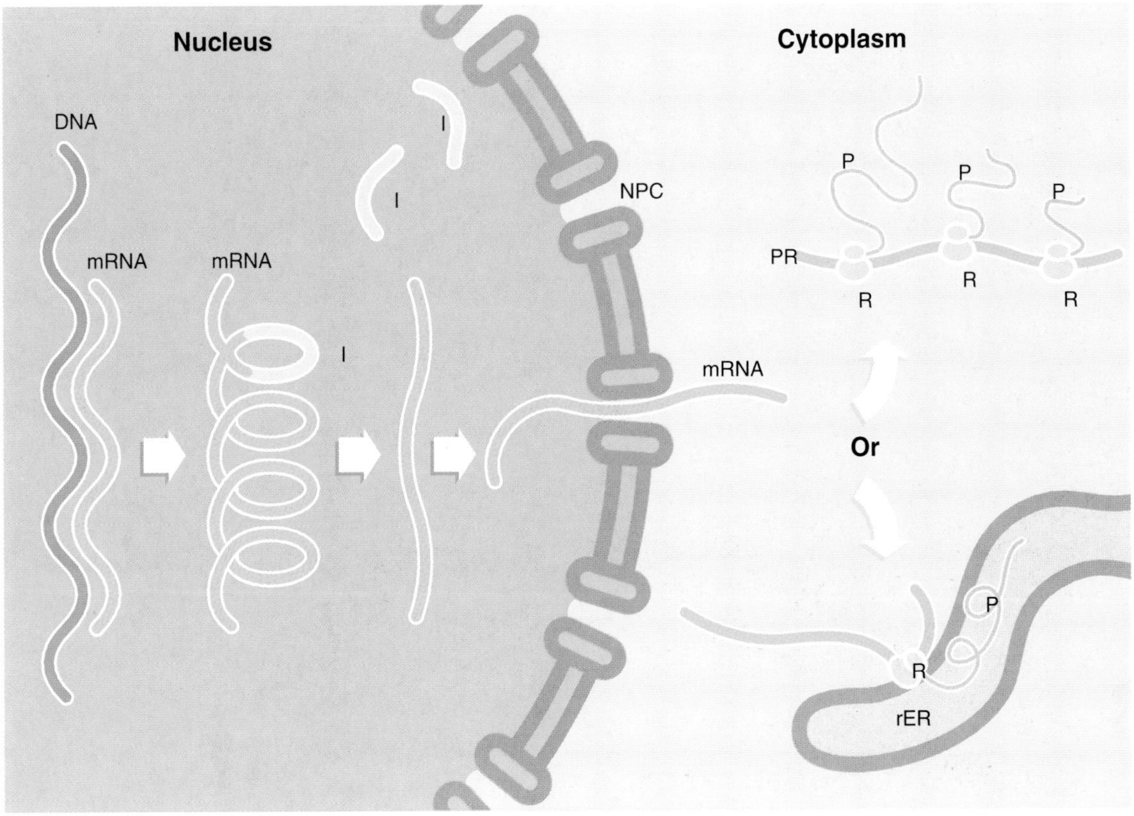

Fig. 1.6 Protein synthesis

Protein synthesis occurs in several steps. First, the DNA template is copied to form a complementary *messenger RNA* **mRNA** copy, a process known as *transcription.* A fairly recent discovery is that the DNA template contains non-coding sequences or *introns* **I** which are spliced out of the mRNA before it passes through the nuclear pore complex **NPC** into the cytoplasm. Here the mRNA binds to *ribosomes* **R**, organelles which read the mRNA sequence and *translate* it into the specific sequence of amino acids which characterises a particular protein.

Ribosomes are minute cytoplasmic organelles, each composed of two subunits of unequal size. Each subunit consists of a strand of RNA (ribosomal RNA, rRNA) with associated ribosomal proteins forming a globular structure. The two subunits together look something like a cottage loaf. Ribosomes align mRNA strands so that

transfer RNA (tRNA) molecules may be brought into position and their amino acids added sequentially to the growing polypeptide chain **P**. Other ribosomal proteins are enzymes which promote peptide bond formation between amino acids. Ribosomes are often found attached to mRNA molecules in small spiral-shaped aggregations called *polyribosomes* or *polysomes* **PR**, formed by a single strand of mRNA with ribosomes attached along its length. Each ribosome in a polyribosome is making a separate molecule of the protein, an example of the amazing efficiency with which cellular resources are often utilised. Ribosomes and polyribosomes may also be attached to the surface of endoplasmic reticulum **rER** (see Fig. 1.7). Further modification of proteins may then occur in the endoplasmic reticulum, e.g. glycosylation, cross-linking of peptide chains by disulphide bonds.

Rough endoplasmic reticulum and ribosomes

The endoplasmic reticulum consists of an interconnecting network of membranous tubules, vesicles and flattened sacs (*cisternae*) which ramifies throughout the cytoplasm. Much of its surface is studded with ribosomes, giving a 'rough' appearance leading to the name *rough endoplasmic reticulum* (**rER**). Proteins which are destined for export, as well as lysosomal proteins, are synthesised by ribosomes attached to the surface of the rER and pass through the membrane into its lumen. Integral membrane proteins are also synthesised on rER and inserted into the membrane at this point, the extracellular part of the protein protruding into the lumen of the rER and the intramembranous part held firmly in place by hydrophobic attraction. It is within the rER that proteins are folded to form their secondary structure, intrachain disulphide bonds are formed and the first steps of glycosylation take place. In contrast, proteins destined for the cytoplasm, nucleus and mitochondria are synthesised on free ribosomes, (i.e. not attached to ER).

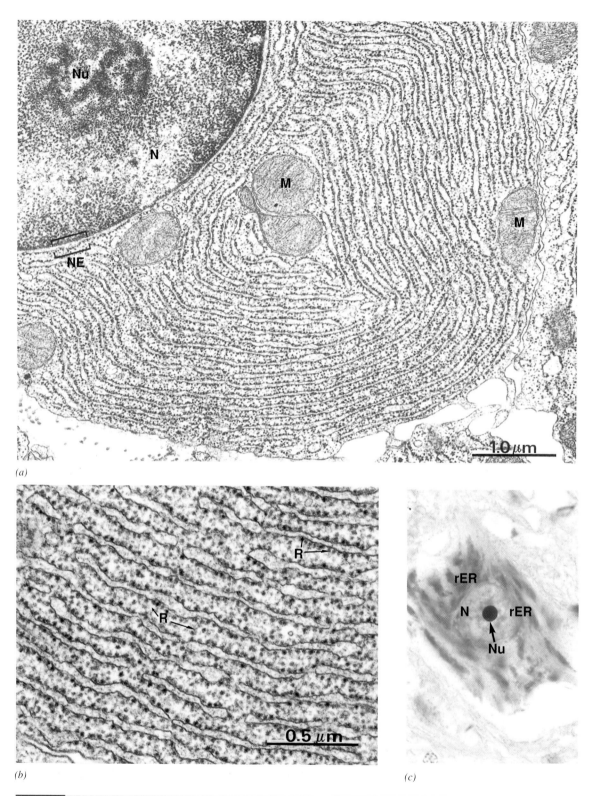

(a)

(b)   *(c)*

Fig. 1.7 **Rough endoplasmic reticulum** (a) EM × 23 000 (b) EM × 50 000 (c) Cresyl violet × 800

These micrographs illustrate rough endoplasmic reticulum in a cell specialised for the synthesis and secretion of protein; in such cells rough endoplasmic reticulum tends to be profuse and to form closely packed parallel laminae of flattened cisternae. In micrograph (a), the dimensions of the rER can be compared with that of mitochondria **M** and the nucleus **N.** The nucleus typically contains a prominent nucleolus **Nu.** Note the close association between the rER and the outer lipid bilayer of the nuclear envelope **NE** with which it is in continuity. The chromatin in the nucleus is mainly dispersed (euchromatin), consistent with prolific protein synthesis.

Micrograph (b) shows part of the rER at high magnification. Numerous ribosomes **R** stud the surface of the membrane system and there are plentiful ribosomes lying free in the intervening cytosol. Micrograph (c) shows a nerve cell at high magnification stained by the basophilic dye, cresyl violet. The basophilic clumps in the cytoplasm represent areas of prolific rough endoplasmic reticulum **rER**. The nuclear envelope can be distinguished due to the basophilia of the numerous ribosomes that stud its outer surface. The nucleus **N** contains a prominent nucleolus **Nu** and dispersed chromatin.

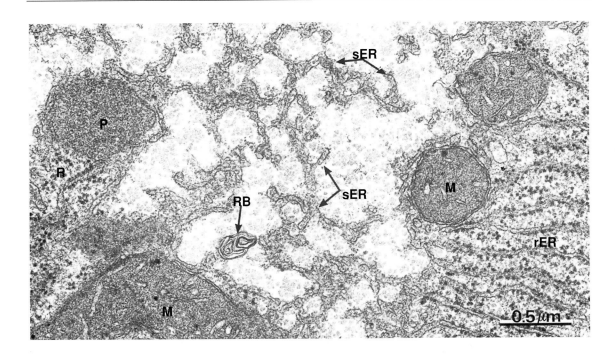

Fig. 1.8 Smooth endoplasmic reticulum EM × 40 000

Smooth endoplasmic reticulum* sER** is continuous with and identical to rER except that it lacks ribosomes. The principal functions of smooth endoplasmic reticulum are lipid biosynthesis and membrane synthesis and repair. Fatty acids and triglycerides are mostly synthesised within the cytosol, whereas cholesterol and phospholipids are synthesised in sER. In liver cells, smooth endoplasmic reticulum is rich in cytochrome P450 and plays a major role in the metabolism of glycogen and detoxification of various noxious metabolic by-products, drugs and alcohol. In muscle cells, where it is called ***sarcoplasmic reticulum, sER is involved in the storage and release of calcium ions which activate the contractile mechanism (see Ch. 6).

Most cells contain only scattered elements of sER interspersed with the other organelles. Cell types with prominent sER include liver cells and those cells specialised for lipid biosynthesis, such as the steroid hormone-secreting cells of the adrenal glands and the gonads. In this micrograph from the liver, most of the membranous elements are smooth endoplasmic reticulum; however, for comparison, rough endoplasmic reticulum **rER** is included in the lower right of the field. Note the continuity of the two forms of ER. This field also includes several mitochondria **M,** a peroxisome **P,** free ribosomes and polyribosomes **R** and a whorl of membrane in a residual body **RB.**

Import, export and intracellular transportation

As discussed above, eukaryotic cells are compartmentalised structures which allow mutually incompatible activities to take place in isolated microenvironments. To facilitate this process, materials must be accurately transported from one compartment to another. For instance, the process of protein synthesis and export which takes place in the rER and Golgi apparatus must be kept separate from the garbage disposal and recycling plant, the *lysosome.* Likewise, microorganisms phagocytosed by cells must be killed and disposed of without damage to normal structures and mechanisms.

Over the past few years, the mechanisms by which materials are moved around the cell have been elucidated. An elegant system has evolved to transport materials between membrane-bound compartments in *coated vesicles.* These transport soluble and membrane proteins from rER to the Golgi apparatus, between the cisternae of the Golgi apparatus, and from the Golgi to the plasma membrane for secretion, *exocytosis.* Transport from the external environment to the interior of the cell is known as *endocytosis,* where materials are transported in similar coated vesicles into the lysosomes. Coated vesicles form when *coat proteins* bind to an area of membrane associated with the material to be transported, forming the membrane into a bud, supported and controlled by the coat proteins. The coated bud then breaks free and becomes a coated vesicle containing, either within its lumen or within its membrane, the materials to be transported to another membrane-bound compartment. The transport vesicle moves to its destination, where the protein coat is shed, before fusing with the destination membrane. In this ingenious system the destination of the package is determined by the protein coat of the vesicle, which is in turn determined by the contents.

It is important to remember that many intracellular proteins are synthesised by free ribosomes in the cytoplasm and are transported within the cells by mechanisms other than transport vesicles.

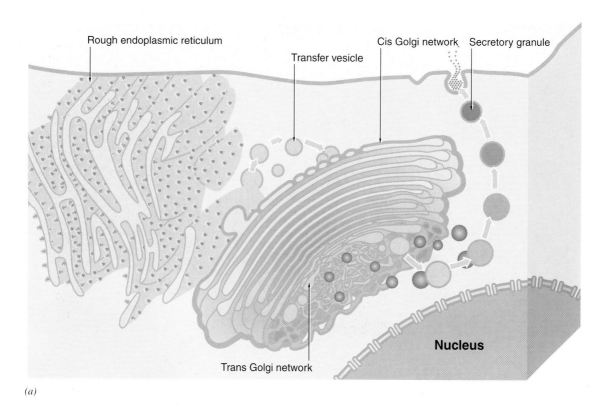

Rough endoplasmic reticulum   Transfer vesicle   Cis Golgi network   Secretory granule

Nucleus

Trans Golgi network

(a)

Fig. 1.9   **Golgi apparatus**   **(a) Schematic diagram (b) EM × 30 000**
(c) Giemsa × 300 (d) Immunoperoxidase × 100 (e) Iron haematoxylin × 400

Diagram (a) illustrates the main structural features of the Golgi apparatus and summarises the mechanism by which secretory products are packaged within membrane-bound vesicles. The Golgi apparatus consists of a system of stacked, saucer-shaped cisternae with the concave surface facing the nucleus. The outermost cisternae are in the form of a network of tubules. Proteins, either within the lumen of a coated vesicle or embedded in its membrane, are transported to the Golgi apparatus from the ER. When they arrive at the convex *forming face* or *cis Golgi network* of the Golgi apparatus, the coat proteins disengage and the vesicles fuse with the membrane of the forming face. In the Golgi apparatus the glycosylation of proteins begun in the ER is completed by sequential addition of sugar residues. It is thought that each cisterna contains the specific enzyme to add a specific sugar and that proteins are passed from cisterna to cisterna by formation of a series of coated vesicles which then fuse with the next cisterna in the stack. On arrival at the concave *maturing face* or *trans Golgi network,* the proteins are accurately sorted into secretory vesicles or lysosomes. Secretory vesicles become increasingly condensed as they migrate through the cytoplasm to form mature *secretory granules*, which are then liberated at the cell surface by exocytosis. A single cell may contain multiple Golgi stacks.

Micrograph (b) illustrates a particularly well developed Golgi apparatus; transfer vesicles **T** and elements of the rough endoplasmic reticulum **rER** are seen adjacent to the forming face. A variety of larger vesicles **V** can be seen in the concavity of the maturing face, some of which appear to be budding from the Golgi cisternae **C**; such vesicles could be either secretory granules or lysosomes.

Note the proximity of the Golgi apparatus to the nucleus **N;** the nuclear membrane **NM** is particularly well demonstrated in this micrograph,

Micrograph (c) illustrates a plasma cell from a bone marrow smear; these cells are responsible for antibody production. The cytoplasm is packed with rough endoplasmic reticulum responsible for protein (antibody) synthesis and is thus strongly basophilic. There is a very well developed Golgi complex **G** which packages the antibody prior to secretion. Since it mainly consists of lipid (membrane), which is dissolved out during preparation, the Golgi remains unstained and appears as a pale area (negative image) adjacent to the nucleus **N.**

Plasma cells **P** are also shown in micrograph (d) which is a section of tonsil. This example of the *immunoperoxidase method* demonstrates plasma cells whose cytoplasm is packed with IgA. Briefly, the tissue section is allowed to react with a solution containing an anti-IgA antibody, an example of an antibody acting as an antigen. The anti-IgA antibody is linked to the enzyme *horseradish peroxidase* which is able to convert a colourless substrate to a brown product which is localised to areas where the the antibody has bound to its antigen, IgA (see Notes on staining techniques, p. 406).

The staining method in micrograph (e) is used here to demonstrate secretory granules in the cells of the pancreas, which secretes digestive enzymes. The secretory cells are grouped around a minute central duct **D**, and the secretory granules, which are stained black, are concentrated towards the luminal aspect of the cell. The nuclei **N** of the secretory cells have dispersed chromatin and prominent nucleoli and are arranged around the periphery of the secretory unit.

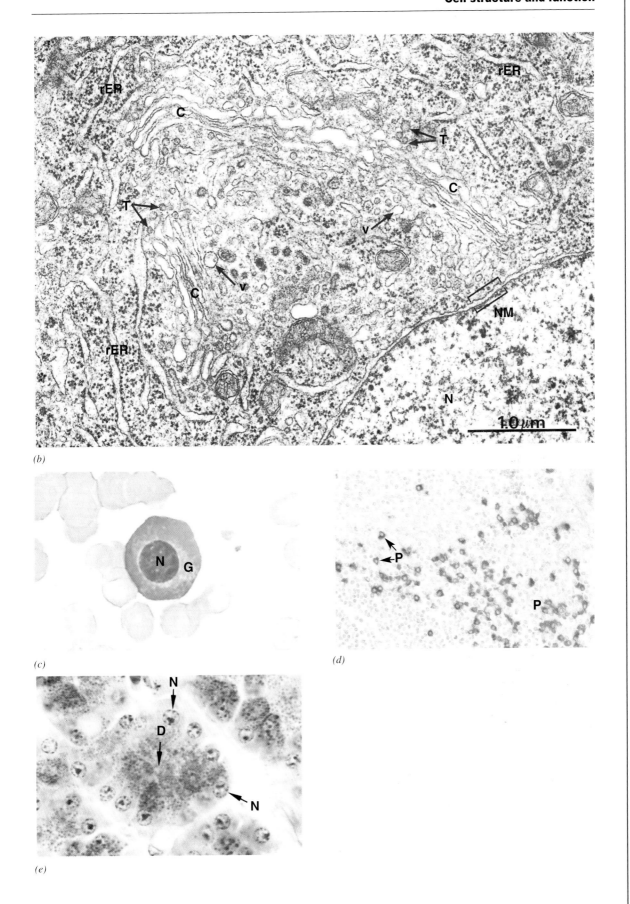

(b)

(c)

(d)

(e)

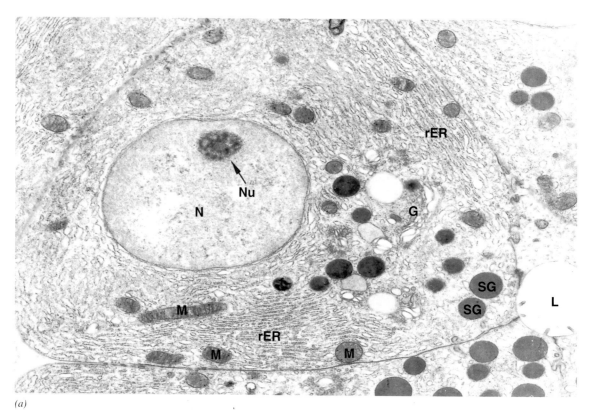

(a)

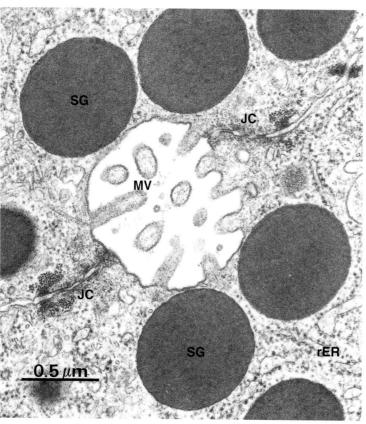

0.5 μm

(b)

Fig. 1.10 Exocytosis
(a) EM × 14 000 (b) EM × 41 500

Micrograph (a) illustrates a typical protein-secreting cell, in this case from the pancreas which secretes a variety of digestive enzymes. In the nucleus **N**, the chromatin is typically dispersed and there is a prominent nucleolus **Nu.** The cytoplasm is packed with rough endoplasmic reticulum **rER,** there is a prominent Golgi apparatus **G** and scattered mitochondria **M.** Secretory granules **SG** become increasingly electron-dense as they are concentrated towards the glandular lumen **L.**

Micrograph (b) shows the apical regions of two pancreatic secretory cells converging on a tiny central excretory duct. Large membrane-bound secretory granules **SG** are seen approaching the lumen.

Note also plentiful rough endoplasmic reticulum **rER,** which is typical of protein-secreting cells. The adjacent cells are joined together by junctional complexes **JC** (see Ch. 3). Stubby microvilli **MV** protrude into the excretory duct.

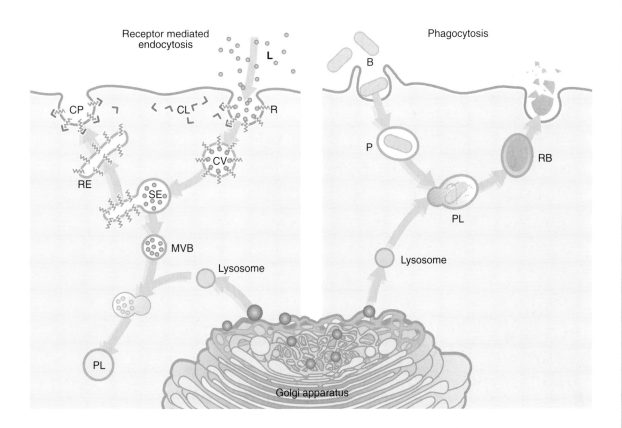

Fig. 1.11 Endocytosis

Particulate matter and large macromolecules are taken up by the cell through a variety of processes collectively known as *endocytosis.* The best known of these mechanisms is *phagocytosis*, which is utilised by cells of the defence system to ingest and kill pathogenic organisms. In recent years the elegant and efficient mechanism of *receptor-mediated endocytosis*, which is probably much more widespread, has been described. *Pinocytosis*, which non-specifically samples the extracellular fluid, and various other types of endocytosis are less well understood. The diagram summarises the main steps of receptor-mediated endocytosis and phagocytosis.

Receptor-mediated endocytosis

Receptor-mediated endocytosis, shown on the left side of the diagram, is used extensively for uptake of specific molecules often referred to as *ligands* **L** because they bind to cell surface receptors **R** (from *ligare*, to bind). The mechanism is somewhat like exocytosis in reverse and uses the coated vesicle mechanism described earlier. First the cell must have the appropriate receptor on its plasma membrane. These are concentrated in preformed *coated pits* **CP**, a well known example being *low-density lipoprotein* (LDL) receptors. The cytoplasmic surface of the pit is coated by a basket-like framework of the protein *clathrin* **CL**. When the receptors bind LDL particles, the coated pit buds off and becomes a *coated vesicle* **CV**. The vesicles very quickly lose their clathrin coat and fuse with *sorting endosomes* **SE**, which are dynamic tubulovesicular structures usually found close to the plasma membrane. The acid pH in the lumen of sorting endosomes encourages dissociation of receptor and ligand; these are then quickly separated so that most of the membrane and its intrinsic receptors are shuttled to *recycling endosomes* **RE** and from there back to the cell surface. Some membrane receptors may go through this whole cycle up to 300 times. The remaining part of

the sorting endosome, which contains the unbound LDL, converts into a *late endosome*, often called a *multivesicular body* **MVB.** Multivesicular bodies are moved towards the Golgi apparatus and there fuse with lysosomes. Degradative enzymes within the lysosomes, now called *phagolysosomes* **PL**, digest the protein component of the LDL, freeing cholesterol for incorporation into membranes.

Phagocytosis

Bacteria **B** are taken up by specialised phagocytic cells, such as neutrophil polymorphs and monocytes, through the process of phagocytosis, shown on the right side of the diagram. The bacterium binds to cell surface receptors, triggering the formation of pseudopodia which extend around the organism until they fuse leaving the engulfed bacterium in a membrane-bound *phagosome* **P** within the cytoplasm. At this stage, recyling of membrane and receptors takes place, although the mechanisms are not yet clear. There may be exchange of materials between early endosomes, recycling endosomes and phagosomes (not shown). The phagosome then fuses with a lysosome to become a *phagolysosome* **PL** (sometimes called a *secondary lysosome*) and the bacterium is subjected to the toxic activities of the lysosomal enzymes. These enzymes also break down the components of the dead bacteria, which may be released into the cytoplasm, expelled from the cell by exocytosis or remain in the cytoplasm as a residual body.

Lysosomes are also involved in the degradation of cellular organelles, many of which have only a finite lifespan and are therefore replaced continuously; this lysosomal function is termed autophagy. Most autophagocytic degradation products accumulate and become indistinguishable from the residual bodies of endocytosis. With advancing age, residual bodies accumulate in the cells of some tissues and appear as brown lipofuscin granules (see Fig. 1.14).

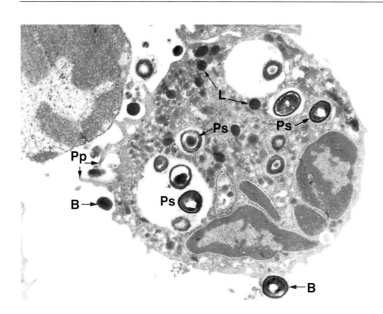

Fig. 1.12 Phagocytosis
EM × 11 750

This micrograph illustrates a highly phagocytic white blood cell, a ***neutrophil***, in the process of engulfing and destroying bacteria **B**. Note the manner in which pseudopodia **Pp** embrace the bacteria before engulfment. Note also phagosomes **Ps** containing bacteria in various stages of degradation. Several lysosomes **L** are also visible.

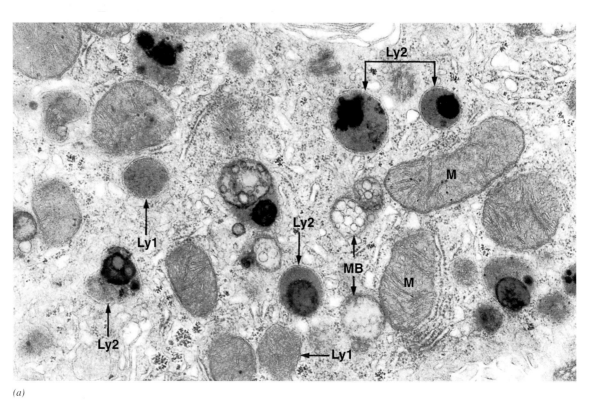

(a)

Fig. 1.13 Lysosomes (a) EM × 27 000 (b) EM × 60 000
   (c) Histochemical method for acid phosphatase: EM × 50 000 (*b and c opposite page, top*)

These micrographs show the typical features of lysosomes and residual bodies. Micrograph (a) shows part of the cytoplasm of a liver cell. Lysosomes **Ly1** vary greatly in size and appearance but are recognised as membrane-bound organelles containing an amorphous granular material. Phagolysosomes or secondary lysosomes **Ly2** are even more variable in appearance but are recognisable by their diverse particulate content, some of which is extremely electron-dense. The distinction between residual bodies and secondary lysosomes is often difficult. Late endosomes or multivesicular bodies **MB** are also seen in this micrograph. Note the size of lysosomes relative to mitochondria **M**.

Micrograph (b) shows two secondary lysosomes at higher magnification, allowing the limiting membrane to be visualised. Both contain electron-dense particulate

material and amorphous granular material.

The lysosomal enzymes comprise more than 40 different acid hydrolases which are optimally active at a pH of about 5.0. This may be a protective mechanism for the cell should lysosomal enzymes escape into the cytosol where they would be less active at the higher pH. Histochemical methods can be used to demonstrate sites of enzyme activity within cells and thus act as markers for organelles that contain these enzymes. Such a method has been used in micrograph (c) to demonstrate the presence of ***acid phosphatase***, a typical lysosomal enzyme; enzyme activity is represented by the electron-dense area within a lysosome **L**. Other organelles remain unstained, but the outline of a mitochondrion **M** and saccules of endoplasmic reticulum **ER** can nevertheless be identified.

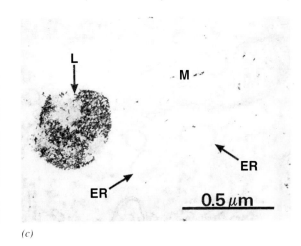

(b) *(c)*

Fig. 1.14 Cellular pigments: lipofuscin and melanin (a) H & E × 320 (b) Modified Azan × 600

In general, mammalian tissues have minimal intrinsic colour when viewed through the microscope: thus the need for staining. A few tissues, however, contain intracellular pigments such as lipofuscin, which probably represents an insoluble degradation product of organelle turnover. With increasing age, it accumulates in the cytoplasm, particularly in sympathetic ganglion cells, as seen in micrograph (a), other neurones and cardiac muscle cells; it is thus sometimes referred to as 'age pigment'. Another natural pigment is melanin, which is mainly responsible for skin colour (see Ch. 9). This brown pigment is also present in nerve cells in certain brain regions such as the substantia nigra, shown in micrograph (b). This specimen has been stained by the Azan method to pick out the nuclei **N** which are stained pale blue with prominent magenta nucleoli.

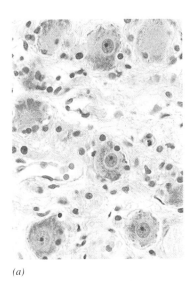

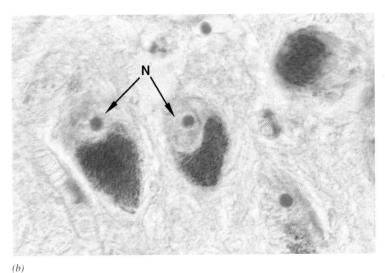

(a) *(b)*

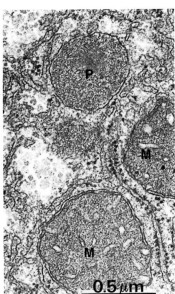

Fig. 1.15 Peroxisomes EM × 40 000

Peroxisomes or *microbodies* are small, spherical, membrane-bound organelles that closely resemble lysosomes in size and ultrastructure. However, they contain an entirely different set of enzymes which can be demonstrated by histochemical techniques. Peroxisomes contain *oxidases* involved in certain catabolic pathways (e.g. beta oxidation of long-chain fatty acids) which result in the formation of hydrogen peroxide, a potentially cytotoxic by-product. Nonetheless, hydrogen peroxide is used by certain phagocytic cells of the defence system to kill ingested microorganisms. Peroxisomes also contain *catalase*, which regulates hydrogen peroxidase concentration, utilising it in the oxidation of a variety of potentially toxic substances including phenols and alcohol.

The peroxisomes of many species have a central crystalloid structure called a *nucleoid* which contains the enzyme *urate oxidase.* This is not present in humans, who thus lack the ability to metabolise urates. The peroxisomes of the liver and kidney are particularly large and abundant, reflecting the functions of these organs in lipid metabolism and management of metabolic waste products.

In this micrograph, note the fine, granular electron-dense contents of a peroxisome **P**, the size of which can be compared to that of adjacent mitochondria **M**.

Energy production and storage

All cellular functions are dependent on a continuous supply of energy, which is derived from the sequential breakdown of organic molecules during the process of *cellular respiration.* The energy released during this process is ultimately stored in the form of ATP molecules. In all cells, ATP forms a pool of readily available energy for all the metabolic functions of the cell. The main substrates for cellular respiration are simple sugars and lipids, particularly glucose and fatty acids. Cellular respiration of glucose (*glycolysis*) begins in the cytosol, where it is partially degraded to form pyruvic acid, yielding a small amount of ATP. Pyruvic acid then diffuses into specialised membranous organelles called *mitochrondria* where, in the presence of oxygen, it is degraded to carbon dioxide and water; this process yields a large quantity of ATP. In contrast, fatty acids pass directly into mitochondria where they are also degraded to carbon dioxide and water; this also generates a large amount of ATP. Glycolysis may occur in the absence of oxygen and is then termed *anaerobic respiration*, whereas mitochondrial respiration is dependent on a continuous supply of oxygen and is therefore termed *aerobic respiration.* Mitochondria are the principal organelles involved in cellular respiration in mammals and are found in large numbers in metabolically active cells, such as those in the liver and skeletal muscle.

Under favourable nutritional conditions, most cells generate and store excess glucose and fatty acids in the relatively insoluble and non-toxic forms, glycogen and triglyceride, respectively. Cells vary greatly in their content of stored carbohydrate and lipid; extreme examples are nerve cells, which contain almost no intracellular glycogen or triglyceride, and fat cells, the cytoplasm of which is almost entirely filled with stored lipid.

Fig. 1.16   Mitochondria

Mitochondria vary considerably in size and shape but are most often elongated, cigar-shaped organelles. They are mobile and tend to localise at intracellular sites of maximum energy requirement. The number of mitochondria in cells is highly variable; liver cells contain as many as 2000 mitochondria, whereas inactive cells contain very few.

Each mitochondrion consists of two layers of membrane. The outer membrane is relatively permeable as it contains a pore-forming protein, known as *porin*, which allows free passage of small molecules. The outer membrane contains enzymes that convert certain lipid substrates into forms that can be metabolised within the mitochondrion. The inner membrane, which is thinner than the outer, is thrown into folds called *cristae* projecting into the inner cavity which is filled with an amorphous matrix. The matrix contains a number of dense *matrix granules*, thought to be binding sites for calcium which is stored in mitochondria. Peripherally, the inner mitochondrial membrane is closely applied to the outer membrane, leaving a narrow *intermembranous space* which extends into each crista. Aerobic respiration takes place within the matrix and on the inner membrane, a process enhanced by the large surface area provided by the cristae. The matrix contains most of the enzymes involved in oxidation of fatty acids and the Krebs cycle. The inner membrane contains the cytochromes, the carrier molecules of the electron transport chain, and the enzymes involved in ATP production. In very high power electron micrographs, some of the enzymes involved in oxidative phosphorylation can be visualised as 'lollipop' structures studding the inner surface of the inner mitochondrial membrane (not illustrated).

As organelles, mitochondria have several highly unusual features. The mitochondrial matrix contains one or more strands of DNA arranged as a circle resembling the chromosomes of bacteria. The matrix also contains ribosomes which have a similar structure to bacterial ribosomes. Mitochondria synthesise 37 of their own constituent proteins, others being synthesised by the usual protein-synthetic mechanisms of the cell. In addition,

mitochondria undergo self-replication in a manner similar to bacterial cell division. It has thus been proposed that mitochondria are derived from bacteria which formed a symbiotic relationship with eukaryotic cells during the process of evolution.

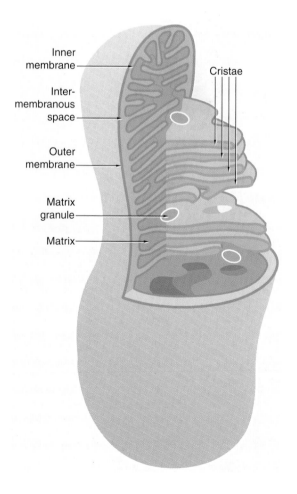

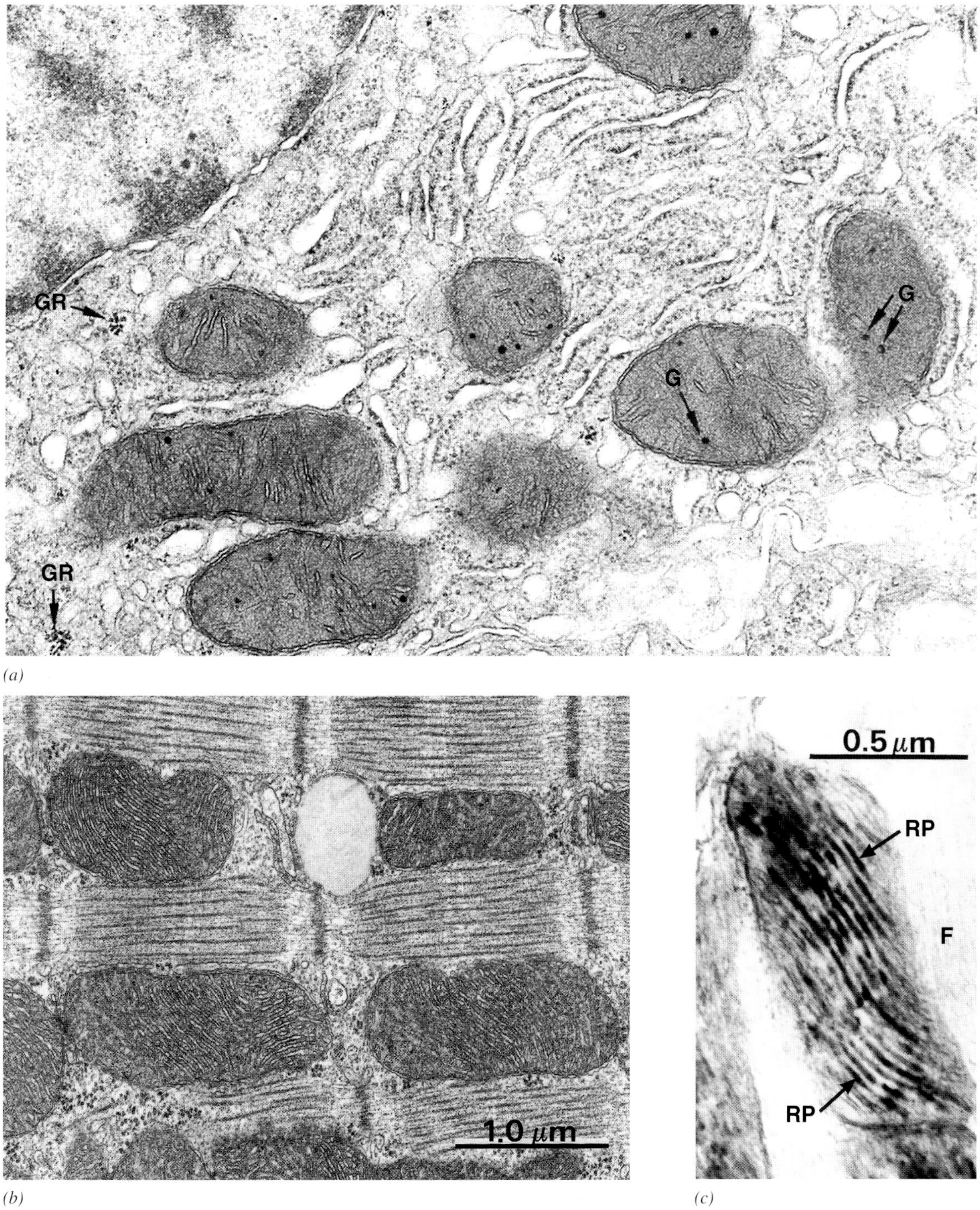

(a)

(b)

(c)

Fig. 1.17 **Mitochondria** **(a) EM × 42 000 (b) EM × 25 000 (c) EM × 50 000**

All mitochondria conform to the same general structure but vary greatly in size, shape and arrangement of cristae; these variations are often characteristic of the cell type. Mitochondria move freely within the cytosol and tend to aggregate in intracellular sites with high energy demands where their shape often conforms to the available space.

Micrograph (a) of liver cell cytoplasm shows the typical appearance of mitochondria when cut in different planes of section; note their relatively dense matrix containing a few matrix granules **G**. *Glycogen rosettes* **GR** are also seen in this micrograph (see Fig. 1.19).

Mitochondria from heart muscle cells can be seen in micrograph (b). The cristae are densely packed, reflecting the metabolic activity of the cell. In some cells the cristae have a characteristic shape, those of heart muscle being laminar. Micrograph (c) uses a histochemical technique to localise a mitochondrial enzyme, cytochrome oxidase. The electron dense reaction product **RP** can be seen in the intermembranous space. The actin and myosin filaments **F** are essentially unstained in this preparation.

THE CELL

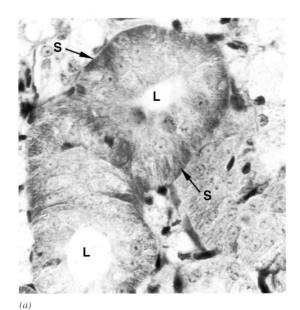

(a)

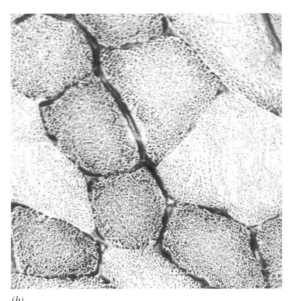

(b)

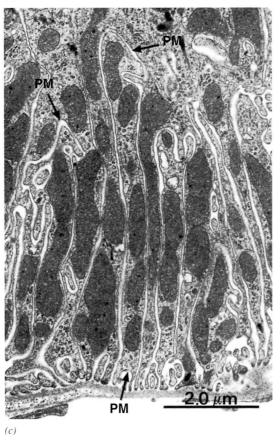

(c)

Fig. 1.18 Mitochondria

(a) Iron haematoxylin × 480 (b) Succinate dehydrogenase × 480 (c) EM × 13 000

Mitochondria are, in general, not seen individually by light microscopy. However, they are acidophilic and with the standard H & E stain are responsible for much of the eosinophilia (pink staining) of cytoplasm. In some cells, the mitochondria are profuse and may be concentrated in one region of the cell where they can be demonstrated directly and indirectly by various staining methods.

Micrograph (a) shows a salivary gland duct made up of cells that are extremely active in secretion and reabsorption of a variety of inorganic ions. This takes place at the base of the cells (i.e. the surface away from the lumen **L**) and is powered by ATP produced by extremely elongated mitochondria associated with numerous basal interdigitations between adjacent cells; a strategy which greatly increases the plasma membrane surface area. The cells have been stained by a modified haematoxylin method, which stains not only basophilic structures (i.e. DNA and RNA) but also acidophilic structures such as mitochondria that can be seen as striations **S** in the basal aspect of the cells.

In specimen (b), which shows skeletal muscle cells in transverse section, an enzyme histochemical method for succinate dehydrogenase has been employed. Succinate dehydrogenase is an enzyme of the citric acid cycle which is exclusive to mitochondria and therefore provides a marker for them. In skeletal muscle there are three muscle fibre types, which differ from each other in mitochondrial concentration. Such a staining method can be used to demonstrate their relative proportions (see also Fig. 6.11).

Micrograph (c) shows the base of an absorptive cell from a kidney tubule where there is intense active transport of ions. The basal plasma membrane **PM** of adjacent cells form interdigitations so as to greatly increase its surface area, and elongated mitochondria are packed into the intervening spaces. Micrographs (a) and (c) demonstrate an example of the same structure, interdigitation of a membrane, being used for the same purpose in two different situations to maximise ion transportation.

THE CELL

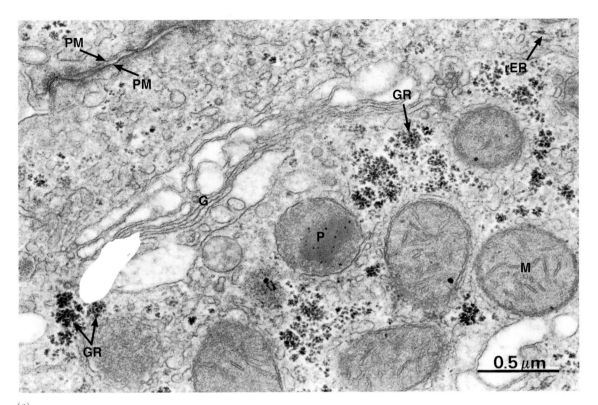

(a)

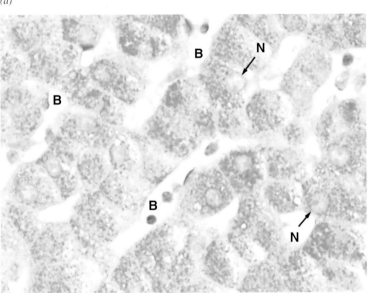

(b)

Fig. 1.19 **Glycogen and lipid droplets** (a) EM × 47 000 (b) PAS/haematoxylin × 600

Glycogen is present in large amounts in liver cells (hepatocytes). In micrograph (a), plentiful glycogen granules are present, appearing either as irregular single granules (called *a particles*) or as aggregations termed *glycogen rosettes* **GR** (also called *b particles*). Compare the size of the ribosomes on the rough endoplasmic reticulum **rER** with glycogen granules, which are slightly larger on average. A prominent Golgi apparatus **G** can be seen near the plasma membrane **PM**. Note that although the Golgi apparatus is classically found near the nucleus it is not at all unusual to find it in other areas of the cytoplasm, especially in cells like hepatocytes which

contain multiple Golgi apparatus. Several mitochondria **M** and a peroxisome **P** can also be seen in this field.

Micrograph (b) has been stained by a histochemical method to demonstrate the presence of glycogen, which is stained magenta. The specimen is of liver, the cytoplasm of each liver cell being packed with glycogen. The section has been counterstained (i.e. stained with a second dye) to demonstrate the liver cell nuclei **N** (blue). It also stains the nuclei of the cells lining the blood channels **B** between the rows of liver cells; these nuclei are smaller and more condensed and hence stain more intensely.

Lipid biosynthesis

Lipids are synthesised by all cells in order to repair and replace damaged or worn membranes. Cells may also synthesise lipid as a means of storing excess energy (as cytoplasmic droplets), for lipid transport (e.g. chylomicron production by cells of the small intestine) and in the form of steroid hormones for sending information to other cells. The precursor molecules (fatty acids, triglycerides and cholesterol) are available to the cell from dietary sources, from mobilisation of lipid stored in other cells or can be synthesised by most cells using simple sources of carbon such as acetyl-CoA and other intermediates of glucose catabolism. Fatty acids and triglycerides are mostly synthesised within the cytosol, whereas cholesterol and phospholipids are synthesised in areas of smooth endoplasmic reticulum.

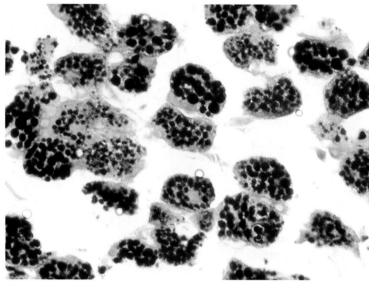

(a) *(b)*

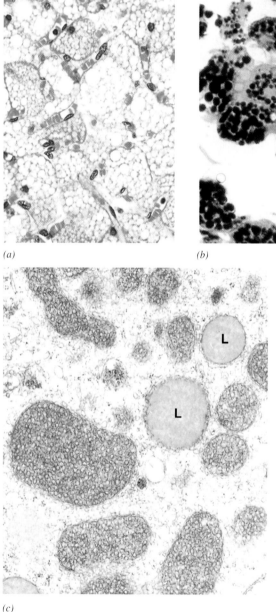

(c)

Fig. 1.20 **Lipid**

(a) H & E × 320 (b) Osmium × 320 (c) EM × 32 400

Routine processing methods for microscopy generally extract lipid from tissues. Therefore lipid droplets within cells appear as unstained vacuoles, as in micrograph (a). Lipids are therefore best demonstrated in frozen sections stained by specific lipid methods such as osmium, as in micrograph (b), with which lipid is stained black. Both micrographs show brown adipose tissue at similar magnifications (see also Fig. 4.13). Lipid droplets **L**, as seen in electron micrograph (c) of the cytoplasm of a liver cell, can be identified as homogeneous, rounded (really spherical in three dimensions) globules of lipid. The lipid forms droplets for the same reason that lipid membranes separate themselves from the cytoplasm, i.e. hydrophobic forces tend to exclude water as in the old saying 'oil and water don't mix'. As lipid droplets accumulate and enlarge, the same hydrophobic forces tend to make them fuse together to form larger droplets which may eventually occupy the entire cytoplasm and push the nucleus to the edge of the cell, as in *adipocytes* (fat cells) (see Fig. 4.11). Note the mitochondria of steroid hormone secreting cells have tubular cristae.

The cytoskeleton and cell movement

Every cell has a supporting framework of minute filaments and tubules, known as the ***cytoskeleton***, which maintains the shape and polarity of the cell. Nevertheless, the cell membrane and intracellular organelles are not rigid or static structures but are in a constant state of movement to accommodate processes such as endocytosis, phagocytosis and secretion. Some cells (e.g. white blood cells) propel themselves about by amoeboid movement; other cells have actively motile membrane specialisations such as cilia and flagella (see Ch. 5); whilst other cells (e.g. muscle cells) are highly specialised for contractility. In addition, cell division is a process which involves extensive reorganisation of cellular constituents. The cytoskeleton incorporates features which accommodate all these dynamic functions.

The cytoskeleton of each cell contains structural elements of three main types, ***microfilaments***, ***microtubules*** and ***intermediate filaments***, as well as many accessory proteins responsible for linking these structures to one another, to the plasma membrane and to the membranes of intracellular organelles.

- **Microfilaments.** Microfilaments are extremely fine strands (approximately 7 nm in diameter) of the protein ***actin.*** Each actin filament consists of two strings of bead-like subunits twisted together like a rope. The globular subunits are stabilised by calcium ions and associated with ATP molecules which provide energy for contractile processes. Actin filaments are best demonstrated histologically in skeletal muscle cells where they form a stable arrangement of bundles with another type of filamentous protein called ***myosin.*** Contraction occurs when the actin and myosin filaments slide relative to one another due to the rearrangement of intermolecular bonds fuelled by the release of energy from associated ATP molecules; this process is described in more detail in Chapter 6. Cells not usually considered to be contractile also contain the globular subunits of actin (***G-actin***) which assemble readily into microfilaments (***F-actin***) and then dissociate, thereby providing a dynamic structural framework for the cell. Membrane specialisations such as ***microvilli*** (see Fig. 5.16) also contain a skeleton of actin filaments which not only provide structural support but also cause the microvilli to shorten and elongate. Beneath the plasma membrane, actin, in association with various transmembrane and linking proteins (predominantly *filamin*), forms a robust supporting meshwork called the ***cell cortex***, which protects against deformation yet can be rearranged to accommodate changes in cell morphology.
- **Intermediate filaments.** Intermediate filaments (10–15 nm in diameter) are, as their name implies, intermediate in size between microfilaments and microtubules. These proteins have a purely structural function and consist of filaments of protein which self-assemble into larger filaments and bind intracellular structures to each other and to plasma membrane proteins. In humans there are more than 50 different types of intermediate filament, but these can be divided into five different classes, with each class expressed in a particular cell type. For example, ***cytokeratin*** intermediate filaments are characteristic of epithelial cells where they form a supporting network within the cytoplasm and are anchored to the plasma membrane at intercellular junctions. Likewise, ***vimentin*** is found in cells of mesodermal origin, ***desmin*** in muscle cells, ***neurofilament proteins*** in nerve cells and ***glial fibrillary acidic protein*** in glial cells.
- **Microtubules.** Microtubules (24 nm in diameter) are much larger than microfilaments but, like them, are made up of globular protein subunits which can readily be assembled and disassembled to provide for alterations in cell shape and position of organelles. The microtubule subunits are of two types, ***alpha*** and ***beta tubulin***, which polymerise to form a hollow tubule; when seen in cross-section, 13 tubulin molecules make up a circle. Microtubules originate from a specialised microtubule organising centre, the ***centriole***, found in the ***centrosome*** (see below), and movement may be effected by the addition or subtraction of tubulin subunits from the microtubules, making them longer or shorter. ***Microtubule-associated proteins (MAPs)*** stabilise the tubular structure and include ***capping proteins***, which stabilise the growing ends of the tubules. Two attachment proteins, ***dynein*** and ***kinesin*** (which can move along the tubules towards and away from the cell centre, respectively), may become attached to membranous organelles (e.g. mitochondria, vesicles), providing a means by which they can be moved about within the cytoplasm rather like an engine pulling cargo along a railway track. The function of the spindle during cell division is a classic example of this process on a large scale (see Fig. 2.3). In cilia, nine pairs of microtubules are disposed in a cylindrical structure, and movement occurs by rearrangement of chemical bonds between adjacent microtubule pairs (see Fig. 5.15).

The organising centre for microtubules, the centrosome, which contains a pair of centrioles, is often found near the nucleus. Each centriole consists of nine triplets of microtubules arranged in a cylindrical manner. The two cylinders are arranged at right angles to one another. The centrosome acts as a nucleation centre for microtubules which radiate from here towards the cell periphery. Centrioles appear to be necessary for microtubular function. For example, prior to cell division the pair of centrioles is duplicated, the pairs migrating towards opposite ends of the cell. Here they act as organising centres for the microtubules of the spindle which controls distribution of chromosomes to the daughter cells. Likewise, a pair of centrioles, known as a basal body, is found attached to the microtubules at the base of cilia.

The elements of the cytoskeleton are attached to one another and to the plasma membrane and the membranes of cytoplasmic organelles by a variety of linking proteins. In addition, some of the metabolic enzyme systems of the cytosol appear to be bound to various elements of the cytoskeleton.

In summary, the cytoskeleton consists of three main structural elements. The microfilaments and microtubules are labile and dynamic structures (except where they perform highly specialised functions such as in muscle and cilia), whereas the intermediate filaments serve a more static supporting function. The functions of the cytoskeleton are fourfold. Firstly, it provides the structural support for the plasma membrane, cellular organelles and some cytosol enzyme systems. Secondly, it provides the means for movement of intracellular organelles, the plasma membrane and other cytosol constituents necessary for the routine functions of all cells. and for cell division. Thirdly, the cytoskeleton provides the locomotor mechanism for amoeboid movements and specialised motile structures such as cilia and flagella. Finally, it is responsible for the property of contractility in the cells of specialised tissues such as muscle.

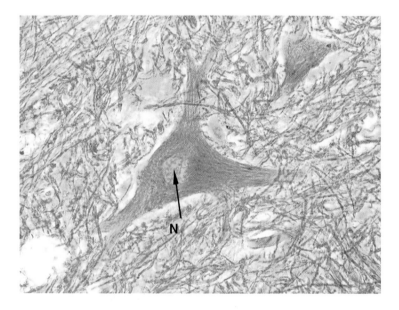

Fig. 1.21 Cytoskeleton

Silver impregnation method × 600

Individual elements of the cytoskeleton are not easily visualised by light microscopy. However, in cells with prominent aggregations of cytoskeletal elements, e.g. nerve cells or cells undergoing division, these can be demonstrated by impregnation with silver or gold. In this micrograph of a nerve cell body, the silver-impregnated cytoskeleton, which appears brown/black in colour, can be seen radiating from the vicinity of the nucleus **N** into various cytoplasmic extensions.

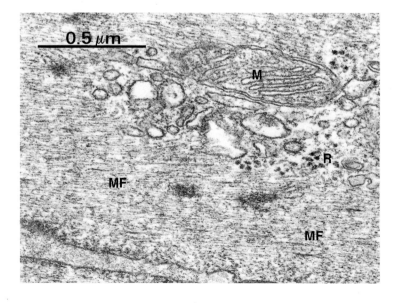

Fig. 1.22 Microfilaments

EM × 76 500

In general, individual microfilaments are difficult to demonstrate because of their small diameter and diffuse arrangement amongst other cytoplasmic components. In this example from a smooth muscle cell, a cell type in which cytoplasmic filaments are a predominant feature, parallel arrays of microfilaments **MF** are readily seen. The diameter of microfilaments may be compared with the diameter of a mitochondrion **M** and ribosomes **R**.

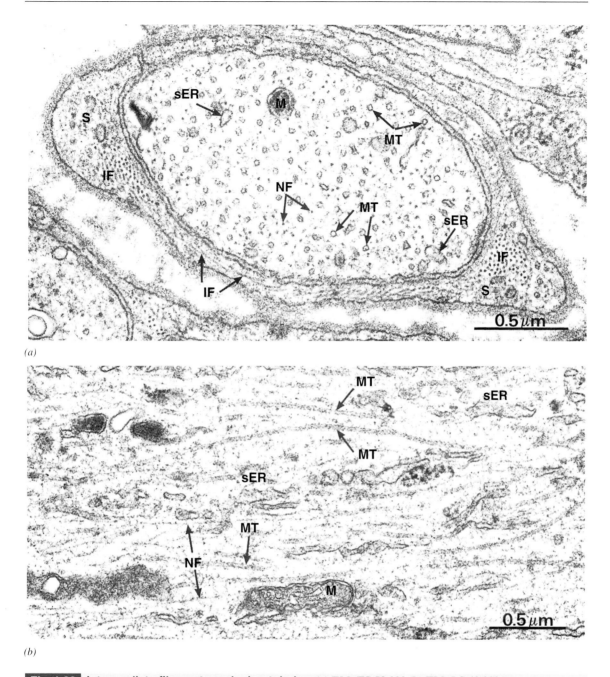

(a)

(b)

Fig. 1.23 Intermediate filaments and microtubules (a) EM: TS 53 000 (b) EM: LS 40 000

These micrographs are taken from nervous tissue; nerve cells contain both intermediate filaments and microtubules, allowing comparison of size and morphology. Each nerve cell has an elongated cytoplasmic extension called an axon (see Ch.7), which in the peripheral nervous system is ensheathed by a supporting Schwann cell. Micrograph (a) shows an axon in transverse section ensheathed by the cytoplasm of a Schwann cell **S.** Micrograph (b) shows part of an axon in longitudinal section. The axonal microtubules provide structural support and transport along the axon.

In longitudinal section, microtubules **MT** appear as straight, unbranched structures, and in transverse section they appear hollow. Their diameter can be compared with small mitochondria **M** and smooth endoplasmic reticulum **sER.**

Intermediate filaments (known as *neurofilaments* in this case) are a prominent feature of nerve cells, providing internal support for the cell by cross-linkage with microtubules and other organelles. The neurofilaments **NF** are dispersed among and in parallel with the microtubules, but are much smaller in diameter and are not hollow in cross-section. Intermediate filaments **IF** are also seen in the Schwann cell cytoplasm in micrograph (a).

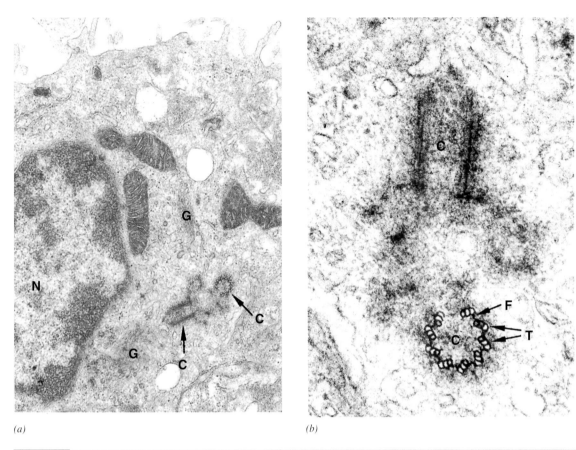

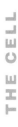

Fig. 1.24 Centrosome (a) EM × 9200 (b) EM × 48 000

The centrosome is a zone of cytoplasm, distinguishable by its different texture, usually centrally located in the cell adjacent to the nucleus **N** and often surrounded by the Golgi apparatus **G.** It contains a pair of *centrioles* **C**, together known as a *diplosome*, and a variable number of small dense bodies called *centriolar satellites.* Centrioles are highly specialised structures, composed of microtubules, which act as a *microtubule organising centre*. Microtubules radiate outwards from the centrioles in a star-like arrangement.

Each centriole is cylindrical in form, consisting of nine triplets of parallel microtubules. In transverse section, as in the lower half of micrograph (b), each triplet **T** is seen to consist of an inner microtubule, which is circular in cross-section, and two further microtubules, which are

C-shaped in cross-section. Each of the inner microtubules is connected to the outermost microtubule of the adjacent triplet by fine filaments **F**, thus forming a cylinder. The two centrioles of each diplosome are arranged with their long axes at right angles to each other, as can be seen in these micrographs.

Structures apparently identical to centrioles form the basal bodies of cilia and flagella (see Figs 5.15, 18.6 and 18.7), both of which are moved by microtubules. Cilia are a cell surface specialisation, each cilium comprising a minute hair-like cytoplasmic extension containing microtubules. Cilia move in a wave-like fashion for the purpose of moving secretions across a tissue surface. Flagella are the long tails responsible for the motility of sperm.

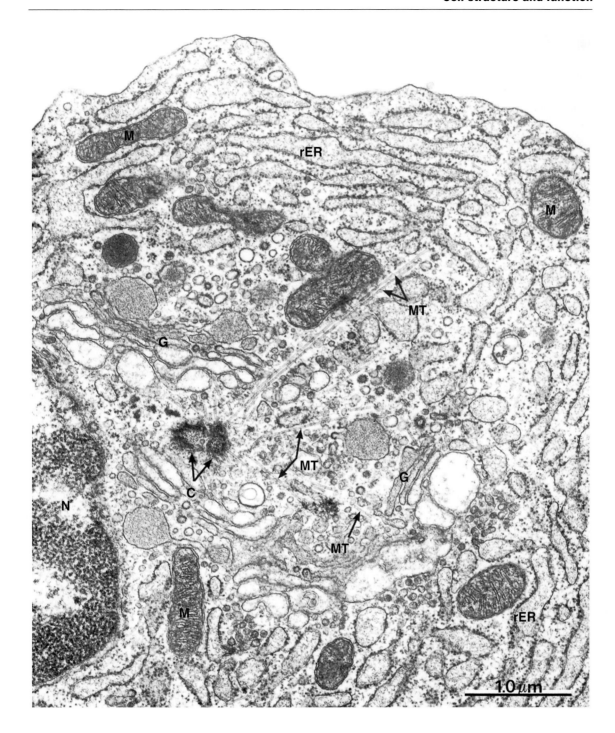

Fig. 1.25 Centrosome and microtubules EM × 30 000

This micrograph shows the centrosome acting as an organising centre for the microtubules of the cytoskeleton. The centrosome consists of two centrioles **C** (both cut somewhat obliquely in this specimen), typically located at the centre of the cell close to the nucleus **N.** Several microtubules **MT** are seen radiating from the centrosome towards the cell periphery.

Other features of this micrograph, which is from an antibody-secreting plasma cell, include profuse rough endoplasmic reticulum **rER** distended with secretory product, several saccular profiles of an extensive Golgi complex **G** and scattered mitochondria **M.**

The integrated function of cells in tissues, organs and organ systems

As mentioned at the outset, cells are the functional units of all living organisms; indeed the most primitive organisms merely consist of single cells. In multicellular organisms, however, individual cells become specialised (*differentiated*) and grouped together to perform specific functions. Cells of similar morphology and function form *tissues* which are relatively homogeneous in overall structure; examples include cartilage, bone and muscle. *Organs* are anatomically discrete collections of tissues which together perform certain specific functions (e.g. liver, kidney, eye, ovary). Tissues and organs may constitute integrated functional systems forming major anatomical entities (e.g. central nervous system, female reproductive tract, gastro-intestinal tract, urinary system) or be more diffusely arranged (e.g. immune defence system, diffuse neuro-endocrine system). Despite the foregoing, the terms tissue, organ and system are not necessarily mutually exclusive and may in some cases be used interchangeably depending on the functional implications. Part 2 of this book describes five basic tissues: blood, supporting/connective tissue, epithelia, muscle and nervous tissues. These are constituents of all organs and organ systems. Many tissues contain a mixture of functionally specialised cells and less specialised supporting tissue, to which the terms *parenchyma* and *stroma* may be applied, respectively.

Within tissues and organs, cells interact with one another in numerous ways during embryological development and growth, maintenance of structural integrity, response to injury (inflammation and repair), integration and control of tissue and organ functions and the maintenance of overall biochemical and metabolic integrity (*homeostasis*). This often involves the elaboration of structural connections between adjacent cells (various types of intercellular junctions) which may also serve as conduits for information exchange in the form of electrical excitation or chemical messengers. Some cells are indirectly bound to one another within tissues by various extracellular elements (e.g. the fibres of supporting/connective tissues). Within tissues, cellular functions are integrated by a great variety of local chemical mediators (*humoral factors*). At the level of systems and the body as a whole, functions are coordinated via circulating chemical messengers (*hormones*) and/or via the nervous system. The great pleasure to be derived from the study of histology is that all structures, from the subcellular to organ systems reflect these functional requirements and interrelationships.

2. Cell cycle and replication

Introduction

The development of a single, fertilised egg cell to form a complex, multicellular organism involves cellular replication, growth and progressive specialisation (*differentiation*) for a variety of functions. The mechanism of cellular replication in all but the male and female germ cells is known as *mitosis*. Mitosis or mitotic division of a single cell results in the production of two daughter cells, each genetically identical to the parent cell. Following mitosis, the daughter cells enter a period of growth and metabolic activity prior to further mitotic division. The time interval between mitotic divisions, the life cycle of an individual cell, is called the *cell cycle*.

As development of the fertilised ovum progresses to produce a multicellular embryo, groups of cells and their progeny become increasingly specialised to form tissues with different specific functions. In the fully developed organism, the differentiated cells of some tissues, such as the neurones of the nervous system, lose the ability to undergo mitosis, such cells being described as *terminally differentiated*. In contrast, the cells of certain other tissues, e.g. the lining cells of gut and skin, undergo continuous cycles of mitotic division throughout the lifespan of the organism. Between these extremes are cells such as liver cells which do not normally undergo mitosis but retain the capacity to undergo mitosis should the need arise (*facultative dividers*).

Cell division and differentiation balanced by cell death both during the development and growth of the immature organism and in the mature adult. In these circumstances, cell death occurs by a mechanism known as *apoptosis*.

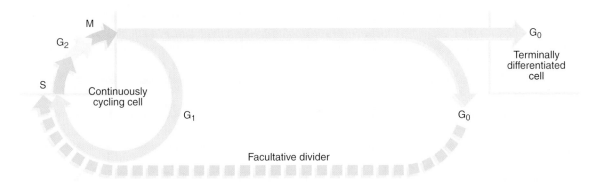

Fig. 2.1 The cell cycle

Historically, only two phases of the cell cycle were recognised: a relatively short mitotic phase (*M phase*) and a non-dividing phase (*interphase*), which usually occupies most of the life cycle of the cell. With the development of radioisotopes, it was found that there is a discrete period during interphase when nuclear DNA is replicated; this phase, described as the synthesis or *S phase*, is completed some time before the onset of mitosis. Thus interphase may be divided into three separate phases. Between the end of the M phase and the beginning of the S phase is the first gap or G_1 *phase*; this is usually much longer than the other phases of the cell cycle. During the G_1 phase, cells differentiate and perform their specialised functions as part of the whole tissue. The interval between the end of the S phase and the beginning of the M phase, the second gap or G_2 *phase*, is relatively short and is the period in which cells prepare for mitotic division.

Some cell types progress continually through the cell cycle to accommodate tissue growth or cell turnover, whereas terminally differentiated cells leave the cell cycle after the M phase and enter a state of continuous differentiated function designated as G_0 *phase*.

Facultative dividers enter the G_0 phase but retain the capacity to re-enter the cell cycle when suitably stimulated. Some liver cells appear to enter a protracted G_2 phase in which they perform their normal differentiated functions despite the presence of a duplicated complement of DNA.

Generally, in tissues with a regular turnover of cells, the cells which actually divide are a group of relatively undifferentiated cells, often called *reserve cells*. Some of the progeny of these cells differentiate to become the various types of mature cells found in the tissue, while others remain undifferentiated to maintain the pool of reserve cells. Such cells may be found in the base of the crypts of the small intestine (Ch. 14) and in the bone marrow where they produce the precursor cells for the formed elements of the blood (Ch. 3). The differentiated mature cells have lost their capacity to divide during the process of maturation.

In general, the S, G and M phases of the cell cycle are relatively constant in duration, each taking up to several hours to complete, whereas the G_1 phase is highly variable, in some cases lasting for several days or even longer. The G_0 phase may last for the entire lifespan of the organism.

Mitosis

Somatic cell division occurs in two phases. Firstly, the chromosomes duplicated in S phase are distributed equally between the two potential daughter cells; this process is known as mitosis. Secondly, the dividing cell is cleaved into genetically identical daughter cells by cytoplasmic division or *cytokinesis*. Although mitosis is always equal and symmetrical, cytokinesis may, in some situations, result in the formation of two daughter cells with grossly unequal amounts of cytoplasm or cytoplasmic organelles. In other circumstances, mitosis may occur in the absence of cytokinesis, as in the formation of binucleate and multinucleate cells.

Fig. 2.2 **Chromosomes during mitosis** *(illustrations opposite)*
(a) Diagrams (b) Chromosome spread: Giemsa × 1200

The nuclei of all cells of an individual, except the germ cells of the gonads, contain the same set complement of DNA, a quantity called the *genome*. This is present in the form of a fixed number of chromosomes, this number being specific to each species. DNA is a very large molecular weight polymer consisting of many deoxyribonucleotides with a double-stranded structure. Each strand consists of a backbone of alternating deoxyribose **S** and phosphate **P** moieties. Each deoxyribose unit is covalently bound to a *purine* or *pyrimidine* base which is in turn non-covalently linked to a complementary base on the other strand, thus linking the strands together. The bases are of four types, *adenine, cytosine, thymine* and *guanine,* with adenine only linking to thymine and cytosine only linking to guanine, thus making each strand complementary to the other (diagram 1). Linked in this way, the strands assume a double helical conformation around a common axis, the internucleotide phosphodiester bonds running in opposite directions (i.e. antiparallel) and the planes of the linked bases lying at right angles to the axis (diagram 2). The sequence of bases in either strand of the DNA molecule forms the genetic code for the individual. The bases are read in groups of three called *codons*, each coding for one amino acid. In human cells, there are 46 chromosomes (the *diploid* number) comprising 23 homologous pairs, the members of each pair having the same length of DNA and coding for the same proteins.

Histologically, individual chromosomes are not visible within the cell nucleus during interphase. During S phase, each chromosome is duplicated (as shown in diagram 3). The resulting identical chromosomes, now known as *chromatids*, remain attached to one another at a point called the *centromere*, and become even more tightly coiled and condensed when they may be visualised with the light microscope.

The extremely long DNA molecule making up each chromosome binds to a range of *histone proteins* which hold the chromosome in a supercoiled and folded conformation, compact enough to be accommodated within the nucleus. Thus the 2 nm diameter double helix is coiled and packed through several orders of three-dimensional complexity to form an elongated structure some 300 nm in diameter and very much shorter in length than the otherwise uncoiled molecule would be. This is the form in which the chromosome is structured during the G_1 and G_0 phases of the cell cycle, during which *gene transcription* (the prerequisite for protein synthesis) occurs.

Diagram 4 shows further detail of the structure of mitotic chromosomes and their supercoiled three-dimensional structure. Note the position of the kinetochore (see Fig. 2.3) which provides attachment for the microtubules of the cell spindle during cell division and seems also to control the progression of mitosis.

Micrograph (b) illustrates the chromosomes of a human cell cultured in vitro and arrested at the onset of mitosis; the preparation has been treated with the enzyme trypsin, and stained to show the cross-banding pattern along the length of each duplicated chromosome. Each duplicated chromosome comprises two chromatids joined at the centromere **C**. Each member of a homologous pair of mitotic chromosomes is identical in length, centromere location and banding pattern. Study of the chromosomes in this fashion, *karyotyping*, can reveal structural and numerical chromosomal abnormalities, known as *cytogenetic abnormalities*.

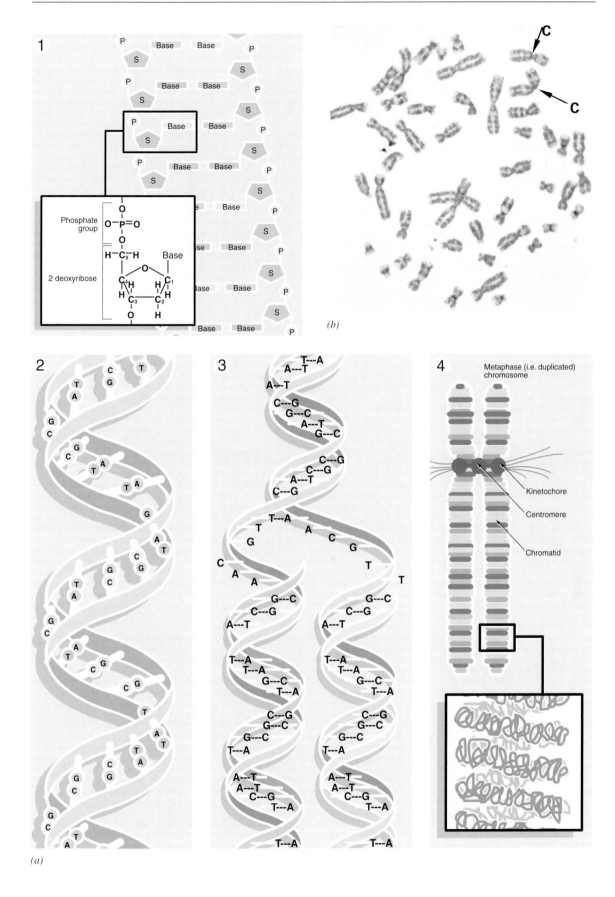

(a)

1

P   Base   Base   P

S   S

P   Base   Base   P

S   S

P   Base   Base   P

S   S

Phosphate group

O
|
O—P=O
|
O
|
H—C5—H   Base
|
O
C4   C1
H   H   H
| |
C3   C2
| |
O   H

2 deoxyribose

(b)

2

3

4   Metaphase (i.e. duplicated) chromosome

Kinetochore

Centromere

Chromatid

C

C

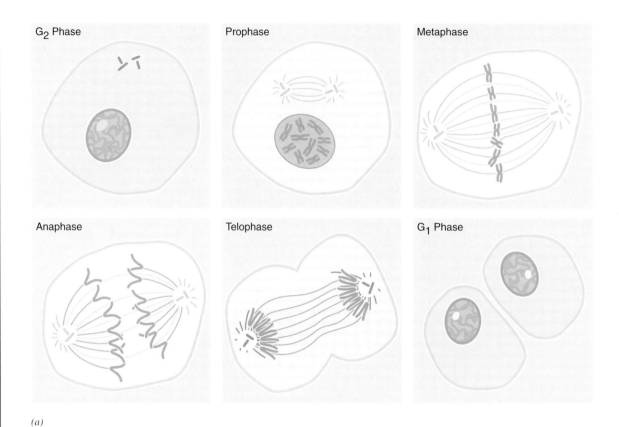

(a)

Fig. 2.3 **Mitosis** (a) Schematic diagram (b) Mitotic series: Giemsa × 800 *(opposite)*

The series of micrographs, shown opposite, illustrates the mitotic process in actively dividing immature blood cells from a smear preparation of human bone marrow.

Mitosis is a continuous process which is traditionally divided into four phases, *prophase, metaphase, anaphase* and *telophase*, each stage being readily recognisable with the light microscope. Cell division requires the presence of a structure called the *mitotic apparatus*, which comprises a spindle of longitudinally arranged microtubules extending between a pair of centrioles (see Fig. 1.24) at each pole of the dividing cell. The mitotic apparatus is visible within the cytoplasm only during the M phase of the cell cycle since it disaggregates shortly after completion of mitosis.

Prophase. The beginning of this stage of mitosis is defined as the moment when the chromosomes (already duplicated during the preceding S phase) first become visible within the nucleus. As prophase continues, the chromosomes become increasingly condensed and shortened and the nucleoli disappear. Dissolution of the nuclear envelope marks the end of prophase.

During prophase, the microfilaments and microtubules of the cytoskeleton disaggregate into their protein subunits. During the preceding interphase, the pair of centrioles in the centrosome has duplicated, and in prophase these migrate towards opposite poles of the cell whilst simultaneously a spindle of microtubules is formed between them (*interpolar microtubules*). As the centriole pairs move apart, the interpolar microtubules progressively elongate by the addition of tubulin subunits.

Metaphase. The nuclear envelope having disintegrated, the mitotic spindle moves into the nuclear area and each duplicated chromosome becomes attached, at a site called the *kinetochore*, to another group of microtubules of the mitotic spindle (*kinetochore* or *chromosome microtubules*). The kinetochore is a DNA and protein structure on each duplicated chromosome, located at the centromere, the structure which binds the duplicated

chromosomes (*chromatids*) together (see also diagram 4, Fig. 2.2). The chromosomes then become arranged in the plane of the spindle equator, known as the equatorial or *metaphase plate*. The kinetochore also appears to control entry of the cell into anaphase so that the process of mitosis does not progress until all chromatid pairs are aligned at the cell equator. This is sometimes called the *metaphase checkpoint* and prevents the formation of daughter cells with unequal numbers of chromosomes.

Anaphase. This stage of mitosis is marked by the splitting of the centromere which binds the chromatids of each duplicated chromosome. The mitotic spindle becomes lengthened by addition of tubulin subunits to its interpolar microtubules; the centrioles are thus pulled apart and the chromatids of each duplicated chromosome are drawn by the kinetochore microtubules to opposite ends of the spindle, thus achieving an exact division of the duplicated genetic material. By the end of anaphase, two groups of identical chromosomes (the former chromatids) are clustered at opposite poles of the cell.

Telophase. During the final phase of mitosis, the chromosomes begin to uncoil and to regain their interphase conformation. The nuclear envelope reassembles and nucleoli again become apparent. The process of cytokinesis also takes place during telophase. The plane of cytoplasmic division is usually defined by the position of the spindle equator, thus producing two cells of equal size. The plasma membrane around the spindle equator becomes indented to form a circumferential furrow around the cell, the *cleavage furrow*, which progressively constricts the cell until it is cleaved into two daughter cells. A ring of microfilaments is present just beneath the surface of the cleavage furrow and cytokinesis occurs as a result of contraction of this filamentous ring. In early G_1 phase, the mitotic spindle disaggregates and in many cell types the single pair of centrioles begins to duplicate in preparation for the next mitotic division.

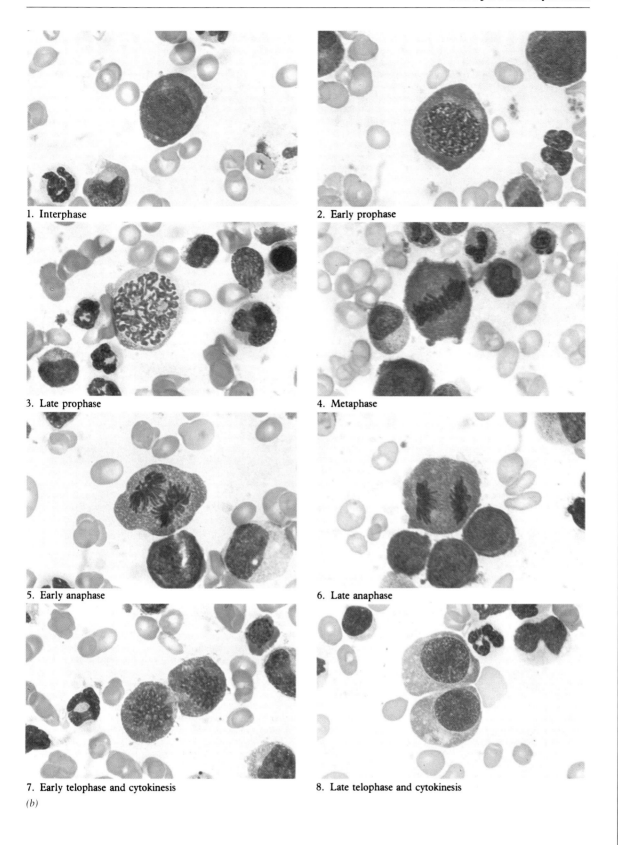

1. Interphase

2. Early prophase

3. Late prophase

4. Metaphase

5. Early anaphase

6. Late anaphase

7. Early telophase and cytokinesis

8. Late telophase and cytokinesis

(b)

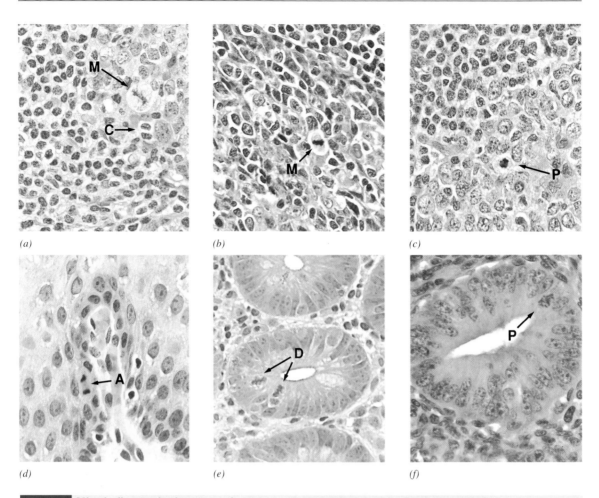

(a)   (b)   (c)

(d)   (e)   (f)

Fig. 2.4 | Mitotic figures in tissue sections (a)–(f) H & E × 400 (g) EM × 30 000 *(opposite)*

This series of six light micrographs shows the appearance of mitotic figures as seen in tissue sections. In smear preparations (as shown in Fig. 2.3) an image of the whole cell is seen making the identification of mitotic cells and the stage of mitosis relatively simple. In contrast, with tissue sections, what is seen depends on the plane of section through the cell and the thickness of the section, whole cells rarely being encompassed within it. Thus mitotic figures are more difficult to identify with certainty and the appearance is much more variable.

Specimens (a), (b) and (c) are from lymphoid tissue in which there is considerable lymphocyte cell division (see Ch. 11). Cells in metaphase **M** and in cytokinesis **C** can be identified with some confidence in micrograph (a). Micrograph (b) shows another good example of a cell in metaphase **M**, whilst micrograph (c) shows a dividing cell in probable late prophase **P**.

Micrograph (d) shows the proliferative basal layer of the epithelium lining the uterine cervix with a good example of a mitotic figure in late anaphase **A**. The proliferating epithelium of a duodenal crypt is illustrated in micrograph (e) and contains two dividing cells **D**; the stage of mitosis cannot be readily determined. Lastly, micrograph (f) shows a gland from the endometrium in the proliferative phase of the menstrual cycle; it contains a mitotic cell in prophase **P**.

Micrograph (g) shows an electron microscopic view of part of a dividing cell, in this case a supporting Schwann cell in the developing nervous system. The plasma membrane **PM** can be identified, but the

nuclear membrane has dissolved and condensed chromatin **C** has spread out into the cytoplasm. Mitochondria **M**, smooth endoplasmic reticulum **sER** and ribosomes **R** are seen in the peripheral cytoplasm. In the centre of the nuclear material, numerous microtubules **MT** can be seen in transverse section representing part of the spindle apparatus. Taken together, these features probably indicate that the cell is in anaphase, the plane of section being through one end of the dividing nuclear material and oriented at right angles to the spindle axis.

Mitotic index

The term mitotic index is used to describe the proportion of cells of a tissue which are in mitosis at a particular point in time. This can be crudely estimated by counting the number of mitotic figures per high-power field and is employed in pathology as a measure of the rate of cellular proliferation in certain malignant tumours. More precise techniques include the use of certain antibodies which react with structures found only in proliferating cell, such as proliferating cell nuclear antigen. Using the immunoperoxidase technique, these can highlight dividing cells in tissue sections, facilitating accurate counts. Under experimental conditions, mitotic index can be estimated accurately by injecting a laboratory animal with radioactive thymidine. This labelled thymidine is incorporated into the replicating DNA of dividing cells which can then be identified by subjecting tissue sections to the process of autoradiography.

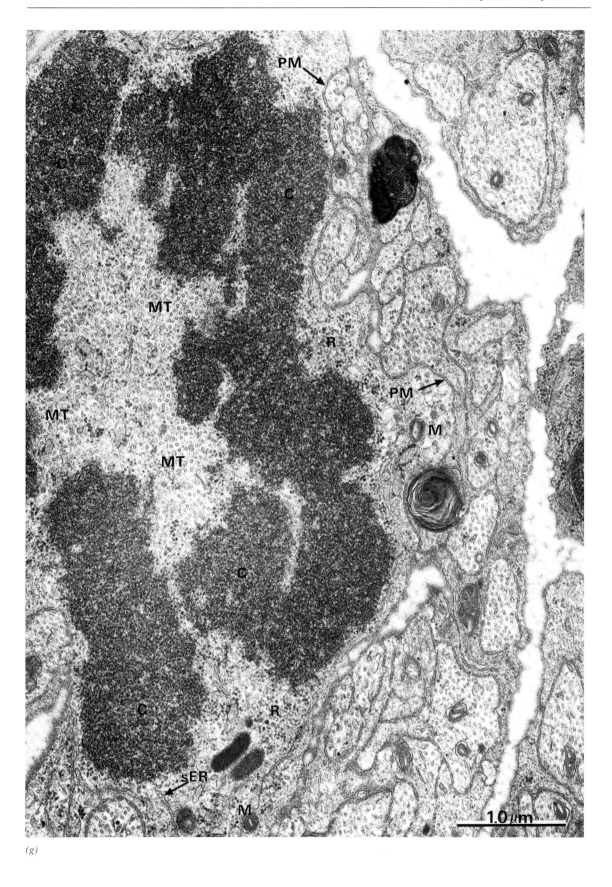

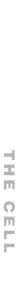

Meiosis

In all somatic cells, cell division (mitosis) results in the formation of two daughter cells, each one genetically identical to the mother cell. Somatic cells contain a full complement of chromosomes (the ***diploid number***) which function as homologous pairs as described earlier. The process of sexual reproduction involves the fusion of specialised male and female cells called ***gametes*** to form a ***zygote*** which has the diploid number of chromosomes. Each gamete thus contains only half the diploid number of chromosmes, known as the ***haploid number*** (23 in humans).

The production of haploid cells involves a unique form of cell division called ***meiosis*** which occurs only in the germ cells of the gonads during the formation of gametes; meiotic cell division is thus also called ***gametogenesis***. Meiosis involves two cell division processes, of which only the first is preceded by duplication of chromosomes.

1. **First meiotic division**. This results in the formation of two daughter cells, the process differing from mitosis in two important respects:

   - In mitosis, each duplicated chromosome divides at the centromere, liberating two chromatids which migrate to opposite ends of the mitotic spindle, whereas in the first meiotic division there is no such separation of the chromatids, but rather one duplicated chromosome of each homologous pair migrates to each end of the spindle. Thus at the end of the first meiotic division, each daughter cell contains a half complement of duplicated chromosomes, one chromosome being derived from each homologous pair of the mother cell.
   - During the first meiotic division, and preceding the process just described, there is an exchange of ***alleles*** (alternate gene forms coding for the same characteristic) between the chromatids of homologous pairs of duplicated chromosomes. This exchange, called ***chiasma formation***, results in chromatids with a different genetic constitution from those of the parent cell.

2. **Second meiotic division**. This merely involves splitting of each rearranged duplicated chromosome at the centromere to liberate chromatids which migrate to opposite poles of the spindle.

Thus, meiotic cell division of a single diploid germ cell gives rise to four haploid gametes. In the male, each of the four gametes undergoes morphological development into a mature ***spermatozoon***. In the female, unequal distribution of the cytoplasm results in one gamete gaining almost all the cytoplasm from the mother cell, whilst the other three acquire almost none; the large gamete matures to form an ***ovum*** and the other three, called ***polar bodies***, degenerate.

During both the first and second meiotic divisions, the cell passes through stages which have many similar features to prophase, metaphase, anaphase and telophase of mitosis. Unlike mitosis, however, the process of meiotic cell division can be suspended for a considerable length of time. For example, in the development of the human female gamete, the germ cells enter prophase of the first meiotic division during the fifth month of fetal life and then remain suspended until some time after sexual maturity; the first meiotic division is thus suspended for between 12 and 45 years!

The primitive germ cells of the male, the ***spermatogonia***, are present only in small numbers in the male gonads before sexual maturity. After this, spermatogonia multiply continuously by mitosis to provide a supply of cells which then undergo meiosis to form male gametes. In contrast, the germ cells of the female, called ***oogonia***, multiply by mitosis only during early fetal development, thereby producing a fixed complement of cells with the potential to undergo gametogenesis.

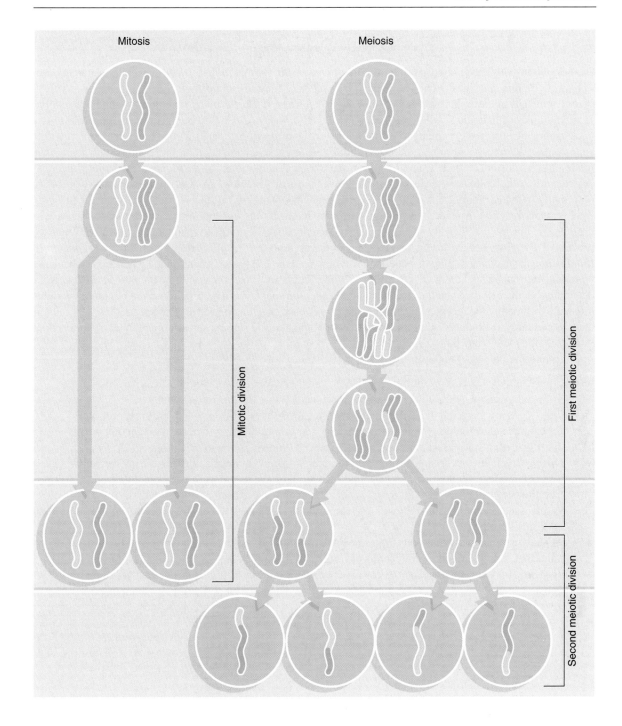

Mitosis   Meiosis

Mitotic division

First meiotic division

Second meiotic division

Fig. 2.5 **Comparison of mitosis and meiosis**

This diagram compares the behaviour of each homologous pair of chromosomes during mitosis and meiosis; the fate of only one homologous pair is represented here. The key differences between the two forms of cell division are as follows:

- Meiosis involves two sequential cell divisions, the first resulting in reduction of the chromosome complement to the haploid state and the second resulting in the production of four haploid daughter cells, the gametes.

- Chiasmata formation occurs in meiosis only. The purpose of chiasma formation is to rearrange alleles such that every gamete is genetically different. In contrast, the products of mitosis are genetically identical.

Cell death balances cell division in normal tissues

Dead and dying single cells are a common finding in tissues. In normal tissues, individual cell death may occur as part of cell turnover, during involution of tissue as part of normal embryological development or as part of cyclical changes in tissues or organs. Death of single cells also occurs in many pathological conditions. All of these examples of individual cell death are known as *apoptosis*, because (although occurring in response to a wide range of triggers) there seems to be a common mechanism of cell death with characteristic microscopic appearances. Apoptosis is brought about by entirely different mechanisms than those that cause *necrosis,* a mode of cell and tissue death which occurs in pathological conditions. A well-known example of necrosis is myocardial infarction, where heart muscle dies as a result of lack of oxygen. While apoptosis occurs in both pathologic and normal conditions, necrosis is always pathological and is usually accompanied by an inflammatory reaction. Apoptosis is an active process requiring the expenditure of energy, while necrosis is characterised by the inability of cells to produce the energy (ATP) required to maintain homeostasis. When the process of apoptosis occurs during development of the embryo or fetus it is often referred to as *programmed cell death*, a name which highlights both its inevitability and the fact that it is controlled by genetic mechanisms.

In both normal and pathological conditions, a wide variety of triggers may initiate the process of apoptosis, depending on the cell type and the situation. The trigger for apoptosis to begin may be the binding of a signal molecule to a membrane receptor, or the lack of a particular signal that is needed to block apoptosis. Within the nucleus certain gene products either inhibit (*bcl-2*) or stimulate (*p53*) apoptosis, depending on their interactions with each other and many other regulators.

Examples of apoptosis include:

- Some cell types have a preset limited lifetime and inevitably undergo apoptosis as part of their life cycle, e.g. keratinocytes in the skin or epithelial cells lining the gastrointestinal tract.
- Other cells are triggered to destroy themselves if they behave in ways which are 'inappropriate'; for example, developing lymphocytes which are capable of reacting to normal body components are triggered to self-destruct in the thymus, a process known as clonal deletion (see Ch. 11).
- During development certain cells are programmed to die by apoptosis, e.g. in humans the webs between the fingers and toes disappear and the tadpole loses its tail as it matures into a frog.
- Certain tissues in adults grow and regress in a cyclical fashion, such as, the growth of ovarian follicles before ovulation in females followed by regression of the corpus luteum by apoptosis to form a corpus albicans (see Ch. 19).
- In many pathological conditions, it has become clear that apoptosis may be triggered to destroy abnormal cells such as those infected by viruses and those with genetic mutations. Failure of normal apoptosis may also be important in certain conditions. It has recently been shown that failure of apoptosis may be as important as unrestricted cell division in cancer. Failure of clonal deletion may also lead to autoimmune disorders.

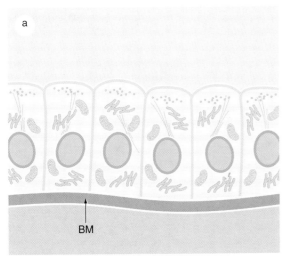

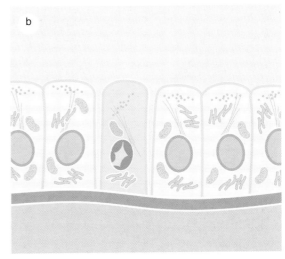

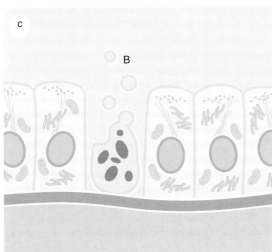

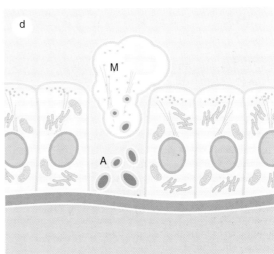

Fig. 2.6 **The mechanism of apoptosis**

Although a variety of extrinsic and intrinsic triggers may initiate apoptosis, at the molecular level the key feature of apoptosis seems to be the slicing of the DNA into short lengths. This is carried out by a set of enzymes which may be present in the cell in inactive form or may be synthesised by the cell when it receives the apoptosis signal. When these enzymes are activated, a series of changes occur in the cell, many of which can be discerned with the light microscope. Some cells are programmed to destruct at a certain phase of their life and are only prevented from doing so by receiving an external signal which stops the process. Other cells require constant positive signals to live (such as growth factors) and if these are withdrawn, they will proceed to apoptosis.

The process of apoptosis is shown in this diagram of simple columnar epithelial cells resting on basement membrane **BM**.

When a normal cell (a) receives a signal to initiate apoptosis, the characteristic change by light microscopy (b) is condensation of the nuclear chromatin (*pyknosis*) to form one or more dark-staining masses found against the nuclear membrane. At the same time the cell shrinks away from its neighbours with loss of cell–cell contacts and increasing eosinophilia (pink staining) of the cytoplasm. The cytoplasmic organelles are still preserved at this stage. As the process continues (c), the nuclear material breaks into fragments (*karyorrhexis*). This is accompanied by dissolution of the nuclear membrane. Cytoplasmic blebs **B** break away from the cell surface and eventually the entire cell breaks up (*karyolysis*) (d) to form membrane-bound fragments, some of which contain nuclear material, known as *apoptotic bodies* **A**. These apoptotic bodies may be phagocytosed by tissue *macrophages* **M**, scavenger cells derived from the bone marrow and found in virtually every tissue in the body. Apoptotic cells may also be phagocytosed by their neighbouring cells.

In some circumstances, part of the cell remains as a normal tissue component after apoptosis. For instance, in the skin, keratinocytes undergo apoptosis as part of their normal life cycle, but for some considerable time after the nucleus has disappeared, the cell cytoplasm filled with keratin intermediate filaments remains as an anucleate 'squame' to form a waterproof coating on the surface of the skin.

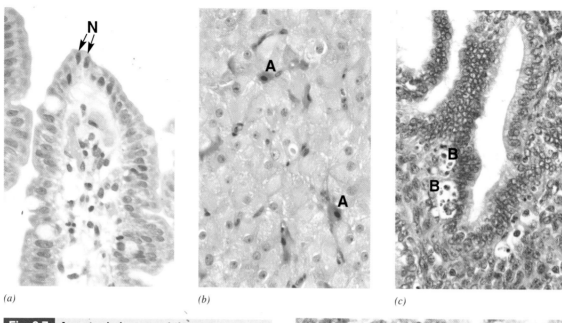

(a)   *(b)*   *(c)*

Fig. 2.7   **Apoptosis in normal tissues**
H & E (a) × 300 (b) × 200 (c) & (d) × 300

These four micrographs illustrate the typical features of apoptotic cells in normal tissues. Specimen (a) shows the tip of a villus in the small intestine. Several nuclei **N** in the epithelial cells at the tip are more darkly stained than the neighbouring cells, indicating that these cells are beginning the process of apoptosis prior to being shed from the surface. Micrograph (b) is a corpus luteum, formed from an ovarian follicle after discharge of an ovum (see Ch. 19). Towards the end of the cycle, pituitary hormones result in involution of the corpus luteum, a process which involves progressive death of its constituent cells. In this micrograph several apoptotic cells **A** can be identified by their condensed nuclei and eosinophilic cytoplasm.

Micrographs (c) and (d) show a later stage of apoptosis. Micrograph (c) shows epithelial cells of endometrial glands at the beginning of menstruation (see Ch. 19). Two cells have undergone apoptosis and reached the stage of forming easily identified apoptotic bodies **B**. The apoptotic bodies have been phagocytosed by adjacent cells, which are themselves about to undergo the same process as the superficial part of the endometrium is shed.

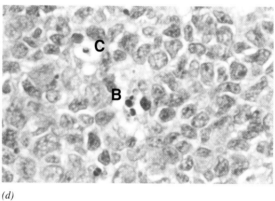

(d)

Micrograph (d) is from a lymph node and shows two apoptotic cells. One of these **C** has a small condensed nucleus with indistinct cytoplasm while the other is represented by a number of apoptotic bodies **B** which have been phagocytosed by a macrophage. This appearance is common in normal lymph node follicles where lymphocytes are induced to proliferate in response to an antigenic stimulus (see Ch. 11).

BASIC TISSUE TYPES

PART TWO

3. Blood *46*

4. Supporting/connective tissue *65*

5. Epithelial tissues *80*

6. Muscle *97*

7. Nervous tissues *116*

3. Blood

Introduction

Blood is a tissue consisting of a variety of cells suspended in a fluid medium called **plasma**. It functions principally as a vehicle for the transport of gases, nutrients, metabolic waste products, cells and hormones throughout the body. Thus any sample of blood is composed not only of cells and molecules involved in transport processes but also cells and molecules in the process of being transported.

Plasma is essentially an aqueous solution of inorganic salts which is constantly exchanged with the extracellular fluid of body tissues. Plasma also contains proteins, the **plasma proteins**, of three main types: **albumins, globulins** and **fibrinogen**. Collectively, the plasma proteins exert a colloidal osmotic pressure within the circulatory system which helps to regulate the exchange of aqueous solution between plasma and extracellular fluid. The albumins, which constitute the bulk of plasma proteins, bind relatively insoluble metabolites such as fatty acids and thus serve as transport proteins. The globulins are a diverse group of proteins which include the antibodies of the immune system (see Ch. 11) and certain proteins responsible for the transport of lipids and some heavy metal ions. Fibrinogen is a soluble protein which polymerises to form the insoluble protein **fibrin** during blood clotting. In general, the molecular components of plasma cannot be demonstrated by light and electron microscopy.

Blood cell types

The cells of blood are of three major functional classes: **red blood cells (erythrocytes), white blood cells (leucocytes)** and **platelets (thrombocytes)**. All are formed in the bone marrow, the process being known as **haemopoiesis**.

Erythrocytes are primarily involved in the transport of oxygen and carbon dioxide and function exclusively within the vascular system. The whole mass of red blood cells and their precursors in the bone marrow is called the **erythron**.

The leucocytes constitute an important part of the defence and immune systems of the body and, as such, act mainly outside blood vessels in the tissues; thus the leucocytes found in circulating blood are merely in transit between their various sites of activity.

Platelets play a vital role in the control of bleeding (**haemostasis**) by plugging defects in blood vessel walls and contributing to the activation of the blood clotting cascade.

Methods used to study blood and bone marrow

The standard method of examination of the blood is to make a **smear** on a glass slide. After fixation, a polychromatic **Romanowsky-type staining technique** such as the **Giemsa, Wright** or **Leishman method** is used for examination with the light microscope. Four distinctive staining characteristics can be identified according to the affinity of the various cellular organelles for the different stains employed in these methods:

- **basophilia** (deep blue) – affinity for the basic dye **methylene blue**; this is a characteristic of DNA in nuclei and RNA in the cytoplasm, i.e. ribosomes
- **azurophilia** (purple) – affinity for azure dyes; this is typical of lysosomes, one of the granule types found in leucocytes
- **eosinophilia** (pink) – affinity for the acidic dye **eosin** (thus also described as **acidophilia**); this is a particular feature of haemoglobin which fills the cytoplasm of erythrocytes
- **neutrophilia** (salmon pink/lilac) – affinity for a dye once erroneously believed to be of neutral pH; characteristic of the specific cytoplasmic granules of neutrophil leucocytes.

Bone marrow is usually studied by taking an aspirate from an active area of haemopoiesis (e.g. sternum, iliac crest). This is made into a smear, fixed and stained as for peripheral blood films. These processes induce marked artefactual alterations from that in vivo, particularly in respect of cell size and morphology, and this must be taken into account when comparing blood or marrow smears with tissue sections and ultrastructural preparations.

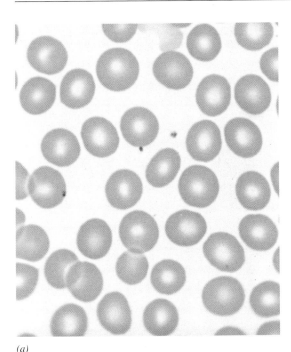

(a)

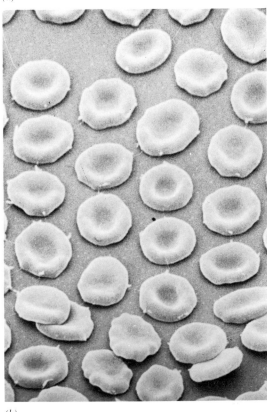

(b)

Fig. 3.1 **Erythrocytes**
(a) Giemsa × 1200 (b) Scanning EM × 2400

The erythrocyte is highly adapted for its principal function of oxygen and carbon dioxide transport. During differentiation in the bone marrow, vast quantities of the iron-containing respiratory pigment *haemoglobin* are synthesised. Before release into the blood circulation, the erythrocyte nucleus is extruded and, by maturity, all cytoplasmic organelles degenerate. The fully differentiated erythrocyte thus consists merely of an outer plasma membrane enclosing haemoglobin and the limited number of enzymes necessary for maintenance of plasma membrane integrity and gaseous transport functions.

Micrograph (a) demonstrates the characteristic appearance of erythrocytes in a stained smear of peripheral blood. The cells are stained pink (eosinophilia/acidophilia) due to their high content of haemoglobin, a basic protein. The pale staining of the central region of the erythrocyte is a result of its biconcave disc shape.

Scanning electron microscopy reveals the biconcave disc shape of erythrocytes which provides a 20–30% greater surface area than a sphere relative to cell volume, thus significantly enhancing gaseous exchange. This shape, along with the fluidity of the plasma membrane, allows the erythrocyte to deform readily, and thus erythrocytes (average diameter 7.2 μm) are able to pass through the smallest capillaries (3–4 μm in diameter).

The erythrocyte plasma membrane is composed of a lipid bilayer incorporating various globular proteins conforming to the standard fluid mosaic model of membrane structure (see Fig. 1.2). Immediately beneath the plasma membrane is a meshwork of proteins forming a cytoskeleton anchored to the membrane by one or more membrane-incorporated proteins; the main skeletal protein is the long fibre-like protein, *spectrin*. The biconcave shape of erythrocytes is determined in part by the cytoskeleton and in part by its water content, the latter being related to the concentration of inorganic ions within the cell.

The binding, transport and delivery of oxygen by haemoglobin are not dependent on erythrocyte metabolism. However, erythrocytes utilise energy in maintenance of normal electrolyte gradients across the plasma membrane, maintenance of the iron atoms of haemoglobin in the divalent form and maintenance of the sulphydryl groups of red cell enzymes and haemoglobin in the reduced, active form. The energy required for this process is derived from anaerobic metabolism of glucose. The absence of mitochondria precludes aerobic energy production and erythrocytes are thus totally dependent on glucose as an energy source.

The lifespan of an erythrocyte averages 120 days and is partly governed by its ability to maintain the biconcave shape. Without the appropriate organelles, erythrocytes are unable to replace deteriorating enzymes and membrane proteins, leading to diminished ability to pump sodium ions from the cell, uptake of water and the assumption of a spheroidal shape. Such cells are removed from the circulation by the spleen and liver (see Ch. 11).

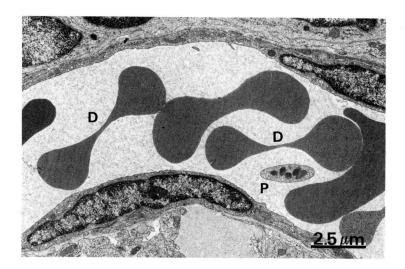

Fig. 3.2 **Erythrocytes**
EM × 6000

This electron micrograph illustrates the erythrocytes within a capillary. The observed shape of the erythrocyte depends on the plane of section through the cell. The classic 'dumb-bell' shape **D** is only seen when the erythrocyte is cut through its thin central zone; more frequently, irregularly shaped erythrocytes are seen reflecting the deformation which occurs in small blood vessels. The high electron density of erythrocytes is due to the iron atoms of haemoglobin. Note the total absence of organelles. A platelet **P** is also seen in this field.

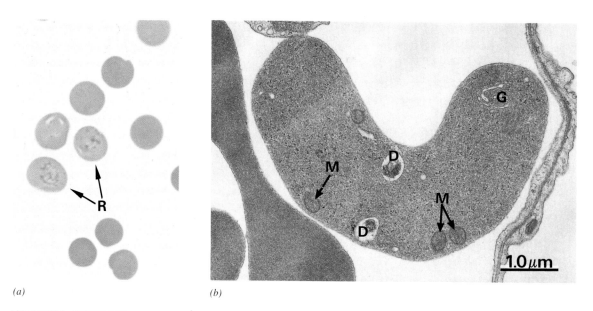

(a)   *(b)*

Fig. 3.3 **Reticulocytes** (a) Cresyl blue/eosin × 1200 (b) EM × 16 000

Reticulocytes are the immature form in which erythrocytes are released into the circulation from the bone marrow. They still contain sufficient mitochondria, ribosomes and Golgi elements to complete the cytoskeleton and the remaining 20% of haemoglobin synthesis. Final maturation into erythrocytes occurs within 24–48 hours of release. The rate of release of reticulocytes into the circulation generally equals the rate of removal of spent erythrocytes by the spleen and liver. Since the lifespan of circulating erythrocytes is about 120 days, reticulocytes constitute slightly less than 1% of circulating red blood cells.

Reticulocytes cannot be easily distinguished from mature erythrocytes in routinely stained blood smears, but when fresh blood is incubated with the basic dye, brilliant cresyl blue, a blue-stained *reticular* precipitate **R** is formed in the reticulocytes due to the interaction of the dye with ribosomal RNA remnants. This technique, called *supravital staining*, is illustrated in micrograph (a).

When severe erythrocyte depletion occurs, such as after haemorrhage or haemolysis, the rate of erythrocyte production in the bone marrow increases and the proportion of reticulocytes in circulating blood rises (*reticulocytosis*). Thus the reticulocyte count provides a convenient measure of the rate of red blood cell formation in the bone marrow. Reticulocytes are slightly larger than mature erythrocytes. Micrograph (b) shows the ultrastructure of a reticulocyte with an adjacent mature erythrocyte for comparison. Overall the cytoplasmic density is lower, due to a lower concentration of haemoglobin. Scattered ribosomes can still be discerned as well as a few mitochondria **M**, a couple of degenerating mitochondria **D** and a small Golgi remnant **G**.

White cell series

Five types of leucocyte are normally present in the circulation. These are traditionally divided into two main groups based on their nuclear shape and cytoplasmic granules:

- **Granulocytes**
  Neutrophils
  Eosinophils
  Basophils
- **Mononuclear leucocytes**
  Lymphocytes
  Monocytes

Granulocytes are so named for their prominent cytoplasmic secretory granules. Each of the three different types of granulocyte has type-specific granules, the names *neutrophil, eosinophil* and *basophil* being derived from the staining characteristics of these *specific granules*. The granulocytes have a single multilobed nucleus which conveyed to early microscopists the erroneous impression that these cells were multinucleate and led to the confusing description of the other main group of leucocytes as mononuclear cells (see below). The multilobed nucleus may assume many morphological shapes leading to the use of the term *polymorphonuclear leucocyte* or *polymorph* as a synonym for the term granulocyte. To confuse matters further, the term polymorph is often used to refer to neutrophils since they exhibit the greatest degree of nuclear polymorphism and are by far the most prolific of the polymorphs. Granulocytes are also referred to as *myeloid cells* due to their exclusive origin from bone marrow; this should not, however, be taken to imply that they are the only white blood cells to be formed in the bone marrow.

Lymphocytes and monocytes have non-lobulated nuclei and were described as mononuclear leucocytes by early microscopists to distinguish them from the polymorphs whose multilobed nuclei were originally believed to represent multiple nuclei. Again, to distinguish this group from the granulocytes, the term *agranulocytes* was also employed since cytoplasmic granules were not readily seen with early microscopic methods; unfortunately this may give the erroneous impression that these cells are devoid of cytoplasmic granules.

Leucocytes constitute an important part of the body's defences against foreign invaders. Neutrophils and monocytes are highly phagocytic and engulf microorganisms, cell debris and particulate matter in a non-specific manner; this activity may be enhanced and directed by immune responses to specific foreign agents (see Ch. 11). Lymphocytes play the key role in all immune responses and, in contrast to the other leucocytes, their activity is always directed against specific foreign agents.

In general, all the leucocytes perform their functions in the tissues and merely use the blood as a vehicle for transit between sites of formation, storage and activity. It follows, therefore, that increased demand for particular leucocytes in various sites is reflected in increased numbers in the circulation. For example, bacterial infections attract neutrophils and this is often reflected in increased numbers of neutrophils in circulating blood (*neutrophilia*). In contrast, viral infections tend to excite a lymphocytic response and an increase in the number and proportion of lymphocytes in the peripheral circulation (*lymphocytosis*).

All leucocytes exhibit amoeboid movement which provides the means for migration in and out of the circulatory system and through the tissues.

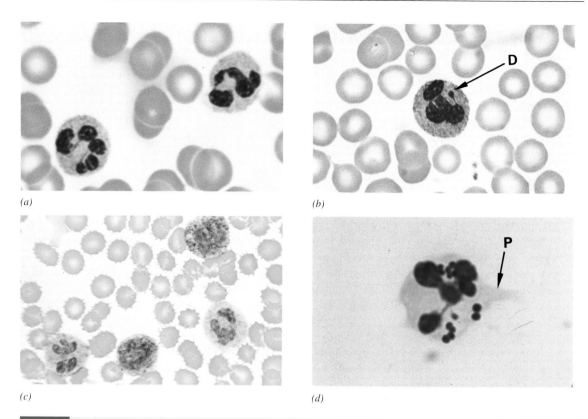

(a)

(b)

(c)

(d)

Fig. 3.4 Neutrophils (a) Giemsa × 1200 (b) Giemsa × 1200
(c) Histochemical method for alkaline phosphatase × 800 (d) Giemsa × 2400

Neutrophils are the most common type of leucocyte in blood and constitute 40–75% of circulating leucocytes. Being highly motile and phagocytic, their principal function is in the acute inflammatory response to tissue injury where they ingest and destroy damaged tissue and invading microorganisms, particularly bacteria.

The most prominent feature of the neutrophil is the highly lobulated nucleus. When mature, there are usually five lobes connected by fine strands of nuclear material. In less mature neutrophils the nucleus is generally not as lobulated. In micrograph (a), two neutrophils in different stages of maturity are illustrated.

In neutrophils of females, the condensed, quiescent X-chromosome or Barr body (see Fig. 1.4) exists in the form of a small drumstick-shaped appendage of one of the nuclear lobes. This is known as the *drumstick chromosome* **D** and is shown in micrograph (b); it is visible in about 3% of neutrophils in peripheral blood films of females.

The cytoplasm of neutrophils is lightly stippled with purplish granules called *azurophilic granules* which are large lysosomes; these are often referred to as *primary granules* as they are the first granules to appear during neutrophil differentiation. These granules contain the usual lysosomal acid hydrolases but also a number of microbicidal agents including *myeloperoxidase*; this can be demonstrated by the peroxidase stain and is used as a

marker for the primary granules and for identification of leukaemias arising in neutrophil precursors.

The most numerous granules in the cytoplasm are the *secondary granules*, which are specific to neutrophils. They are much smaller than primary granules (0.2–0.8 μm) and are barely visible by light microscopy. These granules contain and secrete substances involved in the acute inflammatory response such as inflammatory mediators and complement activators. These substances are released into the extracellular space during inflammation.

Small *tertiary granules* contain enzymes which are released into the extracellular space, including gelatinase (which breaks down damaged collagen). They also insert adhesion molecules into cell membranes, thus possibly facilitating phagocytosis.

Alkaline phosphatase activity has been traditionally used as a histochemical marker for the specific granules of neutrophils as seen in micrograph (c). Enzyme activity is indicated by a brown, granular deposit in the neutrophil cytoplasm; immature neutrophils, recognisable by their less lobulated nuclei, exhibit less enzyme activity.

Micrograph (d) illustrates a neutrophil which has engulfed some coccoid bacteria; note the pseudopodium **P**, a typical feature of highly motile cells. This specimen was obtained experimentally by incubating fresh blood with bacteria. In vivo, neutrophils die after engulfing bacteria and do not re-enter the circulation.

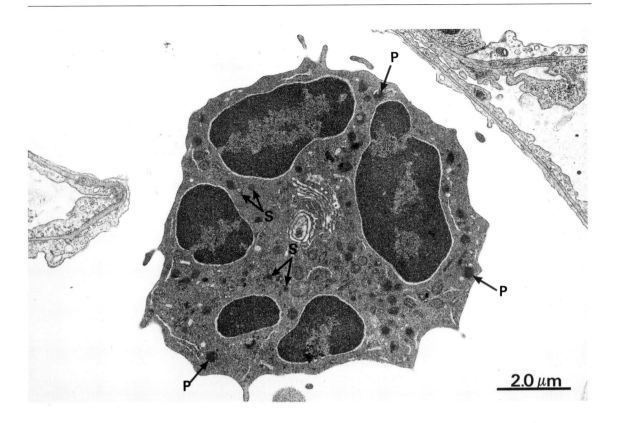

Fig. 3.5 Neutrophil EM × 10 000

With electron microscopy, neutrophils have three distinguishing features. Firstly, the nucleus has up to five lobes which in section may appear as separate nuclei. The chromatin is highly condensed reflecting a low degree of protein synthesis. Secondly, the cytoplasm contains a considerable number of membrane-bound granules. The primary granules **P** are large, spheroidal and electron-dense, similar to the lysosomes of other cell types. The secondary granules **S** are more numerous, small and often rod-like, and of variable density and shape. Tertiary granules cannot be readily identified. Thirdly, all other cytoplasmic organelles are scarce although the cytoplasm is particularly rich in dispersed glycogen.

Since the mature neutrophil has few appropriate organelles for protein synthesis, it has very limited capacity to regenerate expended lysosomal and specific enzymes which are rapidly depleted by phagocytic activity. The neutrophil is thus incapable of continuous function and degenerates after a single burst of activity. Defunct neutrophils are the main cellular constituent of *pus* and are therefore sometimes referred to as *pus cells*.

The paucity of mitochondria and the abundance of glycogen in neutrophils reflect the importance of the anaerobic mode of metabolism. Energy production via glycolysis permits neutrophils to function in the poorly oxygenated environment of damaged tissues whilst the hexose monophosphate pathway generates microbicidal oxidants.

Neutrophils are highly motile cells moving through the extracellular spaces in a crawling fashion with an undulating pseudopodium typically thrust out in the line of advance (see Fig. 3.4d). Motility and intense endocytotic activity are reflected in a large content of the contractile proteins, actin and myosin, tubulin and microtubule-associated proteins.

Neutrophil function

Neutrophils in the circulation are attracted by the presence of organisms, particularly bacteria. This process is mediated by chemotactic factors (*chemotaxins*) released from damaged tissue and generated by the interaction of antibodies with antigens on the surface of the microorganisms (see Ch. 11). The coating of organisms with antibodies and complement greatly enhances neutrophilic phagocytic activity, the phenomenon being known as *opsonisation*. Organisms which do not generate chemotaxins or become opsonised are thus relatively resistant to neutrophil phagocytosis and are thus highly pathogenic.

As the first step in phagocytosis, the organism is surrounded by pseudopodia which then fuse to completely enclose it in an endocytotic vesicle called a *phagosome*. This then fuses with cytoplasmic granules, in particular the primary granules, which discharge their contents exposing the organism to a potent mixture of lysosomal enzymes. Killing is greatly enhanced by the generation of hydrogen peroxide and superoxide by enzymatic reduction of oxygen. A by-product of this powerful destructive capacity is considerable damage to the surrounding tissues in the event of leakage of the granule contents into the extracellular environment.

An important precursor to granule discharge is a phenomenon known as *neutrophil stimulation*. This involves the binding of complement fraction C5a to a significant proportion of receptors on the neutrophil plasma membrane; C5a is the most potent neutrophil chemotaxin and induces chemotaxis, degranulation and generation of hydrogen peroxide and superoxide.

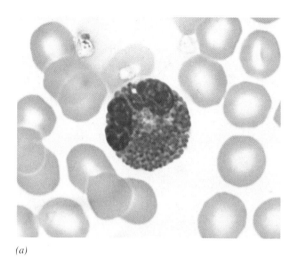

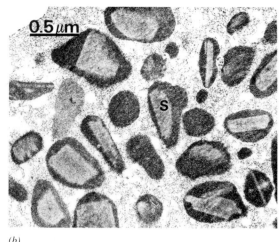

(a)   *(b)*

Fig. 3.6 **Eosinophils** (a) Giemsa × 1600 (b) Human EM × 25 000
(c) Mouse EM × 20 000 *(opposite)* (d) Rat EM × 25 000 *(opposite)*

Eosinophils account for 1–6% of leucocytes in circulating blood; their numbers exhibit a marked diurnal variation, being greatest in the morning and least in the afternoon. Eosinophils remain in the bone marrow for several days after production, then circulate for about 3–8 hours; the majority then enter the skin, pulmonary or gastrointestinal mucosae from which they may migrate into local secretions. The fate and lifespan of eosinophils are not known, although few if any appear to re-enter the circulation.

Increased numbers of circulating eosinophils (*eosinophilia*) are found in many types of parasitic disease and defence against parasites appears to be one of their principal functions. Eosinophil numbers are also increased in the tissues in some allergic disorders (e.g. in the nasal and bronchial mucosae in hay fever and asthma) although their function in this context is poorly understood.

The eosinophil (12–17 μm in diameter) is larger than the neutrophil and is easily recognised by its large specific granules which stain bright red with eosin and a more brick-red with Romanowsky methods. Most cells have a bilobed nucleus but, as seen in micrograph (a), this is often partly obscured by the densely packed cytoplasmic granules.

The most characteristic ultrastructural feature of eosinophils is the large, ovoid, specific granules **S**, each containing an elongated crystalloid. In humans, as illustrated in micrograph (b), the crystalloids are relatively electron-lucent and irregular in form but in many other mammals they have a more regular, discoid shape. Micrograph (c) shows an eosinophil within the tissues of a mouse; in this species the crystalloids are also relatively electron-lucent. Micrograph (d) shows the specific granules of a rat eosinophil, the crystalloids of which are very electron-dense.

The specific granules are membrane-bound and of uniform size and the matrix contains a variety of hydrolytic enzymes including *histaminase*. The crystalloid has a cubic lattice structure and consists of an extremely alkaline (i.e. basic) protein called the *major basic protein*, other basic proteins, hydrolytic lysosomal enzymes and a peroxidase different from the myeloperoxidase of neutrophils.

Smaller granules are also present in mature eosinophils and contain *aryl sulphatase* and *acid phosphatase*; the

concentration of the former is eight times greater in eosinophils than in other white cells and appears to be secreted independently of phagocytosis and degranulation.

As seen in micrograph (c), the characteristic bilobed nucleus **N** is readily seen with the electron microscope. The cytoplasm contains a fairly extensive smooth endoplasmic reticulum **sER**, clusters of ribosomes **R** and a little rough endoplasmic reticulum **rER**. Glycogen is abundant and there is a scattering of mitochondria **M**.

Eosinophil function

Eosinophils are phagocytic cells with a similar metabolism to neutrophils but with a greater oxidative capacity via the hexose monophosphate shunt; nevertheless, eosinophils appear less microbicidal than neutrophils. They have, however, a particular phagocytic affinity for antigen–antibody complexes.

The eosinophil plasma membrane has different immunoglobulin and complement receptors from other leucocytes. All eosinophils have receptors for IgE which may be important in the destruction of parasites; this is not present on neutrophils.

Eosinophils undergo chemotaxis in response to bacterial products and complement components; however, they are preferentially attracted by substances released from basophils and mast cells, notably histamine and *eosinophil chemotactic factor of anaphylaxis (ECF-A)*, as well as activated lymphocytes.

Phagocytosis occurs in the usual manner, but if the object is too large to be engulfed (e.g. a parasite), the eosinophil appears to release its granule contents into the external environment; schistosomes appear to be injured in this way. Killing is mediated by antibody and complement (see Ch. 11).

Eosinophils may have a role in ameliorating some aspects of hypersensitivity reactions as they neutralise histamine and also produce a factor called *eosinophil-derived inhibitor* which is thought to inhibit mast cell degranulation. SRS-A, a vasoactive substance produced by basophils and mast cells (see Fig. 3.7), is inhibited by activated eosinophils. The role of aryl sulphatase (see above) is not understood; however, it is not involved in the inhibition of SRS-A as once thought.

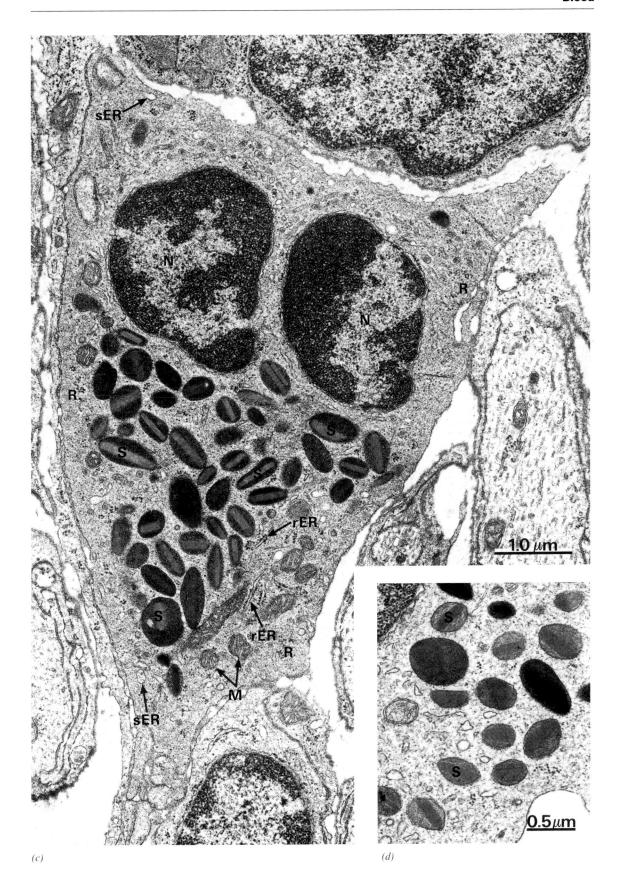

(c)

(d)

sER

N

N

R

R

S

S

S

S

rER

rER

R

M

sER

1.0 μm

S

S

0.5μm

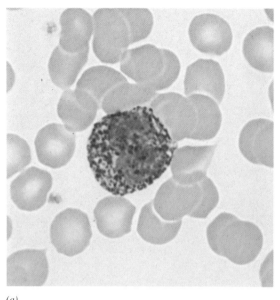

(a)

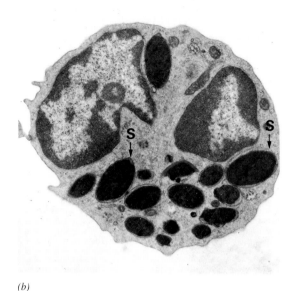

(b)

Fig. 3.7   **Basophils**   (a) Giemsa × 1500 (b) EM × 10 500

Basophils are the least common leucocyte and constitute less than 1% of leucocytes in circulating blood. Characterised by large intensely basophilic cytoplasmic granules, they share many structural and functional similarities with tissue mast cells (see Fig. 4.14). Basophils are the precursors of mast cells en route to peripheral tissues.

Basophils are formed in the bone marrow, sharing a common precursor with the other granulocytes up to the myeloblast stage; from here, development proceeds through analogous stages as for neutrophils and eosinophils. The lifespan of basophils is unknown.

The basophil (14–16 μm in diameter) is intermediate in size between the neutrophil and eosinophil. Like the latter, it has a bilobed nucleus but this is usually obscured by numerous large, densely basophilic (deep blue) specific granules which are larger, but fewer in number, than those of eosinophils. The granules are highly soluble in water and tend to be dissolved away during common blood smear preparation, thus adding to the difficulty of identifying basophils in blood smears. Special techniques of fixation, embedding and staining may thus need to be used. When stained with the basic dye, *toluidine blue*, the granules bind the dye which changes colour to red, a phenomenon described as *metachromasia* (see Fig. 4.14).

With electron microscopy, the characteristic bilobed nucleus of the basophil is easily seen. The large specific granules **S** are membrane-bound, round or oval in shape and filled with closely packed, electron-dense material; the granules of basophils are larger and fewer in number than those of mast cells.

A small population of smaller granules is also found near the nucleus. The cytoplasm also contains free ribosomes, mitochondria and glycogen whilst the plasma membrane exhibits blunt, irregularly spaced surface projections.

Basophil function

The cytoplasmic granules of basophils and mast cells contain proteoglycans consisting of sulphated glycosaminoglycans linked to a protein core; this accounts for their metachromatic staining property. The proteoglycans are a variable mixture of *heparin* and *chondroitin sulphate*. The granules also contain *histamine* and many other mediators of inflammatory processes, e.g. *slow reacting substance of anaphylaxis (SRS-A), eosinophil chemotactic factor of anaphylaxis (ECF-A)*.

Basophil infiltration, mast cell proliferation and degranulation are features of a variety of immunological and other disorders; however, the principal function of basophils and mast cells is probably in immunological responses to certain parasites.

Basophils and mast cells have membrane receptors highly specific for the Fc segment of IgE which is produced by plasma cells in response to a variety of environmental antigens (allergens). Exposure to allergen results in the antigen forming bridges between adjacent IgE molecules which triggers rapid exocytosis of granule contents (degranulation). The release of histamine and other vasoactive mediators is thus responsible for the so-called *immediate hypersensitivity (anaphylactoid) reaction* characteristic of allergic rhinitis (hay fever), some forms of asthma, urticaria and anaphylactic shock. Nevertheless, there are other IgE-independent stimuli for mast cell degranulation.

Basophils may also account for up to 15% of infiltrating cells in allergic dermatitis and skin allograft rejection, a phenomenon known as *cutaneous basophil hypersensitivity*; this is induced by sensitised lymphocytes and is thus a type of cell-mediated hypersensitivity (see Ch. 11). In this case degranulation is slow rather than rapid as in immediate hypersensitivity reactions.

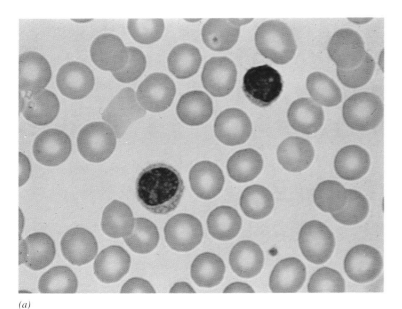

(a)

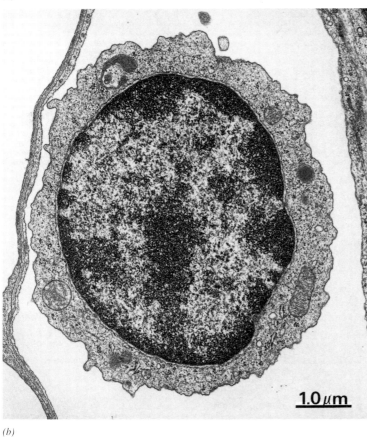

1.0 μm

(b)

Fig. 3.8 Lymphocytes
(a) Giemsa × 800 (b) EM × 15 000

Lymphocytes are the smallest cells in the white cell series, being only slightly larger than erythrocytes. They are the second most common leucocyte in circulating blood and make up 20–50% of the differential white cell count; increased numbers are commonly seen during viral infections.

Lymphocytes play the central role in all immunological defence mechanisms and are thus described in detail in Chapter 11. Blood provides the medium in which lymphocytes circulate between the various lymphoid tissues and all other tissues of the body. Most of the lymphocytes in the circulation are in a relatively inactive functional and metabolic state.

Lymphocytes are characterised by a round, densely stained nucleus and a relatively small amount of pale basophilic, non-granular cytoplasm. The amount of cytoplasm depends upon the state of activity of the lymphocyte, and in circulating blood there is a predominance of 'small' inactive lymphocytes (6–9 μm in diameter). 'Large' lymphocytes (9–15 μm in diameter) make up about 3% of lymphocytes in peripheral blood. Large lymphocytes represent activated B lymphocytes en route to the tissues where they will become antibody-secreting plasma cells; they also include *natural killer cells* (see Ch. 11).

Micrograph (a) illustrates small and large lymphocytes. In the large lymphocyte, the cytoplasm is readily visible but in the small lymphocyte the cytoplasm is almost too sparse to be seen.

Micrograph (b) shows a small circulating B lymphocyte in a pulmonary capillary. The nucleus is typically rounded but slightly indented and the chromatin is moderately condensed; nucleoli are not usually present. The sparse cytoplasm contains a few mitochondria, a rudimentary Golgi apparatus, minimal endoplasmic reticulum and a comparatively large number of free ribosomes which account for the basophilia of light microscopy. The plasma membrane exhibits small cytoplasmic projections which, with the scanning electron microscope, appear as short microvilli.

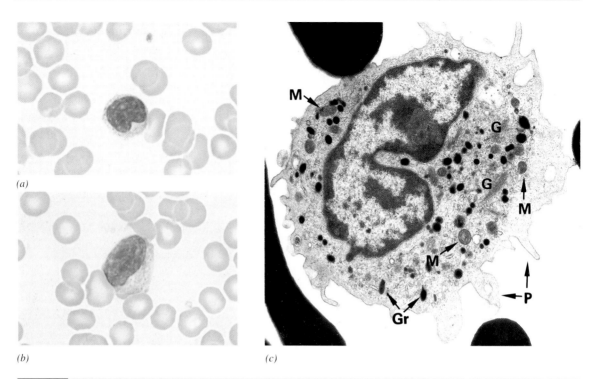

Fig. 3.9 **Monocytes** (a) Giemsa × 1000 (b) Giemsa × 1000 (c) EM × 20 000

Monocytes are the largest of the white cells (up to 20 μm in diameter) and constitute from 2 to 10% of leucocytes in peripheral blood. They are highly motile and phagocytic cells and are the precursors of *macrophages*, large phagocytic cells of various types found in peripheral tissues and lymphoid organs.

Monocytes are characterised by a large, eccentrically placed nucleus which is stained less intensely than that of other leucocytes. As seen in these light micrographs, nuclear shape is variable but there is often a deep indentation of that aspect of the nucleus adjacent to the centre of the cell; nuclear indentation tends to become more pronounced as the cell matures, so as to give a horseshoe appearance. Two or more nucleoli may be visible. The extensive cytoplasm stains pale greyish blue with Romanowsky methods and contains numerous small pink-purple stained lysosomal granules and cytoplasmic vacuoles which may confer a 'frosted-glass' appearance.

With the electron microscope, the cytoplasm is seen to contain a variable number of ribosomes and polyribosomes and relatively little rough endoplasmic reticulum. The Golgi apparatus **G** is well developed and located with the centrosome in the vicinity of the nuclear indentation. Small elongated mitochondria **M** are prolific. Numerous small pseudopodia **P** extend from the cell, reflecting phagocytic ability and amoeboid movement.

The cytoplasmic granules **Gr** of monocytes are electron-dense, homogeneous and membrane-bound. Histochemical studies show them to be of two types. One type represents primary lysosomes and contains acid phosphatase, aryl sulphatase and peroxidase; these are analogous to the primary (azurophilic) granules of neutrophils. The content of the other granule type is not known.

In contrast to neutrophils, monocytes are capable of continuous lysosomal activity and regeneration which utilises aerobic and anaerobic metabolic pathways depending on the availability of oxygen in the tissues.

Monocytes–macrophage system
Monocytes migrate to peripheral tissues where they assume the role of macrophages. This has led to the concept of a single functional unit, the *monocyte–macrophage system (mononuclear phagocyte system)*, consisting of circulating monocytes, their bone marrow precursors, and tissue macrophages both free and fixed (*histiocytes*). Included in the system are the Kupffer cells of the liver, microglia of the CNS, Langerhans cells of the skin, antigen-presenting cells of the lymphoid organs and the osteoclasts of bone. *Multinucleate giant cells* may form by fusion of macrophages or nuclear reduplication. The system does not include vascular endothelial cells or the reticular cells and fibroblasts of lymphoid organs which may exhibit some phagocytic activity; these were included in the now obsolete concept of the *reticuloendothelial system*.

Monocyte function
Monocytes appear to have little function in circulating blood. They respond to the presence of necrotic material (*necrotaxis*), invading microorganisms (*chemotaxis*) and inflammation by migration into the tissues and differentiation into macrophages; with their great capacity for phagocytosis and a large content of hydrolytic enzymes, the macrophages engulf and destroy tissue debris and foreign material as part of the process of healing and restoration of normal function.

Some of these functions form an integral part of immunological mechanisms, e.g. antigen presentation, final destruction of antigen; in this case, lymphocyte activation results in the production of factors which enhance macrophage phagocytic activity.

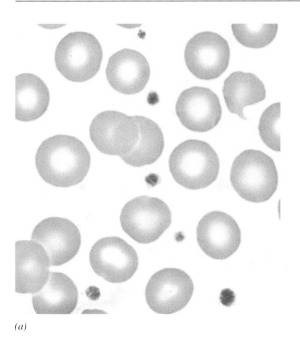
(a)

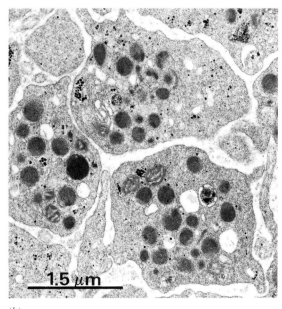
(b)

Fig. 3.10 **Platelets** **(a) Giemsa × 1600 (b) EM × 18 000**

Platelets (thrombocytes) are small, non-nucleated cells formed in the bone marrow from the cytoplasm of huge cells called *megakaryocytes*. Their numbers in circulating blood range from 150 000 to 400 000/mL. Platelets have a variety of functions essential to the normal process of haemostasis. Firstly, they form plugs to occlude sites of vascular damage by adhering to collagenous tissue at the margin of the wound; later the platelet plug is replaced by fibrin. Secondly, they promote clot formation by providing a surface for the assembly of coagulation protein complexes that are responsible for thrombin generation. Thirdly, platelets secrete factors that are involved in vascular repair.

Platelets are round or oval, biconvex discs varying in size from about 1.5 to 3.5 μm in diameter. In blood smears, as in micrograph (a), their shape is not clearly seen and they are often partially clumped together. The cytoplasm has a purple-stained, granular appearance due to their numerous organelles which are concentrated towards the centre of the cell; the peripheral cytoplasm is very poorly stained and therefore barely visible.

Platelets contain most of the cytoplasmic organelles of other cells including mitochondria, microtubules, glycogen granules, occasional Golgi elements and ribosomes as well as enzyme systems for both aerobic and anaerobic respiration. The most conspicuous organelles, as seen in micrograph (b), are the electron-dense granules which constitute about 20% of platelet volume and are of four types:

- **Alpha granules** are variable in size and shape and contain two *platelet exclusive proteins*, namely *platelet factor 4* (regulates vascular permeability, calcium mobilisation from bone, chemotaxis of monocytes and neutrophils) and *beta thromboglobulin* (function unknown, but serum level is used to monitor platelet activation in various disease states); these granules also contain coagulation factors (fibrinogen, factor V, factor VIII/von Willebrand factor) and other proteins including *fibronectin, thrombospondin, platelet-derived growth factor* (may be involved in repair of damaged blood vessels) and other growth factors.

- **Dense granules** are very electron-dense and appear to contain *serotonin*; serotonin is not synthesised by platelets or their precursors but is absorbed from the plasma having been produced by enterochromaffin cells of the gut (see Ch. 17).
- **Lysosomes** are membrane-bound vesicles distinct from the alpha granules and contain lysosomal enzymes.
- **Microperoxisomes** are small in number and have peroxidase activity, probably catalase.

The platelet plasma membrane has three unusual features relating to adherence to foreign or altered blood vessels surfaces. Firstly, it has the ability to form fibrillar bridges between one platelet and another. Secondly, a very thick, filamentous glycocalyx rich in acid mucopolysaccharides gives substance to the fibrillar bridges. Thirdly, twice as many membrane proteins are exposed to the external environment as face inwards; this is the reverse of the situation in all other cells and is as if the membrane is turned inside out.

Platelets contain a well developed cytoskeleton. Beneath the cell periphery is a *marginal band of microtubules* which depolymerise at the onset of platelet aggregation. The cytoplasm is rich in the contractile proteins actin and myosin (previously called *thrombosthenin*) and other filamentous elements, all probably involved in the functions of clot retraction and extrusion of granule contents.

Located deep to the marginal band of microtubules and also scattered throughout the cytoplasm is the *dense tubular system* (*DTS*) consisting of narrow membranous tubules which contain a homogeneous electron-opaque substance; this contains an isoenzyme of peroxidase that is specific for platelets. The function of the DTS is poorly understood but there is evidence that it may be the site of prostaglandin synthesis.

Platelets contain a system of interconnected membrane channels which are in continuity with the external environment via external pits, the cytoplasmic aspect of these membranes being associated with elements of the cytoskeleton. The function of this *canalicular membrane system* is not understood but it may be involved in the secretion of the contents of alpha granules.

Haemopoiesis

Haemopoiesis is the process by which mature blood cells develop from precursor cells. In the human adult, haemopoiesis takes place in the bone marrow mainly of the skull, ribs, sternum, vertebral column, pelvis and the proximal ends of the femurs. Before maturity, however, haemopoiesis occurs in other sites at different stages in development. In the early embryo, primitive blood cells arise in the yolk sac and, later, the liver. From the third to seventh months, the spleen is the major site of haemopoietic activity. As the bones develop during the fourth and fifth months of intrauterine life, granulocyte and platelet formation begins in the marrow cavities with erythropoiesis becoming established by the seventh month. By birth, haemopoiesis is almost exclusive to the bone marrow although the liver and spleen may resume activity in times of need. From birth to maturity, the number of active sites of haemopoiesis in bone marrow diminishes although all bone marrow retains haemopoietic potential.

The lineage of each blood cell type has been the subject of numerous theories but only one has gained substantial experimental support, the ***monophyletic theory***. This proposes that all blood cell types are derived from a single primitive stem cell type called a ***multipotential (pluripotential) stem cell***. The multipotential cells replicate at a slow rate differentiating into five discrete types of ***unipotential stem cells***, each committed to a different developmental lineage: erythrocytes, granulocytes, lymphocytes, monocytes and platelets. Unipotential stem cells (which are not readily distinguishable from each other histologically) divide at a rapid rate to provide histologically recognisable precursors of the mature cell types.

In vitro culture systems are used to study haemopoiesis, progenitor cells being described as ***colony forming units*** (***CFU***). The rate of division of these cells is modulated by hormones called ***poietins (***e.g. erythropoietin) and locally produced ***colony stimulating factors*** and ***interleukins***.

Bone marrow

Bone marrow consists of a meshwork of vascular sinuses and highly branched fibroblasts (see Ch. 4) with the interstices packed with haemopoietic cells. The production of blood cells by the bone marrow is astronomical with an estimated daily output of about 2.5 billion erythrocytes, a comparable number of platelets, some 50–100 billion granulocytes (1.0 billion/kg body weight per day) as well as large numbers of monocytes and immunologically naive lymphocytes. In addition to its haemopoietic function, the bone marrow, along with the spleen and liver, is one of the major sites of removal of aged and defective erythrocytes from the circulation. The bone marrow also plays a central role in the immune system, being the site of B lymphocyte differentiation (the mammalian equivalent of the bursa of Fabricius of birds) as well as containing large numbers of antibody-secreting plasma cells (see Ch. 11).

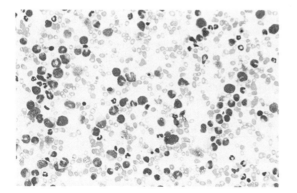

Fig. 3.11 **Bone marrow smear** Giemsa × 640

This micrograph shows the general appearance of a smear made from an aspirate of bone marrow. Nucleate cells of developing erythrocyte and leucocyte cell lines make up a considerable proportion of the cells, in contrast to smears of peripheral blood where nucleate cells (i.e. mature leucocytes) are few and far between. Cells of the same lineage are relatively easy to identify as they tend to be drawn out into trails from the various colony forming units in the marrow; this is better seen at lower magnification than shown here.

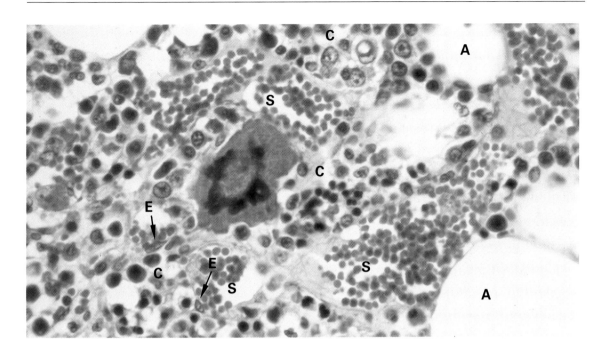

Fig. 3.12 Bone marrow H & E × 300

Active bone marrow is crammed with dividing stem cells and the precursors of mature blood cells, the predominance of maturing erythrocytes conferring a deep red colour: hence the name *red marrow*. With increasing age, the marrow of peripheral long bones becomes less active and is progressively dominated by fat cells, so that in mature mammals much of the marrow is inactive and yellow in colour; *yellow marrow* may, however, be reactivated if the need arises for increased haemopoiesis.

Active bone marrow consists of two main components: a framework of reticulin (see Fig. 4.8) and specialised fibroblasts (reticular cells) which supports the developing blood cells; and a system of interconnected blood sinusoids which drain towards the central vein.

The bone marrow sinuses are of the continuous endothelium type (see Ch. 8) but an unusual feature is that the underlying basement membrane is discontinuous. The sinus endothelial cells are active in endocytosis and probably control passage of all materials into and out of the haemopoietic compartment. In places, the endothelial cytoplasm is so thin that the endothelial barrier is little more than the inner and outer layers of plasma membrane, and such sites may provide the route of exit of mature blood cells into the circulation.

Beyond the endothelium and its basement membrane is a discontinuous layer of fibroblasts (reticular cells) with extensive branched cytoplasmic processes which embrace the outer surface of the sinus wall as well as ramifying throughout the haemopoietic spaces. The reticular cells

synthesise reticulin fibres which, along with the cytoplasmic processes, form a meshwork which supports the haemopoietic cells. By the accumulation of lipid, the reticular cells also give rise to the fat cells (adipocytes) characteristically found in the bone marrow. Macrophages are also present within the haemopoietic cords and are involved in phagocytosis of cellular debris. The haemopoietic compartment also contains typical non-cellular supporting elements (see Ch. 4) including collagen fibres and the large molecular weight proteins laminin and fibronectin which bind the haemopoietic cells to the fibrous elements of the marrow stroma. Ground substance proteoglycans may have the function of binding growth factors and other modulators of haemopoiesis.

This micrograph illustrates haemopoietic cords **C** separated by broad sinusoids **S** which are filled with erythrocytes and occasional leucocytes. Note the nuclei of occasional flattened endothelial cells **E** which line the sinusoids. Of the haemopoietic cells, only one can be reliably identified, namely a huge megakaryocyte (responsible for platelet formation) near the centre of the field. Note also a few scattered adipocytes **A**.

The functional relationship between bone and bone marrow is obscure. Bone may merely provide protection and support for the delicate bone marrow tissue or there may be some specific metabolic relationship between the two tissues. In support of the latter, it has been observed that transplanted bone marrow is unable to survive in sites other than the medullary cavities of bone marrow.

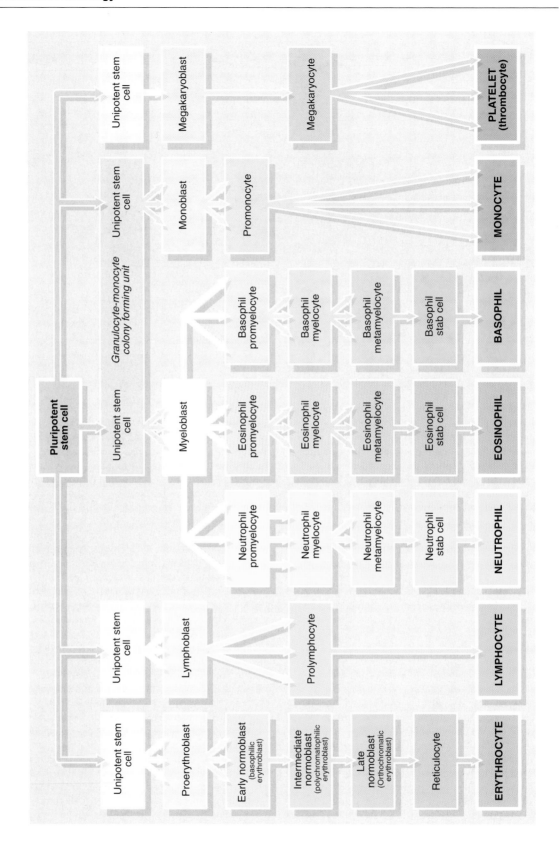

Fig. 3.13 Haemopoiesis *(illustration opposite)*

This diagram summarises the main developmental stages in blood cell formation. Such a classification is somewhat arbitrary since the process of haemopoiesis is a continuum of proliferation and progressive differentiation from stem cell to the mature form found in circulating blood.

Red cell formation (erythropoiesis). The process of erythropoiesis is directed towards producing a cell devoid of organelles but packed with haemoglobin. The first recognisable erythrocyte precursor is known as the *proerythroblast*, a large cell with numerous cytoplasmic organelles and no haemoglobin. Further stages of differentiation are characterised by three main features:

- decreasing cell size
- progressive loss of organelles; the presence of numerous ribosomes at early stages accounts for the marked cytoplasmic basophilia (blue staining) which steadily decreases as the number of ribosomes falls
- progressive increase in the cytoplasmic haemoglobin content; this accounts for the increasing eosinophilia (pink staining) of the cytoplasm towards maturity.

Haemoglobin synthesis begins during the *early normoblast (basophilic erythroblast)* stage and is complete by the end of the reticulocyte stage. Cell division ceases with the early normoblast stage, after which the nucleus progressively condenses and is finally extruded at the *late normoblast (orthochromatic erythroblast)* stage. The early normoblast stage also marks the beginning of the progressive loss of cytoplasmic organelles, only remnants of which remain by the reticulocyte stage. This process, accompanied by progressive haemoglobin synthesis, is represented morphologically by the transition from basophilia through polychromasia (intermediate normoblast) to the eosinophilia (orthochromasia) of the mature erythrocyte.

The process of erythropoiesis from stem cell to erythrocyte takes about 1 week. The rate of erythropoiesis is controlled by the hormone erythropoietin secreted by the kidney and by the availability of red cell components, particularly iron, folic acid, vitamin B_{12} and protein precursors.

The *erythroblastic island* is the unit of erythropoiesis within the bone marrow and consists of one or two macrophages surrounded by erythrocyte progenitor cells. In bone marrow aspirates, the erythroblastic islands are broken up and ultrastructural studies of bone marrow sections are required to demonstrate their structure. The plasma membranes of the macrophages exhibit long cytoplasmic processes and deep invaginations which accommodate the dividing erythroid cells. As the erythroid cell differentiates, it migrates outwards along the cytoplasmic process of the macrophage leaving less mature cells in its wake.

Approaching maturity, the erythroblast makes contact with the nearby sinusoidal endothelium and passes through its cytoplasm to enter the circulation. The nucleus is extruded prior to entry into the bloodstream and is phagocytosed by perisinusoidal macrophages. Cell culture studies indicate that endothelial cells, macrophages and fibroblasts are all essential for erythropoiesis, the fibroblasts being responsible for the production of various growth factors.

Granulocyte formation (granulopoiesis). The *myeloblast* is the earliest recognisable stage in granulopoiesis, the inappropriate name of myeloblast being derived from an outdated view that granulocytes were the only white cells formed in *myeloid tissue* (bone marrow). Myeloblasts give rise to *promyelocytes* which are characterised by the development of azurophilic granules; since the azurophilic granules develop before the specific granules, they are referred to as primary granules. As described earlier, the primary granules are merely large lysosomes.

The next stage in differentiation is the *myelocyte* which is marked by the development of specific granules, the process continuing through a further three cell divisions. The relative number and proportion of primary granules progressively decreases and the proportion of specific (secondary) granules progressively increases. From the myelocyte state through the *metamyelocyte* stage to the mature granulocyte forms, the nucleus becomes increasingly segmented. The immediate precursors of mature granulocytes tend to have an irregular horseshoe or sometimes ring-shaped nucleus and are termed *stab cells* or *band forms*.

On reaching maturity, neutrophils enter the bloodstream where some appear to circulate whilst others become adherent to the endothelial walls of small vessels (*marginated pool*) entering the circulating pool in response to exercise and stress; exit from the circulation appears to occur in a random manner. The bone marrow contains a huge pool of stored neutrophils which can be rapidly mobilised should the need arise. Corticosteroids increase the rate of release from the bone marrow and reduce the rate of exit from the circulation.

Lymphocyte formation (lymphopoiesis). Only two precursor stages, the *lymphoblast* and the *prolymphocyte*, are recognisable in the development of lymphocytes. The main feature of lymphopoiesis is a progressive diminution in cell size.

Unlike other blood cell types, lymphocytes also proliferate outside the bone marrow. This occurs in the tissues of the immune system in response to specific immunological stimulation (see Ch. 11).

Monocyte formation (monopoiesis). There is considerable evidence that monocytes and granulocytes have a common progenitor, the *granulocyte-monocyte colony forming unit (CFU-GM)* and that growth of colonies requires the presence of *colony stimulating factors (CSFs)* with functions analogous to that of erythropoietin in erythropoiesis.

Two morphological precursors of monocytes are recognised, *monoblasts* and *promonocytes*, with at least three cell divisions occurring before the mature monocyte stage is reached. Monopoiesis is characterised by a reduction in cell size and progressive indentation of the nucleus. Mature monocytes leave the bone marrow soon after their formation and there is no reserve pool as for neutrophils. Monocytes spend an average of 3 days in the circulation before migrating by diapedesis into the tissues in an apparently random fashion after which they are unable to re-enter the circulation.

Platelet formation (thrombopoiesis). See Fig. 3.16. In bone marrow smears, the earlier phases of haemopoiesis may be recognisable only with great difficulty, the characteristic, detailed features of each stage having been described using techniques of fixation and staining which are rarely applied in routine haematological practice. The recognition of such stages is of little practical value except in certain pathological conditions under which circumstances the classic characteristics of each cell type are often distorted.

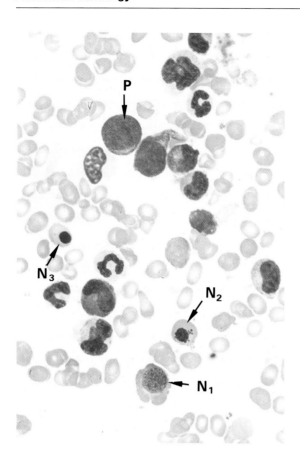

Fig. 3.14 Erythropoiesis Giemsa × 1200

This bone marrow smear illustrates several stages in erythropoiesis. The proerythroblast **P** is the first recognisable erythrocyte precursor; the cell has a large, intensely stained, granular nucleus containing one or more paler nucleoli. The sparse cytoplasm is strongly basophilic due to its high content of RNA and lack of haemoglobin. A narrow, pale zone of cytoplasm close to the nucleus represents the Golgi apparatus.

Three increasingly differentiated normoblast forms can also be recognised. An early normoblast (basophilic erythroblast) N_1 can be distinguished from the proerythroblast stage by its smaller size and smaller nucleus which has more condensed chromatin. More advanced in the maturation sequence is an intermediate normoblast (polychromatophilic erythroblast) N_2, the cytoplasm of which exhibits both basophilia and eosinophilia (i.e. polychromasia), the latter due to increasing haemoglobin content. The nucleus is also condensed and is accompanied by several small fragments called *Howell–Jolly bodies*, an unusual finding in normal erythropoiesis. With further haemoglobin synthesis and degeneration of cytoplasmic ribosomes, the late normoblast (orthochromatic erythroblast) stage N_3 is reached and by this time the nucleus is extremely condensed prior to being extruded from the cell.

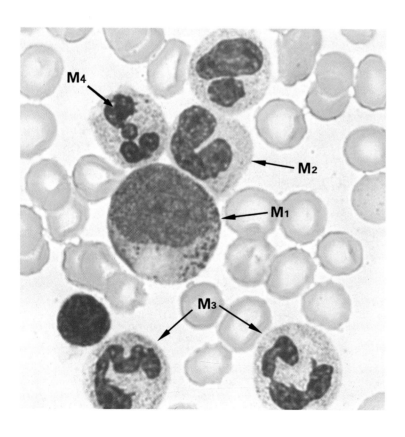

Fig. 3.15 Granulocyte precursors Giemsa × 1600

This micrograph illustrates three phases of neutrophil granulocyte development. A neutrophil myelocyte M_1 is recognised by its large, eccentrically located nucleus, a prominent Golgi apparatus (negative image) and cytoplasm containing many azurophilic (primary) granules. The next stage towards maturity, the metamyelocyte M_2, is a smaller cell characterised by indentation of the nucleus and loss of prominence of the azurophilic granules. The final stage before maturity, the stab cell M_3, has a more highly segmented nucleus approaching that of the mature neutrophil M_4.

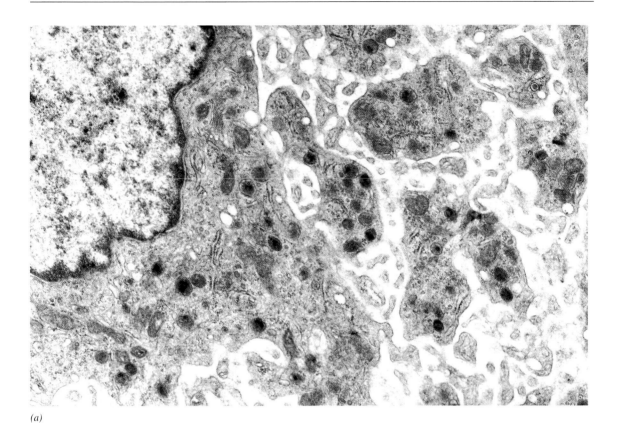

(a)

Fig. 3.16 **Megakaryocytes and platelet formation** (a) EM × 22 500 (b) Giemsa × 800

Megakaryocytes are responsible for platelet production and are the largest cells seen in bone marrow aspirates (30–100 μm in diameter).

These huge polyploid cells have a large irregular, multilobular nucleus containing clumped dispersed chromatin and devoid of nucleoli. The extensive cytoplasm is filled with fine basophilic granules reflecting the profusion of cytoplasmic organelles. With light microscopy, the margin of the cell is often difficult to define clearly due to numerous disaggregating platelets **P**, cytoplasmic processes, ruffles and blebs.

The precursor of the megakaryocyte in the bone marrow is the *megakaryoblast* which undergoes as many as seven reduplications of nuclear and cytoplasmic constituents without cell division (*endomitosis*), each associated with increasing ploidy, nuclear lobulation and cell size.

Cytoplasmic maturation involves the elaboration of granules, vesicles and *demarcation membranes* and progressive loss of free ribosomes and rough endoplasmic reticulum.

The megakaryocyte cytoplasm is divided into three zones:

- *A perinuclear zone* contains the Golgi apparatus and associated vesicles, rough and smooth endoplasmic reticulum, developing granules, centrioles and spindle tubules; the zone remains attached to the nucleus after platelet shedding.
- *The intermediate zone* contains an extensive system of interconnected vesicles and tubules known as the *demarcation membrane system* (*DMS*) which is in continuity with the plasma membrane and has the

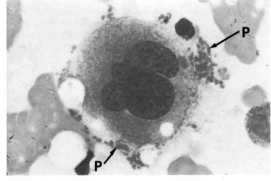

(b)

function of delineating developing platelet fields (i.e. potential platelets); at least some of the DMS appears to be derived from the Golgi.

- *The outer marginal zone* is filled with cytoskeletal filaments and is traversed by membranes connecting with the demarcation membrane system.

Platelets are formed not by budding, as often described, but rather by fragmentation of the megakaryocyte cytoplasm with the release of demarcated platelet fields; like platelets, they are very uneven in size. Platelets appear to be released in at least two different ways. In the bone marrow, megakaryocytes exude pseudopodia called *proplatelets* into the sinusoidal lumens, each representing a string of platelet fields which then fragment in the circulation. Mature megakaryocytes also appear to enter the bone marrow sinusoids intact and pass to the pulmonary vascular bed where they fragment into platelets.

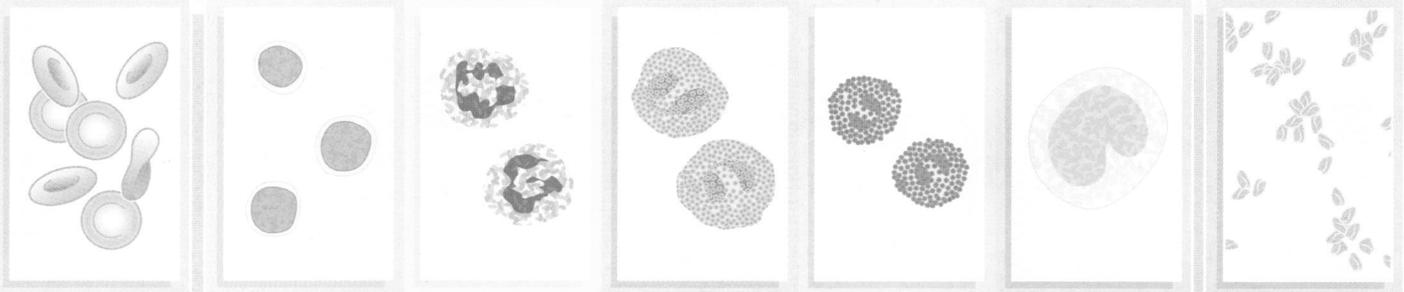

Functional Histology

BASIC TISSUE TYPES

Cell type	Erythrocyte	Lymphocyte	Neutrophil	Eosinophil	Basophil	Monocyte	Platelets
Size	6.7 – 7.7 µm	6 – 15 µm	12 – 14 µm	12 – 17 µm	14 – 16 µm	16 – 20 µm	1.5 – 3.5 µm
Number per litre	$3.9 – 6.5 \times 10^{12}$	$0 – 0.1 \times 10^{9}$	$2 – 7.5 \times 10^{9}$	$1.3 – 3.5 \times 10^{9}$	$0 – 0.44 \times 10^{9}$	$0.2 – 0.8 \times 10^{9}$	$150 – 400 \times 10^{9}$
Differential leucocyte count	—	20 – 50 %	40 – 75 %	1 – 6 %	< 1 %	2 – 10 %	—
Duration of development	5 – 7 days	1 – 2 days	6 – 9 days	6 – 9 days	3 – 7 days	2 – 3 days	4 – 5 days
Lifespan of mature cell	120 days	?	6 hours to a few days	8 – 12 days	?	Months to years	8 – 12 days

Fig. 3.17 Mature cell types in circulating blood

4. Supporting/connective tissues

Introduction

Connective tissue is the term traditionally applied to a basic type of tissue of mesodermal origin which provides structural and metabolic support for other tissues and organs throughout the body. Connective tissues usually contain blood vessels and mediate the exchange of nutrients, metabolites and waste products between tissues and the circulatory system. The traditional term 'connective tissue' thus hardly does justice to the wide range of functions of this type of tissue and it is now probably more appropriate to use the term supporting tissue.

Supporting tissues occur in many different forms with diverse physical properties. In most organs, loose supporting tissues act as a biological packing material between cells and other tissues with more specific functions. Dense forms of supporting tissue provide tough physical support in the dermis of the skin, comprise the robust capsules of organs such as the liver and spleen, and are the source of great tensile strength in ligaments and tendons. Cartilage and bone, the major skeletal components, are highly specialised forms of supporting tissue. The function of the skeletal tissues is, however, so specialised that they are considered separately in Chapter 10. Supporting tissues have important metabolic roles such as the storage of fat (white adipose tissue) and the regulation of body temperature in the newborn (brown adipose tissue). Cells of the immune system enter support tissues where they assist in defence against pathogenic microorganisms. The processes of tissue repair are largely a function of supporting tissues.

All supporting/connective tissues have two major constituents, *cells* and *extracellular matrix*. The extracellular matrix is generally the dominant component and determines the physical properties of each type of supporting tissue. Extracellular material consists of a matrix of organic material called *ground substance* within which are embedded a variety of *fibres*. A group of *structural glycoproteins* comprises the third constituent of the extracellular matrix and mediates the interaction of cells with the other constituents.

The cells of supporting/connective tissue

The cells of supporting tissue may be divided into several types according to their basic function:

- Cells responsible for synthesis and maintenance of the extracellular material are derived from precursor cells in primitive supporting tissue (*mesenchyme*). The most common support cell is termed the fibroblast. Fibroblasts with additional contractile function are found in some tissues and are known as *myofibroblasts*. It is customary to describe a precursor or immature cell by the suffix 'blast' as in erythroblast (see Fig. 3.17) and the mature form by the suffix 'cyte' as in erythrocyte. This convention, however, is not commonly used in respect of supporting tissues, where the term 'fibrocyte' would be a more appropriate term than fibroblast for the mature cell form.
- Cells responsible for the storage and metabolism of fat are known as *adipocytes* and may collectively form *adipose tissue*.
- Cells with defence and immune functions are commonly encountered in the support tissues. These cells are also derived from mesenchyme. This group of cells includes the mast cells and tissue macrophages as well as all types of white blood cells.

Ground substance

Ground substance derived its name from being an amorphous transparent material which has the properties of a semi-fluid gel. Tissue fluid is loosely associated with ground substance, thereby forming the medium for passage of molecules throughout supporting tissues and for the exchange of metabolites with the circulatory system.

Ground substance consists of a mixture of long, unbranched polysaccharide chains of seven different types, each composed of repeating disaccharide units. One of the disaccharide units is usually a uronic acid and the other an amino sugar (either N-acetyl glucosamine or N-acetyl galactosamine) thus giving rise to the modern term *glycosaminoglycans* (*GAGs*); these were formerly called *mucopolysaccharides*. The glycosaminoglycans are acidic (negatively charged) due to the presence of hydroxyl, carboxyl and sulphate side groups on the disaccharide units.

Hyaluronic acid is the predominant GAG in the loose supporting tissues and is the only one without sulphate side groups; the other GAGs (*chondroitin-4-sulphate, chondroitin-6-sulphate, dermatan sulphate, heparan sulphate, heparin sulphate* and *keratan sulphate*) differ from hyaluronic acid in that they are co-valently linked to a variety of protein molecules to form proteoglycans (formerly known as *mucoproteins*); these proteoglycans are huge molecules consisting of 90–95% carbohydrate. Further, the proteoglycans may form non-covalent links with hyaluronic acid chains to form even larger molecular complexes.

Unlike many proteins, GAG molecules are not flexible enough to form globular aggregates but remain in an expanded form, thus occupying a huge volume for relatively small mass. In addition, their highly charged side groups render them extremely hydrophilic, thus attracting a large volume of water and positive ions, particularly sodium, which constitute *extracellular fluid*. The extracellular fluid imparts the characteristic turgor of supporting tissue.

In summary, ground substance is basically composed of glycosaminoglycans in the form of hyaluronic acid and proteoglycans. These huge molecules are entangled and electrostatically linked to one another and their water of hydration, to form a flexible gel through which metabolites may diffuse. The size of the spaces between the GAG molecules and the nature of electrostatic changes determine the permeability characteristics of any particular supporting tissue, a fact of particular significance in the structure of basement membranes (see p. 67). The mechanical properties of ground substance are reinforced by the fibrous proteins of the extra-cellular tissue to which the components of ground substance are also bound.

The fibres of supporting/connective tissue

The fibrous components of supporting tissue are of two main types: *collagen* (including *reticulin* which was formerly considered a separate fibre type) and *elastin*.

Collagen

Collagen is the main fibre type found in most supporting tissues and is the most abundant protein in the human body. Its most notable function is the provision of tensile strength. Collagen is secreted into the extracellular matrix in the form of *tropocollagen* which consists of three polypeptide chains (alpha chains) bound together to form a helical structure 300 nm long and 1.5 nm in diameter. In the extracellular matrix, the tropocollagen molecules polymerise to form collagen. At least 19 different types of collagen (designated by Roman numerals I–XIX) have now been delineated on the basis of morphology, amino acid composition and physical properties.

- *Type I collagen* is found in fibrous supporting tissue, the dermis of the skin, tendon, ligaments and bone, in a variable arrangement from loose to dense according to the mechanical support required. The tropocollagen molecules are aggregated to form fibrils strengthened by numerous intermolecular bonds. Parallel collagen fibrils are further arranged into strong bundles 2–10 μm in diameter which confer great tensile strength to the tissue; these bundles are visible with the light microscope.
- *Type II collagen* is found in hyaline cartilage and consists of fine fibrils which are dispersed in the ground substance.
- *Type III collagen* makes up the fibre type known as reticulin which was previously thought to represent a separate species of fibre because of its affinity for silver salts. Reticulin fibres form the delicate branched 'reticular' supporting meshwork in highly cellular tissues such as the liver, bone marrow and lymphoid organs.
- *Type IV collagen* does not form fibrils but rather a mesh-like structure and is an important constituent of basement membranes.
- *Type VII collagen* forms anchoring fibrils that link to basement membrane.

The remaining collagen types are present in various specialised situations.

Elastin

Elastin is an important structural protein which is arranged as fibres and/or discontinuous sheets in the extra-cellular matrix particularly of skin, lung and blood vessels where it confers the properties of stretching and elastic recoil. Elastin is synthesised by fibroblasts in a precursor form known as *tropoelastin* which undergoes polymerisation in the extracellular tissues. Deposition of elastin in the form of fibres requires the presence of microfibrils of the structural glycoprotein *fibrillin* (see below) which become incorporated around and within the elastic fibres.

The structural glycoproteins

The structural glycoproteins are a group of molecules composed principally of protein chains bound to branched polysaccharides; much has yet to be learned about their role in the function of extracellular material. The structural glycoproteins include two fibril-forming molecules, *fibrillin* and *fibronectin*, and a number of non-filamentous proteins including *laminin, entactin* and *tenascin* which function as links between cells and extracellular matrix.

Fibrillin forms microfibrils 8–12 nm in diameter which, in certain specialised situations, e.g. the mesangium of the kidney (see Ch. 16), appear to enhance adhesion between other extracellular constituents. As mentioned earlier, fibrillin is a constituent of elastic fibres where it appears to play a role in the orderly deposition of the fibres.

Fibronectin plays a part in controlling the deposition and orientation of collagen in extracellular matrix and the binding of the cell to the extracellular material. Cell membranes incorporate a group of transmembrane protein complexes called *integrins* which act as *cell adhesion molecules*. One of these, the *fibronectin receptor*, establishes bonds within the cell to the actin filaments of the cytoskeleton and binds with fibronectin externally. The fibronectin in turn binds with collagen and the glycosaminoglycan, heparin sulphate, thus establishing structural continuity between the cytoskeleton and the extracellular matrix.

Laminin is a major component of basement membranes, binding with specific cell adhesion molecules so as to form links between cell membranes and other constituents of the basement membrane. Entactin, another non-fibrillary protein, has the function of binding laminin to type IV collagen in basement membranes. Tenascin also binds to integrins and is important in the embryo where it appears to be involved in control of nerve cell growth.

Basement membranes

Basement membranes are sheet-like arrangements of extracellular matrix proteins which act as an interface between the support tissues and parenchymal cells. Such basement membranes are associated with epithelial and muscle cells, as well as forming a limiting membrane around the central nervous system. The term derives from the fact that the first basement membranes to be recognised were those lying beneath the basal cells of surface epithelia. In the context of muscle and nervous tissue, the term *external lamina* may also be applied.

Epithelia in particular are almost entirely composed of closely packed cells with minimal intercellular material between them. The basement membrane provides structural support as well as binding the epithelium to the underlying supporting tissue. Basement membrane is also involved in the control of epithelial growth and differentiation, forming an impenetrable barrier to downward epithelial growth; this is only breached if epithelia undergo malignant transformation. Epithelium is devoid of blood vessels and the basement membrane must therefore permit the flow of nutrients, metabolites and other molecules to and from the epithelium. Where an epithelium acts as a selective barrier to the passage of molecules from one compartment to another (e.g. between the lumen of blood vessels and surrounding tissues), the basement membrane assumes a critical role in regulating permeability. This reaches an extreme of sophistication in the kidney where the glomerular basement membrane is part of the highly selective filter for molecules passing from the bloodstream into the urine. Critical association of basement membranes with epithelial structure and function was thus responsible for the basement membrane being traditionally discussed as if it were a uniquely epithelial structure. Increasing understanding demands that it be considered as one of the supporting tissues.

The main constituents of basement membranes and external laminae are the glycosaminoglycan *heparan sulphate*, the fibrous protein *collagen type IV*, and the structural glycoproteins *fibronectin, laminin* and *entactin*. Fibronectin appears to be produced by fibroblasts of the supporting tissue but the remainder are at least partly, if not exclusively, elaborated by the tissues being supported.

With the electron microscope, the basement membrane is seen to consist of three layers. A relatively electron-lucent layer, the *lamina lucida* (ranging from 10 to 50 nm in width), abuts the basal cell membrane of the parenchymal tissue. The intermediate layer is electron-dense and is thus known as the *lamina densa*; depending on the tissue, this varies from 20 to 300 μm in thickness. Beyond the lamina densa is a broad, relatively electron-lucent layer known as the *lamina fibroreticularis* which merges with the underlying supporting tissue.

The electron-dense material of both lamina lucida and lamina densa represents a fine meshwork of collagen type IV which is exclusive to basement membranes. Another major constituent of these layers is laminin which binds the type IV collagen to the other basement membrane constituents and to laminin receptors in the parenchymal basal plasma membranes. Entactin mediates the binding of laminin to type IV collagen. The fibroreticular layer probably represents a condensation of the underlying supporting tissue. Its collagen content is mainly of type III (reticulin) which, via the fibrillar glycoprotein fibronectin, is also bound to integrins in the parenchymal basal plasma membrane.

BASIC TISSUE TYPES

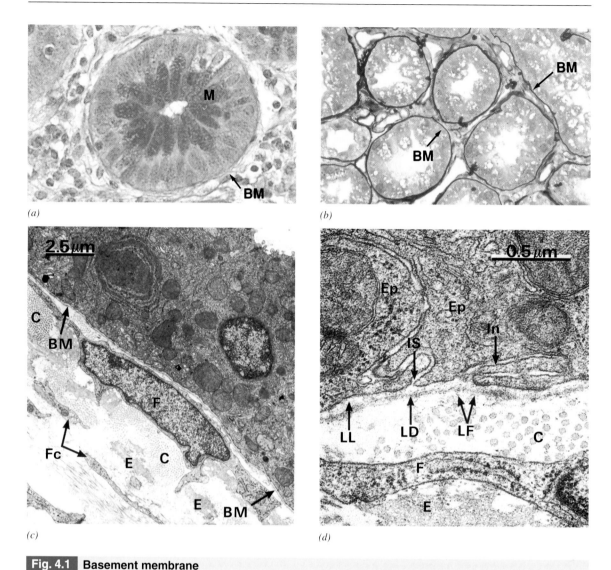

Fig. 4.1 Basement membrane

(a) PAS/haematoxylin × 400 (b) Jones' methenamine silver × 100 (c) EM × 5000 (d) EM × 45 000

With the light microscope, basement membranes can be seen beneath certain epithelial tissues where they happen to be relatively thick or where histochemical or other methods have been employed which are specific for particular basement membrane constituents. Micrograph (a) shows a duodenal crypt lined by mucus-secreting cells and is stained by the PAS method. This has affinity for the complex carbohydrates of the proteoglycans in the basement membrane **BM** as well as the mucus **M** at the luminal aspect of the crypt lining cells. In micrograph (b), a silver impregnation method which has affinity for reticulin demonstrates the basement membrane **BM** of the renal tubules.

Micrograph (c) shows the epithelial lining of mouse trachea. A basement membrane **BM** can be clearly seen separating it from the underlying supporting tissue which contains the cell body and nucleus of a fibroblast **F**, numerous fine fibroblastic cytoplasmic processes **Fc**, bundles of collagen fibrils **C** (cut in transverse section) and elastin fibres **E**.

At higher magnification in micrograph (d), the three layers of the basement membrane can be seen. The relatively electron-lucent *lamina lucida* **LL** abuts the basal epithelial cell membrane. The intermediate layer is electron-dense and represents the *lamina densa* **LD**. Beyond the lamina densa is the broad, relatively electron-lucent *lamina fibroreticularis* **LF** which merges with the fibrous and fibrillary (reticular) components of the underlying supporting tissue. In this field, note collagen fibrils **C**, part of a fibroblast **F** and elastin **E**. The basement membrane typically passes uninterrupted beneath the intercellular space **IS** between two epithelial cells **Ep** and beneath a basal invagination **In** of one of these cells.

The lamina densa was formerly known as the *basal lamina*. The terms *basal lamina* and *basement membrane* were often used interchangeably until it was realised that all three layers seen with the electron microscope represent the single layer seen with the light microscope. This has led to considerable terminological confusion and, if used, the term basal lamina should be confined to its meaning as lamina densa.

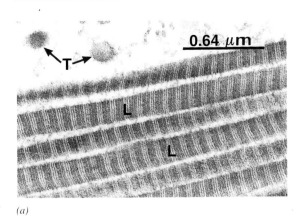
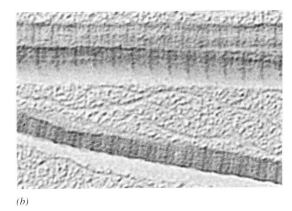

(a)   *(b)*

Fig. 4.2   Collagen   (a) EM × 32 000 (b) SEM × 32 000 (teased preparation)

The typical appearance of type I collagen, the most common variety, is shown in these specimens. The characteristic feature is a pattern of cross-banding with a periodicity of approximately 64 nm which results from the polymerisation of tropocollagen molecules (300 nm in length) such that each molecule overlaps the next by approximately one-quarter of its length. In micrograph (a) collagen fibres are shown in traverse **T** and longitudinal **L** section.

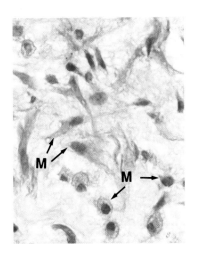

Fig. 4.3   Primitive mesenchyme   H & E × 400

Primitive mesenchyme is the embryological tissue from which all types of supporting connective tissue, including that of the skeleton, are derived. Mesenchymal cells are relatively unspecialised and are capable of differentiation into all the cell types found in mature supporting tissue. Some mesenchymal cells remain in fully mature supporting tissue and provide a pluripotential source of cells as the need arises for replacement or repair.

Mesenchymal cells **M** have an irregular, star (stellate) or spindle (fusiform) shape with delicate branching cytoplasmic extensions which form an interlacing network throughout the tissue. The oval nuclei have dispersed chromatin and visible nucleoli. The extracellular material consists almost exclusively of ground substance and does not contain mature fibres. Thus, mesenchyme represents a very loose variant of supporting tissue. The circulatory system of the embryo is poorly developed until a late stage and mesenchyme permits free diffusion of metabolites to and from developing tissues.

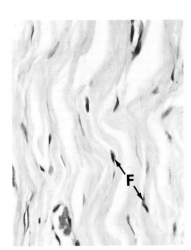

Fig. 4.4   Mature fibroblasts   H & E × 320

This micrograph demonstrates the typical histological appearance of mature fibroblasts in a relatively loose type of supporting tissue; collagen fibres are stained pink in this preparation. The fibroblast nuclei **F** are condensed and elongated in the direction of the collagen fibres. The cytoplasm is greatly reduced in volume, the cell being long and thin with fine cytoplasmic processes extending into the matrix to meet up with those of other fibroblasts; these are usually very difficult to see with the light microscope. The main function of fibroblasts is to maintain the integrity of supporting tissues by continuous slow turnover of the extracellular matrix constituents.

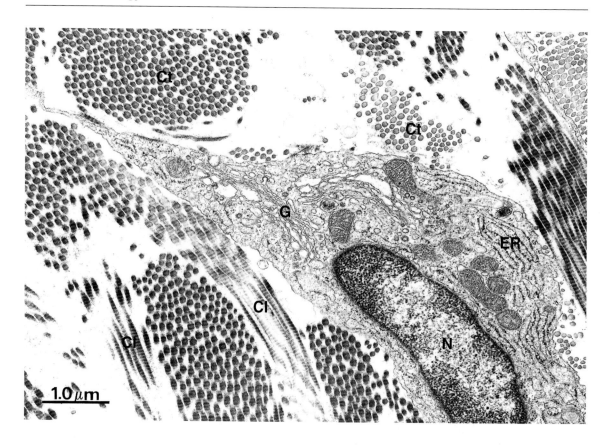

Fig. 4.5 Fibroblasts EM × 18 500

This micrograph illustrates the body of a mature fibroblast within loose collagenous supporting tissue. The nucleus **N** is moderately condensed, and nucleoli are not a prominent feature. The small quantity of cytoplasm is mostly occupied by rough endoplasmic reticulum **rER**, reflecting the dominant protein-secreting function of this type of cell. The Golgi apparatus **G** is visible and a few mitochondria are present.

Bundles of collagen fibres are seen in transverse **Ct** and longitudinal section **Cl** in the extracellular matrix.

During active synthesis of extracellular fibres, the fibroblast cytoplasm becomes much expanded and the rough endoplasmic reticulum and Golgi apparatus become much more prominent features. Fibroblasts synthesise and secrete the precursors of the glycosaminoglycans, collagen, elastin and all other extracellular constituents; however, in the mature, relatively inactive fibroblast, few secretory vesicles are found.

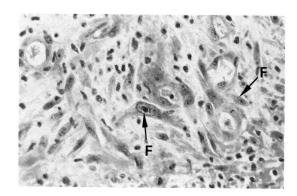

Fig. 4.6 Active fibroblasts: healing wound
H & E × 400

Active fibroblasts **F** are readily demonstrated in healing wounds, as in this micrograph. The nuclei are large and rounded in shape with prominent nucleoli reflecting active protein synthesis. The cytoplasm is extensive and its strongly stained, granular appearance is evidence of an extensive system of rough endoplasmic reticulum involved in protein synthesis. The relative absence of formed fibres in the extracellular matrix permits the meshwork of cytoplasmic extensions between fibroblasts to be visualised somewhat more easily than in less active supporting tissues.

Fibroblasts with a contractile function (myofibroblasts) play an important role in contraction and shrinkage of the resultant scar tissue.

BASIC TISSUE TYPES

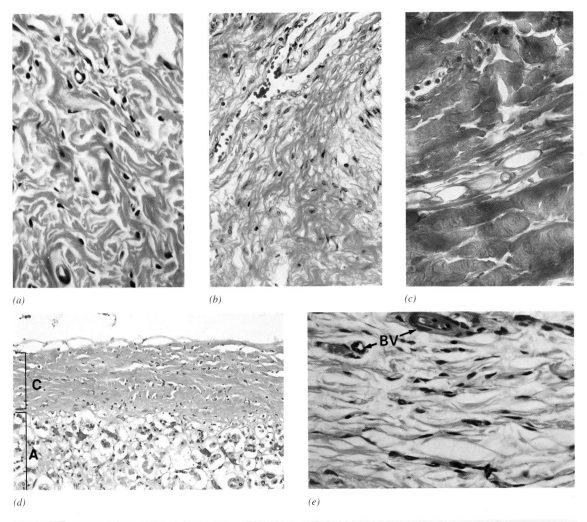

(a)　　　　　　　　　(b)　　　　　　　　　(c)

(d)　　　　　　　　　(e)

Fig. 4.7 Common forms of supporting tissue

(a) H & E × 320 (b) Masson's trichrome × 320 (c) Azan × 320 (d) H & E × 100 (e) H & E × 320

These micrographs illustrate a variety of common forms of supporting tissue. In the past, rather rigid descriptive classifications have been employed, e.g. 'dense regular connective tissue', 'dense irregular connective tissue', 'loose (areolar) connective tissue' etc., but in reality supporting tissues exhibit a great diversity of density and regularity and such rigid descriptions have outlived their usefulness.

The first three micrographs show collagen fibres stained by three common histological methods. Collagen is acidophilic due to its positively charged side groups; thus in standard H & E preparations, collagen is eosinophilic (i.e. pink-stained). With the trichrome stain, collagen stains green or blue (depending on the variant of the stain used) and with the Azan staining method, collagen is deep blue. These three specimens are of the dense supporting tissue of the skin (dermis) where the collagen fibres are arranged in coarse irregular interwoven bundles which confer great tensile strength. Fibroblasts are recognised by their highly condensed nuclei (stained red with Azan).

Micrograph (d) shows the capsule **C** of the adrenal gland **A** demonstrating again the typical dense arrangement of collagen fibres where mechanical support is the primary function. The collagen fibres are elongated and arranged in a regular manner to provide a well organised and robust enveloping capsule. Similar capsules invest the liver, spleen, lymph nodes, salivary glands, gonads and other encapsulated organs. Fibroblast nuclei are elongated in the direction of the collagen fibres.

Loose collagenous tissue supports the epithelial linings of the gastrointestinal, respiratory and urinary tracts, forms the deeper layers of the skin and occurs as a loose interstitial packing in many other organs. Such supporting tissue is illustrated in micrograph (e). The collagen fibres are loosely arranged and pursue a wave-like course in unstretched preparations. The open (*areolar*) spaces between collagen fibres are filled with ground substance which is not stained in this type of preparation since it is dissolved away during tissue processing. Several small blood vessels **BV** are seen. This type of tissue is traditionally referred to as ***areolar tissue***.

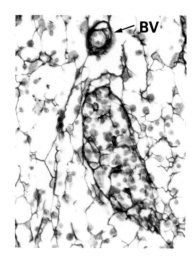

Fig. 4.8 Reticulin fibres

Silver impregnation method/haematoxylin × 800

Reticular tissue forms a delicate supporting framework for many highly cellular organs such as endocrine glands, lymph nodes and the liver. In such organs, a fine network of branching fibres ramifies throughout the parenchyma usually anchored to a dense, collagenous capsule and septae which traverse the tissue. Reticulin is a non-banded form of collagen designated collagen type III.

Reticulin fibres are usually poorly stained in common preparations but are able to absorb metallic silver by which they are stained black. This phenomenon led early histologists to believe that reticulin had a completely different chemical composition from that of collagen. Reticulin is the earliest type of collagen fibre to be produced during the development of all supporting tissues and is also present in varying quantities in most mature supporting tissues.

This micrograph shows the fine reticular architecture of part of a lymph node; the framework provides loose support for lymphoid cells, the nuclei of which have been counterstained blue. Reticulin is also a major component of the walls of small blood vessels **BV** as seen at the top of the field.

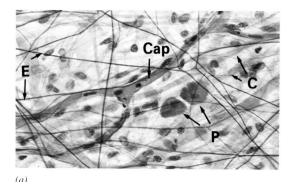
(a)

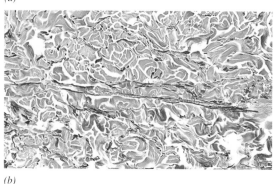
(b)

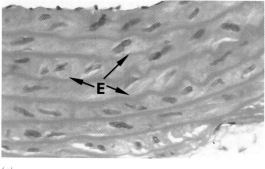
(c)

Fig. 4.9 Elastin fibres

(a) Spread preparation, elastin/H & E × 320
(b) Elastic van Gieson × 100 (c) H & E × 400

Elastin is found in varying proportions in most supporting tissues conferring elasticity to enable recovery of tissue shape following normal physiological deformation. Elastin is thus present in large amounts in tissues such as lung, skin and urinary bladder. It is also important as a constituent of the wall of blood vessels.

In most tissues, elastin occurs as short branching fibres which form an irregular network throughout the tissue. This is not easily seen in tissue sections but is better demonstrated in ***spread preparations*** such as in micrograph (a) in which elastin fibres **E** are stained black, collagen fibres **C** are stained pink and nuclei are stained blue. A branched capillary **Cap** crosses the field and two densely stained plasma cells **P** are also seen (see Ch. 11).

Micrograph (b) shows a histological section stained specifically for elastin; with this method, elastin is stained black and collagen is stained red. The specimen is of the dermis of the skin. The dominant feature is the coarse, closely packed, interwoven bundles of collagen between which are dispersed numerous finer elastic fibres. Most of the elastic fibres are cut in transverse or oblique section but some are cut in longitudinal section making them readily identifiable.

Micrograph (c) shows the wall of a large artery, this being made up mainly of smooth muscle cells, collagen and thick sheets of elastin (see Ch. 8). Like the collagen and smooth muscle cytoplasm, the elastin **E** is eosinophilic; it is only recognisable in this situation because the elastin sheets are very thick and because the elastin has a relaxed wave-like conformation due to collapse of the vessel wall.

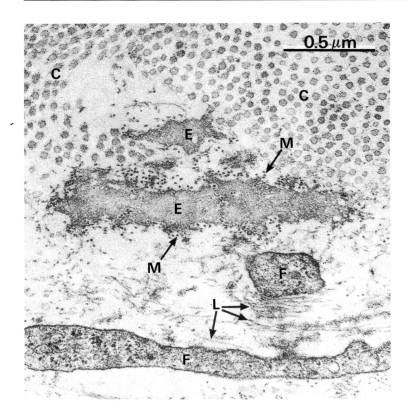

Fig. 4.10 Elastin EM × 50 000

This micrograph shows elastin **E** in the delicate supporting tissue underlying the epithelium of mouse trachea. The field also contains collagen fibrils **C** (cut in transverse section) and the fine cytoplasmic extensions of fibroblasts **F** responsible for elaboration of the extracellular constituents.

The elastin is not made up of fibrils but rather is an amorphous mass of polymerised tropoelastin. Microfibrils **M** of the structural glycoprotein fibrillin, which is involved in the process of elastin deposition, can just be discerned at this magnification (in transverse section) lying within and around the elastin. Microfibrils can also be seen in the lower part of the field cut in longitudinal section **L** in association with small amounts of elastin.

Adipose tissue

Most supporting tissues contain cells which are adapted for the storage of fat; these cells, called *adipocytes*, are derived from primitive mesenchyme where they develop as *lipoblasts*. Adipocytes are found in isolation or in clumps throughout loose supporting tissues or may constitute the main cell type as in adipose tissue.

Stored fat within adipocytes is derived from three main sources: dietary fat circulating in the bloodstream as chylomicrons; triglycerides synthesised in the liver and transported in blood; and triglycerides synthesised from glucose within adipocytes. Adipose tissue is often regarded as an inactive energy store, however it is an extremely important participant in general metabolic processes in that it acts as a temporary store of substrate for the energy-deriving processes of almost all tissues. Adipose tissue, therefore, generally has a rich blood supply. The rate of fat deposition and utilisation within adipose tissue is largely determined by dietary intake and energy expenditure, but a number of hormones and the sympathetic nervous system profoundly influence the fat metabolism of adipocytes.

There are two main types of adipose tissue:

- **White adipose tissue**. This type of adipose tissue comprises up to 20% of total body weight in normal, well-nourished male adults and up to 25% in females. It is distributed throughout the body particularly in the deep layers of the skin (see Ch. 9). In addition to being an important energy store, white adipose tissue acts as a thermal insulator under the skin and functions as a cushion against mechanical shock in such sites as around the kidneys.
- **Brown adipose tissue.** This highly specialised type of adipose tissue is found in newborn mammals and some hibernating animals, where it plays an important part in body temperature regulation. Only small amounts of brown adipose tissue are found in human adults and, although previously thought to contribute little to thermoregulation, there is now increasing evidence that (at least in some individuals) brown adipose tissue may play a role in burning off excess energy thus preventing obesity.

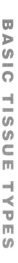

BASIC TISSUE TYPES

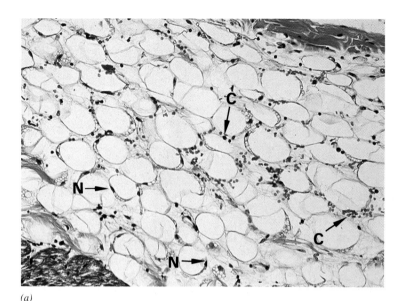

(a)

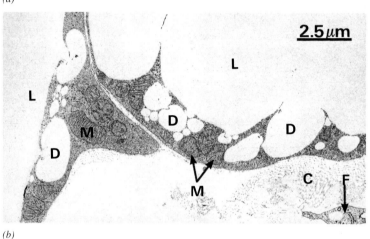

2.5μm

(b)

Fig. 4.11 White adipose tissue (a) Masson's trichrome × 480 (b) EM × 6000

The typical appearance of white adipose tissue is illustrated in micrograph (a). Fat stored in adipocytes accumulates as lipid droplets which fuse to form a single large droplet which distends and occupies most of the cytoplasm. The adipocyte nucleus **N** is compressed and displaced to one side of the stored lipid droplet and the cytoplasm is reduced to a small rim around the periphery. In routine histological sections, the lipid content of adipocytes is extracted during tissue processing, leaving a large unstained space within each cell. Note the minute dimensions of blood capillaries **C** compared with the size of the surrounding adipocytes.

The electron micrograph (b) shows the periphery of two adjacent adipocytes. Contrary to the impression given by light microscopy, the main lipid droplet **L** in each cell has an irregular outline with numerous tiny droplets **D** at the periphery in the process of fusion with the main droplet. The lipid is not bounded by a membrane. The thin rim of cytoplasm contains the usual organelles, most notably mitochondria **M**. Each adipocyte is surrounded by an external lamina. In the adjacent extracellular tissue can be seen a fibroblastic cytoplasmic process **F** and collagen fibrils **C**.

Adipocytes have receptors for insulin, glucocorticoids, growth hormone and noradrenaline that modulate uptake and release of fat. Adipocytes secrete the hormone leptin that is involved in regulation of appetite.

Fig. 4.12 Fibrofatty tissue H & E × 200

This micrograph demonstrates the typical appearance of adipocytes **A** scattered within loose, collagenous supporting tissue. Adipocytes occur either singly or in groups, particularly in the tissues supporting the lining of the gastrointestinal tract as shown here. Like the adipocytes of white adipose tissue, the size of adipocytes in loose supporting tissue depends on the equilibrium between dietary fat intake and energy expenditure.

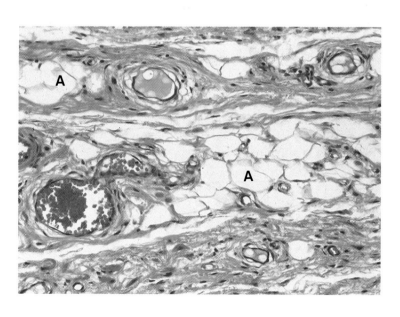

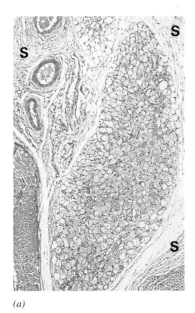

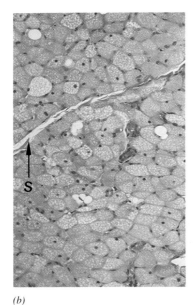

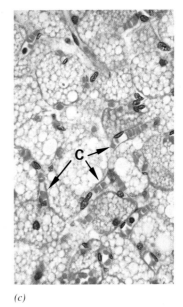

(a)   *(b)*   *(c)*

Fig. 4.13   Brown adipose tissue
(a) H & E × 100 (b) H & E × 200
(c) H & E × 320 (d) Rabbit, EM × 4070

These micrographs demonstrate the typical histological appearance of brown adipose tissue. As seen in micrographs (a) and (b), brown adipose tissue is arranged in lobules separated by fibrous septae **S** which convey blood vessels and sympathetic nerve fibres. Within the cytoplasm, lipid is stored in the form of multiple small droplets, giving the cytoplasm a vacuolated appearance. The cytoplasm is relatively copious and stains strongly due to the presence of numerous mitochondria.

At high magnification in micrograph (c), the nuclei of brown adipocytes are seen to be eccentrically located within the cell but, unlike those of white adipocytes, the nuclei are plump and surrounded by a significant quantity of strongly eosinophilic cytoplasm. The stored lipid is contained within multiple droplets, all of which have been dissolved away during tissue processing. A frozen section of brown adipose tissue stained for lipid is shown in Figure 1.20b. Note the rich network of capillaries **C** between the brown adipocytes.

The electron micrograph (d) shows brown adipose tissue taken from a newborn rabbit and readily demonstrates the multilocular nature of stored lipid **L**. The cytoplasm of brown adipocytes is crammed with mitochondria **M** which have numerous, closely packed cristae. These mitochondria are extremely rich in cytochromes, molecules involved in oxidative energy production; this accounts for the brown colour of brown adipose tissue when examined macroscopically.

Unlike the metabolism of other tissues, in brown adipose cells the process of electron transport is readily uncoupled from the phosphorylation of ADP to form ATP. The energy derived from oxidation of lipids, and energy released by electron transport in the uncoupled state, is dissipated as heat which is rapidly conducted to the rest of the body by the rich vascular network of brown adipose

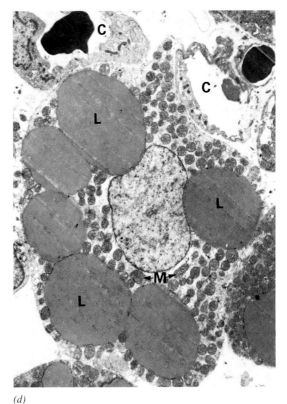

(d)

tissue. Note the intimate association of capillaries **C** with the brown adipocyte in this micrograph.

Using these metabolic processes, neonatal humans and other mammals utilise brown adipose tissue to generate body heat during the vulnerable period after birth. Brown adipose tissue undergoes involution in early infancy and in adult humans is found only in odd sites such as around the adrenal gland and great vessels. The production of heat by brown adipose tissue is controlled directly by the sympathetic nervous system.

The defence cells of supporting tissue

The supporting tissues not only contain cells responsible for their synthesis, maintenance and metabolic activity, but also a variety of cells with defence and immune functions. Traditionally, these cells have been divided into two categories: fixed (intrinsic) cells and wandering (extrinsic) cells.

The intrinsic defence cells of supporting tissue are the *tissue-fixed macrophages* (*histiocytes*) and *mast cells*. Tissue-fixed macrophages are now generally believed to be derived from circulating monocytes (see Fig. 3.9) which have become at least temporarily resident in supporting tissues. Mast cells are functionally analogous to basophils (see Fig. 3.7) but there are structural differences which suggest that mast cells are not merely basophils resident in the tissues.

The wandering category of defence and immune cells includes all the remaining members of the white blood cell series (see Ch. 3). Although leucocytes are usually considered as a constituent of blood, their principal site of activity is outside the blood circulation, particularly within loose supporting tissues. Leucocytes are normally found only in relatively small numbers, but in response to tissue injury and other disease processes their numbers increase greatly. The supporting tissues of those regions of the body which are subject to the constant threat of pathogenic invasion, such as the gastrointestinal and respiratory tracts, contain a large population of leucocytes, maintaining constant surveillance.

The reticuloendothelial concept

The term *reticuloendothelial system* has long been used to describe a diverse group of cells found in many tissues but in particular the bone marrow, liver, spleen, lymph nodes and thymus. The principal functional characteristic of such cells is their ability to phagocytose particulate matter and effete (worn out or dead) cells, e.g. old blood cells. Such phagocytic cells are found lining certain blood- and lymph-filled spaces, such as the sinusoids of the liver (see Fig. 15.8), bone marrow (see Fig. 3.12) and spleen (see Fig. 11.25), and in this context they have some features in common with the *endothelial cells* which line all blood and lymphatic vessels (see Ch. 8).

Certain highly cellular tissues, such as lymph nodes and the haemopoietic cords of bone marrow, have a supporting framework of reticulin fibres (see Fig. 4.8) upon which are draped cells with long cytoplasmic processes morphologically similar to primitive mesenchymal cells (see Fig. 4.3); these cells are traditionally described as *reticulum* or *reticular cells*. Some if not all of these cells are probably responsible for synthesis of the reticulin framework, being thus analogous to fibroblasts; many of these cells, if not all, may also exhibit considerable phagocytic activity.

Because of the close structural and functional association of these cell types with the haemopoietic, macrophage–monocyte (see Fig. 3.9) and immune systems, they were thought to represent some common functional denominator. Consequently, 'reticuloendothelial' and related terms became widely and often indiscriminately applied to tissues and cells within these systems. Scientific advances have rendered the concept so imprecise as to serve little purpose and it should now be considered of historical interest only.

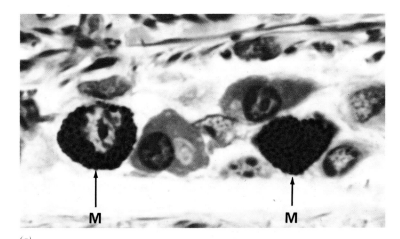

(a)

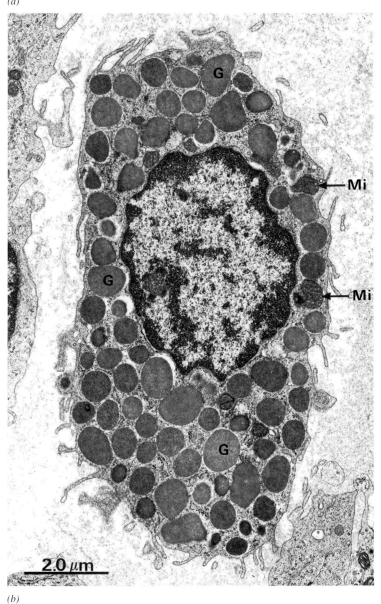

2.0 μm

(b)

Fig. 4.14 **Mast cells**
**(a) Thin section, toluidine blue
× 1200 (b) EM × 12 000**

Mast cells are found in all supporting tissues but are particularly prevalent in the skin, gastrointestinal lining, the serosal lining of the peritoneal cavity and around blood vessels. Their major constituents and functions are very similar to those of basophils from which they may be derived and which are described in detail with Figure 3.7. Mast cells are long-lived with the ability to proliferate in the tissues. Mast cell degranulation results in the release of histamine and other vasoactive mediators which induce the immediate hypersensitivity (anaphylactoid) response (characteristic of urticaria, allergic rhinitis and asthma) and anaphylactic shock.

Mast cells are not readily identified in routine histological sections due to the water solubility of their densely basophilic granules which tend to be lost during preparation. Thus special techniques of fixation, embedding and staining must be employed. With suitable staining, however, the characteristic feature of mast cells is an extensive cytoplasm packed with large granules which are nevertheless smaller in size, though more numerous, than those of basophils. When stained with certain blue basic dyes such as *toluidine blue*, the granules bind to the dye changing its colour to red. This property is known as *metachromasia*.

The light micrograph (a) demonstrates two mast cells **M** in the supporting tissue underlying the tracheal surface. A pale nucleus can be seen in one cell but the plane of section is outside the nucleus of the other. Note the large, densely packed granules which exhibit metachromasia.

In the electron micrograph (b), mast cell granules **G** are seen to be membrane-bound and to contain a dense amorphous material. The granules are liberated from the cell by exocytosis when stimulated during an inflammatory or allergic response. The cytoplasm contains a few rounded mitochondria **Mi** and a little rough endoplasmic reticulum. The non-segmented nucleus has less condensed chromatin than that of basophils. Other differences from basophils include a more uniform distribution of their thin surface processes, a greater number of cytoplasmic filaments and a lack of glycogen granules.

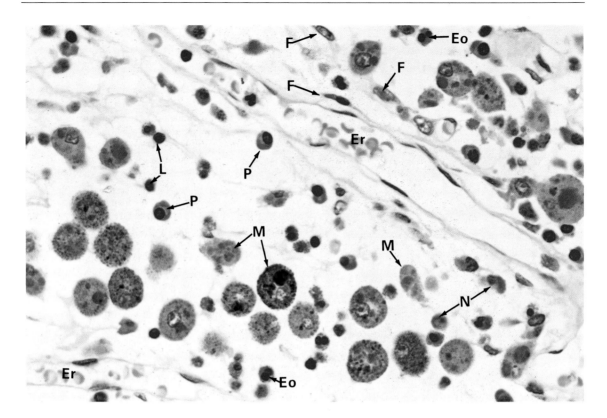

Fig. 4.15 Leucocytes in loose supporting tissue H & E × 640

The appearance of leucocytes within tissue sections differs greatly from the appearance seen in blood smears (see Ch. 3). In this micrograph, a variety of leucocytes are seen in the loose supporting tissue beneath the lining of the large intestine, a site which is normally rich in such cells even in the absence of inflammation.

Fibroblasts **F** are identified by their relatively large, elongated nuclei. Erythrocytes **Er** within small blood vessels are intensely eosinophilic (red stained); the presence of erythrocytes (approximate diameter 7 μm) provides a reference for the size of other cells of the granulocyte series (see Ch. 3).

Of the granulocytes, neutrophils are only rarely seen in the tissues except in acute or chronic inflammation. Neutrophils **N** are recognised by their multilobed nuclei and poorly stained cytoplasm. Eosinophils **Eo** are present in large numbers in normal supporting tissues and are recognised by their bilobed nuclei and strongly eosinophilic cytoplasmic granules. Basophils, and their analogues mast cells, are poorly stained in H & E preparations and are therefore difficult to recognise.

Lymphocytes **L** are easily recognised by their small, densely stained nuclei and a thin halo of poorly stained cytoplasm. Plasma cells **P**, responsible for antibody synthesis (see Ch. 11), are recognised by their large

granular nuclei and extensive amphophilic (purple stained) cytoplasm containing a pale stained perinuclear area which represents a well developed and active Golgi apparatus. The amphophilia of plasma cells is attributable to large amounts of rough endoplasmic reticulum (basophilic) and of protein (antibody acidophilic) resulting in a purple colour.

Large mononuclear phagocytes, analogous to the monocytes of blood, are distributed throughout all supporting tissues where they may exhibit intense phagocytic activity; these cells are also known as macrophages, tissue-fixed macrophages, and histiocytes when present in supporting tissue. Inactive macrophages are small and drape themselves on the fibres of the extracellular matrix and may be difficult to distinguish from fibroblasts. In contrast, actively phagocytic macrophages are plump and may move in an amoeboid manner through the ground substance. When actively phagocytic, macrophages may be easily recognised by their large size and content of engulfed material; note, however, that active macrophages have an extremely variable appearance, depending on the nature of their phagocytic activity. Most of the cytoplasmic detail of the macrophages **M** shown in this preparation is obscured by engulfed material which appears brown.

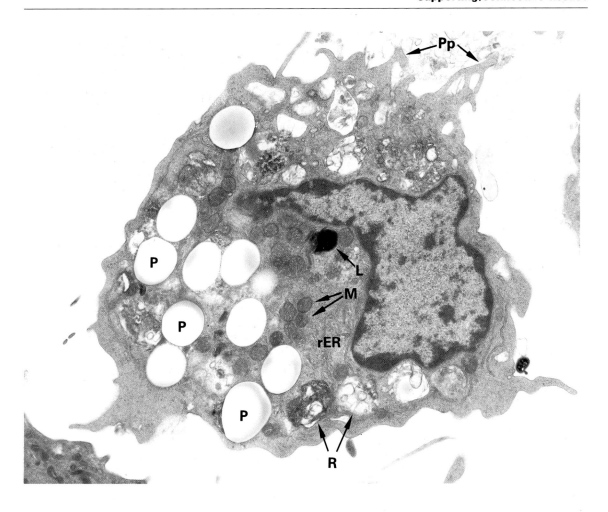

Fig. 4.16 **Macrophage** EM × 11 600

The ultrastructural features of macrophages vary widely according to their state of activity and tissue location. This micrograph shows an active macrophage obtained from the peritoneum of a rat which had previously been injected intraperitoneally with latex particles; a number of particles **P** have been engulfed by the macrophage.

The macrophage nucleus is irregular with heterochromatin typically clumped around the nuclear envelope. The cytoplasm contains a few mitochondria **M** and a variable amount of free ribosomes and rough endoplasmic reticulum **rER**. In quiescent macrophages, lysosomes **L** are abundant but their number is much reduced in actively phagocytic cells; lysosomes are later regenerated by the Golgi apparatus. The macrophage cytoplasm contains an assortment of phagosomes and residual bodies **R**. Residual material may be released from the macrophage by exocytosis. Such material may remain sequestered in the tissues, as occurs with the dyes used in tattooing of the skin, or the material may be returned to the circulation for excretion or re-use in biosynthetic processes. Actively phagocytic cells exhibit irregular cytoplasmic projections or pseudopodia **Pp** which are involved in amoeboid movement and phagocytosis.

In addition to their role as tissue scavengers, macrophages play an important role in immune mechanisms (see Ch. 11) since they are often the first cells to make contact with antigens. Macrophages process antigenic material in some way before presenting it to lymphocytes; lymphocytes are then stimulated to undergo specific immune responses. Macrophages involved in this way are described as ***antigen presenting cells***. As a result of various immune mechanisms, antigenic material may become combined or coated with substances such as antibodies and complement which are then collectively known as ***opsonins***. Opsonins greatly enhance the phagocytic ability of macrophages and other phagocytes such as neutrophils (see Ch. 3), a process which is known as ***opsonisation***. Other substances such as ***lymphokines***, which are released during the immune response, act directly upon macrophages to increase greatly their metabolic and phagocytic activity.

BASIC TISSUE TYPES

5. Epithelial tissues

Introduction

The epithelia are a diverse group of tissues which, with rare exceptions, cover or line all body surfaces, cavities and tubes. Epithelia thus function as interfaces between different biological compartments. As such, epithelia mediate a wide range of activities such as selective diffusion, absorption and/or secretion, physical protection and containment; all these major functions may be exhibited at a single epithelial surface. For example, the epithelial lining of the small intestine is primarily involved in absorption of the products of digestion, but the epithelium also protects itself from noxious intestinal contents by the secretion of a surface coating of mucus.

Surface epithelia form continuous sheets comprising one or more layers of cells. The cells are separated by a minute quantity of intercellular material which may represent the fused glycocalyces of adjacent cells (see Ch. 1). Epithelial cells are closely bound to one another by a variety of membrane specialisations called *cell junctions* which provide physical strength and mediate exchange of 'information' and metabolites.

All epithelia are supported by a *basement membrane* of variable thickness. Basement membranes separate epithelia from underlying supporting tissues and are never penetrated by blood vessels; epithelia are thus dependent on the diffusion of oxygen and metabolites from adjacent supporting tissues. The structure of basement membranes is described in detail in Chapter 4.

Classification of epithelia

Epithelia are traditionally classified according to three morphological characteristics:

- The number of cell layers: a single layer of epithelial cells is termed *simple epithelium*, whereas epithelia composed of several layers are termed *stratified epithelia*.
- The shape of the component cells: this is based on the appearance in sections taken at right angles to the epithelial surface. In stratified epithelia the shape of the outermost layer of cells determines the descriptive classification. Cellular outlines are often difficult to distinguish, but the shape of epithelial cells is usually reflected in the shape of their nuclei.
- The presence of surface specialisations such as cilia and keratin: an example is the epithelial surface of skin which is classified as 'stratified squamous keratinising epithelium' since it consists of many layers of cells, the surface cells of which are flattened (squamous) in shape and covered by an outer layer of the proteinaceous material, keratin (see Fig. 5.7).

Epithelia may be derived from ectoderm, mesoderm or endoderm although in the past it was thought that true epithelia were only of ectodermal or endodermal origin. Two types of epithelia derived from mesoderm, i.e. the lining of blood and lymphatic vessels and the linings of the serous body cavities, were not considered to be epithelia and were termed *endothelium* and *mesothelium,* respectively. By both morphological and functional criteria, such distinction has little practical value; nevertheless, the terms endothelium and mesothelium are still used to describe these types of epithelium.

Glandular epithelia

Epithelium which is primarily involved in secretion is often arranged into structures called *glands*. Glands are merely invaginations of epithelial surfaces which are formed during embryonic development by proliferation of epithelium into the underlying tissues. Glands which maintain their continuity with the epithelial surface, discharging their secretions onto the free surface via a duct, are called *exocrine glands*.

Several of the solid organs are composed of epithelial cells arranged in sheets or tubules, e.g. the kidneys and the liver.

In some situations epithelial tissue forms solid organs or isolated islands of epithelial secretory tissue lie deep within other tissues. The secretory products of such glands, known as *endocrine* or *ductless glands*, pass into the bloodstream; their secretions are known as *hormones* (see Ch. 17).

The majority of epithelial cells contain cytokeratin intermediate filaments, and this can be used to recognise an epithelial phenotype using immunohistochemistry.

Simple epithelia

Simple epithelia are defined as surface epithelia consisting of a single layer of cells. Simple epithelia are almost always found at interfaces involved in selective diffusion, absorption or secretion. They provide little protection against mechanical abrasion and thus are not found on surfaces subject to such stresses. The cells comprising simple epithelia range in shape from extremely flattened to tall columnar, depending on their function. For example, flattened simple epithelia are ideally suited to diffusion and are therefore found in the air sacs of the lung (alveoli), the lining of blood vessels (endothelium) and lining body cavities (mesothelium). In contrast, highly active epithelial cells, such as the cells lining the small intestine, are generally tall since they must accommodate the appropriate organelles. Simple epithelia may exhibit a variety of surface specialisations, such as microvilli and cilia, which facilitate their specific surface functions.

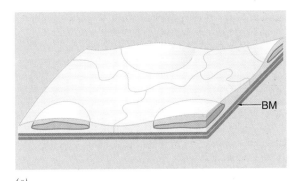

(a)

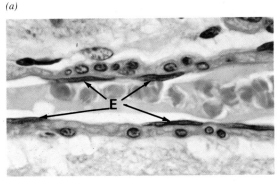

(b)

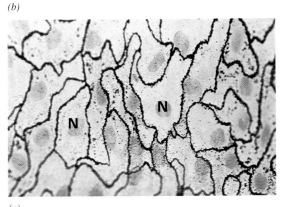

(c)

Fig. 5.1 Simple squamous epithelium
(a) Diagram (b) H & E × 800 (c) Spread preparation, silver method/neutral red × 320

Simple squamous epithelium is composed of flattened, irregularly shaped cells forming a continuous surface which may be referred to as *pavemented epithelium*; the term 'squamous' derives from the comparison of the cells to the scales of a fish. Like all epithelia, this delicate lining is supported by an underlying basement membrane **BM** as shown diagrammatically, although this is rarely thick enough to be seen with routine light microscopy.

Simple squamous epithelium is found lining surfaces involved in passive transport (diffusion) of either gases (as in the lungs) or fluids (as in the walls of blood capillaries). Simple squamous epithelium also forms the delicate lining of the pleural, pericardial and peritoneal cavities where it permits passage of tissue fluid into and out of these cavities. Although these cells appear simple in form they have a wide variety of important roles. The cells frequently have specalised surface receptors that control secretion of locally acting chemical messengers.

Micrograph (b) shows a small blood vessel and illustrates the typical appearance of simple squamous epithelium in section. The epithelial lining cells **E** (known as endothelium in the circulatory system) are so flattened that they can only be recognised by their nuclei which bulge into the vessel lumen. The supporting basement membrane is thin and, in H & E stained preparations, has similar staining properties to the endothelial cell cytoplasm; hence it cannot be seen in this micrograph.

In the preparation used in micrograph (c), the mesothelial lining of the peritoneal cavity has been stripped from the underlying tissues and spread onto a slide thus permitting a surface view of simple squamous epithelium. The intercellular substance has been stained with silver thereby outlining the closely interdigitating and highly irregular cell boundaries. The nuclei **N** are stained red.

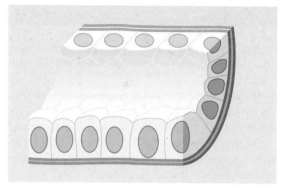
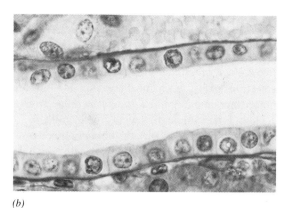

(a) *(b)*

Fig. 5.2 Simple cuboidal epithelium (a) Diagram (b) Azan × 400

Simple cuboidal epithelium represents an intermediate form between simple squamous and simple columnar epithelium; the distinction between tall cuboidal and low columnar is often arbitrary and is of descriptive value only. In section perpendicular to the basement membrane, the epithelial cells appear square, leading to its traditional description as cuboidal epithelium; on surface view, however, the cells are actually polygonal in shape. The nucleus is usually round and located in the centre of the cell.

Simple cuboidal epithelium usually lines small ducts and tubules which may have excretory, secretory or absorptive functions; examples are the small collecting ducts of the kidney, salivary glands and pancreas.

The micrograph shows the cells lining a small collecting tubule in the kidney. Although the boundaries between individual cells are indistinct, the nuclear shape provides an approximate indication of the cell size and shape. Reflecting the considerable metabolic activity of these cells, the nuclear chromatin is relatively dispersed and nucleoli are prominent. The underlying basement membrane appears as a prominent blue line with the Azan staining method.

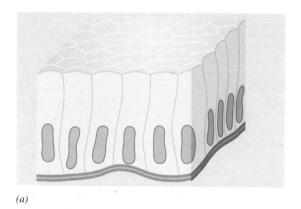
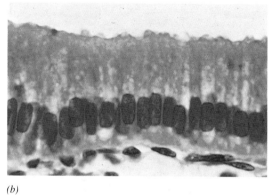

(a) *(b)*

Fig. 5.3 Simple columnar epithelium (a) Diagram (b) H & E × 800

Simple columnar epithelium is similar to simple cuboidal epithelium except that the cells are taller and appear columnar in sections at right angles to the basement membrane. The height of the cells may vary from low to tall columnar depending on the site and/or degree of functional activity. The nuclei are elongated and may be located towards the base, the centre or occasionally the apex of the cytoplasm; this is known as *polarity*. Simple columnar epithelium is most often found on highly absorptive surfaces such as in the small intestine, although it may constitute the lining of highly secretory surfaces such as that of the stomach.

The micrograph illustrates an unusually tall example of simple columnar epithelium and is taken from the lining of the gall bladder where it has the function of absorbing water, thus concentrating bile. Note the typically elongated nuclei which in this location exhibit basal polarity.

The luminal plasma membranes of highly absorptive epithelial cells are often arranged into numerous, minute, finger-like projections called *microvilli* which greatly increase the surface area of the absorptive interface. Microvilli are far too small to be resolved individually by light microscopy although they may collectively give the appearance of a *striated* or *brush border* at the luminal surface (see Fig. 5.16).

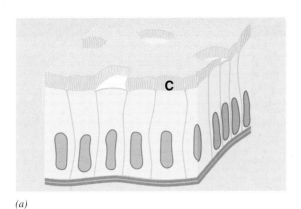

(a)

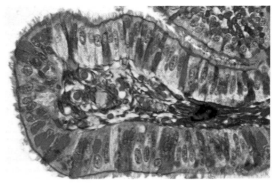

(b)

Fig. 5.4　**Simple columnar ciliated epithelium**　(a) Diagram (b) Azan × 320

This type of simple columnar epithelium is traditionally described as a separate entity because of the presence of surface specialisations called cilia **C** on the majority of the cells. Among the ciliated cells are scattered non-ciliated cells which usually have a secretory function.

Cilia are much larger than microvilli and are readily visible with the light microscope. Each cilium consists of a finger-like projection of the plasma membrane, its cytoplasm containing a motile specialisation of the cytoskeleton (see Fig. 5.15). Each cell may have up to 300 cilia which, along with those of other cells, beat in a wave-like manner, generating a current which propels fluid or minute particles over the epithelial surface. Simple columnar ciliated epithelium

is not common in humans except in the female reproductive tract.

This micrograph taken from the Fallopian tube (oviduct) shows one of its numerous folds covered by simple columnar ciliated epithelium. The predominant cell type in this epithelium is tall columnar and ciliated, the nuclei being located towards the luminal aspect of the cells. The less numerous, blue stained cells with basally located nuclei are not ciliated and have a secretory function. Ciliary action facilitates transport of the ovum from the ovary towards the uterus. As in this preparation, cilia are often stuck together in clumps by surface secretions or they may become flattened during tissue processing and therefore difficult to distinguish.

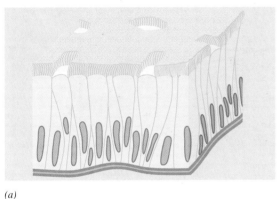

(a)

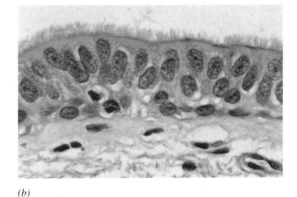

(b)

Fig. 5.5　**Pseudostratified columnar ciliated epithelium**　(a) Diagram (b) H & E × 600

Another variant of simple columnar epithelium is described in which the majority of cells are also usually ciliated. The term *pseudostratified* is derived from the appearance of this epithelium in section which conveys the erroneous impression that there is more than one layer of cells. In fact, this is a true simple epithelium since all the cells rest on the basement membrane. The nuclei of these cells, however, are disposed at different levels, thus creating the illusion of cellular stratification. Not all the ciliated cells extend to the luminal surface; such cells are capable of cell division providing replacements for cells lost or damaged.

Pseudostratified columnar ciliated epithelium may be distinguished from true stratified epithelia by two

characteristics. Firstly, the individual cells of the pseudostratified epithelium exhibit polarity, with nuclei being mainly confined to the basal two-thirds of the epithelium. Secondly, cilia are never present on stratified epithelia.

Pseudostratified epithelium is almost exclusively confined to the larger airways of the respiratory system in mammals and is therefore often referred to as *respiratory epithelium*. Micrograph (b) illustrates the lining of a bronchus. In the respiratory tract, the cilia propel a surface layer of mucus containing entrapped particles towards the pharynx in what is often described as the *mucociliary escalator*.

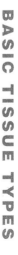

Stratified epithelia

Stratified epithelia are defined as epithelia consisting of two or more layers of cells. Stratified epithelia have mainly a protective function and the degree and nature of the stratification are related to the kinds of physical stresses to which the surface is exposed. In general, stratified epithelia are poorly suited for the functions of absorption and secretion by virtue of their thickness, although some stratified surfaces are moderately permeable to water and other small molecules. The classification of stratified epithelia is based on the shape and structure of the surface cells since cells of the basal layer are usually cuboidal in shape.

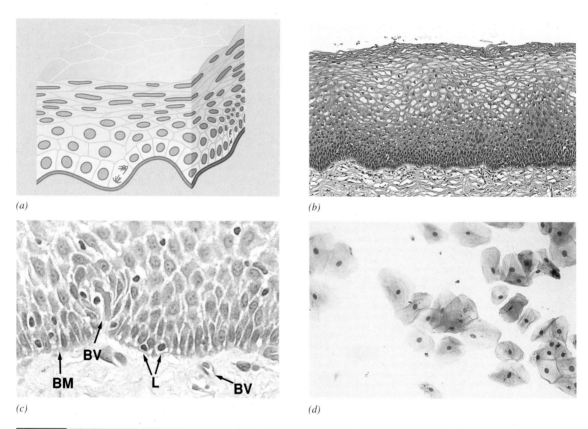

(a)   *(b)*

(c)   *(d)*

Fig. 5.6   **Stratified squamous epithelium**
(a) Diagram (b) H & E × 100 (c) H & E × 400 (d) Papanicolou × 400

Stratified squamous epithelium consists of a variable number of cells layers which exhibit transition from a cuboidal basal layer to a flattened surface layer. The basal cells divide continuously, their offspring being progressively pushed towards the free surface where they are ultimately shed. During the process, the cells undergo first maturation, then degeneration, the surface cells showing overt signs of degeneration; this is particularly evident in the nuclei which become progressively condensed (pyknotic) and flattened, before ultimately disintegrating.

Stratified squamous epithelium is well adapted to withstand abrasion since loss of surface cells does not compromise the underlying tissue; it is poorly adapted to withstand desiccation. This type of epithelium lines the oral cavity, pharynx, oesophagus, anal canal, uterine cervix and vagina, sites which are subject to mechanical abrasion but which are kept moist by glandular secretions.

The epithelium demonstrated in micrograph (b) is from the uterine cervix. Note the highly cellular basal layer and the transformation through the large polygonal cells of the intermediate layers to the degenerate superficial squamous cells. The junction between epithelium and underlying supporting tissue is irregular, enhancing the adhesion of the epithelium to the underlying tissues.

Micrograph (c) shows the deep layers at high magnification; a few lymphocytes **L** are scattered at this level. The basement membrane **BM** is quite thick and, as in all epithelia, blood vessels **BV** do not extend beyond the basement membrane.

Micrograph (d) shows a smear made from cells scraped from the uterine cervix as it projects into the vagina. The degenerate, scaly superficial cells stain pink with this staining method, the living cells from deeper layers staining blue.

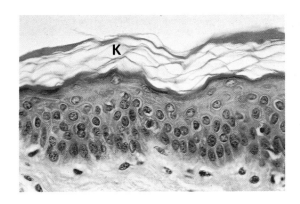

Fig. 5.7 **Stratified squamous keratinising epithelium** H & E × 320

This specialised form of stratified squamous epithelium constitutes the epithelial surface of the skin (epidermis) and is adapted to withstand the constant abrasion and desiccation to which the body surface is exposed. During maturation, the epithelial cells accumulate cross-linked cytoskeletal proteins in a process called *keratinisation* resulting in the formation of a tough, non-living surface layer consisting of the protein *keratin* **K** (see Ch. 9). Keratinisation may be induced in normally non-keratinising stratified squamous epithelium such as that of the oral cavity when exposed to excessive abrasion or desiccation.

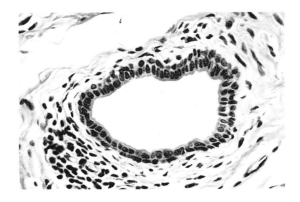

Fig. 5.8 **Stratified cuboidal epithelium** H & E × 320

Stratified cuboidal epithelium is a thin, stratified epithelium which usually consists of only two or three layers of cuboidal or low columnar cells. This type of epithelium is usually confined to the lining of the larger excretory ducts of exocrine glands such as the salivary glands. Stratified cuboidal epithelium is probably not involved in significant absorptive or secretory activity but merely provides a more robust lining than would be afforded by a simple epithelium.

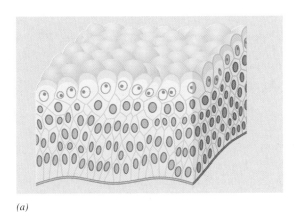

(a)

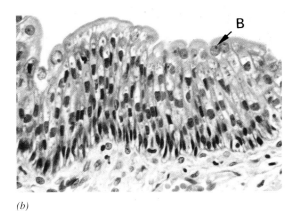

(b)

Fig. 5.9 **Transitional epithelium** (a) Diagram (b) H & E × 320

Transitional epithelium is a form of stratified epithelium almost exclusively confined to the urinary tract in mammals where it is highly specialised to accommodate a great degree of stretch and to withstand the toxicity of urine. This epithelial type is so named because it has some features which are intermediate (transitional) between stratified cuboidal and stratified squamous epithelia. In the relaxed (contracted) state, transitional epithelium appears to be about four to five cell layers thick. The basal cells are roughly cuboidal, the intermediate cells are polygonal and the surface cells are large and rounded and may contain two nuclei. In the stretched state, transitional epithelium often appears only two or three cells thick (although the actual number of

layers remains constant) and the intermediate and surface layers are extremely flattened.

The micrograph shows the appearance of transitional epithelium from the lining of a contracted bladder. The shape and apparent size of the basal and intermediate cells vary considerably depending on the degree of distension, but the cells of the surface layer usually retain several characteristic features. Firstly, the surface cells are large and pale stained and present a scalloped surface outline. Secondly, the luminal surface of the cells appears thickened and more densely stained. Thirdly, the nuclei of the surface cells are large and round, and often exhibit prominent nucleoli; some surface cells are binucleate **B**.

Membrane specialisations of epithelia

The intercellular, luminal and basal surfaces of epithelial cells exhibit a variety of specialisations.

Intercellular surfaces

The apposed surfaces of epithelial cells are linked by several different types of membrane and cytoskeletal specialisations. These *cell junctions* permit epithelia to form a continuous cohesive layer in which all of the cells 'communicate' and cooperate to achieve the particular functional requirements of the epithelium.

Cell junctions are of three functional types:

- *Occluding junctions*, also known as *tight junctions*, are located immediately beneath the luminal surface of simple columnar epithelium (e.g. intestinal lining) where they seal the intercellular spaces so that luminal contents cannot penetrate between the lining cells. Each tight junction forms a continuous circumferential band or zonule around the cell and is thus also known as a *zonula occludens*.

- *Adhering junctions* tightly bind the constituent cells of the epithelium together and act as anchorage sites for the cytoskeleton of each cell so that cytoskeletons of all cells are effectively linked into a single functional unit. Adhering junctions are of two morphological types. Deep to the tight junctions of columnar epithelial cells, an adhering junction forms a continuous band (*zonula adherens*) around the cell providing structural reinforcement to the occluding junction. Secondly, adhering junctions in the form of small circular patches or spots called *desmosomes* (*macula adherens*) are circumferentially arranged around columnar cells deep to the continuous adhering junction. The combination of zonula occludens, zonula adherens and circumferentially arranged desmosomes is known as a *junctional complex*. Desmosomes (spot-adhering junctions) are also widely scattered elsewhere in epithelial intercellular interfaces, binding the whole epithelial mass into a structurally coherent whole.

- *Communicating junctions*, also known as *gap* or *nexus junctions* due to their ultrastructural appearance, are circular intercellular contact areas containing hundreds of tiny pores which permit passage of small molecules between adjacent cells. Molecules involved in such cytoplasmic interchange include ions responsible for electrical excitation of cell membranes, nutrients and chemical signalling agents.

Adhering junctions and communicating junctions are not exclusive to epithelia and are also present in cardiac and visceral muscle where they appear to serve similar functions.

Luminal surfaces

The luminal surfaces of epithelial cells may incorporate three main types of specialisation: *cilia, microvilli* and *stereocilia*. Cilia are relatively long, motile structures which are easily resolved by light microscopy. In contrast, microvilli are short, often extremely numerous projections of the plasma membrane which cannot be individually resolved with the light microscope. Stereocilia are merely extremely long microvilli usually found only singly or in small numbers in odd sites such as the male reproductive tract; stereocilia are not motile and thus quite inappropriately named.

Basal surfaces

The interface between all epithelia and underlying supporting tissues is marked by a non-cellular structure known as the *basement membrane* which provides structural support for epithelia and constitutes a selective barrier to the passage of materials between epithelium and supporting tissue. Details of basement membrane structure are provided in the introduction of Chapter 4 and illustrated in Figure 4.1. The basal plasma membranes of some simple epithelia which are very active in ion transport (e.g. the cells of the kidney tubules) exhibit extensive basal interdigitations or folds. These greatly enhance surface area and provide an arrangement by which the energy-providing mitochondria can be situated in intimate association with the plasma membrane; an example is shown in Figure 1.18c. *Hemidesmosomes* are present on the inner aspect of the basal plasma membrane adjacent to basement membrane and provide a means of anchorage of the cell via its cytoskeleton to the basement membrane and underlying supporting tissue.

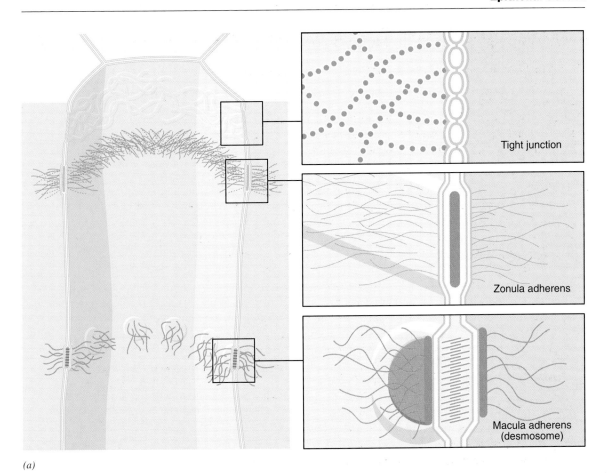

(a)

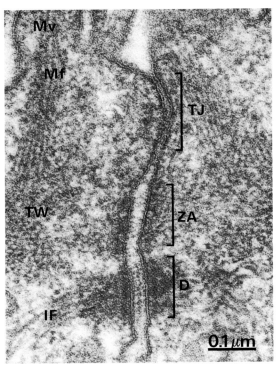

(b)

Fig. 5.10 **Intercellular junctions** **(a) Schematic diagram (b) Junctional complex, EM × 125 000**

The illustration (a) demonstrates, in a highly schematic manner, the three-dimensional (circumferential) arrangement of the junctional complex with respect to the cell surface and the detailed structure of the various types of intercellular junction of which it is comprised.

Between the cells of simple cuboidal and simple columnar epithelia, a junctional complex encircles each cell preventing access of luminal contents to the intercellular spaces and strengthening the luminal surface against cellular disaggregation.

As seen in the micrograph of intestinal columnar epithelium, the junctional complex begins immediately below the luminal surface and is made up of three components: a *tight junction* **TJ** (*zonula occludens*), *a continuous adhering junction* or *zonula adherens* **ZA** and a row of *spot-adhering junctions* or *desmosomes* **D**.

In this field, the bases of microvilli **Mv** which cover the surface of small intestinal lining cells can be identified. As described in Figure 5.16, each microvillus contains a core of cytoskeletal microfilaments **Mf** which insert into a zone of condensed intermediate and microfilaments lying just beneath the cell surface, the *terminal web* **TW**; this finds anchorage in the zonula adherens. The desmosome **D** is the anchorage point for intermediate filaments of **IF** of the cytoskeleton.

BASIC TISSUE TYPES

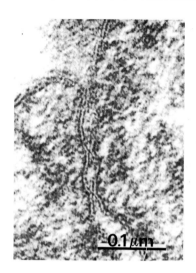

Fig. 5.11 Occluding (tight) junctions EM × 190 000

The occluding or tight junction (zonula occludens) forms a collar around each cell immediately beneath the cell surface, sealing the intercellular space from ingress of luminal contents. As seen in this electron micrograph, the outer electron-dense layers of opposing cell membranes are seen to come extremely close together with minimal intercellular material between them. In places, the plasma membranes appear to fuse completely, these sites being represented at the molecular level by the opposed membranes exhibiting a system of fine matching ridges known as *sealing strands* which 'stitch' the membranes together in the manner of two pieces of cloth haphazardly stitched together on a sewing machine (see Fig. 5.10a). Continuing this analogy, each 'stitch' comprises a pair of membrane proteins, one an integral part of each opposing plasma membrane, linked tightly together.

As well as sealing the intercellular space from the luminal environment, tight junctions may prevent migration of 'floating' membrane proteins from their appropriate domains on the cell surface (e.g. luminal surface proteins are confined to that surface).

Structurally similar but discontinuous strips of tight junction called *fascia occludens* are found between the endothelial cells lining blood vessels, except in the vessels of the brain where they are of the continuous (zonula occludens) type.

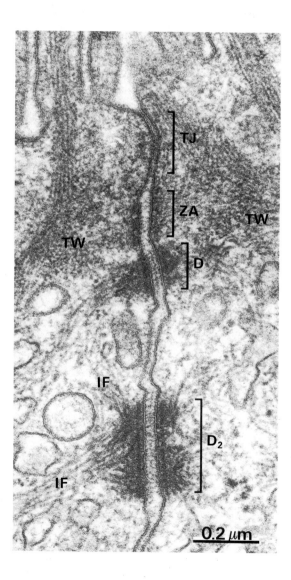

Fig. 5.12 Adhering junctions EM × 95 000

As previously described, adhering junctions provide anchorage points for cytoskeletal elements, in effect linking the cytoskeletons of individual cells into a strong transcellular network. These junctions are of two forms, the continuous belt (zonula adherens) and the spot or patch type (macula adherens or desmosome). The zonula adherens (also known as a belt desmosome) forms a single continuous band lying deep to the zonula occludens (tight junction) beneath the cell surface of certain columnar lining epithelia. A row of desmosomes is also disposed circumferentially around the apical aspect of columnar epithelium, forming the third component of the junctional complex. Larger desmosomes are also scattered over the intercellular surfaces of all epithelial cells. This micrograph from the intestinal lining illustrates a junctional complex comprising tight junction **TJ**, zonula adherens **ZA** and desmosome **D**. At a deeper level, a larger desmosome D_2 represents one of the scattered intercellular adhering junctions.

At the zonula adherens, opposing plasma membranes diverge and the intercellular space contains a relatively electron-lucent material of unknown composition which forms a strong bond between the opposing membrane surfaces. The cytoplasmic aspect of the membrane provides anchorage for the fine meshwork of microfilaments making up the terminal web **TW**. Contraction of the terminal web probably regulates tension at the epithelial surface. It may also provide for small lateral movements, thus keeping the microvilli in a state of gentle agitation, maximising contact of microvilli with molecules in the luminal contents and preventing clogging.

Desmosomes have a somewhat different structure. The widened space between opposed plasma membranes contains numerous fine transverse filaments called *transmembrane linkers* which appear to form an electron-dense line where they link up midway across the intercellular space. Within the cells, intermediate filaments **IF** insert into an electron-dense plaque on the inner aspect of the desmosome (see also Fig. 5.10a). Desmosome numbers are greatest in stratified squamous epithelia, reflecting their role in providing structural integrity at surfaces subject to considerable mechanical stress, e.g. friction. Many of the proteins in the desmosome are now well characterised.

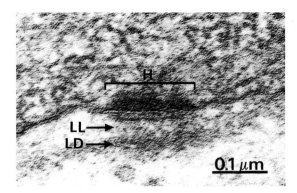

Fig. 5.13 **Hemidesmosome** EM × 150 000

Hemidesmosomes **H** are found along the basal plasma membranes of certain epithelia providing anchorage of the intermediate filament cytoskeleton to the plasma membrane at the base of the cell and to the underlying basement membrane.

On the cytoplasmic aspect of the plasma membrane is a protein plaque containing $\alpha_6\beta_4$ integrin into which insert intermediate filaments. The underlying lamina densa **LD** is thickened and more electron-dense as is the lamina lucida **LL** which contains an electron-dense line. This appearance is the result of anchoring filaments that link the membrane integrins to the extracellular matrix.

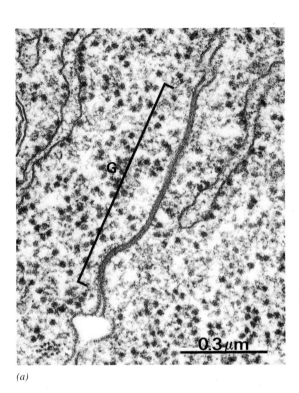

(a)

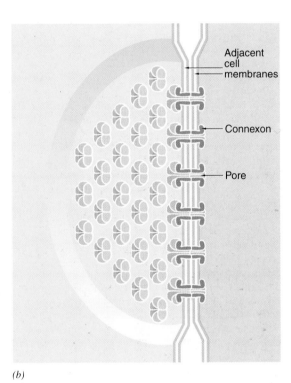

(b)

Fig. 5.14 **Communicating (gap, nexus) junctions** (a) EM × 80 000 (b) Diagram

Communicating junctions are broad patches where adjacent plasma membranes are closely opposed leaving a narrow intervening gap (hence the name gap junction). A gap junction **G** is demonstrated in the electron micrograph which is taken from intestinal epithelium.

As seen in the diagram, each gap junction contains numerous pores which permit the passage of positively charged ions and other small molecules (less than 2 nm in diameter) from the cytoplasm of one cell to another. Large molecules and negatively charged ions are denied access. Thus they serve as sites for exchange of metabolites, control molecules for growth, development, cell recognition and differentiation. Gap junctions also provide the means of electrical coupling of visceral and cardiac muscle cells permitting synchronous contraction.

Each pore consists of a minute tubular structure called a ***connexon*** which traverses the intercellular gap. The connexon comprises a pair of grommet-like cylinders,

one penetrating each of the opposing cell membranes. Each cylinder is made up of six transmembrane protein molecules as indicated in the diagram. Tubal patency is maintained by the proteins being arranged in a slightly twisted conformation. This is highly sensitive to the intracellular concentration of calcium ions which, if increased, results in closure of the pores. A rise in intracellular calcium concentration is a feature of cell death and this mechanism appears to provide a means of sealing off apoptotic cells and their potentially noxious contents from adjacent viable cells.

Communicating junctions are more numerous in embryonic epithelia where they appear to be involved in exchange of chemical messengers, in cell recognition, differentiation and control of cell position. They are also probably involved in the passage of nutrients from cells deep in the epithelium (adjacent to supporting tissues and blood vessels) to cells more remote from the nutritional supply.

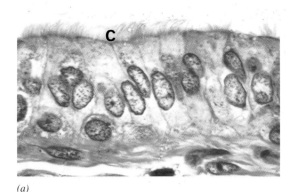

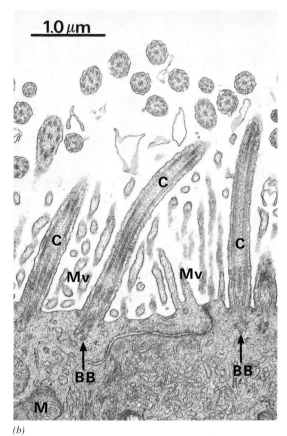

(a)

(b)

Fig. 5.15 Cilia (a) Thin section, toluidine blue × 800 (b) EM × 20 000 (c) Schematic diagram

Cilia are motile structures which project in parallel rows from certain epithelial surfaces, notably in the respiratory and female reproductive tracts. Cilia beat with a wave-like synchronous rhythm propelling surface films of mucus or fluid in a consistent direction over the epithelial surface. In the airways, mucus traps debris from inspired air, the cilia moving the mucus upwards towards the throat where it is swallowed thus keeping the airways clean. In the oviducts, ciliary action helps to transport the ovum from the ovary towards the uterus.

Cilia measure from about 7 to 10 μm in length and may therefore be around half the length of the cell (depending on cell size). A single epithelial cell may have up to 300 cilia usually of similar length.

Micrographs (a) and (b) show ciliated cells from the respiratory tract. Cilia **C** are readily visible with light microscopy although during processing they often become matted together and flattened making them less conspicuous. In micrograph (b), the proximal parts of three cilia **C** are seen in longitudinal section and, more superficially, the tips of a number of others otherwise lying outside the plane of section. Note the internal microtubular contents. Small surface microvilli **Mv** are seen between the cilia providing a useful size comparison.

Each cilium is bounded by an evagination of the luminal plasma membrane and, as shown diagrammatically, contains a central core called the *axoneme* consisting of 20 microtubules arranged as a central pair surrounded by nine peripheral doublets. At its base, the axoneme inserts into a structure called a *basal body* which has a microtubular arrangement identical to that of a centriole, i.e. nine triplets of microtubules forming a short cylinder (see Fig. 1.24). Each peripheral doublet of the cilium axoneme is continuous with the two inner microtubules of the corresponding triplet of the basal body. Basal bodies **BB** can be readily identified in micrograph (b).

Each axoneme doublet consists of one tubule of circular cross-section closely applied to another incomplete tubule which is C-shaped in cross-section. From each complete tubule, pairs of 'arms' consisting of the protein *dynein*, which has ATPase activity, extend towards the incomplete tubule of the adjacent doublet as well as towards the central microtubule pair. Ciliary action results from longitudinal movement of the doublets relative to one another, energy for the process being provided in the form of ATP by mitochondria **M** in the subjacent cytoplasm as in micrograph (b).

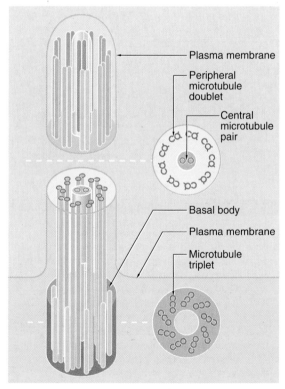

Plasma membrane

Peripheral microtubule doublet

Central microtubule pair

Basal body

Plasma membrane

Microtubule triplet

(c)

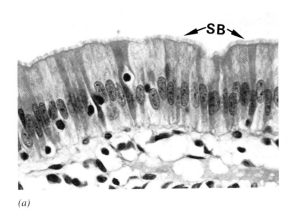

(a)

Fig. 5.16 Microvilli
(a) H & E × 320 (b) EM × 4000 (c) EM × 30 000

Microvilli are minute finger-like projections of the luminal plasma membrane found in many epithelia, particularly those specialised for absorption where their presence may increase the surface area as much as 30-fold. Microvilli are only 0.5–1.0 μm in length and are thus very short in relation to the size of the cell, a feature contrasting markedly with cilia (see Fig. 5.15). Furthermore, individual microvilli are too small to be resolved by light microscopy.

Some epithelia have only a small number of irregular microvilli. However, epithelia in such highly absorptive sites as in the small intestine and proximal renal tubules have up to 3000 regular microvilli per cell; collectively these can be seen with the light microscope as so-called *striated* or *brush borders*. Micrographs (a) and (b) illustrate the typical features of microvilli constituting the striated border **SB** of cells lining the small intestine.

As seen at very high magnification in micrograph (c), the cytoplasmic core of each microvillus contains fine actin filaments **F** which insert into the terminal web, a specialisation of the actin cytoskeleton lying immediately beneath the cell surface; at the periphery of the cell the terminal web is anchored to the zonula adherens (see Fig. 5.12) enhancing the surface stability of the epithelium. At the tip of the microvillus, the filaments attach to an electron-dense part of the plasma membrane. The filaments, of which the principal constituent is actin, maintain stability of microvilli and may also mediate some contraction and elongation of the microvilli, thus preventing clogging.

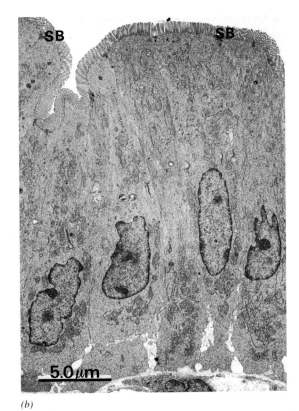

(b)

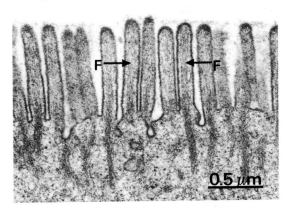

(c)

Fig. 5.17 Stereocilia H & E × 320

Extremely long microvilli, readily visible with light microscopy, are found in small numbers in parts of the male reproductive tract such as the epididymis (shown in this micrograph) and other odd sites. Originally, these structures were thought to be an unusual form of cilia and were termed stereocilia; however, electron microscopy has shown that they do not have the internal structure of cilia but merely a filamentous skeleton like that of microvilli. Stereocilia **S** are thought to facilitate absorptive processes in the epididymis but the reason for their unusual form is not known.

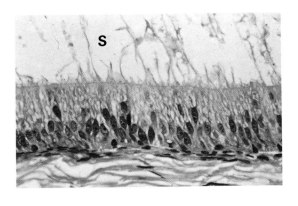

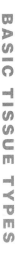

BASIC TISSUE TYPES

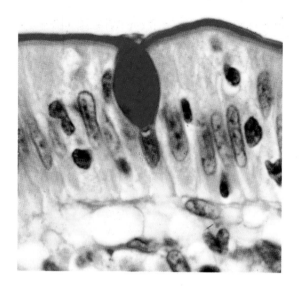

Fig. 5.18 Goblet cell PAS/haematoxylin × 800

Goblet cells are modified columnar epithelial cells which synthesise and secrete mucus. Goblet cells are scattered amongst the cells of many simple epithelial linings, particularly those of the respiratory and gastrointestinal tracts, and are named for their resemblance to drinking goblets.

The distended apical cytoplasm contains a dense aggregation of *mucigen granules* which, when released by exocytosis, combine with water to form the viscid secretion called mucus. Mucigen is composed of a mixture of neutral and acidic proteoglycans (mucopolysaccharides) and therefore can be readily demonstrated by the PAS method which stains carbohydrates magenta. The 'stem' of the goblet cell is occupied by a condensed, basal nucleus and is crammed with other organelles involved in mucigen synthesis.

In this example from the lining of the small intestine, note the tall columnar nature of the surrounding absorptive cells. The PAS-positive surface coating is not only due to secreted mucus but also to the presence of a thick glycocalyx (see Ch. 1) on the numerous microvilli which characterise small intestine absorptive cells.

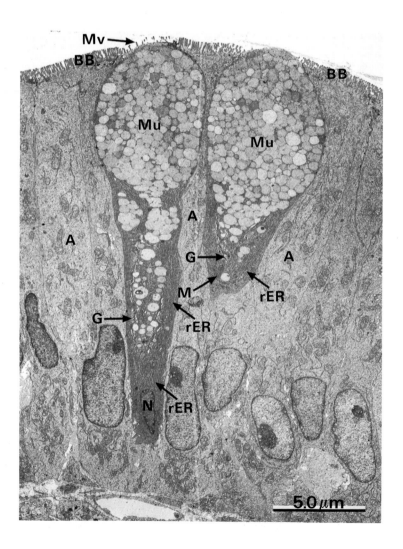

Fig. 5.19 Goblet cell
EM × 5000

This micrograph shows two goblet cells amongst columnar absorptive cells **A** of the small intestine; the nucleus of the goblet cell on the right is outside the plane of section, the nucleus **N** of the other being typically highly condensed. The cytoplasm is packed with rough endoplasmic reticulum **rER**; a few mitochondria **M** are present. A prominent Golgi apparatus **G** is found in the supranuclear region.

The protein component of mucigen is synthesised by the rough endoplasmic reticulum and passed to the Golgi apparatus where it is combined with carbohydrate and packaged into membrane-bound, secretory vacuoles containing mucigen **Mu**. Goblet cells secrete at a steady basal rate and may be stimulated by local irritation to release their entire mucigen contents. Sparse microvilli **Mv** are seen at the surface of the goblet cell and may be associated with the secretory process. Note the microvilli forming the brush border **BB** of the absorptive cells.

Mucus has a variety of functions. In the upper gastrointestinal tract it protects the intestinal lining cells from autodigestion whilst in the lower tract it lubricates the passage of faeces. In the respiratory tract it protects the lining from drying, contributes to the humidification of inspired air and acts as a sticky surface trap for fine dust particles and microorganisms.

Exocrine glands

Exocrine glands discharge their secretory product via a duct onto an epithelial surface. The cells of which they are composed are highly specialised epithelial cells, the internal structure of the cells reflecting the nature of the secretory product and the mode of secretion (see Ch. 1).

Exocrine glands may be classified according to two major characteristics, which are described below.

The morphology of the gland

Exocrine glands may be broadly divided into simple and compound glands. **Simple glands** are defined as those with a single, unbranched duct. The secretory portions of simple glands have two main forms, tubular or acinar (spherical), which may be coiled and/or branched. **Compound glands** have a branched duct system and their secretory portions have similar morphological forms to those of simple glands.

The means of discharge of secretory products from the cells. This occurs in three ways:

- **Merocrine secretion** (also called **eccrine** secretion) involves the process of exocytosis and is the most common form of secretion; proteins are usually the major secretory product.
- **Apocrine secretion** involves the discharge of free, unbroken, membrane-bound vesicles containing secretory product; this is an unusual mode of secretion and applies to lipid secretory products in the breasts and some sweat glands.
- **Holocrine secretion** involves the discharge of whole secretory cells with subsequent disintegration of the cells to release the secretory product. Holocrine secretion occurs principally in sebaceous glands.

In general, all glands have a continuous basal rate of secretion which is modulated by nervous and hormonal influences. The secretory portions of some exocrine glands are embraced by contractile cells which lie between the secretory cells and the basement membrane. The contractile mechanism of these cells is thought to be similar to that of muscle cells and has given rise to the term **myoepithelial cells**.

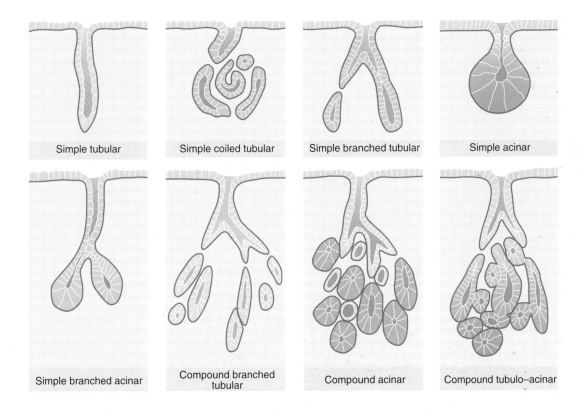

Simple tubular · Simple coiled tubular · Simple branched tubular · Simple acinar

Simple branched acinar · Compound branched tubular · Compound acinar · Compound tubulo–acinar

Fig. 5.20 **Exocrine gland types**

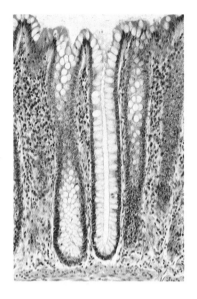

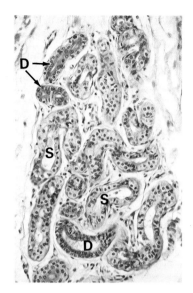

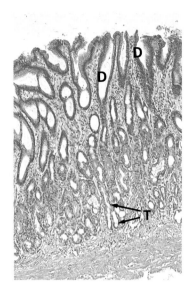

Fig. 5.21 Simple tubular glands H & E × 50

This example of simple tubular glands is taken from the large intestine. This type of gland has a single, straight tubular lumen into which the secretory products are discharged. In this example, the entire duct is lined by secretory cells; the secretory cells are goblet cells. In other sites mucus is secreted by columnar cells which do not have the classic goblet shape but nonetheless function in a similar manner.

Fig. 5.22 Simple coiled tubular glands H & E × 80

Sweat glands are almost the only example of simple coiled tubular glands. Each consists of a single tube which is tightly coiled in three dimensions; portions of the gland are thus seen in various planes of section. Sweat glands have a terminal secretory portion **S** lined by simple cuboidal epithelium which gives way to a non-secretory (excretory) duct **D** lined by stratified cuboidal epithelium.

Fig. 5.23 Simple branched tubular glands H & E × 60

Simple branched tubular glands are found mainly in the stomach. The mucus-secreting glands of the pyloric part of the stomach are shown in this example. Each gland consists of several tubular secretory portions **T** which converge onto a single, unbranched duct **D** of wider diameter; this is also lined by mucus-secreting cells. Unlike those of the large intestine (see Fig. 5.21), these mucous cells do not have a goblet shape.

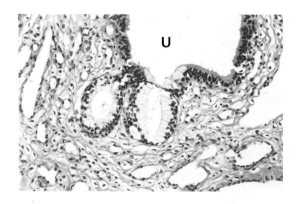

Fig. 5.24 Simple acinar glands H & E × 128

Simple acinar glands occur in the form of pockets in epithelial surfaces and are lined by secretory cells. In this example of the mucus-secreting glands of the penile urethra, the secretory cells are pale stained compared to the non-secretory cells lining the urethra **U**. Note that the term *acinus* can be used to describe any rounded exocrine secretory unit.

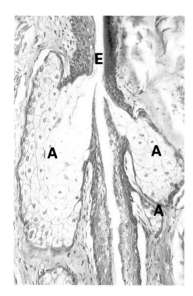

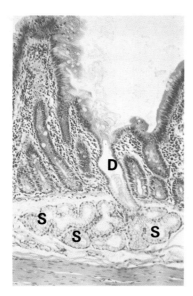

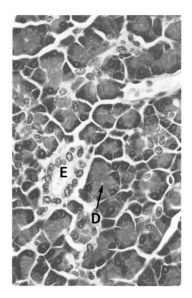

Fig. 5.25 Simple branched acinar gland Masson's trichrome × 80

Sebaceous glands provide a good example of simple branched acinar glands. Each gland consists of several secretory acini **A** which empty into a single excretory duct; the excretory duct **E** is formed by the stratified epithelium surrounding the hair shaft. The mode of secretion of sebaceous glands is holocrine, i.e. the secretory product, sebum, accumulates within the secretory cells and is discharged by degeneration of the cells.

Fig. 5.26 Compound branched tubular gland H & E × 20

Brunner's glands of the duodenum, as shown in this example, are described as compound branched tubular glands. Although difficult to visualise here, the duct system **D** is branched, thus defining the glands as compound glands; the secretory portions **S** have a tubular form which is branched and coiled.

Fig. 5.27 Compound acinar gland Chrome alum haematoxylin/phloxine × 320

Compound acinar glands are those in which the secretory units are acinar in form and drain into a branched duct system. The pancreas shown in this micrograph consists of numerous acini, each of which drains into a minute duct. These minute ducts **D**, which are just discernible in the centre of some acini, drain into a system of branched excretory ducts **E** of increasing diameter and lined by simple cuboidal epithelium.

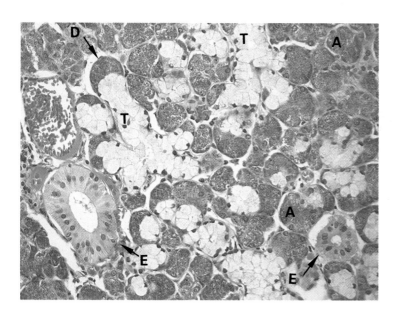

Fig. 5.28 Compound tubulo-acinar gland H & E × 200

Compound tubulo-acinar glands have three types of secretory units, namely branched tubular, branched acinar and branched tubular with acinar end-pieces called *demilunes*. The submandibular salivary gland shown here is the classic example. It contains two types of secretory cells, mucus-secreting cells and serous cells; the former are poorly stained but the latter, which have a protein-rich secretion (digestive enzymes), stain strongly due to their large content of rough endoplasmic reticulum. Generally, the mucous cells form tubular components **T** whereas the serous cells form acinar components **A** and demilunes **D**. Two excretory ducts **E** are also seen.

Endocrine glands

Endocrine glands are ductless glands, the secretory products diffusing directly into the bloodstream. The secretory products are known as hormones and control the activity of cells and tissues usually far removed from the site of secretion.

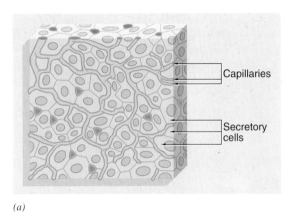

(a)

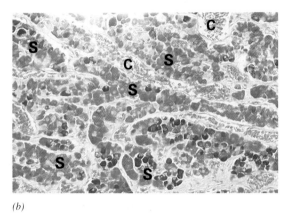

(b)

Fig. 5.29   **Endocrine gland** (a) Diagram (b) Isamine blue eosin × 128

Most endocrine glands consist of clumps or cords of secretory cells surrounded by a rich network of small blood vessels. Each clump of endocrine cells is surrounded by a basement membrane, reflecting its epithelial origin. Endocrine cells release hormones into the intercellular spaces from which they diffuse rapidly into surrounding blood vessels.

The micrograph of the pituitary gland shows the typical features of endocrine glands. The secretory cells **S** are arranged in cords and clumps and are surrounded by delicate supporting tissue containing a rich network of broad capillaries **C**. The basement membrane surrounding each clump of endocrine cells is not visible at this magnification. Like many other endocrine glands, the secretory cells of the pituitary are of several different types; in this case, the majority are eosinophilic (red stained), some stain blue and some stain very little.

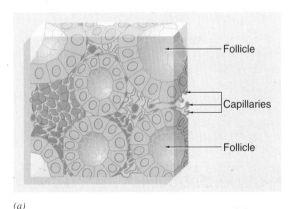

(a)

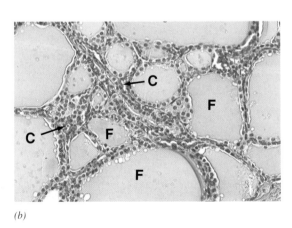

(b)

Fig. 5.30   **Follicular endocrine gland** (a) Diagram (b) H & E × 150

The thyroid gland is an unusual endocrine gland which stores hormone within spheroidal cavities enclosed by the secretory cells; these spheroidal units are called *follicles*. Secretion of stored hormone involves reabsorption of hormone from the follicular lumen, release into the surrounding interstitial spaces, and then diffusion into the rich capillary network which embraces each follicle.

The micrograph shows typical thyroid follicles **F** of variable size. The secretory cells lining the follicles are of flattened cuboidal shape. Stored thyroid hormone is bound to a glycoprotein which is strongly eosinophilic. The relatively sparse interfollicular supporting tissue is mainly occupied by capillaries **C** which can be identified by the strongly eosinophilic (pink stained) erythrocytes within them.

6. Muscle

Introduction

Although all cells are capable of some sort of movement, the dominant function of several cell types is to generate motile forces through contraction. In these specialised contractile cells, motile forces are generated by the interaction of the proteins actin and myosin (contractile proteins). Certain forms of contractile cell function as single-cell contractile units:

- *Myoepithelial cells* are an important component of certain secretory glands (Ch. 5) where they function to expel secretions from glandular acini.
- *Pericytes* are smooth muscle-like cells that surround blood vessels (Ch. 8).
- *Myofibroblasts* are cells that have a contractile role in addition to being able to secrete collagen. This type of cell is generally inconspicuous in normal tissues but comes to be a dominant cell type when tissues undergo repair after damage in the formation of a scar.

Other forms of contractile cell function by forming multicellular contractile units termed muscles. Such muscle cells can be divided into three types:

- **Skeletal muscle** is responsible for the movement of the skeleton and organs such as the globe of the eye and the tongue. Skeletal muscle is often referred to as *voluntary muscle* since it is capable of voluntary (conscious) control. The arrangement of the contractile proteins gives rise to the appearance of prominent cross-striations in some histological preparations and hence the name *striated muscle* is often applied to skeletal muscle. The highly developed functions of the cytoplasmic organelles of muscle cells has led to the use of a special terminology for some muscle cell components: plasma membrane or plasmalemma = *sarcolemma*; cytoplasm = *sarcoplasm*; endoplasmic reticulum = *sarcoplasmic reticulum*.
- **Smooth muscle** is so named because, unlike other forms of muscle, the arrangement of contractile proteins does not give the histological appearance of cross-striations. This type of muscle forms the muscular component of visceral structures such as blood vessels, the gastrointestinal tract, the uterus and the urinary bladder, giving rise to the alternative name of *visceral muscle*. Since smooth muscle is under inherent autonomic and hormonal control, it is also described as *involuntary muscle*.
- **Cardiac muscle** has many structural and functional characteristics intermediate between those of skeletal and smooth muscle and provides for the continuous, rhythmic contractility of the heart. Although striated in appearance, cardiac muscle is readily distinguishable from skeletal muscle and should not be referred to by the term 'striated muscle'

Muscle cells of all three types are surrounded by an external lamina (see Ch. 4). In all muscle cell types, contractile forces developed from the internal contractile proteins are transmitted to the external lamina via link proteins which span the muscle cell membrane. The external lamina binds individual muscle cells into a single functional mass.

Skeletal muscle

Skeletal muscles have a wide variety of morphological forms and modes of action; nevertheless all have the same basic structure. Skeletal muscle is composed of extremely elongated, multinucleate contractile cells, often described as *muscle fibres*, bound together by collagenous supporting tissue. Individual muscle fibres vary considerably in diameter from 10 to 100 μm and may extend throughout the whole length of a muscle reaching up to 35 cm in length.

Skeletal muscle contraction is controlled by large motor nerves, individual nerve fibres branching within the muscle to supply a group of muscle fibres, collectively described as a *motor unit*. Excitation of any one motor nerve results in simultaneous contraction of all the muscle fibres of the corresponding motor unit. The structure of neuromuscular junctions is described in Figure 7.12. The vitality of skeletal muscle fibres is dependent on the maintenance of their nerve supply which, if damaged, results in atrophy of the fibres. Skeletal muscle contains highly specialised stretch receptors known as neuromuscular spindles which are shown in Figure 7.30.

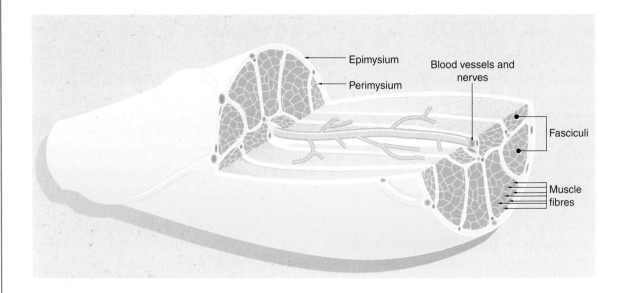

Fig. 6.1 Skeletal muscle

This diagram illustrates the arrangement of the basic components which make up a typical skeletal muscle.

The individual muscle cells (muscle fibres) are grouped together into elongated bundles called *fasciculi* with delicate supporting tissue called *endomysium* occupying the spaces between individual muscle fibres.

Each fascicle is surrounded by loose collagenous tissue called *perimysium*. Most muscles are made up of many fasciculi and the whole muscle mass is invested in a dense collagenous sheath called the *epimysium*. Large blood vessels and nerves enter the epimysium and divide to ramify throughout the muscle in the perimysium and endomysium.

The size of the fasciculi reflects the function of the particular muscle concerned. Muscles responsible for fine, highly controlled movements, e.g. the external muscles of the eye, have small fasciculi and a relatively greater proportion of perimysial supporting tissue. In contrast, muscles responsible for gross movements only, e.g. the muscle of the buttocks, have large fasciculi and relatively little perimysial tissue. Muscle fibres are anchored to the support tissue so that contractile forces can be transmitted. The connective tissue framework contains both collagen and elastic fibres. This connective tissue becomes continuous with that of the tendons and muscle attachments (see Ch. 10) which distribute and direct the motive forces of the muscle to bone, skin etc. as appropriate.

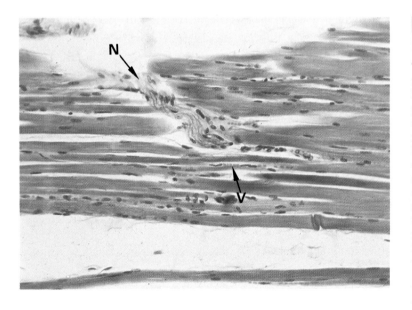

Fig. 6.2 Skeletal muscle
Trichrome stain × 150

This micrograph shows part of a fasciculus of a skeletal muscle at high magnification. The individual purple stained muscle cells (fibres) are highly elongated and arranged in parallel, the spaces between them being occupied by small amounts of endomysial supporting tissue. The endomysium, which consists mainly of reticulin fibres (unstained) and a small amount of collagen (stained blue in this preparation), conveys numerous small blood vessels, lymphatics and nerves throughout the muscle. In this micrograph, a small nerve bundle **N** is seen; tiny blood vessels **V** can be identified by the rows of erythrocytes contained within them.

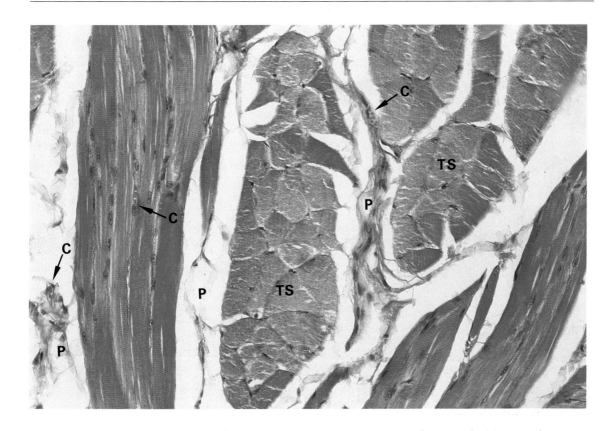

Skeletal muscle Masson's trichrome × 300

This micrograph shows the skeletal muscle of the tongue which is made up of numerous small fasciculi oriented in various different directions. This staining method clearly distinguishes skeletal muscle cells, stained red, from supporting tissue, the collagen of which is stained blue.

In the centre and at the upper right of the field are fasciculi cut in transverse section **TS**, the remaining fasciculi being cut longitudinally. The spaces between the fasciculi are filled with loose collagenous tissue, the

perimysium **P**, which is continuous with the delicate endomysium, separating individual muscle fibres in each fasciculus. The supporting tissue of skeletal muscle also contains elastin fibres (not distinguishable in this preparation) which are most numerous in muscles attached to soft tissues as in the tongue and face. Note the rich network of capillaries **C** in the endomysium and perimysium.

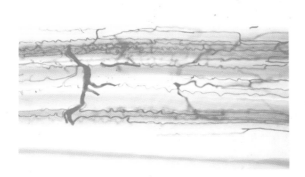

Fig. 6.4 **Skeletal muscle blood supply**
Perfusion method × 128

This specimen was prepared by perfusing the blood supply of a skeletal muscle with a red dye; the muscle fibres were then teased apart to reveal the endomysial capillary bed.

Large blood vessels enter the epimysium and divide to ramify throughout the muscle in the perimysium. Fine branches arise from the perimysial arteries and pass between the muscle fibres transversely to their long axes. These give rise to numerous capillaries which run longitudinally through the endomysium. Frequent transverse anastomoses between the capillaries result in a fine, elongated capillary network surrounding each muscle fibre.

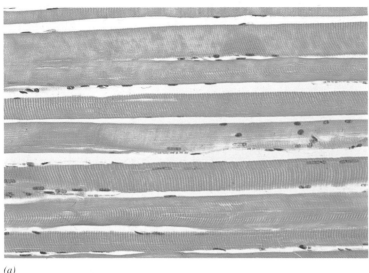

(a)

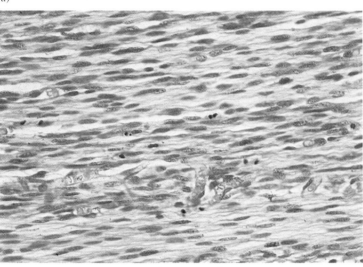

(b)

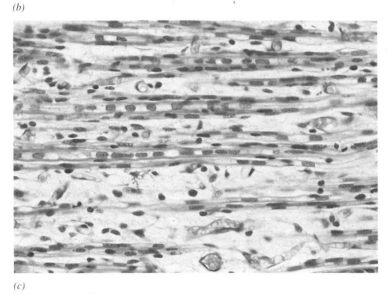

(c)

Fig. 6.5 Skeletal muscle and its embryogenesis (a) Mature skeletal muscle, H & E × 320 (b) Myoblasts, H & E × 150 (c) Myotubes, H & E × 150

Micrograph (a) demonstrates the characteristic histological features of skeletal muscle fibres in longitudinal section. Skeletal muscle fibres are extremely elongated, unbranched cylindrical cells with numerous flattened nuclei located at fairly regular intervals just beneath the sarcolemma (plasma membrane).

During embryological development, certain mesenchymal cells in each myotome differentiate into long, mononuclear skeletal muscle precursors called *myoblasts* which then proliferate by mitosis; this is shown in micrograph (b). Subsequently, the myoblasts fuse end to end forming progressively elongated multinucleate cells called *myotubes*, seen in micrograph (c), which may eventually contain up to 100 nuclei.

Synthesis of the contractile proteins begins after myoblast fusion, the proteins being laid down initially in the central axis of the myotube, the nuclei being displaced peripherally as more contractile protein is formed. Most of the process of muscle development is completed by the time of birth along with the process of innervation. Thereafter, growth occurs by increase in bulk of the muscle cell cytoplasm.

Mature muscle cells can regenerate if damaged by proliferation of stem cells which remain in adult muscles. These muscle stem cells resemble myoblasts and are called *satellite cells*. They enter mitosis after muscle damage and several fuse to form differentiated muscle fibres. Muscle fibres which are the result of regeneration after damage have nuclei in the centre of the fibre rather than at the periphery.

Regular cross-striations are the characteristic feature of skeletal muscle fibres and can be seen in longitudinal sections as in micrograph (a). The cross-striations result from the arrangement of the contractile proteins as described later.

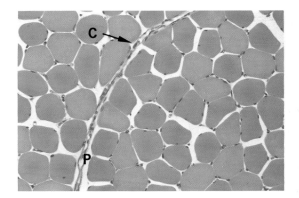

Fig. 6.6 Skeletal muscle TS, H & E × 320

This micrograph of skeletal muscle cut in transverse section shows the extreme peripheral location of the nuclei of skeletal muscle fibres. In cross-section muscle fibres appear polyhedral with flattening of adjacent cells. In normal muscle the cross-sectional areas of individual fibres are approximately the same. The wide endomysial spaces are a shrinkage artefact.

In the endomysial spaces, note the numerous minute capillaries **C** recognisable by the eosinophilic erythrocytes contained within them. Compare the huge diameter of the muscle fibres which may be as great as 0.1 mm in diameter with that of the capillaries, the latter being approximately 7 μm across. Note also a strand of perimysial tissue **P** cutting across the field separating two fasciculi from one another.

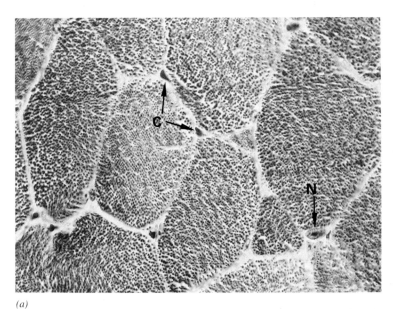

(a)

Fig. 6.7 Skeletal muscle
(a) TS, iron haematoxylin × 1200
(b) Schematic diagram

Micrograph (a) shows a transverse section through several skeletal muscle fibres at very high magnification. The plane of section includes only one skeletal muscle nucleus **N**. Note the presence of erythrocytes in endomysial capillaries **C**.

In some preparations such as this, the transversely sectioned muscle fibres are seen to be packed with numerous dark dots. These represent the cut ends of *myofibrils*, elongated cylindrical structures which lie parallel to one another in the sarcoplasm.

As shown diagrammatically in (b), each myofibril exhibits a repeating pattern of cross-striations which is a product of the highly ordered arrangement of the contractile proteins within it; this can only be seen with electron microscopy (see Fig. 6.8). Furthermore, the parallel myofibrils are arranged with their cross-striations in register, giving rise to the regular striations seen with light microscopy in longitudinal sections of skeletal muscle as in Fig. 6.5.

Muscle fibre   Myofibrils

(b)

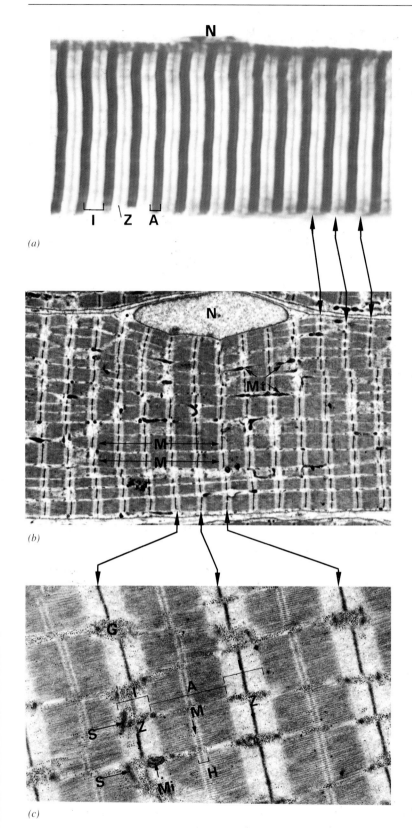

(a)

(b)

(c)

Fig. 6.8 Skeletal muscle
(a) Heidenhain's haematoxylin
× 1200 (b) EM × 2860
(c) EM × 18 700

This series of micrographs shows the arrangement of the contractile proteins within skeletal muscle and explains the striations seen with light microscopy.

Micrograph (a) shows the striations of a skeletal muscle fibre at a magnification close to the limit of resolution. They are composed of alternating broad light **I** bands (isotropic in polarised light) and dark (anisotropic) **A** bands. Fine dark lines called **Z** bands (Zwischenscheiben) can be seen bisecting the light I bands. Note the nucleus **N** at the extreme periphery of the cell.

Micrograph (b) shows the electron microscopic appearance of muscle with a nucleus **N** situated in a similar position. The sarcoplasm is filled with myofibrils **M** oriented parallel to the long axis of the cell. These are separated by a small amount of sarcoplasm containing rows of mitochondria **Mt** in a similar orientation.

Each myofibril has prominent regular cross-striations arranged in register with those of the other myofibrils and corresponding to the I, A and Z bands seen in light microscopy. The Z bands are the most electron-dense and divide each myofibril into numerous contractile units, called *sarcomeres*, arranged end to end.

With further magnification in (c), the arrangement of the contractile proteins (*myofilaments*) may be seen in each sarcomere. The dark **A** band is bisected by the lighter **H** (heller) band, which is further bisected by a more dense **M** (Mittelscheibe) band. Irrespective of the degree of contraction of the muscle fibre, the A band remains constant in width. In contrast, the I and H bands narrow during contraction and the Z bands are drawn closer together. These findings are explained by the *sliding filament theory* (Fig. 6.9).

Mitochondria **Mi** and numerous glycogen granules **G** provide a rich energy source in the scanty cytoplasm between the myofibrils. The mature muscle cell contains little rough endoplasmic reticulum; it contains, however, a smooth membranous system **S** which is involved in activation of the contractile mechanism (see Figs. 6.10–6.12).

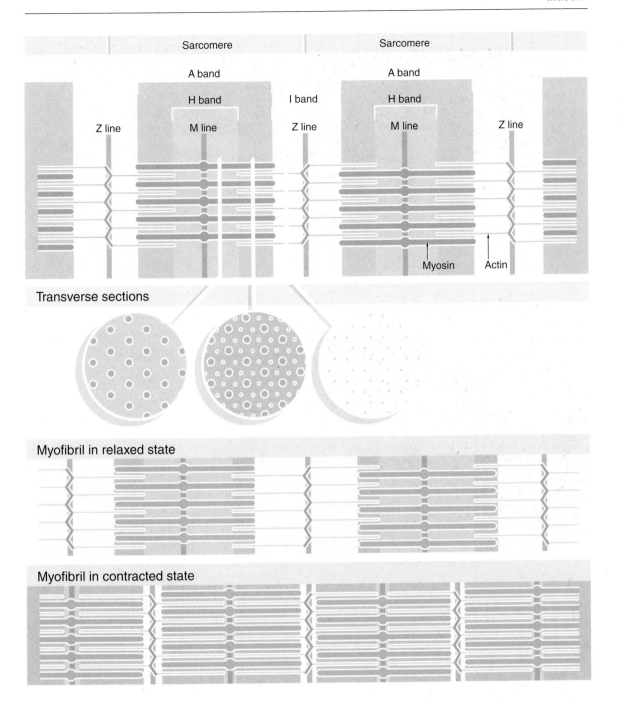

Transverse sections

Myofibril in relaxed state

Myofibril in contracted state

Fig. 6.9 **The arrangement of myofilaments in the sarcomere**

The sarcomere consists of two types of myofilaments, *thick filaments* and *thin filaments*. Each type remains constant in length irrespective of the state of contraction of the muscle. The thick filaments, which are composed mainly of the protein myosin, are maintained in register by their attachment to a disc-like zone represented by the M line. Similarly the thin filaments, which are composed mainly of the protein *actin*, are attached to a disc-like

zone represented by the Z line. The I and H bands, both areas of low electron density, represent areas where the thick and thin filaments do not overlap one another.

The widely accepted sliding filament theory proposes that under the influence of energy released from ATP, the thick and thin filaments slide over one another, thus causing shortening of the sarcomere.

BASIC TISSUE TYPES

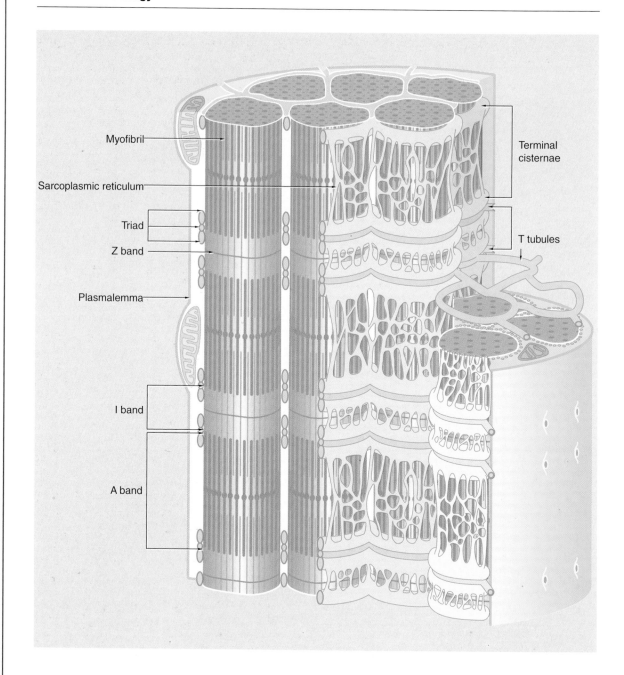

Myofibril

Sarcoplasmic reticulum

Triad

Z band

Plasmalemma

I band

A band

Terminal cisternae

T tubules

Fig. 6.10 The conducting system for contractile stimuli

To permit the synchronous contraction of all sarcomeres in the muscle fibre, a system of tubular extensions of the muscle cell plasma membrane (sarcolemma) extends transversely into the muscle cell to surround each myofibril at the region of the junction of the A and I bands. Known as the *T system*, its lumen is continuous with the extracellular space. (In amphibian skeletal muscle, which was the first to be studied, the T tubules are disposed at the Z bands; the same applies in cardiac muscle.)

Between the T tubules, a second membrane system derived from smooth endoplasmic reticulum, the *sarcoplasmic reticulum*, forms a membranous network which embraces each myofibril. On either side of each

T tubule, the sarcoplasmic reticulum exhibits a flattened cisternal arrangement, each pair of *terminal cisternae* and a T tubule forming a *triad* near the junction of the I and A bands of each sarcomere.

Calcium ions are concentrated within the lumen of the *sarcoplasmic reticulum*. Depolarisation of the sarcolemma of the muscle fibre is rapidly disseminated throughout the sarcoplasm by the T tubule system. This promotes the release of calcium ions from the sarcoplasmic reticulum into the sarcoplasm surrounding the myofilaments. Calcium ions activate the sliding filament mechanism resulting in muscle contraction.

BASIC TISSUE TYPES

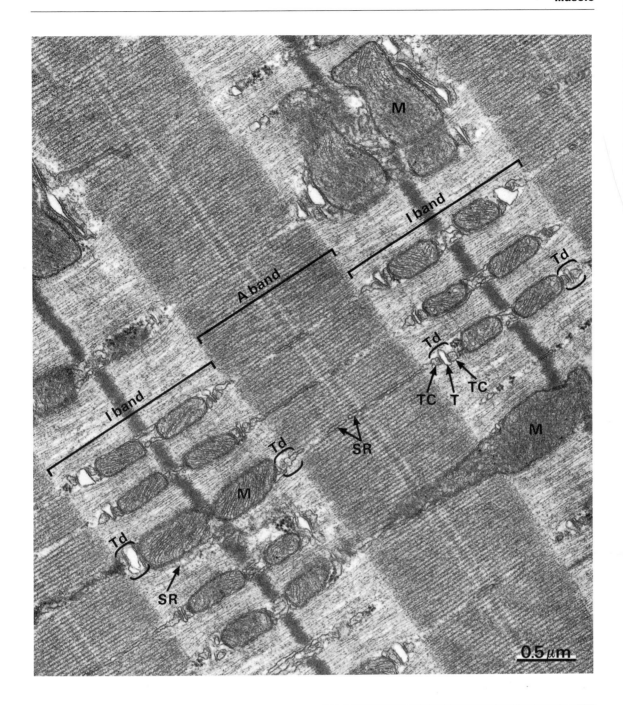

Fig. 6.11 Skeletal muscle EM × 33 000

This electron micrograph of mammalian skeletal muscle cut in longitudinal section demonstrates the main elements of the conducting system. In the vicinity of the junction of the **A** and **I bands** (and depending on the state of contraction) are tubular triads **Td** each comprising a central flattened tubule of the T system **T** and a pair of terminal cisternae **TC** of the sarcoplasmic reticulum. Within the A bands can be seen tubular elements of the sarcoplasmic reticulum **SR** connecting the terminal cisternae. Likewise within the I bands, similar though less regular longitudinal tubular profiles of sarcoplasmic reticulum are seen. The conducting system of 'slow-twitch' (red) fibres as shown here (see Fig. 6.13) is more regular than that of 'fast-twitch' (white) fibres where this pattern is more difficult to discern. Note the distribution of mitochondria **M**, regularly arranged between the sarcomeres within the I bands in immediate association with those parts of the actin and myosin filaments which interact during the process of contraction. The reason for this appearance is evident in the following micrograph.

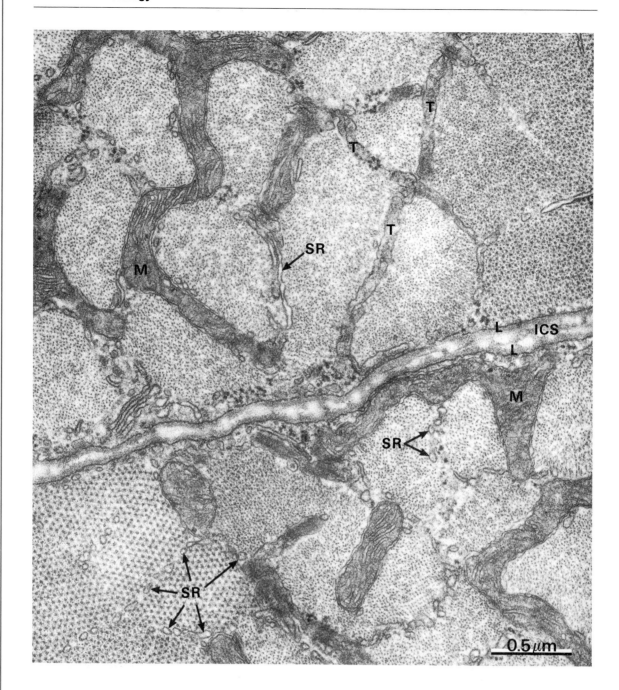

Fig. 6.12 Skeletal muscle EM × 44 000

This micrograph shows parts of two skeletal muscle cells cut in transverse section in the vicinity of the junction of A and I bands; the intercellular space **ICS** bisects the field. Note the external lamina **L** adjacent to the plasmalemma. Sarcomeres at the upper right and lower left of this field have been sectioned through the end part of the A band and thus show both actin and myosin filaments. The remaining sarcomeres are cut through the I band and contain only actin filaments. This results from the fact that the bands of all sarcomeres within any one muscle cell are not exactly in register with one another.

Each sarcomere is ensheathed by a network of tubules of the sarcoplasmic reticulum **SR**. The plane of section has also included a part of a broader diameter T tubule system **T** which branches to encompass several different sarcomeres. Direct communication of T tubules with the intercellular space is difficult to visualise as the tubules appear to ramify into a complex tubular system just beneath the plasmalemma; the continuity of T tubule lumen and the intercellular space has been convincingly demonstrated, however, by experimental techniques. Note the extraordinary serpentine branched mitochondria **M** which lie between the sarcomeres within the I bands, giving rise to the mitochondrial appearance seen in longitudinal section in the previous micrograph.

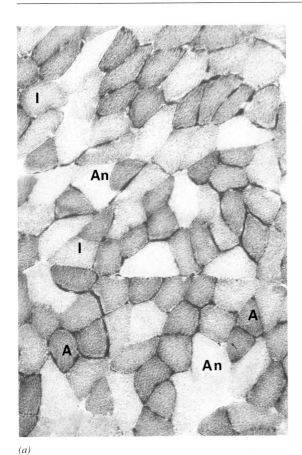 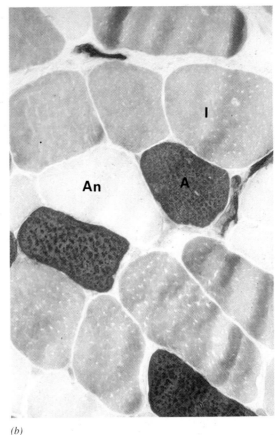

(a)   (b)

Fig. 6.13 Skeletal muscle TS: histochemical techniques (a) Succinate dehydrogenase × 200 (b) ATPase × 600

The mode of activity of skeletal muscle varies from one part of the body to another. Some muscles, such as those involved in the maintenance of posture, are required to contract almost continuously whilst others, such as the extra-ocular muscles, make rapid short-lived movements. In humans, distinction between these types cannot be made on gross examination of the muscle. In domestic poultry, however, the extremes are easily identified by a difference in colours; for example, leg muscles are red and flight (breast) muscles are white.

Correspondingly, 'slow-twitch' and 'fast-twitch' muscle fibre types can be demonstrated by nerve stimulation studies. The metabolic requirements of each fibre type differ markedly, the slow red fibres mainly relying on aerobic metabolism and the fast white fibres using predominantly anaerobic pathways. Most muscles actually contain a mixture of these extreme fibre types as well as an intermediate type.

Aerobic (*type I*) muscle fibres are small in cross-section and contain abundant mitochondria. They also contain a large content of *myoglobin*, an oxygen-storage molecule analogous to haemoglobin, which accounts for the red colour of such fibres. In addition these fibres have a rich blood supply.

In contrast, anaerobic (*type II*) muscle fibres are large in cross-section, contain few mitochondria and relatively little myoglobin; they also have a relatively poor blood supply. These muscle fibres are, however, rich in

glycogen and glycolytic enzymes. These characteristics account for the 'white' colour of such fibres. Anaerobic fibres predominate in muscles responsible for intense but sporadic contraction such as the biceps and triceps of the arms.

The activity of the specific mitochondrial enzyme *succinate dehydrogenase*, which catalyses one of the stages of Krebs' cycle, demonstrates the relative proportions of mitochondria within the muscle fibres. In micrograph (a), note the presence of intensely stained small-diameter aerobic fibres **A**, poorly stained large-diameter anaerobic fibres **An** and intermediate fibres **I**.

Type I and II fibres can also be identified by the nature of their myosin ATPase, which differs in its protein structure between different fibre types. In the preparation in micrograph (b), type I fibres are dark **A** and type II fibres are light **An**; intermediately stained fibres **I** can also be seen.

The type of metabolism of each fibre is determined by the frequency of impulses in its motor nerve supply. Any one motor nerve supplies fibres of one type only and all the fibres of a particular motor unit are of the same metabolic type. Indeed, if the motor nerve supply to one type of fibre is experimentally transplanted to supply another fibre type, this fibre type will become converted to the metabolic pattern of the former.

BASIC TISSUE TYPES

Smooth muscle

In contrast to skeletal muscle, which is specialised for relatively forceful contractions of short duration and under fine voluntary control, smooth muscle is specialised for continuous contractions of relatively low force, producing diffuse movements resulting in contraction of the whole muscle mass rather than contraction of individual motor units. Contractility is an inherent property of smooth muscle, occurring independently of neurological innervation often in a rhythmic or wave-like fashion. Superimposed on this inherent contractility are the influences of the autonomic nervous system, hormones and local metabolites which modulate contractility to accommodate changing functional demands. For example, the smooth muscle of the intestinal wall undergoes continuous rhythmic contractions which result in waves of constriction passing along the bowel, propelling the luminal contents distally. This activity is enhanced by parasympathetic stimulation and influenced by a variety of hormones released in response to changes in the nature and volume of the gut contents. The structure of autonomic neuromuscular junctions is described in Chapter 7.

The cells of smooth muscle are relatively small with only a single nucleus. The fibres are bound together in irregular branching fasciculi, the arrangement varying considerably from one organ to another according to functional requirements.

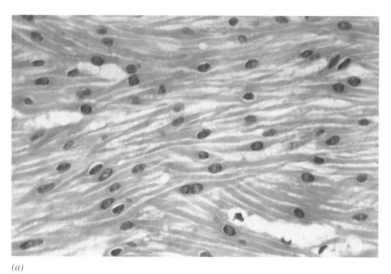

(a)

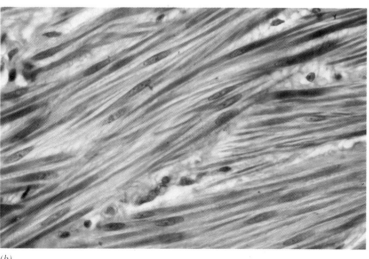

(b)

Fig. 6.14 Smooth muscle
(a) LS, H & E × 480
(b) LS, Masson's trichrome × 480

As seen in these micrographs, smooth muscle fibres are elongated, spindle-shaped cells with tapered ends which may occasionally be bifurcated. Smooth muscle fibres are generally much shorter than skeletal muscle fibres and contain only one nucleus which is elongated and centrally located in the cytoplasm at the widest part of the cell; however, depending on the contractile state of the fibres at fixation, the nuclei may sometimes appear to be spiral-shaped.

Smooth muscle fibres are bound together in irregular, branching fasciculi and these fasciculi, rather than individual fibres, are the functional contractile units. Within the fasciculi, individual muscle fibres are arranged roughly parallel to one another with the thickest part of one cell lying against the thin parts of adjacent cells.

The contractile proteins of smooth muscle are not arranged in myofibrils as in skeletal and cardiac muscle, and thus visceral muscle cells are not striated.

Between individual muscle fibres and between fasciculi is a network of supporting collagenous tissue; this is well demonstrated in micrograph (b) in which the collagen is stained blue.

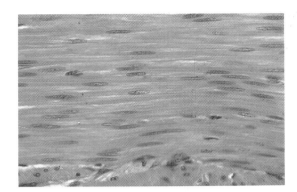

Fig. 6.15 Smooth muscle LS, H & E × 320

This micrograph illustrates smooth muscle from the bowel wall cut in longitudinal section. In this case, the fibres are arranged in a highly regular manner and packed so closely that it is difficult to identify individual cell outlines although cell shape can be deduced from that of the nuclei.

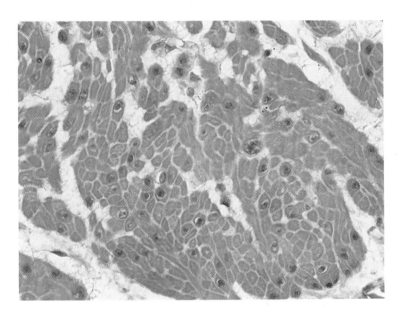

Fig. 6.16 Smooth muscle TS, H & E × 600

This micrograph shows smooth muscle in transverse section at very high magnification. The spindle-shaped cells are sectioned at various different points along their length which gives the erroneous impression that they are of differing diameters. Nuclei are only included in the plane of section where fibres have been cut through their widest diameter. Note the plump nuclear shape and central location of nuclei within the cytoplasm.

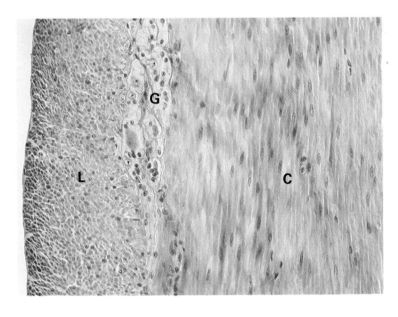

Fig. 6.17 Smooth muscle Masson's trichrome × 150

In many tubular visceral structures, such as the ileum seen in this micrograph, smooth muscle is disposed in layers with the cells of one layer arranged at right angles to those of the adjacent layer. This arrangement permits a wave of contraction to pass down the tube, propelling the contents forward; this action is called *peristalsis*.

Typically, the longitudinal smooth outer muscle layer **L** is closely applied to the inner circular layer **C** with only a minimal amount of supporting tissue between; in this specimen the collagen is stained blue. The supporting tissue contains clumps of large cells with pale nuclei which represent parasympathetic ganglia **G** (see Fig. 7.19).

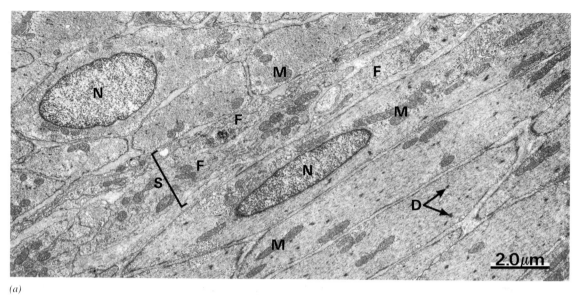

(a)

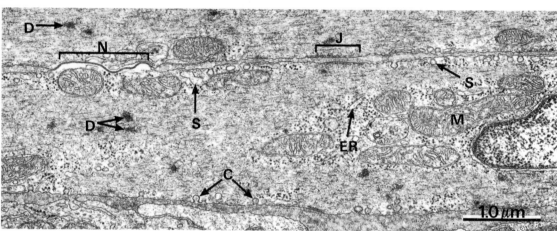

(b)

Fig. 6.18   **Smooth muscle** (a) EM × 8 000 (b) EM × 21 000

At low magnification, micrograph (a) demonstrates the spindle-shaped and elongated central nuclei **N** of smooth muscle cells. The cells at the lower right are cut longitudinally and those at the upper left transversely. Between them is a band of supporting tissue **S** containing the cytoplasmic processes of fibroblasts **F**. Note the relative sparsity of mitochondria **M** and other intracellular organelles.

At high magnification in micrograph (b), details of the plasma membrane and endomembrane system can be seen. The plasma membrane contains numerous flask-shaped invaginations. In some areas these are irregular in shape and size and may be involved in pinocytosis. In other areas, the invaginations are regular in shape and distribution and are called *caveolae* **C**.

The endomembrane system contains some elements which represent a poorly developed Golgi and endoplasmic reticulum **ER**. Other vesicular and tubular structures **S** are seen near the plasma membrane, often in association with caveolae; these probably constitute a system analogous to the sarcoplasmic reticulum of skeletal muscle, with the caveolae being analogous to the T tubule system.

Thick and thin filaments of myosin and actin criss-cross the cytoplasm of each cell and are anchored to the cell membrane at attachment junctions **J**. Filaments are also attached within the cytoplasm to dense bodies **D** which are believed to hold filaments in register.

The narrow intercellular spaces are of almost uniform width but at numerous sites the plasma membranes of adjacent cells form specialised cell junctions. Nexus (gap) junctions **N** mediate spread of excitation throughout visceral muscle (see Fig. 5.14).

Smooth muscle contraction

Smooth muscle does not show the longitudinally organised system of contractile proteins that is seen in striated muscle, but has an arrangement where bundles of contractile proteins criss-cross the cell, being inserted into anchoring points (*focal densities*) within the cytoplasm as well as anchoring to the cell membrane.

Tension generated by contraction is transmitted through anchoring densities in the cell membrane to the surrounding external lamina, thus allowing a mass of smooth muscle cells to function as one unit. The abundant intermediate filaments of smooth muscle, desmin, are also inserted into the focal densities (Fig 6.19).

The contraction mechanism of smooth muscle differs from that for striated muscle. Because the contractile proteins are arranged in a criss-cross lattice inserted around the cell membrane, contraction results in shortening of the cell, which assumes a globular shape in contrast to its elongated shape in the relaxed state (Fig. 6.19).

The mechanism of smooth muscle contraction is as follows:

- Thin filaments of actin are associated with tropomyosin.
- Thick filaments composed of myosin only bind to actin if one chain is phosphorylated.
- Ca^{2+} ions in the cytosol of smooth muscle cells cause contraction as in striated muscle, but the control of Ca^{2+} ion movements is different. In relaxed smooth muscle, free Ca^{2+} ions are normally sequestered in sarcoplasmic reticulum throughout the cell. On membrane excitation, free Ca^{2+} ions are released into the cytoplasm and bind to a protein called *calmodulin* (a calcium-binding protein). The calcium–calmodulin complex then activates an enzyme called *myosin light-chain kinase*, which phosphorylates myosin and permits it to bind to actin. Actin and myosin subsequently interact by filament sliding to produce contraction in a similar way to that for skeletal muscle.
- Contraction of smooth muscle can be modulated by surface receptors activating internal secondary messenger systems. Expression of different receptors allows smooth muscle in different sites to respond to several different hormones.
- Compared with skeletal muscle, smooth muscle is able to maintain a high force of contraction for very little ATP usage.

Most smooth muscle is present in the walls of hollow viscera (e.g. gut, ureter, Fallopian tube) where it is arranged in sheets with cells aligned circumferentially or longitudinally, with contraction resulting in reduction of the lumen diameter.

In these so-called *unitary smooth muscles*, cells tend to generate their own low level of rhythmic contraction, which may also be stimulated by stretch and is transmitted from cell to cell via the gap junctions. Such smooth muscle is richly innervated by the autonomic nervous system (see Ch. 7), which increases or decreases levels of spontaneous contraction rather than actually initiating it. Physiologically, this is termed tonic smooth muscle and is characterised by slow contraction, no action potentials and a low content of fast myosin.

A second arrangement of smooth muscle is typified by that in the iris of the eye. Here, rather than simply modulating spontaneous activity, autonomic innervation precisely controls contraction, resulting in opening and closing of the pupil. Similar neurally controlled or multi-unit smooth muscle is found in the vas deferens and some large arteries. Physiologically, this is termed *phasic smooth muscle* and is characterised by rapid contraction associated with an action potential.

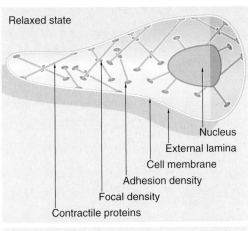

Relaxed state

Nucleus
External lamina
Cell membrane
Adhesion density
Focal density
Contractile proteins

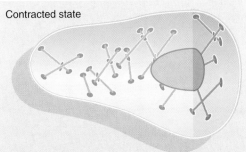

Contracted state

Fig. 6.19 Smooth muscle contraction

Contractile proteins are inserted into focal densities and anchoring densities around the cell membrane. In the relaxed state the cell is elongated. With contraction the smooth muscle adopts a globular shape.

Cardiac muscle

Cardiac muscle exhibits many structural and functional characteristics intermediate between those of skeletal and visceral muscle. Like the former, its contractions are strong and utilise a great deal of energy, and like the latter the contractions are continuous and initiated by inherent mechanisms, although they are modulated by external autonomic and hormonal stimuli.

Cardiac muscle fibres are essentially long cylindrical cells with one or at most two nuclei, centrally located within the cell. The ends of the fibres are split longitudinally into a small number of branches, the ends of which abut onto similar branches of adjacent cells giving the impression of a continuous three-dimensional cytoplasmic network; this was formerly described as a *syncytium* before the discrete intercellular boundaries were recognised.

Between the muscle fibres, delicate collagenous tissue analogous to the endomysium of skeletal muscle supports the extremely rich capillary network necessary to meet the high metabolic demands of strong continuous activity.

Cardiac muscle fibres have an arrangement of contractile proteins similar to that of skeletal muscle and are consequently striated in a similar manner. However, this is often difficult to visualise with light microscopy due to the irregular branching shape of the cells and their myofibrils. Cardiac muscle fibres also have a system of T tubules and sarcoplasmic reticulum analogous to that of skeletal muscles. In the case of cardiac muscle, however, there is a slow leak of calcium ions into the cytoplasm from the sarcoplasmic reticulum after recovery from the preceding contraction; this causes a succession of automatic contractions independent of external stimuli. The rate of this inherent rhythm is then modulated by external autonomic and hormonal stimuli.

Between the ends of adjacent cardiac muscle cells are specialised intercellular junctions called *intercalated discs* which not only provide points of anchorage for the myofibrils but also permit extremely rapid spread of contractile stimuli from one cell to another. Thus, adjacent fibres are caused to contract almost simultaneously, thereby acting as a functional syncytium. In addition, a system of highly modified cardiac muscle cells constitutes the pacemaker regions of the heart and ramifies throughout the organ as the Purkinje system, thus coordinating contraction of the myocardium as a whole in each cardiac cycle; this is illustrated and described in more detail in Chapter 8.

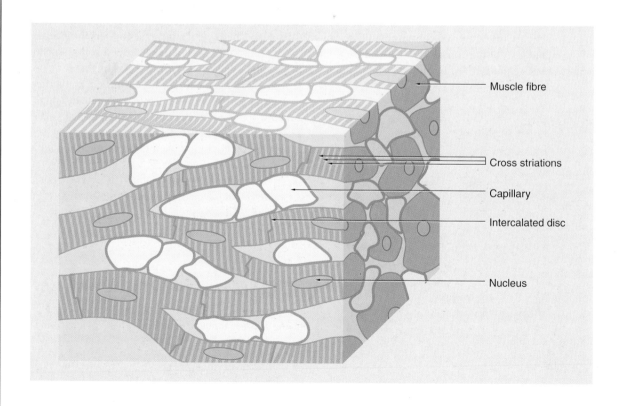

Fig. 6.20   Cardiac muscle

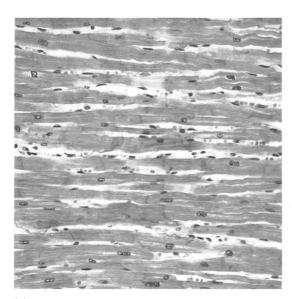

(a)

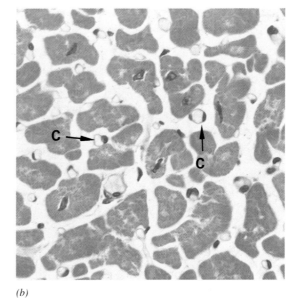

(b)

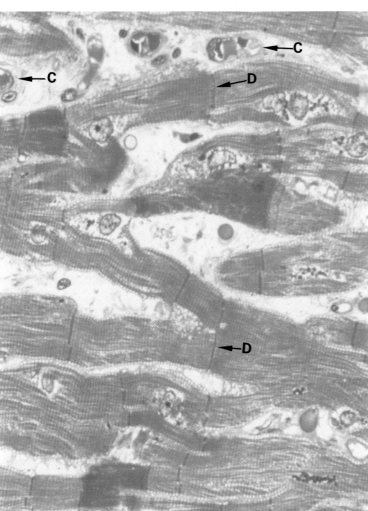

(c)

Fig. 6.21 Cardiac muscle
**(a) LS, H & E × 198 (b) TS,
H & E × 480 (c) Thin section,
toluidine blue × 640**

In longitudinal section in micrograph (a), cardiac muscle cells are seen to contain one or two nuclei and an extensive cytoplasm which branches to give the appearance of a continuous three-dimensional network. In routine H & E preparation such as this, the cross-striations are not readily visible. The elongated nuclei are mainly centrally located, a characteristic well demonstrated in transverse section as in micrograph (b).

Micrograph (c) illustrates an extremely thin resin-embedded section at very high magnification. The branching cytoplasmic network is readily seen with prominent intercalated discs **D** marking the intercellular boundaries. Note the typical cross-striations.

In each of these specimens, note the delicate supporting tissue filling the intercellular spaces and containing an extensive network of blood capillaries **C**.

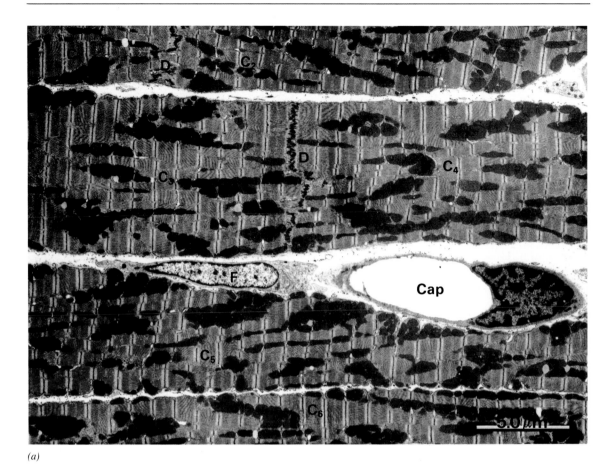

(a)

(b)

Fig. 6.22 **Cardiac muscle**
(a) EM × 5000 (b) EM × 38 000

Micrograph (a) illustrates portions of six cardiac muscle cells labelled C_1 to C_6. None of their nuclei are included in the plane of section. Cells C_1 and C_2 abut one another end to end and are demarcated by an intercalated disc **D**. Cells C_3 and C_4 are demarcated in a similar fashion. The intercellular space contains a capillary **Cap** and a fibroblast **F**.

The sarcomeres of cardiac muscle have an identical banding pattern to that of skeletal muscle. The sarcomeres are not, however, arranged into single columns making up cylindrical myofibrils as in skeletal muscle, but form a branching myofibrillar network continuous in three dimensions throughout the cytoplasm. The branching columns of sarcomeres are separated by sarcoplasm containing rows of mitochondria and sarcoplasmic reticulum. The great abundance of mitochondria in cardiac muscle reflects the enormous metabolic demands of continuous cardiac muscle activity.

Conduction of excitatory stimuli to the sarcomeres of cardiac muscle is mediated by a system of T tubules and sarcoplasmic reticulum essentially similar in arrangement to that of skeletal muscle. The T tubules, however, ramify throughout the cardiac muscle cytoplasm at the Z lines and their origins are seen as indentations in the sarcolemma which thus has a somewhat scalloped outline.

The conducting system can be seen at high magnification in micrograph (b). T tubules **T** and sarcoplasmic reticulum **SR** form poorly defined triads compared with those of skeletal muscle. Note the typical closely packed cristae of the mitochondria **M**, a lipid droplet **L** and glycogen granules **G**.

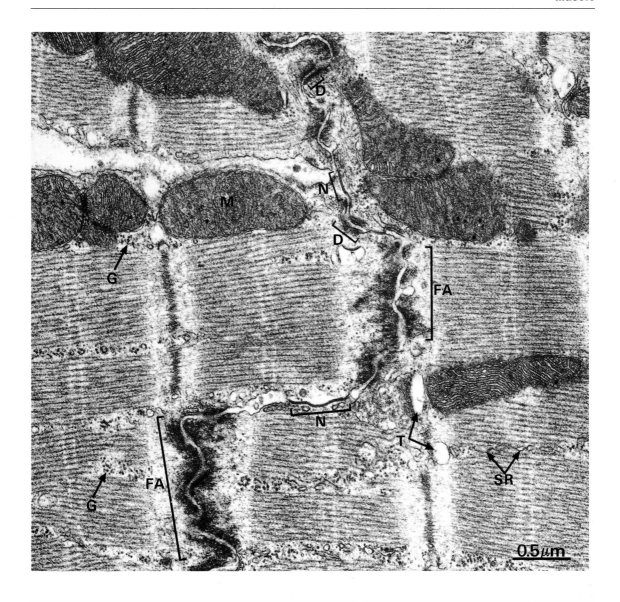

Fig. 6.23 **Cardiac muscle: intercalated disc** EM × 31 000

Intercalated discs are specialised transverse junctions between cardiac muscle cells at sites where they meet end to end; they always coincide with the Z lines. Intercalated discs bind the cells, transmit forces of contraction and provide areas of low electrical resistance for the rapid spread of excitation throughout the myocardium.

The intercalated disc is an interdigitating junction and consists of three types of membrane-to-membrane contact. The predominant type of contact, the *fascia adherens* **FA**, resembles the zonula adherens of epithelial junctional complexes (see Fig. 5.12) but is more extensive and less regular. The actin filaments at the ends of terminal sarcomeres insert into the fasciae adherentes

and thereby transmit contractile forces from cell to cell. *Desmosomes* **D** occur less frequently and provide anchorage for intermediate filaments of the cytoskeleton. Gap (nexus) junctions **N** (see Fig. 5.14) are present mainly in the longitudinal portions of the interdigitations and are sites of low electrical resistance through which excitation passes from cell to cell.

Note the similarity of the sarcomeres of cardiac and skeletal muscle (see Fig. 6.8). The mitochondria **M** are elongated or spheroidal and have abundant closely packed cristae rich in oxidative enzyme systems. The sarcoplasm within and between the sarcomeres is rich in glycogen granules **G**. Lace-like profiles of sarcoplasmic reticulum **SR** and parts of T tubules **T** can be identified.

7. Nervous tissues

Introduction

The function of the nervous system is to receive stimuli from both the internal and external environments which are then analysed and integrated to produce appropriate, coordinated responses in various effector organs. The nervous system is composed of an intercommunicating network of specialised cells called *neurones* which constitute most sensory receptors, the conducting pathways, and the sites of integration and analysis.

The functions of the nervous system depend on a fundamental property of neurones called *excitability*. As in all cells, the resting neurone maintains an ionic gradient across its plasma membrane thereby creating an electrical potential. Excitability involves a change in membrane permeability in response to appropriate stimuli such that the ionic gradient is reversed and the plasma membrane becomes *depolarised*; a wave of depolarisation, known as an *action potential*, then spreads along the plasma membrane. This is followed by the process of *repolarisation* in which the membrane rapidly re-establishes its resting potential. At *synapses*, the sites of intercommunication between adjacent neurones, depolarisation of one neurone causes it to release chemical transmitter substances, *neurotransmitters*, which initiate an action potential in the adjacent neurone.

Within the nervous system, neurones are arranged to form pathways for the conduction of action potentials from receptors to effector organs via integrating neurones. Neurotransmitters not only mediate neurone-to-neurone transmission but also act as chemical intermediates between the nervous system and effector organs which also exhibit the property of excitability. The effector organs of voluntary nervous pathways are generally skeletal muscle whilst those of involuntary pathways are usually smooth muscle, cardiac muscle and muscle-like epithelial cells (myoepithelial cells) within some exocrine glands.

The nervous system is divided anatomically into the *central nervous system* (CNS), comprising the brain and spinal cord, and the *peripheral nervous system* (PNS) which constitutes all nervous tissue outside the CNS. Functionally, the nervous system is divided into the *somatic nervous system* which is involved in voluntary functions, and the *autonomic nervous system* which exerts control over many involuntary functions. Histologically, however, the entire nervous system merely consists of variations in the arrangement of neurones and their supporting tissues.

This chapter encompasses the cell and tissue types found in the nervous system and includes the structure of the peripheral nervous system and relatively simple types of sensory receptor. Details of the arrangement of nervous tissue in the central nervous system are the subject of Chapter 20 whilst the structure of the highly specialised organs of sensory reception associated with the cranial nerves, e.g. eye and ear, is presented in Chapter 21.

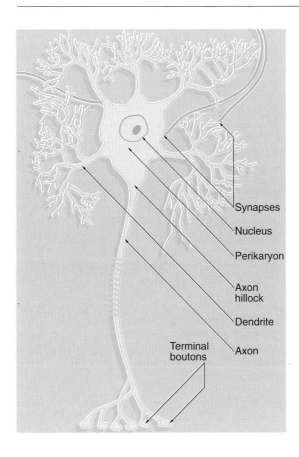

Synapses

Nucleus

Perikaryon

Axon
hillock

Dendrite

Terminal
boutons

Axon

Fig. 7.1   The neurone

Despite great variation in size and shape in different parts of the nervous system, all neurones have the same basic structure as shown in this idealised diagram. The neurone consists of a large *cell body* containing the nucleus surrounded by cytoplasm known as the *perikaryon*. Processes of two types extend from the cell body, namely a single *axon* and one or more *dendrites*.

Dendrites are highly branched, tapering processes which either end in specialised sensory receptors (as in primary sensory neurones) or form synapses with neighbouring neurones from which they receive stimuli. In general, dendrites function as the major sites of information input into the neurone.

Each neurone has a single axon arising from a cone-shaped portion of the cell body called the *axon hillock*. The axon is a cylindrical process up to 1 metre in length terminating on other neurones or effector organs by way of a variable number of small branches which end in small swellings called *terminal boutons*.

Action potentials arise in the cell body as a result of integration of afferent (incoming) stimuli; action potentials are then conducted along the axon to influence other neurones or effector organs. Axons are commonly referred to as *nerve fibres*.

In general, the cell bodies of all neurones are located in the central nervous system; exceptions are the cell bodies of most primary sensory neurones and the terminal effector neurones of the autonomic nervous system where, in both cases, the cell bodies lie in aggregations called *ganglia* in peripheral sites.

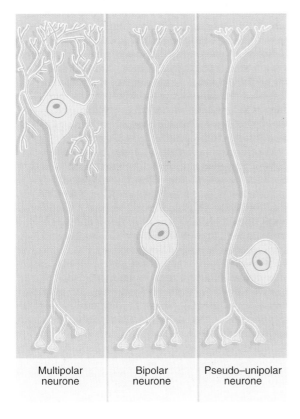

Multipolar
neurone

Bipolar
neurone

Pseudo–unipolar
neurone

Fig. 7.2   Basic neurone types

Throughout the nervous system, neurones have a wide variety of shapes which fall into three main patterns according to the arrangement of the axon and dendrites with respect to the cell body.

The most common form is the *multipolar neurone* in which numerous dendrites project from the cell body; the dendrites may all arise from one pole of the cell body or may extend from all parts of the cell body. In general, intermediate, integratory and motor neurones conform to this pattern.

Bipolar neurones have only a single dendrite which arises from the pole of the cell body opposite to the origin of the axon. These unusual neurones act as receptor neurones for the senses of smell, sight and balance.

Most other primary sensory neurones are described as *pseudo-unipolar neurones* since a single dendrite and the axon arise from a common stem of the cell body; this stem is formed by the fusion of the first part of the dendrite and axon of a bipolar type of neurone during embryological development.

As a general rule, neurone impulses are conveyed along dendrites towards the nerve cell body (afferent) whilst axons usually convey impulses away from the nerve cell body (efferent).

Neurones are terminally differentiated cells that, for all practical purposes, do not regenerate in the event of cell death. Studies have shown cell division in neurones in the adult brain, although the biological significance of this remains uncertain. However, regeneration of axons and dendrites can occur in the event of damage, provided the neurone cell body remains viable. This is the basis of nerve grafting used to treat peripheral nerve injuries.

BASIC TISSUE TYPES

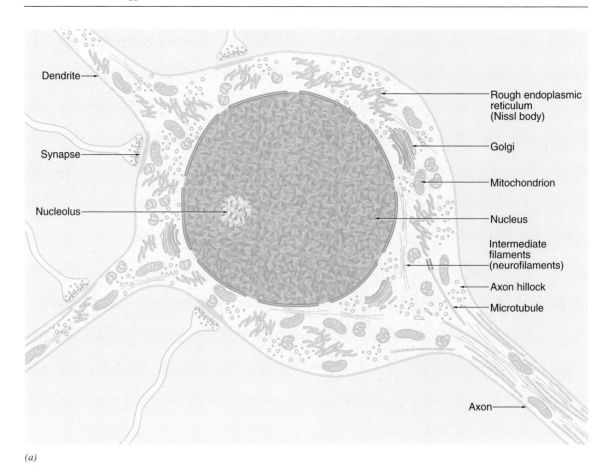

Dendrite

Synapse

Nucleolus

Rough endoplasmic
reticulum
(Nissl body)

Golgi

Mitochondrion

Nucleus

Intermediate
filaments
(neurofilaments)

Axon hillock

Microtubule

Axon

(a)

Fig. 7.3 **Ultrastructure of the neurone** (a) Schematic diagram (b) EM × 19 000 *(opposite)*

The diagram (a) illustrates the main ultrastructural features of the neurone, in this case a multipolar neurone with an axon and two dendrites. The nucleus is large, round or ovoid and usually centrally located within the perikaryon. Reflecting the intense metabolic activity of the neurone (and consequent need to replace damaged proteins), the chromatin is completely dispersed and the nucleolus is a conspicuous feature.

The cytoplasm of the cell body contains large aggregations of rough endoplasmic reticulum which correspond to the *Nissl substance* of light microscopy (see Fig. 7.4); the rough endoplasmic reticulum extends into the dendrites but not into the axon hillock or axon. Rough endoplasmic reticulum is a much more prominent feature in large neurones, such as somatic motor neurones, than in smaller neurones such as those of the autonomic nervous system. A diffuse Golgi apparatus is found adjacent to the nucleus. Smooth endoplasmic reticulum is not a prominent feature of the perikaryon, but tubules, cisternae and vesicles are prominent in the axon and dendrites. The mitochondria of the perikaryon are numerous and have the usual rod-like appearances; those of the axon are extremely slender and elongated.

Neurones are very metabolically active and expend much energy in maintaining ionic gradients across the plasma membrane. Neurones synthesise neurotransmitter substances or their precursors in the perikaryon from where they are transported along the axon to the synapse to be released when appropriately stimulated.

Numerous intermediate filaments (neurofilaments) and microtubules are arranged in parallel bundles throughout the perikaryon and along the length of the axon and dendrites. The intermediate filaments provide structural support and the microtubules are involved in axonal transport of neurotransmitter substances, enzymes, membrane and other cellular constituents.

The electron micrograph (b) shows part of the cell body of a neurone and includes a portion of the nucleus **N**. At the lower right, part of the neuronal plasma membrane **PM** is seen including a synapse **S** with the terminal bouton **TB** of an adjacent neurone. Features of the cytoplasm of the perikaryon are areas of rough endoplasmic reticulum **rER**, free ribosomes **R** and scattered mitochondria **M**. An extensive Golgi complex **G** is represented by several stacks of flattened membranous cisternae. Associated with the Golgi are several multivesicular bodies **MB** involved in transport to other organelles including lysosomes **L**. Microtubules **T** can be identified in oblique section but neurofilaments are not readily identifiable.

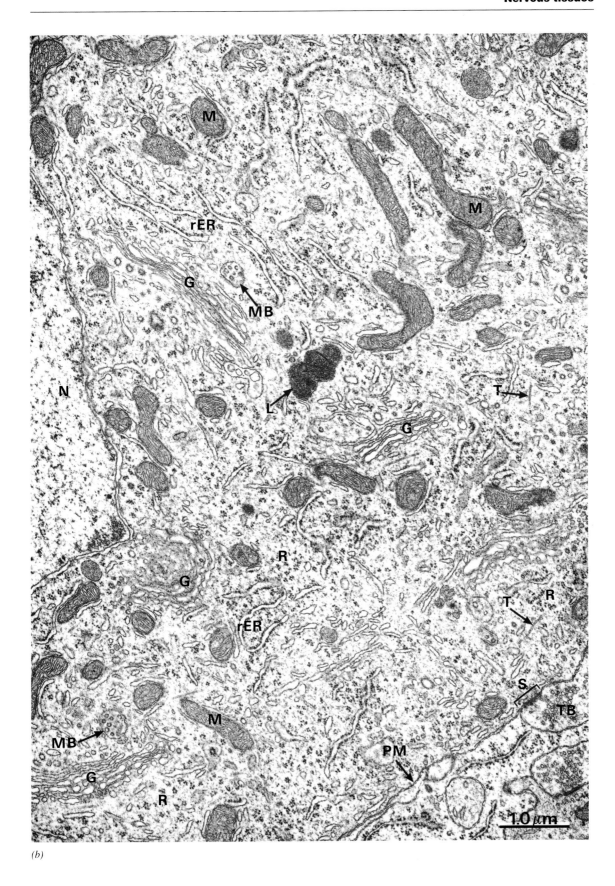

(b)

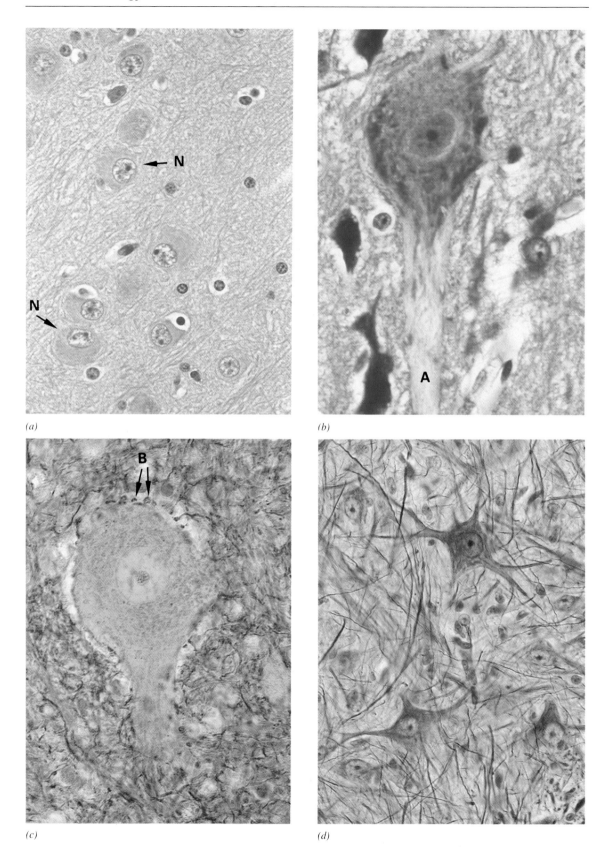

(a)

(b)

(c)

(d)

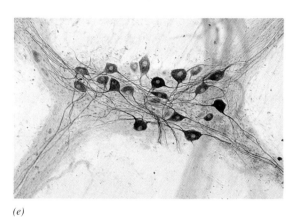

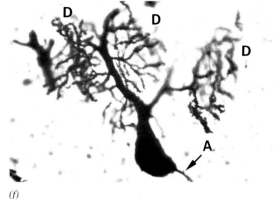

(e)   *(f)*

Fig. 7.4 **Neurones and methods of study with light microscopy** *(micrographs (a) to (d) opposite)*
(a) H & E × 480 (b) Nissl method × 1200 (c) Gold method × 1200 (d) Gold/toluidine blue × 600
(e) Spread preparation, gold method × 320 (f) Golgi–Cox × 320

The large size and complex morphology of neurones, the extreme elongation of axons, and the need to study neuronal interconnections have resulted in an extensive range of techniques being employed in neurohistology.

Methods which demonstrate nuclei, cell bodies and their cytoplasmic contents include routine stains such as H & E and more specific techniques for demonstrating particular cytoplasmic elements such as the Nissl method for RNA; however, these methods are of limited use in the study of axons and dendrites.

Heavy metal impregnation techniques with gold and silver are valuable in the study of neurone morphology, including axons and dendrites, and were widely employed by the pioneers of neuro-anatomy such as Cajal and Golgi from whom they take their names. Thick sections are often used with such methods as there is then a much greater chance of whole cells being included in the plane of section. Likewise, *spread preparations* often permit the examination of complete neurones and their cytoplasmic processes. Heavy metals are also deposited in the neuronal microtubules thus permitting study of the cytoskeleton.

Immunohistochemistry can also be used to identify neurone-specific proteins, e.g. neurofilament protein, and γγ enolase (neurone-specific enolase).

Micrograph (a), stained with H & E, shows neurones **N** in the brain; the nuclei are huge in comparison with those of surrounding support cells; dispersed chromatin and prominent nucleoli reflect a high level of protein (enzyme) synthesis. The extensive cytoplasm is basophilic (blue stained) due to extensive ribosomal RNA. No detail can be seen of cytoplasmic processes.

In micrograph (b), the Nissl method stains RNA, identifying the rER (Nissl substance) as dark blue material giving the neuronal cytoplasm a granular appearance; DNA in the nucleus and nucleoli has similar staining properties. In this specimen, note the axon **A** which is devoid of Nissl substance beyond the axon hillock.

A very similar neurone is shown in micrograph (c) using a heavy metal impregnation technique. Virtually the only intracellular detail that can be seen is the cytoskeleton and a negative image of the nucleus. Note the numerous axons with tiny terminal boutons **B** making synapses with the cell body.

Micrograph (d) employs another gold method which provides excellent detail of neuronal shape and shows the presence of the cytoskeleton in the dendrites and axons; the blue counter-stain demonstrates the nuclei of surrounding support cells. Note that detail of neuronal processes is lost when these pass out of the plane of section.

Spread preparations, as shown in micrograph (e), overcome this problem to a certain extent. This example shows neurones in a small peripheral ganglion, their main cytoplasmic processes being very clearly delineated.

Finally, micrograph (f) illustrates a very thick section stained by a silver impregnation method and shows a Purkinje cell in the cerebellar cortex. These cells have a single small axon **A** at one pole and an extraordinary, finely branching dendritic tree **D** at the other pole. Note that the base of the dendritic system (arrowed) is in this case much larger than that of the axon.

Myelinated and non-myelinated nerve fibres

In the peripheral nervous system, all axons are enveloped by highly specialised cells called *Schwann cells* which provide both structural and metabolic support. In general, small diameter axons (e.g. those of the autonomic nervous system and small pain fibres) are simply enveloped by the cytoplasm of Schwann cells; these nerve fibres are said to be *non-myelinated*. Large diameter fibres are wrapped by a variable number of concentric layers of the Schwann cell plasma membrane forming a *myelin sheath*; such nerve fibres are said to be *myelinated*. Within the central nervous system, myelination is similar to that in the peripheral nervous system except that the myelin sheaths are formed by cells called *oligodendrocytes* (see Fig. 7.22).

In all nerve fibres, the rate of conduction of action potentials is proportional to the diameter of the axon; myelination greatly increases axon conduction velocity compared with that of a non-myelinated fibre of the same diameter.

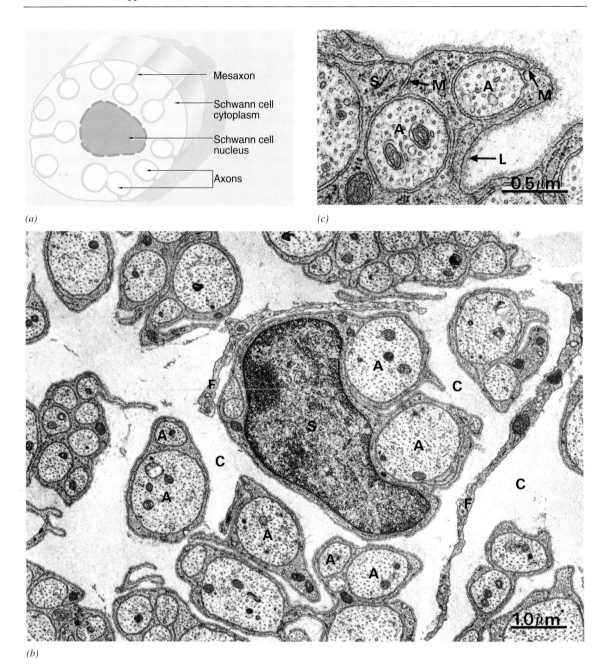

(a)

(c)

(b)

Fig. 7.5 **Non-myelinated nerve fibres** (a) Diagram (b) EM × 15 000 (c) EM × 36 000

The relationship of non-myelinated axons with their supporting Schwann cell is illustrated in diagram (a). One or more axons become longitudinally invaginated into the Schwann cell so that each axon is embedded in a channel, invested by the Schwann cell plasma membrane and cytoplasm. The Schwann cell plasma membrane becomes apposed to itself along the opening of the channel, thus effectively sealing the axon within an extracellular compartment bounded by the Schwann cell. The zone of apposition of the Schwann cell membrane is called the ***mesaxon***. Note that more than one axon may occupy a single channel within the Schwann cell. Each Schwann cell extends for only a short distance along the nerve tract and at its termination the ensheathment is continued by another Schwann cell with which it interdigitates closely end to end.

At low magnification in micrograph (b), non-myelinated axons **A** of various sizes are seen ensheathed by Schwann cells; one of the Schwann cells has been sectioned transversely through its nucleus **S**. Note the variable number of axons enclosed by each Schwann cell. Delicate cytoplasmic extensions of fibroblasts **F** and collagen fibrils **C** cut in cross-section can be seen in the endoneurium.

At high magnification in micrograph (c), part of the cytoplasm of a Schwann cell **S** is shown ensheathing several axons **A**; axons are readily identified by their content of smooth endoplasmic reticulum and microtubules, seen in cross-section. Several mesaxons **M** can be seen. The external surface of the Schwann cell is bounded by an external lamina **L** equivalent to basement membrane in epithelia.

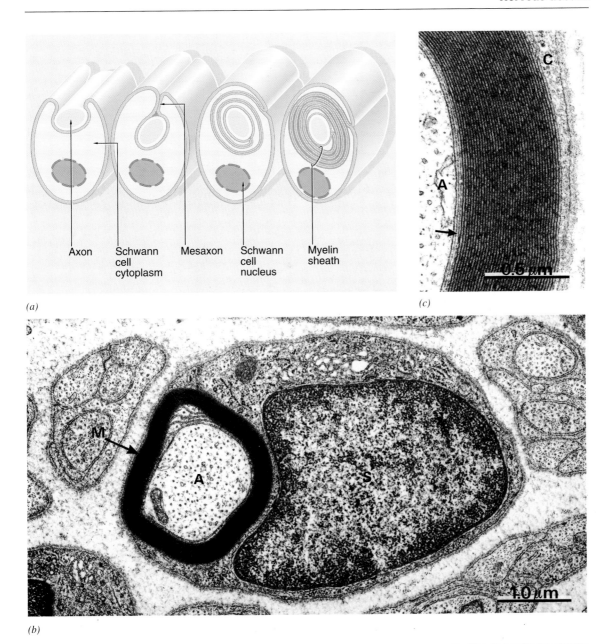

(a)

(c)

(b)

Fig. 7.6 **Myelinated nerve fibre** (a) Diagram (b) EM × 20 000 (c) EM × 46 000

In peripheral nerves, myelination begins with the invagination of a single nerve axon into a Schwann cell; a mesaxon is then formed. As myelination proceeds, the mesaxon rotates around the axon thereby enveloping the axon in concentric layers of Schwann cell cytoplasm and plasma membrane. The cytoplasm is then excluded so that the inner leaflets of plasma membrane fuse with each other and the axon becomes surrounded by multiple layers of membrane which together constitute the myelin sheath. The single segment of myelin produced by each Schwann cell is termed an *internode*; this ensheaths the axon between one node of Ranvier and the next (see Fig. 7.7).

In the CNS, oligodendrocytes are responsible for the process of myelination which follows a similar pattern; a single oligodendrocyte, however, forms multiple myelin internodes, which contribute to the ensheathment of as many as 50 individual axons (see Fig. 7.22).

In micrograph (b), a myelinated nerve fibre from the PNS is sectioned transversely at the level of the nucleus of an ensheathing Schwann cell **S**. The single axon **A** is enveloped by many layers of fused Schwann cell plasma membrane forming the myelin sheath **M**.

Micrograph (c) shows that Schwann cell cytoplasm is absent within the compact myelin sheath which consists of many regular layers of membrane. The darker lines, termed the *major dense lines*, arise by fusion of cytoplasmic leaflets. The intervening *intraperiod* lines represent closely apposed external membrane leaflets. The substantial lipid content of these modified membrane layers insulate the underlying axon **A**, preventing ion fluxes across the axonal plasma membrane except at the nodes of Ranvier. The main bulk of the Schwann cell cytoplasm **C** encircles the myelin sheath. However, a thin layer of Schwann cell cytoplasm also persists immediately surrounding the axon (arrowed).

BASIC TISSUE TYPES

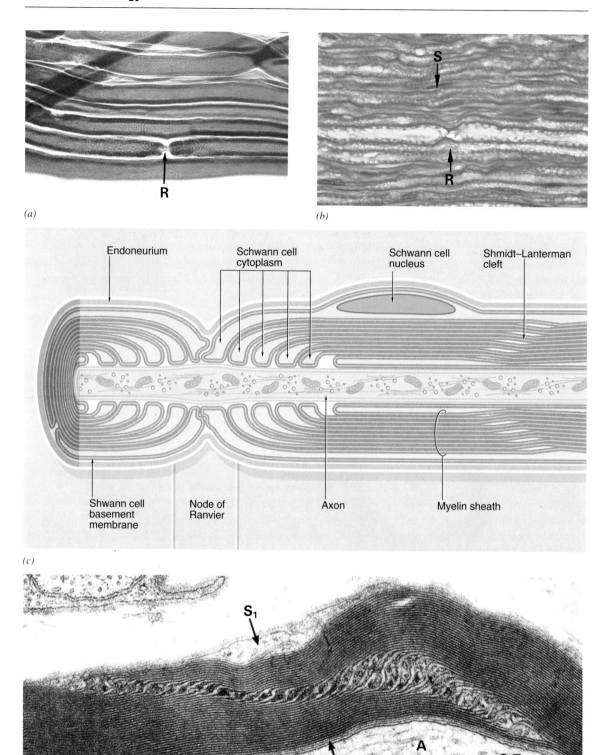

(a)

(b)

(c)

Endoneurium

Schwann cell cytoplasm

Schwann cell nucleus

Shmidt–Lanterman cleft

Shwann cell basement membrane

Node of Ranvier

Axon

Myelin sheath

(d)

0.5 μm

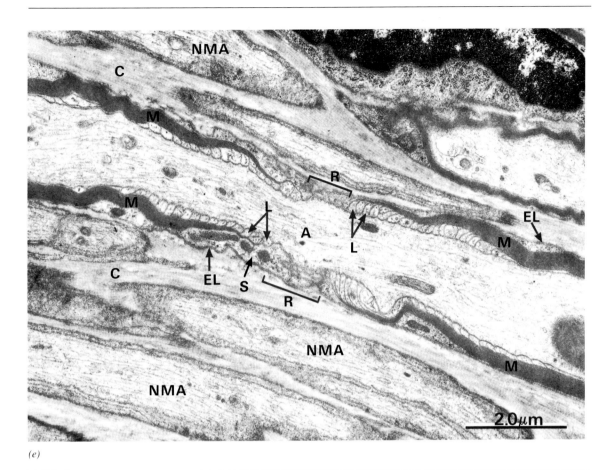

(e)

Fig. 7.7 **Nodes of Ranvier and Schmidt–Lanterman incisures** *(illustrations (a) to (d) opposite)* **(a) Teased preparation, Sudan black × 320 (b) H & E × 320 (c) Schematic diagram (d) EM × 42 000 (e) EM × 14 000**

The myelin sheath of an individual axon is provided by many Schwann cells (oligodendrocytes in the CNS), each Schwann cell covering only a segment of the axon. Between the Schwann cells there are short intervals at which the axon is not covered by a myelin sheath; these points are known as *nodes of Ranvier*.

Micrograph (a) shows a node of Ranvier **R** in a teased preparation of myelinated axons. With this method, only the lipid of the myelin has been stained, and thus Schwann cell nuclei are not seen.

Micrograph (b) shows axons in longitudinal section stained with H & E. Due to a fixation artefact, myelin sheaths appear 'bubbly'; the lipid is mostly dissolved out during preparation and is therefore unstained. A node of Ranvier **R** is identifiable in the large axon in midfield. Several Schwann cell nuclei **S** can also be seen.

Diagram (c) illustrates the manner in which Schwann cells terminate at the node of Ranvier, so exposing the axon to the surrounding environment. Note the manner in which cytoplasmic processes of adjacent Schwann cells interdigitate at the node; also note the continuation of the Schwann cell basement membrane (external lamina) across the node. The myelin sheath prevents the nerve action potential from being propagated continuously along the axon and the action potential travels by jumping from node to node. This mode of conduction, known as *saltatory conduction*, greatly enhances the conduction velocity of axons. The internodal length is related to the diameter of the axon and may be up to 1.5 mm in the largest fibres.

Micrograph (e) illustrates the ultrastructure of a node of Ranvier **R**. The axon **A** is characterised by numerous neurofilaments, microtubules and elongated mitochondria. A myelin sheath **M** can be identified at each end of the field, the myelin becoming progressively thinner as it approaches the node. This is because, as it approaches the node, each compact major dense line expands to form a small membrane loop **L** containing Schwann cell cytoplasm, the loops directly abutting the axonal plasma membrane. Externally, a broader layer of Schwann cell cytoplasm **S** containing mitochondria envelops the nodal area. Note the external lamina **EL** of the Schwann cell and collagen fibrils **C** in surrounding endoneurium. Several non-myelinated axons **NMA** are seen nearby.

At certain points within the internodal myelin sheath, narrow channels of cytoplasm are retained and connect the main bulk of the Schwann cell cytoplasm peripherally to the narrow zone of Schwann cell cytoplasm adjacent to the axon. These uncompacted regions are known as *Schmidt–Lanterman incisures* or *clefts*; in longitudinal section, as in electron micrograph (d), the incisure passes obliquely across the width of the compact sheath. The axon is marked **A**, the peripheral Schwann cell cytoplasm S_1 and the periaxonal Schwann cell cytoplasm S_2. It has been suggested that the clefts are not static but rather continually moving their position providing periodic exposure of the inner faces of the myelin membranes to cytoplasm for the purpose of maintenance and molecular replacement.

Synapses and neuromuscular junctions

Synapses are highly specialised intercellular junctions which link the neurones of each nervous pathway. Similar intercellular junctions link neurones and their effector cells such as muscle fibres; where neurones synapse with skeletal muscle they are referred to as **neuromuscular junctions** or **motor end plates**. Individual neurones intercommunicate via a widely variable number of synapses depending on their location and function within the nervous system. Classically, the axon of one neurone synapses with the dendrite of another neurone (**axodendritic synapse**), but axons may synapse with the cell bodies of other neurones (**axosomatic synapses**) or other axons (**axoaxonic synapses**); dendrite-to-dendrite and cell body-to-cell body synapses have also been described. For a given synapse, the conduction of an impulse is unidirectional but the response may be either excitatory or inhibitory depending on the specific functional nature of the synapse and its location.

The mechanism of conduction of the nerve impulse involves the release from one neurone of a chemical neurotransmitter which then diffuses across a narrow intercellular space to induce excitation or inhibition in the other neurone or effector cell of that synapse. Neurotransmitters mediate their effects by interacting with specific receptors incorporated in the opposing plasma membrane.

The chemical nature of neurotransmitters and the morphology of synapses are highly variable in different parts of the nervous system, but the principles of synaptic transmission and the basic structure of synapses are similar throughout the nervous system.

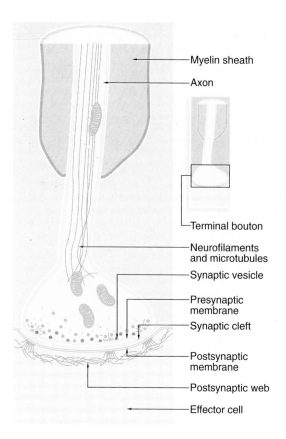

Myelin sheath
Axon

Terminal bouton

Neurofilaments and microtubules
Synaptic vesicle
Presynaptic membrane
Synaptic cleft
Postsynaptic membrane
Postsynaptic web
Effector cell

Fig. 7.8 Synapse

This diagram illustrates the general structure of the synapse. The axon responsible for propagating the stimulus terminates at a bulbous swelling or **terminal bouton**; this is separated from the plasma membrane of the opposed neurone or effector cell by a narrow intercellular gap of uniform width (20–30 nm) called the **synaptic cleft**. The terminal boutons are not myelinated. The boutons contain mitochondria and membrane-bound vesicles of neurotransmitter substance known as **synaptic vesicles** which are approximately 50 nm in diameter.

Although many types of neurotransmitter substance occur in the CNS, only two types are known in the peripheral nervous system: acetylcholine and noradrenaline (norepinephrine). Acetylcholine precursors, acetate and choline, are synthesised in the perikaryon and transported to the synapse where they are conjugated. Noradrenaline synthesis takes place in both the perikaryon and the terminal bouton. Synaptic vesicles are transported into the synaptic bouton down the axon from the cell body. Vesicles can also be formed in the synaptic bouton by recycling of vesicle membrane.

Synaptic vesicles aggregate towards the **presynaptic membrane** and, on arrival of an action potential, dock with the membrane and release their contents into the synaptic cleft by exocytosis. The neurotransmitter diffuses across the synaptic cleft to stimulate receptors in the **postsynaptic membrane**. Associated with synapses are a variety of biochemical mechanisms such as hydrolytic and oxidative enzymes which inactivate the released neurotransmitter between successive nerve impulses. Transmitter may also be taken up back into the terminal bouton and be recycled into new synaptic vesicles. The cytoplasm beneath the postsynaptic membrane often contains a feltwork of fine fibrils, the **postsynaptic web**, which may be associated with desmosome-like structures in maintaining the integrity of the synapse.

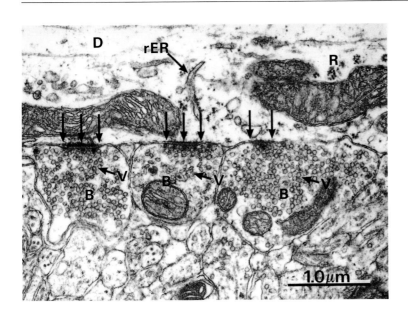

Fig. 7.9 **Axodendritic synapse** EM × 22 000

This micrograph from the CNS illustrates three terminal boutons **B** (probably from different axons) forming synapses with a dendrite **D**. The dendrite can be identified as such by its content of ribosomes **R** and rough endoplasmic reticulum **rER** (which are not present in axons). Note the presence of numerous uniform-sized synaptic vesicles **V** and a few mitochondria within the terminal boutons. The *postsynaptic density* (arrowed) contributes to the structural stability of the closely apposed pre- and postsynaptic membranes.

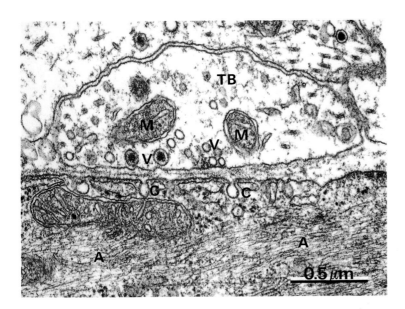

Fig. 7.10 **Autonomic synapse** EM × 42 000

This micrograph illustrates a synapse between an autonomic axon and a smooth muscle cell in the intestine. The terminal bouton **TB** contains mitochondria **M** and a number of synaptic vesicles **V** some of which contain a dense central core probably representing an electron-dense carrier protein; such *dense-cored vesicles* are a feature of autonomic synapses. Frequently more than one neurotransmitter substance is present in individual autonomic neurones.

The postsynaptic membrane exhibits flask-like invaginations **C** which may represent caveolae (see Fig. 6.18). Note the uniform width of the synaptic cleft between the pre- and postsynaptic membranes. The smooth muscle cell contains numerous fine actin microfilaments **A**.

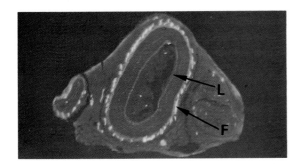

Fig. 7.11 **Sympathetic nerve endings** Formalin-induced fluorescence × 80

Noradrenaline is the main postganglionic neurotransmitter in the sympathetic nervous system. When noradrenaline combines with formalin (and some other compounds) it becomes fluorescent and can be visualised by fluorescence microscopy.

This micrograph illustrates formalin-induced fluorescence **F** in the outer layer of large and small arteries, corresponding to the presence of sympathetic noradrenergic nerve endings. Background autofluorescence outlines the general structure; note that the internal elastic lamina **L** (see Fig. 8.8) of the large artery in midfield is particularly autofluorescent.

BASIC TISSUE TYPES

128 | **Functional Histology**

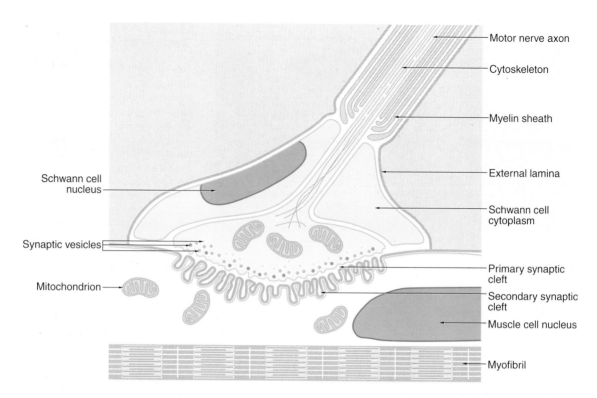

Motor nerve axon

Cytoskeleton

Myelin sheath

External lamina

Schwann cell cytoplasm

Primary synaptic cleft

Secondary synaptic cleft

Muscle cell nucleus

Myofibril

Schwann cell nucleus

Synaptic vesicles

Mitochondrion

(a)

Fig. 7.12 **Motor end plates** *(illustrations (b) to (e) opposite)* **(a) Schematic diagram (b) Teased preparation, gold method** × 320 **(c) Teased preparation, gold method** × 800 **(d) Histochemical method for acetylcholinesterase** × 320 **(e) EM** × 26 000

The motor end plates of skeletal muscle have the same basic structure as other synapses with the addition of several important features. Firstly, one motor neurone may innervate from a few to more than a thousand muscle fibres depending on the precision of movement of the muscle; the motor neurone and the muscle fibres which it supplies together constitute a **motor unit**.

At low magnification in micrograph (b), the terminal part of the axon of a motor neurone is seen dividing into several branches, each terminating as a motor end plate on a different skeletal muscle fibre near to its midpoint. Micrograph (c) shows the lowermost of these motor end plates at higher magnification. The axonal branch is seen to lose its myelin sheath and divides to form a cluster of small bulbous swellings (terminal boutons) on the muscle fibre surface.

As seen in the diagram, the motor end plate occupies a recess in the muscle cell surface, described as the **sole plate**, and is covered by an extension of the cytoplasm of the last Schwann cell surrounding the axon. The external lamina (basement membrane) of the Schwann cell merges with that of the muscle fibre, and the delicate collagenous tissue investing the nerve (endoneurium) becomes continuous with the endomysium of the muscle fibre (not illustrated).

Each of the terminal swellings of the cluster making up the motor end plate has the same basic structure as the synapse shown in Figure 7.8, but the postsynaptic membrane of the neuromuscular junction is deeply folded to form parallel **secondary synaptic clefts**. The overlying presynaptic membrane is also irregular and the cytoplasm

immediately adjacent contains numerous synaptic vesicles. The remaining cytoplasm of the terminal bulb contains many mitochondria and a membrane compartment for recycling secretory vesicles. The sole plate of the muscle fibre also contains a concentration of mitochondria and an aggregation of muscle cell nuclei.

The neurotransmitter of somatic neuromuscular junctions is acetycholine, the receptors for which are concentrated at the margins of the secondary synaptic clefts. The hydrolytic enzyme acetylcholinesterase is present deeper in the clefts associated with the external lamina and is involved in deactivation of the neurotransmitter between successive nerve impulses. The histochemical technique shown in micrograph (d) defines the location of motor end plates by demonstrating acetylcholinesterase activity which appears as a brown deposit.

Micrograph (e) demonstrates the ultrastructure of a motor end plate, the terminal bouton **TB** typically lying in a depression in the skeletal muscle surface and invested externally by Schwann cell cytoplasm **S** and its external lamina **L**. Note the uniform width of the primary synaptic cleft **C₁** and the branching nature of the numerous secondary synaptic clefts **C₂**. The underlying cytoplasm is packed with mitochondria **M**. Myofibrils **Mf** are seen in transverse section at the lower right of the field. The terminal bouton contains numerous synaptic vesicles **V** of uniform size, other membranous elements representing part of the endoplasmic reticulum and a few mitochondria.

BASIC TISSUE TYPES

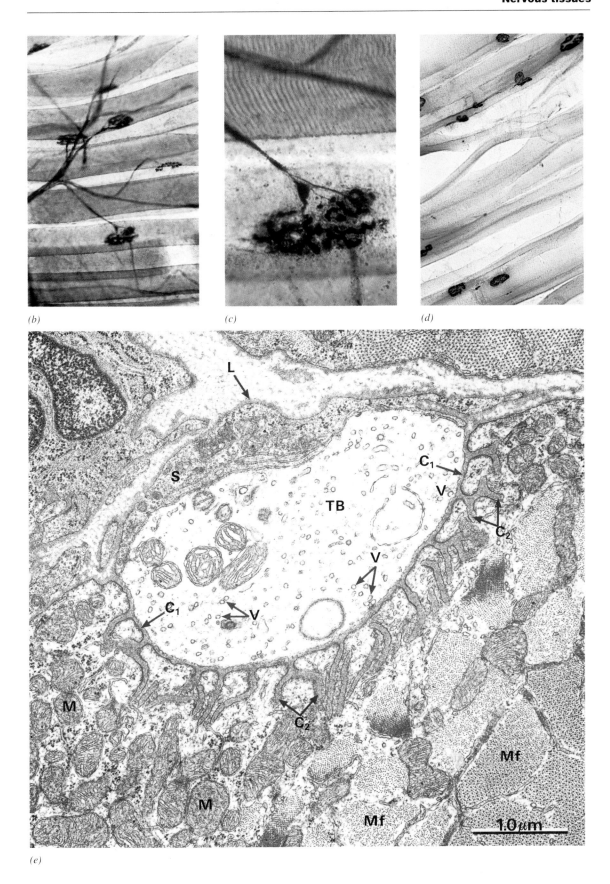

(b)

(c)

(d)

(e)

Peripheral nervous tissues

Peripheral nerves are anatomical structures which may contain any combination of afferent or efferent nerve fibres of either the somatic or autonomic nervous systems. The cell bodies of fibres coursing in peripheral nerves are located either in the CNS or in ganglia in peripheral sites.

Each peripheral nerve is composed of one or more bundles (*fascicles*) of nerve fibres. Within the fascicles, each individual nerve fibre, with its investing Schwann cell, is surrounded by a delicate packing of loose vascular supporting tissue called *endoneurium*. Each fascicle is surrounded by a condensed layer of robust collagenous tissue invested by a layer of flat epithelial cells called the *perineurium*. In peripheral nerves consisting of more than one fascicle, a further layer of loose collagenous tissue called the *epineurium* binds the fascicles together and is condensed peripherally to form a strong cylindrical sheath. Peripheral nerves receive a rich blood supply via numerous penetrating vessels from surrounding tissues and accompanying arteries. Larger vessels course longitudinally within the compartments bounded by the perineurium and epineurium with a rich capillary network in the endoneurium. Extensive anastomoses ensure adequate supply under normal circumstances although this can be put at risk during surgical procedures if too great a length of nerve is dissected from surrounding structures.

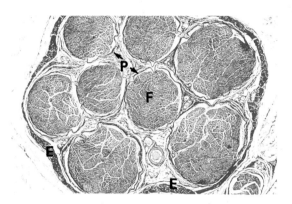

Fig. 7.13 **Peripheral nerve** van Gieson × 20

This micrograph illustrates the typical appearance of a medium-sized peripheral nerve in transverse section. This specimen consists of eight fascicles **F**, each of which contains many nerve fibres. Each fascicle is invested by seven to eight concentric layers of flattened epithelial cells separated by condensed layers of collagen, the perineurium **P**, and the nerve as a whole is encased in a loose collagenous tissue sheath, the epineurium **E**, which is condensed at its outermost aspect. Blood vessels of various sizes can be seen in the epineurial connective tissue.

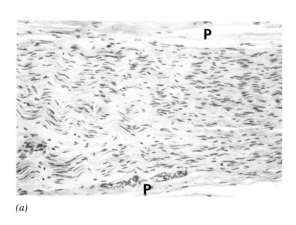

(a)

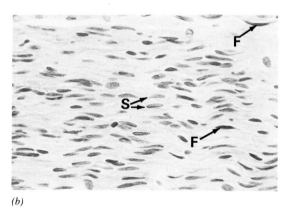

(b)

Fig. 7.14 **Peripheral nerve** (a) H & E × 128 (b) H & E × 320

The peripheral nerve shown in longitudinal section in micrograph (a) consists of a single fascicle invested by the perineurium **P**. Most of the nuclei seen within the fascicle are those of Schwann cells which mark the course of individual axons; axons are not readily visible in this type of preparation. Fibroblasts of the endoneurium are scattered amongst the much more numerous Schwann cells. A striking feature of peripheral nerves is that the fibres follow a zigzag longitudinal course which permits stretching during movement.

At higher magnification in micrograph (b), Schwann cell nuclei **S** are seen to be elongated in the long axis of the nerve. The relatively sparse fibroblasts **F** are distinguished by their more slender, condensed nuclei.

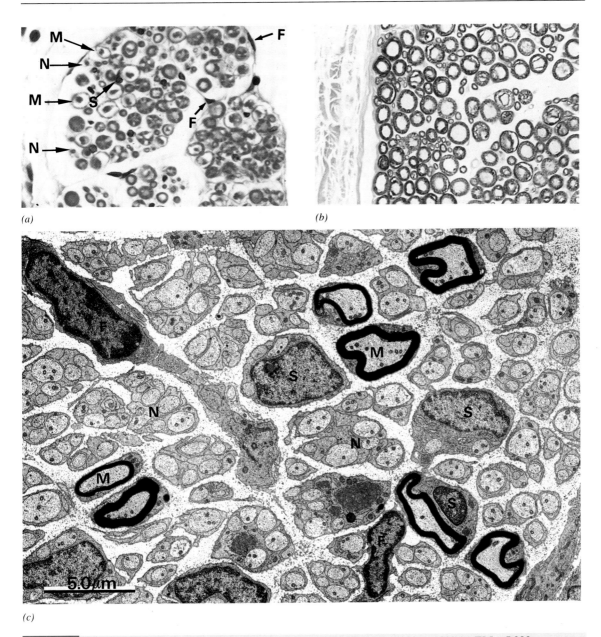

(a)

(b)

(c)

Fig. 7.15 **Peripheral nerve** (a) H & E × 480 (b) Osmium fixation, van Gieson × 800 (c) EM × 5 000

In routinely fixed and stained preparations, myelin is poorly preserved since it is largely composed of lipid material. Schwann cell cytoplasm is, however, well-preserved and has eosinophilic staining properties.

Micrograph (a) shows a peripheral nerve cut transversely and stained with H & E; the nerve contains axons of many different types and calibre, some of which are myelinated. Heavily myelinated fibres **M** can be identified by an unstained ring representing the myelin sheath, the centrally located axon and peripheral rim of Schwann cell cytoplasm being stained pink. Small non-myelinated fibres **N** can also be easily identified. Between these extremes are fibres of various sizes with 'bubbly', artefactually distorted myelin sheaths. Note the nuclei of Schwann cells **S** distributed among the nerve fibres. Several flattened nuclei **F** are also seen in the perineurium.

In osmium fixed preparations as shown in micrograph (b), the lipid constituents of myelin are well preserved and are stained black. Note the wide variation in axon diameter. The collagen of the delicate endoneurium between the individual nerve fibres and in the condensed perineurium surrounding the fascicle is stained red by the van Gieson method.

The ultrastructural features of a typical peripheral nerve are seen in micrograph (c); it contains both myelinated axons **M** and more numerous non-myelinated axons **N**, both ensheathed by Schwann cells **S**. The endoneurium mainly consists of loosely arranged collagen fibrils (difficult to identify at this magnification) lying parallel to the nerve fibres. The nuclei of two fibroblasts **F** can be identified and fibroblast processes extend through the endoneurium.

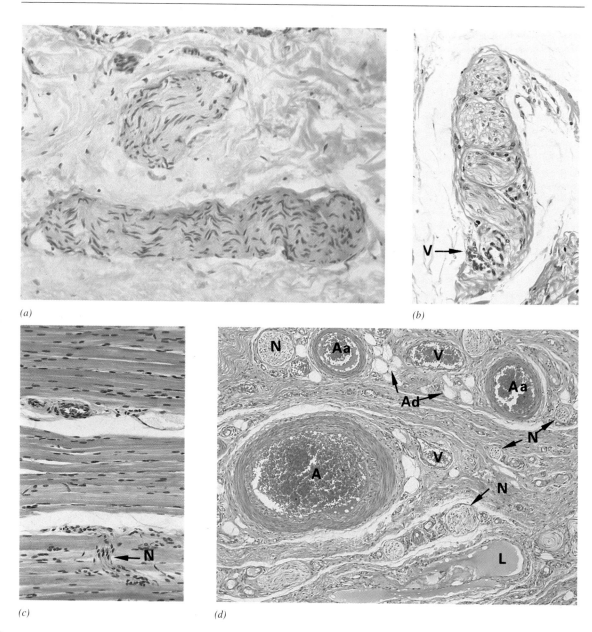

(a)

(b)

(c)

(d)

Fig. 7.16 **Small peripheral nerves**
(a) H & E × 480 (b) Masson's trichrome × 320 (c) Masson's trichrome × 100 (d) H & E × 150

These micrographs illustrate the appearance of a variety of small peripheral nerves in the tissues.

Micrograph (a) shows two small nerves in the dermis of the skin, each nerve consisting of a single fascicle of fibres. The nerve at the bottom of the field is cut in longitudinal section; the wavy shape of the Schwann cell nuclei reflects the course of the axons which are thereby protected from damage when the skin is stretched. The nerve in the upper part of the field is cut in oblique section. Note the dense irregular collagenous dermal tissue surrounding the nerves in this specimen.

Micrograph (b) shows a very small peripheral nerve in the loose fatty hypodermis of the skin. In contrast to the first specimen, with this technique collagen is stained

blue-green. This nerve runs a zigzag course in the skin and the plane of section has cut it in such a way as to show it in four transverse-oblique views. Note small associated blood vessels **V** containing red stained erythrocytes.

Micrograph (c) shows a tiny nerve bundle **N** (probably a motor nerve) in skeletal muscle. A nerve bundle of this size would be almost unrecognisable but for its numerous Schwann cell nuclei.

Finally, a neurovascular bundle from the vulva is the subject of micrograph (d). It contains a small artery **A**, arterioles **Aa**, venules **V**, a lymphatic **L**, several small peripheral nerves **N** cut in transverse section and scattered adipocytes **Ad**.

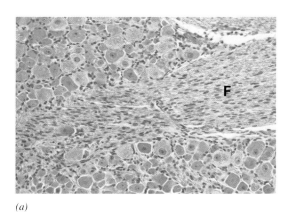

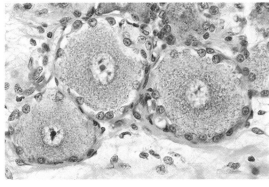

(a)   (b)

Fig. 7.17   Spinal ganglion   (a) H & E × 128 (b) H & E × 800

Ganglia are discrete aggregations of neurone cell bodies located outside the CNS. The spinal ganglia lie on the posterior nerve roots of the spinal cord as they pass through the intervertebral foramina; they contain the cell bodies of primary sensory neurones which are of the pseudo-unipolar form (see Fig. 7.2).

At low magnification in micrograph (a), note the fascicle **F** of nerve fibres passing to the centre of the ganglion, the ganglion cells being located peripherally.

At high magnification in micrograph (b), each cell body is seen to be surrounded by a layer of flattened *satellite cells* which provide structural and metabolic support and have similar embryological origin to the Schwann cells (neural crest).

The whole ganglion is encapsulated by condensed supporting tissue which is continuous with the perineurial and epineurial sheaths of the associated peripheral nerve.

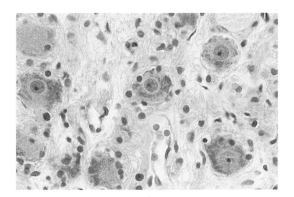

Fig. 7.18   Sympathetic ganglion   H & E × 400

Sympathetic ganglia have a similar structure to that of somatic sensory ganglia with a few minor differences. The ganglion cells are multipolar and thus more widely spaced, being separated by numerous axons and dendrites, many of which pass through the ganglion without being involved in synapses. As seen in this micrograph, the nuclei of the ganglion cells tend to be eccentrically located and the peripheral cytoplasm contains a variable quantity of brown stained lipofuscin granules representing cellular debris sequestered in residual bodies. The satellite cells are smaller in number and irregularly placed due to the numerous dendritic processes of the ganglion cells.

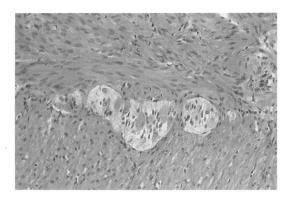

Fig. 7.19   Parasympathetic ganglion
H & E × 320

The cell bodies of the terminal effector neurones of the parasympathetic nervous system are usually located within or near the effector organs. The cell bodies may form well-organised ganglia of moderate size (as in the otic ganglion) but more commonly a few cell bodies are clumped together to form tiny ganglia scattered in the supporting tissue.

This micrograph shows a minute ganglion between two smooth muscle layers in the wall of the gastrointestinal tract. Like all neurones, the ganglion cells are recognised by their large nuclei, with dispersed chromatin and prominent nucleoli, and extensive basophilic cytoplasm. As in other ganglia, the neurones are surrounded by numerous small support cells and afferent and efferent nerve fibres.

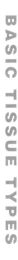

BASIC TISSUE TYPES

Central nervous tissues

The central nervous system consists of the brain and spinal cord, each of which can be divided macroscopically into areas of **grey matter** and **white matter**. Grey matter contains almost all the neurone cell bodies and their associated fibres (axons). White matter consists of tracts of nerve fibres in which a substantial number of the axons are myelinated, myelin appearing white in fresh tissue.

Central nervous tissue consists of a vast number of neurones and their processes embedded in a mass of support cells, collectively known as **neuroglia**, which comprise all the non-neural cells of the CNS. Central nervous tissue proper is devoid of collagenous supporting tissue which is confined to the immediate vicinity of penetrating blood vessels and to the **meninges** which invest the outer surface of the brain. The neuroglia, which form almost half the total mass of the CNS, are highly branched cells which occupy the spaces between neurones; the CNS contains little extracellular material. The neuroglia have intimate functional relationships with neurones providing both mechanical and metabolic support.

Four principal types of neuroglia are recognised: **oligodendrocytes, astrocytes, microglia** and **ependymal cells**. Oligodendrocytes are the CNS equivalent of the Schwann cells of the peripheral nervous system and are responsible for the elaboration of myelin sheaths in the CNS. Astrocytes are highly branched cells which pack the interstices between the neurones, their processes and oligodendrocytes. They provide mechanical support as well as mediating the exchange of metabolites between neurones and the vascular system. They also form part of the blood–brain barrier. Astrocytes also play an important role in repair of CNS tissue after injury or damage by disease. Microglia are the CNS representatives of the monocyte–macrophage system and have defence and immunological functions. Ependymal cells make up a specialised epithelium which lines the ventricles and spinal canal.

Although each functional zone of the CNS has its own peculiar histological appearance, the basic organisation of grey and white matter remains consistent throughout; only the principles of organisation are discussed in this chapter. The various regions of the central nervous system are the subject of Chapter 20.

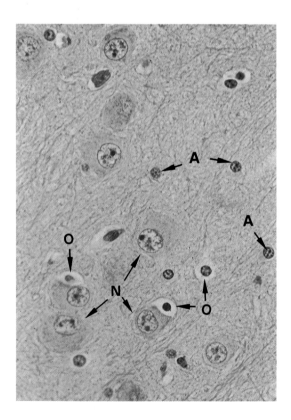

Fig. 7.20 **Grey matter** H & E × 480

Common staining methods usually permit neurones **N** to be readily distinguished from glial cells. Although the size and morphology of neurones vary greatly in different regions of the brain, they are usually recognisable by their large nuclei, with prominent nucleoli and dispersed chromatin, and extensive basophilic granular cytoplasm, one or more processes of which may be visible.

Neuroglia are difficult to differentiate with certainty by common staining methods. In the mature CNS, as in this specimen, oligodendroglia have small round condensed nuclei; their cytoplasm is unstained by routine methods including H & E. As described later, in grey matter oligodendrocytes are not only scattered between the nerve cell bodies along with the astrocytes but also tend to be aggregated around the neurone cell bodies. Thus the cells marked **O** can be presumed to be oligodendrocytes. Others marked **A** are probably astrocytes.

The nuclei of both neurones and neuroglia are surrounded by a feltwork of axons and dendrites arising from and converging upon the neurones. This is described as the **neuropil**. Most neuropil fibres are devoid of myelin (being so close to the neurone cell bodies) accounting for the eosinophilia of neuropil.

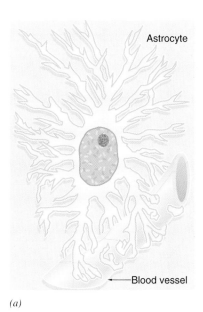

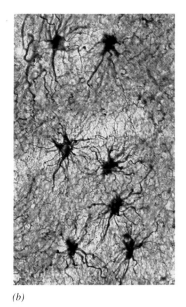

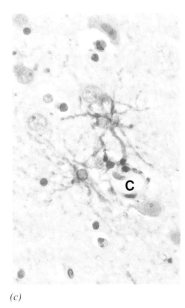

(a) (b) (c)

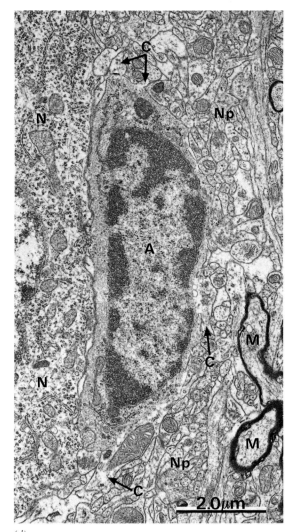

2.0 μm

(d)

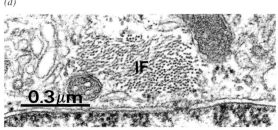

0.3 μm

(e)

Fig. 7.21 **Astrocytes** (a) Diagram
(b) Cajal method × 400 (c) Immunoperoxidase
method for glial fibrillary acidic protein × 400
(d) EM × 12 000 (e) EM × 57 500

Classical heavy metal impregnation methods such as that seen in micrograph (b) identify the presence of star-shaped neuroglia, the astrocytes. These cells, which are the most numerous glial cells in grey matter, have long branched processes which occupy most of the interneuronal spaces. In grey matter, many of the astrocyte processes end in terminal expansions adjacent to the non-synaptic regions of neurones. Other processes of the same astrocytes terminate upon the basement membranes of capillaries, these *perivascular feet* covering most of the surface of the capillary basement membranes. Similar foot processes invest the basement membrane that lies between the CNS and the innermost layer of the meninges, the pia mater (see Fig. 7.26) forming a relatively impermeable barrier called the *glia limitans*.

In grey matter, astrocytes thus mediate metabolic exchange between neurones and blood and regulate the composition of the intercellular environment of the CNS.

All astrocytes contain bundles of intracellular filaments and microtubules. These are particularly prominent in the astrocytes of white matter which have relatively few, straight cytoplasmic processes and are known as *fibrous astrocytes*. By contrast, those of grey matter have numerous short highly branched cytoplasmic processes and are described as *protoplasmic astrocytes*. The intermediate filaments consist of a protein characteristic of astrocytes called *glial fibrillary acidic protein* (*GFAP*) which is demonstrated in micrograph (c); note the capillary **C** being embraced by astrocytic perivascular feet.

Micrograph (d) shows an astrocyte **A** lying adjacent to a nerve cell body **N** in the cerebral cortex. The astrocyte cytoplasm contains many ribosomes, a little rough ER, and a few small mitochondria and lysosomes. The origins of several cytoplasmic extensions **C** can be identified. The cytoplasm appears moderately electron-dense due to its content of intermediate filaments **IF**, which can be seen at higher magnification in micrograph (e). Typically of CNS grey matter, the adjacent neuropil **Np** contains numerous neuronal and glial processes in various planes of section; some myelinated axons **M** are included in the field.

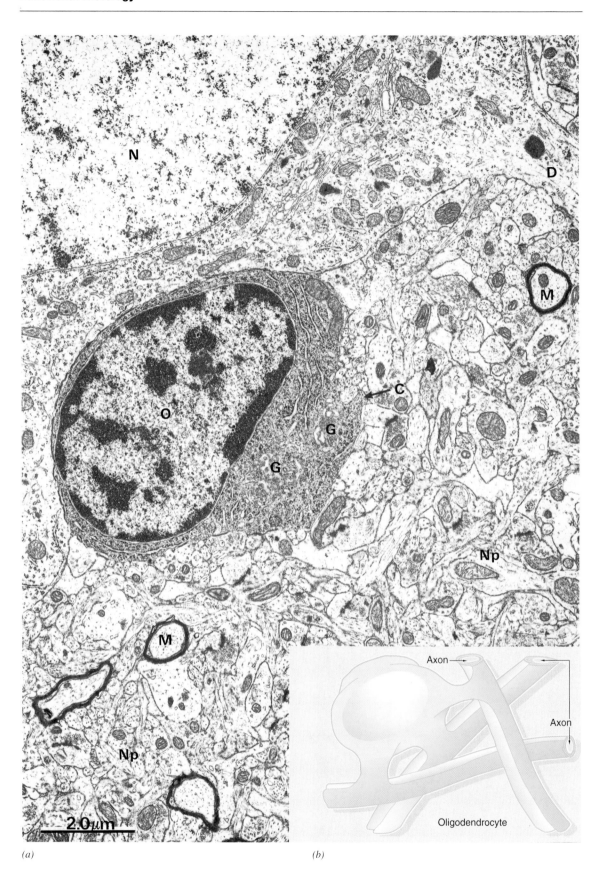

(a)   *(b)*

Fig. 7.22 **Oligodendrocytes** *(illustrations opposite)* **(a) EM × 13 000 (b) Schematic diagram**

Oligodendrocytes were named by the early neurohistologists using classical heavy metal impregnation methods which showed that they had a small number of short, branched processes (Greek: *oligos* = few, *dendron* = tree). It is now known that oligodendrocytes are the cells responsible for myelination of axons in the CNS and the dendrites previously described are the short pedicles that connect the cell body to the myelin sheaths.

In fact, a single oligodendrocyte can contribute to the myelination of up to 50 axons which may belong to the same or different fibre tracts. Conversely, any one axon will require the services of numerous different oligodendrocytes since the myelin internodes along its length are synthesised by different cells. The mechanism of myelin sheath formation is very similar to that of Schwann cells in peripheral nerve (see Fig. 7.6). Oligodendrocytes are thus the predominant type of neuroglia in white matter as well as being abundant in grey matter. Oligodendrocytes also aggregate closely around nerve cell bodies in the grey matter where they are thought to have a support function analogous to that of the satellite cells which surround nerve cell bodies in peripheral ganglia (see Fig. 7.17).

Myelin sheath formation begins in the CNS of the human embryo at about 4 months gestational age with the formation of most sheaths at least commenced by about the age of 1 year. From this time, successive layers continue to be laid down, with final myelin sheath thickness being achieved by the time of physical maturity.

Three types of oligodendrocytes are described, namely *light*, *medium* and *dark* oligodendrocytes according to their staining density with special light microscopic methods and electron microscopy. Light oligodendrocytes are capable of cell division and are highly active in myelin sheath formation and thus predominate in the fetus and neonate, whereas dark oligodendrocytes are the main form in the mature CNS. Medium oligodendrocytes represent the immature form involved in myelin sheath growth and maturation. Some light and medium forms are found in the mature CNS, suggesting that there is some slow constant cell turnover and capacity for remyelination should the need arise (e.g. after demyelinating diseases such as multiple sclerosis). Reflecting their intense biosynthetic activity, light oligodendrocytes are relatively large cells with dispersed nuclear chromatin and prominent nucleoli. The cytoplasm contains numerous ribosomes, microtubules and a large Golgi apparatus. In contrast, the dark oligodendrocyte is smaller with a condensed nucleus. This micrograph shows an intermediate oligodendrocyte **O** lying adjacent to a nerve cell body **N** with a neuronal dendrite **D** at the upper right. The oligodendrocyte contains prominent rough endoplasmic reticulum, ribosomes and Golgi stacks **G**. The commencement of one cytoplasmic process **C** is seen. The remainder of the field shows the complexity of the neuropil **Np** comprising glial and neuronal processes, including some myelinated axons **M**.

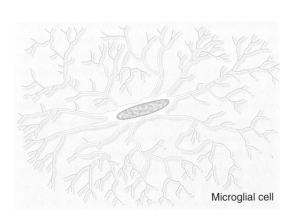

Microglial cell

Fig. 7.23 **Microglia**

Microglia are small cells, derived from cells of mesenchymal origin which invade the CNS at a late stage of fetal development. Microglia have small elongated irregular nuclei and relatively little cytoplasm which forms fine, highly branched processes. In consequence, they are difficult to identify in conventional preparations for light microscopy. In response to tissue damage, microglia transform into large amoeboid phagocytic cells and are thus considered to be the CNS representatives of the macrophage–monocyte defence system (see Fig. 3.12).

In normal circumstances there is only a very small traffic of lymphocytes through the CNS, but this is greatly increased with inflammatory diseases. Considerable numbers of macrophages are, however, present in the space surrounding the CNS capillaries but separated from the CNS compartment proper by the perivascular feet of astrocytes.

Fig. 7.24 **Ependyma** **H & E × 400**

Ependymal cells form the simple epithelial lining of the ventricles and spinal canal. Cuboidal or low columnar in shape, the cells are tightly bound together at their luminal surfaces by the usual epithelial junctional complexes. Unlike other epithelia, however, ependymal cells do not rest on a basement membrane but, rather, the bases of the cells taper and then break up into fine branches which ramify into an underlying layer of processes derived from astrocytes. At the luminal surface, there is a variable number of cilia, which may be involved in propulsion of cerebrospinal fluid within the ventricles. Microvilli are also present and probably have absorptive and secretory functions. It has recently been suggested that some ependymal cells may be stem cells in the adult CNS.

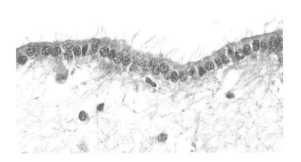

BASIC TISSUE TYPES

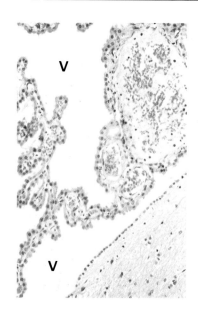

Fig. 7.25 Choroid plexus H & E × 128

The choroid plexus is a vascular structure arising from the wall of each of the four ventricles of the brain and responsible for the production of cerebrospinal fluid (CSF). CSF drains from the interconnected ventricular cavities via three channels connecting the fourth ventricle with the subarachnoid space which surrounds the CNS. CSF is produced at a constant rate and is reabsorbed from the subarachnoid space into the superior sagittal venous sinus via finger-like projections called *arachnoid villi*. Thus the CNS is suspended in a constantly circulating fluid medium which acts as a shock absorber.

Each choroid plexus consists of a mass of capillaries projecting into the ventricle **V** and invested by modified ependymal cells which are separated from the underlying capillaries and delicate supporting tissue by a basement membrane. Long, bulbous microvilli project from the luminal surfaces of the choroid epithelial cells and the cytoplasm contains numerous mitochondria, features which suggest that the elaboration of CSF is an active process. The capillaries of the choroid plexus are large, thin-walled and sometimes fenestrated. The mode of CSF secretion involves active secretion of sodium ions by choroid epithelial cells into the CSF, followed by passive movement of water from the choroid capillaries. Continuous tight junctions (zonula occludens) from a *blood–CSF barrier* preventing ingress of almost all other molecules. Glucose (at about 70% plasma concentration) and small amounts of proteins are normal constituents of CSF but the mode of their passage into the CSF is unknown.

The brain and spinal cord are invested by three layers of supporting tissue collectively called the meninges. The surface of the nervous tissue is covered by a delicate layer called the *pia mater* containing collagen fibres, fine elastin fibres and occasional fibroblasts separated from the processes of underlying astrocytes by a basement membrane. The basement membrane is completely invested by astrocytic processes, the two layers forming the impermeable glia limitans (see also Fig. 7.21). Overlying the pia mater is a thicker fibrous layer, the *arachnoid mater*, which derives its name from the presence of cobweb-like strands which connect it to the underlying pia mater; since the pia and arachnoid are structurally continuous, they are often considered as a single unit, the *pia-arachnoid* or *leptomeninges*. The space between the pia and arachnoid layers is called the *subarachnoid space* and in places forms large cisterns. The subarachnoid space is connected with the ventricular system by three foramina and CSF circulates continuously from the ventricles into the subarachnoid space. The subarachnoid space (i.e. apposed surfaces of the pia and arachnoid layers, and their interconnecting fibres) is lined by flattened arachnoidal cells. The outer surface of the arachnoid mater is also lined by flat cells.

As shown in the diagram, arteries and veins passing to and from the CNS pass in the subarachnoid space loosely attached to the pia mater and invested by subarachnoid mesothelium. As the larger vessels extend into the nervous tissue, they are surrounded by a delicate sleeve of pia mater. Between the penetrating vessels and the pia there is a *perivascular space* which is continuous with the subarachnoid space in some animals but not in humans. In humans, the epithelium of the pia blends with the adventitia of the vessel as it penetrates the brain, separating the perivascular space from the subarachnoid space.

External to the arachnoid mater is a dense fibroelastic layer called the *dura mater* which is lined on its internal surface by flat cells. The dura is closely applied to, but not connected with, the arachnoid layer and a potential space, the *subdural space*, can develop between the two layers. In the cranium, the dura mater merges with the periosteum of the skull, whereas around the spinal cord the dura is suspended from the periosteum of the spinal canal by the *denticulate ligaments*, the intervening *epidural space* being filled with loose, fibrofatty tissue and a venous plexus.

The pia and arachnoid layers of the brain meninges are illustrated in micrographs (b) and (c), the dura mater typically remaining adherent to the skull when the brain is removed from the cranial cavity. The pia mater **P** is attached to the surface of the brain and continues into the sulci **S** and around the penetrating vessels. The arachnoid mater **A** appears to be a completely separate layer and bridges the sulci. Meningeal vessels lie in the subarachnoid space. At high magnification in micrograph (c), delicate fibrous strands **F** can be discerned traversing the subarachnoid space **SS** to connect the pia and arachnoid layers. Two small vessels **V** can be seen in the subarachnoid space. A penetrating vessel is also seen surrounded by a perivascular space **PVS**. The perivascular space is extremely narrow although it often appears artefactually wider as in this micrograph. The CNS contains no lymphatics and interstitial fluid is thought to drain outwards from the brain substance to join the subarachnoid CSF via the perivascular spaces and to contribute as much as 20% of its volume.

As seen in micrograph (d), the capillaries of the CNS are similar to those elsewhere in the body with flattened endothelial cells resting on a basement membrane. The endothelial cells are not fenestrated and are bound together by continuous tight intercellular junctions (zonula occludens) except in the choroid plexus where this is discontinuous. Externally, the basement

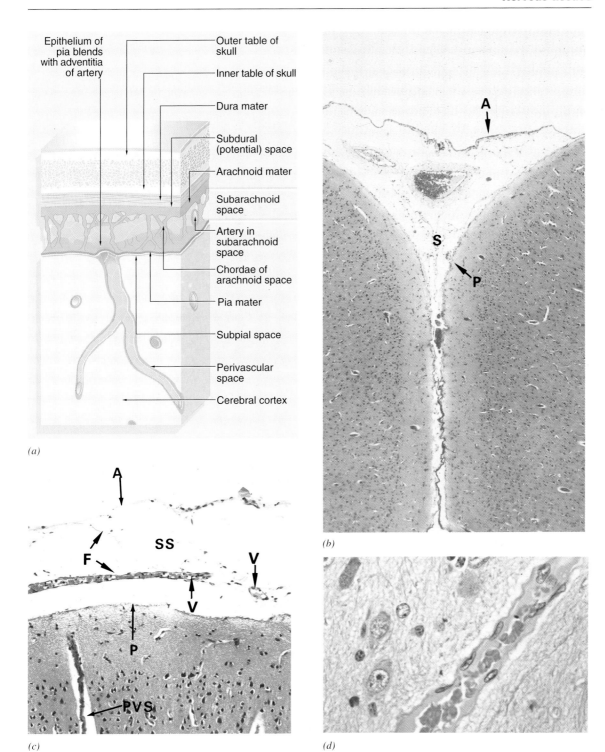

(a)

(b)

(c)

(d)

membranes are completely covered by the perivascular foot processes of astrocytes (see Fig. 7.21). A thin layer of the pia mater extends down into the CNS around smaller arteries, veins, arterioles and venules but is not present around the capillaries of the CNS.

Perfusion studies show that the CNS capillaries are impermeable to certain plasma constituents, especially larger molecules, forming a ***blood–brain barrier***. The capillary endothelium plays the central role since junctions between endothelial cells are sealed; the endothelial cells exhibit little or no pinocytosis. Luminal surface membranes contain various enzymes which

destroy neurotoxic metabolites and neuroactive humoral substances. Maintenance of barrier-type endothelium appears to be under the control of astrocyte foot processes. The blood–brain barrier provides neurones with a relatively constant biochemical and metabolic environment, protection against endogenous and exogenous toxins and infective agents and insulates the neurones from circulating neurotransmitters and other humoral agents. The capillaries of the choroid plexus, the pituitary and pineal glands and the vomiting centre of the hypothalamus are, however, devoid of this barrier as befits their various functions.

Sensory receptors

Sensory receptors are nerve endings or specialised cells which convert (transduce) stimuli from the external or internal environments into afferent nerve impulses; the impulses pass into the CNS where they initiate appropriate voluntary or involuntary responses.

No classification system for sensory receptors has yet been devised which adequately incorporates either functional or morphological features. A widely used functional classification divides sensory receptors into three groups: *exteroceptors, proprioceptors* and *interoceptors*. Exteroceptors are those which respond to stimuli from outside the body and include receptors for touch, light pressure, deep pressure, cutaneous pain, temperature, smell, taste, sight and hearing. Proprioceptors are located within the skeletal system and provide conscious and unconscious information about orientation, skeletal position, tension and movement; such receptors include the vestibular apparatus of the ear, tendon organs and neuromuscular spindles. Interoceptors respond to stimuli from the viscera and include the chemoreceptors of blood, vascular (pressure) baro-receptors, the receptors for the state of distension of hollow viscera such as the gastrointestinal tract and urinary bladder, and receptors for such nebulous senses as visceral pain, hunger, thirst, well-being and malaise.

The structure of the receptors involved in some of these sensory modalities is poorly understood. Sensory receptors may be classified morphologically into two groups, *simple* and *compound*. Simple receptors are merely free, branched or unbranched nerve endings such as those responsible for cutaneous pain and temperature; they are rarely visible with the light microscope unless special staining methods are employed. Compound receptors involve organisation of associated non-neural tissues to complement the function of the neural receptors. The degree of organisation may range from mere encapsulation to highly sophisticated arrangements such as in the eye and ear. By tradition, the eye, ear and receptors for the senses of smell and taste are described as the *organs of special sense*; they are the subject of Chapter 21.

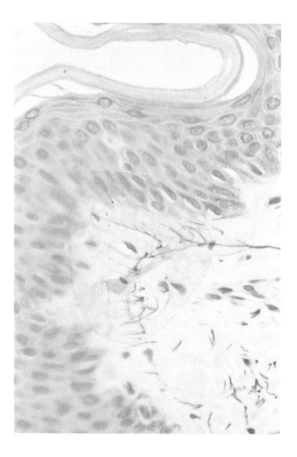

Fig. 7.27 Free nerve endings
Silver/haematoxylin × 480

Free nerve endings are the simplest form of sensory receptor, merely consisting of numerous small terminal branches of afferent nerve fibres. Such free nerve endings are found in supporting tissues throughout the body subserving a variety of relatively unsophisticated sensory modalities such as temperature, touch and pain. The afferent fibres are of relatively small diameter with slow rates of conduction; although some of these fibres are myelinated, the nerve endings are devoid of myelin.

In the skin, free nerve endings are found along the dermo-epidermal junction. Some exhibit a terminal expansion which is intimately associated with non-neuronal cells called *Merkel cells* scattered in the basal layers of the epidermis (see Fig. 9.4). The adjacent Merkel cell cytoplasm contains vesicles with ultrastructural features similar to those found in synapses but no neurotransmitter has yet been demonstrated. Merkel nerve endings are served by large-diameter myelinated fibres and are thought to be responsible for the sensation of touch. A variety of different arrangements of free nerve endings is also incorporated in the follicles of fine and coarse hairs acting as touch receptors, the most sophisticated type being those associated with the whiskers of animals such as cats and rodents.

This thick section of skin stained by a heavy metal impregnation method shows a nerve fibre with many fine terminal branches extending as free nerve endings into the dermo-epidermal junction; Merkel cells cannot be readily identified.

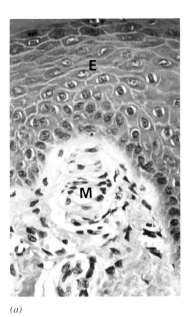

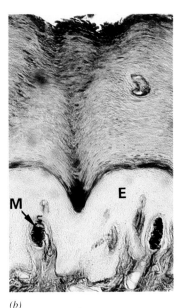

(a)   *(b)*

Fig. 7.28   **Meissner's corpuscles** (a) H & E × 320 (b) Silver method × 150

Meissner's corpuscles are small, encapsulated, sensory receptors found in the dermis of the skin, particularly of the fingertips, soles of the feet, nipples, eyelids, lips and genitalia. They are involved in the reception of light discriminatory touch, the degree of discrimination depending on the proximity of receptors to one another.

As seen in micrograph (a), Meissner's corpuscles **M** are oval in shape and are usually located in the dermal papillae immediately beneath the epidermis **E**. The receptors consist of a delicate collagenous tissue capsule surrounding a mass of plump, oval cells arranged transversely and probably representing specialised Schwann cells. Non-myelinated branches of large myelinated sensory fibres ramify throughout the cell mass in a helical manner as shown by the heavy metal impregnation technique in micrograph (b).

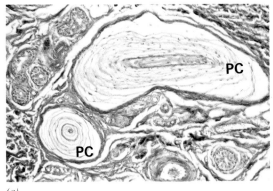

(a)

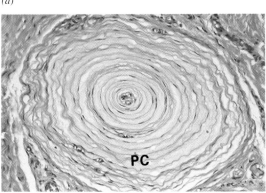

(b)

Fig. 7.29   **Pacinian corpuscles** (a) Masson's trichrome × 80 (b) H & E × 100

Pacinian corpuscles **PC** are large encapsulated sensory receptors responsive to pressure or coarse touch, vibration and tension, and are found in the deeper layers of the skin, ligaments and joint capsules, in some serous membranes, mesenteries, some viscera and in some erogenous areas.

Pacinian corpuscles range from 1 to 4 mm in length and in section have the appearance of an onion. These organs consist of a delicate capsule enclosing many concentric lamellae of flattened cells (probably modified Schwann cells) separated by interstitial fluid spaces and delicate collagen fibres. Towards the centre of the corpuscle the lamellae become closely packed and the core contains a single large unbranched non-myelinated nerve fibre with several club-like terminals which becomes myelinated as it leaves the corpuscle. Distortion of the Pacinian corpuscle produces an amplified mechanical stimulus in the core which is transduced into an action potential in the sensory neurone.

Two other simple encapsulated mechanoreceptors are described. *Ruffini corpuscles* are robust spindle-shaped structures found particularly in the soles of the feet. *Krause end bulbs* are delicate receptors found in the lining of the oropharynx and the conjunctiva of the eye.

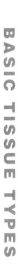

BASIC TISSUE TYPES

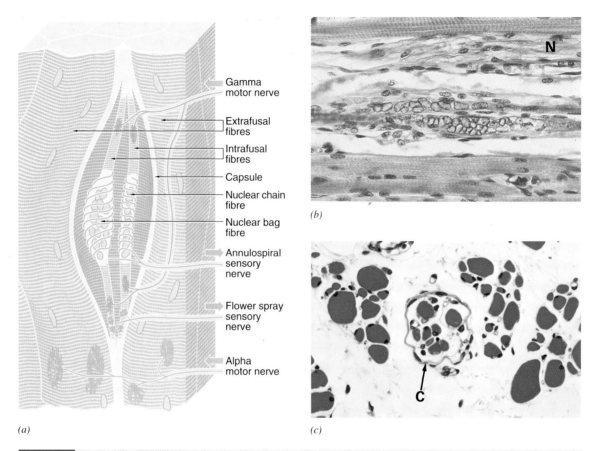

(a)

(b)

(c)

Fig. 7.30 **Neuromuscular spindle**
(a) Schematic diagram (b) LS, H & E × 320 (c) TS, Masson's trichrome × 320

Neuromuscular spindles are stretch receptor organs within skeletal muscles which are responsible for the regulation of muscle tone via the spinal stretch reflex. These receptors are particularly numerous in muscles involved in fine, precision movements such as the intrinsic muscles of the hand and the external muscles of the eye.

Neuromuscular spindles are encapsulated, lymph filled, fusiform structures up to 6 mm long but less than 1 mm in diameter. They lie parallel to the muscle fibres, embedded in endomysium or perimysium. Each spindle contains from two to 10 modified skeletal muscle fibres called *intrafusal fibres* which are much smaller than skeletal muscle fibres proper (*extrafusal fibres*). The intrafusal fibres have a central non-striated area in which their nuclei tend to be concentrated. Two types of intrafusal fibres are recognised. In one type, the central nuclear area is dilated, these fibres being known as *nuclear bag fibres*. In the other type, there is no dilatation and the nuclei are arranged in a single row giving rise to the name *nuclear chain fibres*.

Associated with both types of intrafusal fibres are sensory receptors of two types. Firstly, branched, non-myelinated endings of large, myelinated sensory fibres are wrapped around the central non-striated area of the intrafusal fibres forming *annulospiral endings*. Secondly, *flower-spray endings* of smaller, myelinated sensory fibres are located on the striated portions of the intrafusal fibres.

Together, these sensory receptors are stimulated by stretching of the intrafusal fibres which occurs when the extrafusal muscle mass is stretched. This stimulus evokes reflex contraction of the extrafusal muscle fibres via large (alpha) motor neurones of a simple two-neurone spinal reflex arc. Contraction of the extrafusal muscle mass thus removes the stretch stimulus from the intrafusal stretch receptors and equilibrium is restored.

The sensitivity of the neuromuscular spindle is modulated by higher centres via small (gamma) motor neurones arising from the extrapyramidal system. These gamma motor neurones innervate the striated portions of the intrafusal fibres thus controlling their state of contraction. Contraction of the intrafusal fibres increases the sensitivity of the intrafusal receptors to stretching of the extrafusal mass.

In any one histological section, it is impossible to demonstrate all the structural features of a neuromuscular spindle, but many of the features of the organ are shown in these micrographs. The most easily recognisable features are the discrete capsule **C** which is continuous with the endomysium of the surrounding muscle, best seen in micrograph (c), and the small size of the intrafusal muscle fibres compared with the surrounding extrafusal fibres. In micrograph (b), note the small bundle of nerve fibres **N** passing to and from the spindle.

ORGAN SYSTEMS

PART THREE

8. **Circulatory system** *144*

9. **Skin** *157*

10. **Skeletal tissues** *172*

11. **Immune system** *193*

12. **Respiratory system** *222*

13. **Oral tissues** *237*

14. **Gastrointestinal tract** *249*

15. **Liver and pancreas** *274*

16. **Urinary system** *286*

17. **The endocrine glands** *310*

18. **Male reproductive system** *328*

19. **Female reproductive system** *341*

20. **Central nervous system** *372*

21. **Special sense organs** *380*

Notes on staining techniques *406*

8. Circulatory system

Introduction

The circulatory system mediates the continuous movement of all body fluids, its principal functions being the transport of oxygen and nutrients to the tissues and transport of carbon dioxide and other metabolic waste products from the tissues. The circulatory system is also involved in temperature regulation and the distribution of molecules such as hormones and cells such as those of the immune system. The circulatory system has two functional components: the blood vascular system and the lymph vascular system.

The *blood vascular system* comprises a circuit of vessels through which flow of blood is maintained by continuous pumping of the heart. The *arterial system* provides a distribution network to the *capillaries* which are the main sites of interchange of gases and metabolites between the tissues and blood. The *venous system* returns blood from the capillaries to the heart. In contrast, the *lymph vascular system* is merely a passive drainage system for returning excess extravascular fluid, the *lymph*, to the blood vascular system. The lymph vascular system has no intrinsic pumping mechanism.

The whole circulatory system has a common basic structure:

- An inner lining comprising a single layer of extremely flattened epithelial cells called *endothelium* supported by a basement membrane and delicate collagenous tissue; this constitutes the *tunica intima*.
- An intermediate muscular layer, the *tunica media*.
- An outer supporting tissue layer called the *tunica adventitia*.

The tissues of the walls of large vessels cannot be sustained by diffusion of nutrients from their lumina and are thus supplied by small arteries called *vasa vasorum* (i.e. 'vessels of vessels') which are derived either from the main vessel itself or from adjacent arteries. The vasa vasorum give rise to a capillary network within the tunica adventitia which may extend into the tunica media.

The muscular layer exhibits the greatest variation from one part of the system to another. For example, it is totally absent in capillaries but comprises almost the whole mass of the heart. Blood flow is predominantly influenced by variation in activity of the muscular layer.

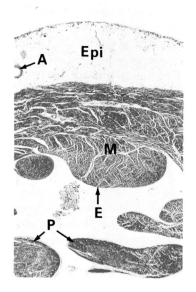

Fig. 8.1 Heart: wall of ventricle (monkey) Masson's trichrome × 20

This micrograph illustrates the three basic layers of the heart wall; monkey tissue has been chosen as that of human is too large to illustrate in this way. The tunica intima of the heart is called the *endocardium* **E** and is difficult to see at this magnification. The tunica media of the heart is called the *myocardium* **M** and is thickest in the ventricular walls. The myocardium is made up of cardiac muscle, the structure of which meets the unique functional requirements of the heart (see Ch. 6).

The tunica adventitia of the heart, the *epicardium* **Epi** (also called *visceral pericardium*), is surrounded by a potential space, the *pericardial cavity*, enclosed by a fibrous sac, the *pericardium* (the *parietal pericardium*), which is not shown in this micrograph. The parietal and visceral layers of the pericardium move freely against one another thus permitting relatively unimpeded movement of the heart.

Note a branch **A** of the coronary arterial system; these arteries represent the vasa vasorum of the heart. Note also *papillary muscles* **P** of the ventricle; these are extensions of the myocardium which, via the *chordae tendinae*, stabilise the cusps of the mitral and tricuspid valves.

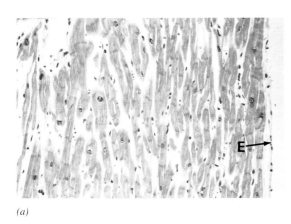

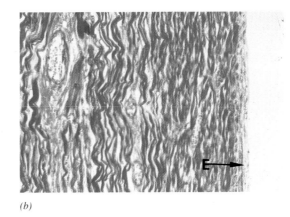

(a)   *(b)*

Fig. 8.2   **Heart: myocardium and endocardium**   (a) H & E × 128 (b) Masson's trichrome × 128

The endocardium, the innermost layer of the heart, consists of an endothelial lining and its supporting tissue. The endothelium **E** is a single layer of flattened epithelial cells, which is continuous with the endothelium of the vessels entering and leaving the heart. The endothelium is supported by a delicate layer of collagenous tissue beneath which lies a more robust fibroelastic layer; this accommodates movement of the myocardium without damage to the endothelium. The deepest aspect of the endocardium may also contain a small amount of adipose tissue.

The subendothelial tissue becomes continuous with the perimysium of the cardiac muscle; this is best demonstrated in micrograph (b) in which collagen is stained blue. The endocardium contains blood vessels, nerves and branches of the conducting system of the heart.

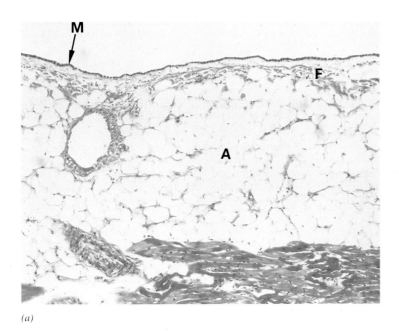

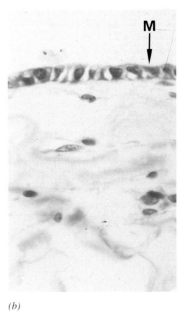

(a)   *(b)*

Fig. 8.3   **Heart: epicardium (visceral pericardium)**   (a) H & E × 200 (b) H & E × 480

The free surface of the epicardium consists of a single layer of flattened epithelial cells, the mesothelium **M**; a similar mesothelial layer lines the opposing parietal pericardial surface. The mesothelial cells secrete a small amount of serous fluid which lubricates the movement of the epicardium on the parietal pericardium.

A thin layer of fibroelastic tissue **F** supports the mesothelium; this layer is connected to the myocardium by a broad layer of adipose tissue **A**. The coronary vessels and autonomic nerves pass in the epicardium to supply the myocardium.

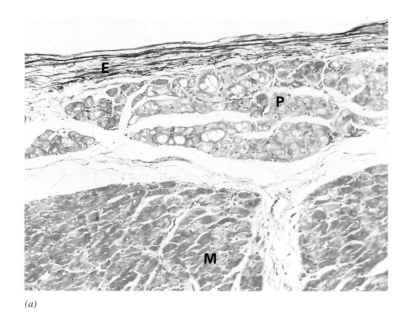

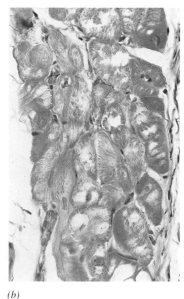

(a)   *(b)*

Fig. 8.4   **Purkinje fibres** (a) H & E/elastin × 150 (b) H & E/elastin × 400

The coordinated contraction of the myocardium during each pumping cycle is mediated by a specialised conducting system of modified cardiac muscle fibres. With each cardiac cycle, a wave of excitation originates in the pacemaker region of the right atrium, the *sinoatrial node*; the excitatory stimuli arise spontaneously at regular intervals, the rate being modulated by the autonomic nervous system. The wave of excitation spreads throughout the atria causing them to contract and thus forcing blood into the ventricles. By this time, the wave of excitation has spread to the *atrioventricular node* from which an excitatory stimulus is passed rapidly throughout the whole ventricular myocardium via the *atrioventricular bundle* or *bundle of His*. This bundle divides within the interventricular septum to give rise to smaller branches called *Purkinje fibres* which pass in the subendocardial supporting tissue before penetrating the ventricular myocardium. This system permits coordinated contraction of the entire ventricular myocardium.

The characteristics of the specialised muscle fibres of the conducting system are demonstrated in these

micrographs. Micrograph (a) illustrates the typical subendocardial location of a bundle of Purkinje fibres **P** and the darkly staining endocardial elastin **E**. Note the broad similarity of the Purkinje bundle to the adjacent myocardium **M**.

As seen in micrograph (b), the conducting cells are larger than myocardial cells and are sometimes binucleate. The extensive pale cytoplasm contains relatively few myofibrils which are arranged in an irregular manner immediately beneath the plasma membrane of the cell. The cytoplasm is rich in glycogen and mitochondria but, in contrast to other cardiac muscle cells, there is no T tubule system. Connections between the Purkinje cells are via desmosomes and gap junctions rather than by intercalated discs as in the rest of the myocardium.

The excitatory cells of the sinoatrial and atrioventricular nodes are small specialised myocardial fibres with electrochemical stimuli being transmitted via gap junctions. The cells contain little contractile protein or glycogen and are embedded in dense vascular collagenous tissue containing numerous autonomic nerve fibres.

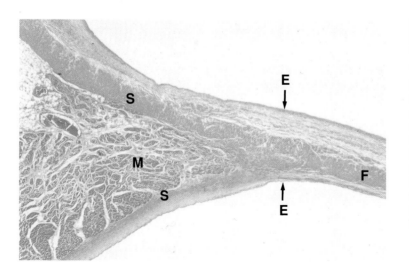

Fig. 8.5   **Heart valve**
H & E × 15

The valves of the heart consist of leaflets of collagenous tissue, the surfaces being invested with a thin endothelial layer continuous with that of the heart chambers and great vessels. This micrograph illustrates the base of a valve arising from the myocardium **M**. The tough central fibrous sheet, the *lamina fibrosa* **F**, represents a merging of the fibroelastic supporting layers **S** beneath the endothelium **E**.

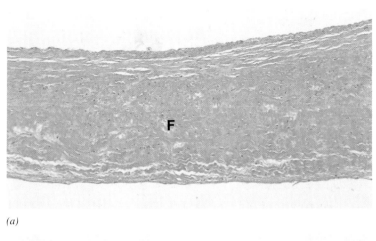

(a)

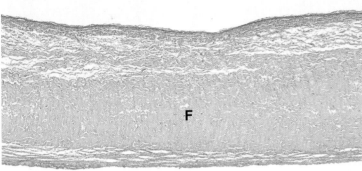

(b)

Fig. 8.6 Heart valve
(a) H & E × 60·
(b) Elastic van Gieson × 60

These sections from the same specimen of heart valve are stained by different methods. The standard H & E section in micrograph (a) highlights the dense collagenous tissue of the lamina fibrosa **F** forming the main bulk of the valve. Micrograph (b) demonstrates the considerable elastin content (stained black) which is particularly concentrated in the less dense subendothelial tissue.

At the attached margins of each valve, the lamina fibrosa becomes condensed to form a fibrous ring (valve annulus) and the rings of the four valves together form a central fibrous cardiac 'skeleton' which is continuous with the collagenous tissue of the myocardium, endocardium and epicardium. The mitral and tricuspid leaflets are connected to the papillary muscles by collagenous strands, the *chordae tendinae*, which also merge with the fibrous lamina of the valve leaflet.

The arterial system

The function of the arterial system is to distribute blood from the heart to capillary beds throughout the body. The cyclical pumping action of the heart produces a pulsatile blood flow in the arterial system. With each contraction of the ventricles (systole), blood is forced into the arterial system causing expansion of the arterial walls; subsequent recoil of the arterial walls assists in maintenance of arterial blood pressure between ventricular beats (diastole). This expansion and recoil is a function of elastic tissue within the walls of the arteries. The flow of blood to various organs and tissues may be regulated by varying the diameter of the distributing vessels. This function is performed by the circumferentially disposed smooth muscle of vessel walls and is principally under the control of the sympathetic nervous system and adrenal medullary hormones.

The walls of the arterial vessels conform to the general three-layered structure of the circulatory system but are characterised by the presence of considerable elastin and the smooth muscle wall is thick relative to the diameter of the lumen. There are three main types of vessel in the arterial system:

- **Elastic arteries**. These comprise the major distribution vessels and include the aorta, the innominate, common carotid and subclavian arteries and most of the pulmonary arterial vessels.
- **Muscular arteries**. These are the main distributing branches of the arterial tree, e.g. the radial, femoral, coronary and cerebral arteries.
- **Arterioles**. These are the terminal branches of the arterial tree which supply the capillary beds.

There is a gradual transition in structure and function between the three types of arterial vessel rather than an abrupt demarcation. In general, the amount of elastic tissue decreases as the vessels become smaller and the smooth muscle component assumes relatively greater prominence.

ORGAN SYSTEMS

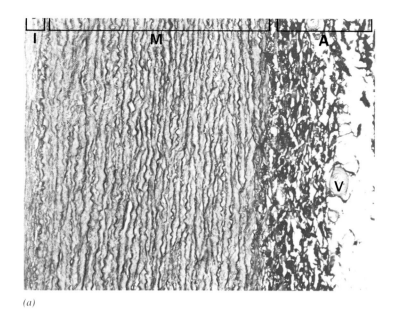

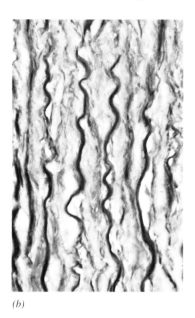

(a)   *(b)*

Fig. 8.7   **Elastic artery: aorta**   **(a) Elastic van Gieson × 33 (b) Elastic van Gieson × 320**

The highly elastic nature of the aortic wall is demonstrated in these preparations in which the elastic fibres are stained black. In micrograph (a), the three basic layers of the wall can be seen: the tunica intima **I**, the broad tunica media **M** and the tunica adventitia **A**.

The tunica intima consists of a single layer of flattened endothelial cells (not seen at this magnification) supported by a layer of collagenous tissue rich in elastin disposed in the form of both fibres and discontinuous sheets. The subendothelial supporting tissue contains scattered fibroblasts and other cells with ultrastructural features akin to smooth muscle cells and known as *myointimal cells*. Both cell types are probably involved in elaboration of the extracellular constituents. The myointimal cells are not invested by basement membrane and are thus not epithelial (myoepithelial) in nature.

With increasing age, the myointimal cells accumulate lipid and the intima progressively thickens; in a more extreme form this represents one of the early changes of atherosclerosis.

The tunica media is particularly broad and extremely elastic. At high magnification in (b), it is seen to consist of concentric fenestrated sheets of elastin (stained black) separated by collagenous tissue (stained red) and relatively few smooth muscle fibres (stained yellow). As seen in micrograph (a), the collagenous tunica adventitia (stained red) contains small vasa vasorum **V** which also penetrate the outer half of the tunica media.

Blood flow within elastic arteries is highly pulsatile; with advancing age the arterial system becomes less elastic thereby increasing peripheral resistance and thus arterial blood pressure.

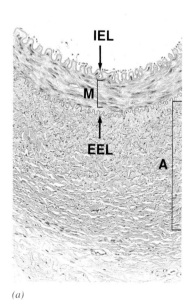

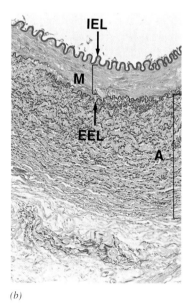

(a)   *(b)*

Fig. 8.8   **Muscular artery**
(a) H & E × 100
(b) Elastic van Gieson × 100

Muscular arteries have the same basic structure as elastic arteries but the elastic tissue is reduced to a well defined, fenestrated elastic sheet, the *internal elastic lamina* **IEL**, separating the tunica intima from the tunica media, and a less defined *external elastic lamina* **EEL** at the junction of the media and the tunica adventitia. Sometimes the internal elastic lamina is duplicated. The intima is often so thin as to be indistinguishable at low magnification. The tunica media **M** comprises a thick layer of circumferentially arranged smooth muscle, stained yellow in micrograph (b). The broad tunica adventitia **A** is mainly composed of collagen with considerable elastin, stained black in micrograph (b).

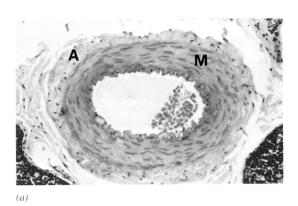

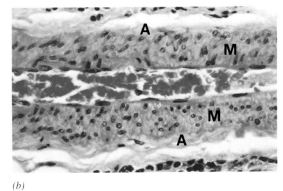

(a)   *(b)*

Fig. 8.9   Small muscular artery/large arteriole   (a) H & E, TS × 128 (b) H & E, LS × 320

Arterioles may be defined as those vessels of the arterial system with a lumen less than 0.3 mm in diameter, although the distinction between small muscular arteries and large arterioles is somewhat artificial. Arterioles are characterised by three main features which are seen in these micrographs.

The tunic intima is very thin and comprises the endothelial lining, a little collagenous supporting tissue and a thin internal elastic lamina. The tunica media **M** is almost entirely composed of smooth muscle cells in six concentric layers or less. The tunica adventitia **A** may be almost as thick as the tunica media and merges with the surrounding collagenous tissues. There is no external elastic lamina.

The flow of blood through capillary beds is regulated mainly by the arterioles which supply them. Contraction of the circularly arranged smooth muscle fibres of the arteriolar wall reduces the diameter of the lumen and hence blood flow. Generalised constriction of arterioles throughout the body markedly increases peripheral resistance to blood flow and the arteriolar compartment of the circulatory system thus has an important role in the regulation of systemic blood pressure.

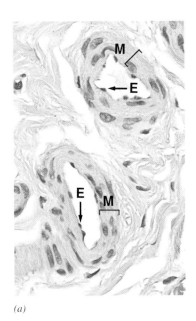

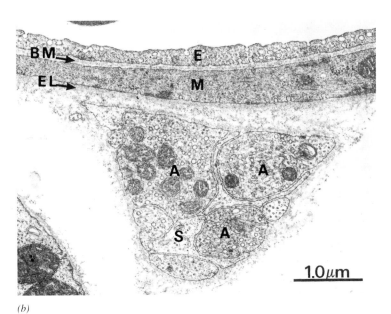

(a)   *(b)*

Fig. 8.10   Small arterioles   (a) H & E × 100 (b) EM × 19 000

Micrograph (a) illustrates two small arterioles in the dense collagenous tissue of the dermis of the skin. The tunica media **M** of each consists of two layers of smooth muscle cells. All that can be seen of the tunica intima are the nuclei of flattened endothelial cells **E**. The adventitia merges imperceptibly with the surrounding supporting tissue. Electron micrograph (b) is an example of the smallest of arterioles having only a single layer of smooth muscle **M** which lies immediately external to the endothelium **E** and its basement membrane **BM**. Note the external lamina **EL** (equivalent to basement membrane) around the smooth muscle cell. The adjacent supporting tissue contains a tiny autonomic nerve bundle including several vesicle-containing sympathetic axons **A** and a supporting Schwann cell **S**. The adventitial layer merges imperceptibly with the surrounding loose collagenous tissue.

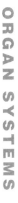

The microcirculation

The microcirculation is that part of the circulatory system concerned with the exchange of gases, fluids, nutrients and metabolic waste products. Exchange occurs mainly within the *capillaries*, extremely thin-walled vessels forming an interconnected network. Blood flow within the capillary bed is controlled by the arterioles and muscular sphincters at the arteriolar-capillary junctions called *precapillary sphincters*. The capillaries drain into a series of vessels of increasing diameter, namely *postcapillary venules, collecting venules* and small *muscular venules* which make up the venous component of the microcirculation.

In different tissues, the structure of the microcirculation varies to meet specific functional requirements. There are four main structural variables:

- **The diameter of the capillaries.** Diameter varies between as little as 3–4 μm (i.e. half the diameter of a red blood cell) and 30–40 μm. Large diameter capillaries are called *sinusoids*; these are found in the liver, spleen, lymph nodes and bone marrow.
- **The nature of the capillary endothelium.** Three types of capillary endothelium are found:
  - *Continuous capillaries:* the endothelial cells form an uninterrupted lining; this is the most common type of capillary.
  - *Fenestrated capillaries:* the endothelial cells contain numerous large pores or *fenestrations*.
  - *Discontinuous endothelium:* the endothelial cells do not form a continuous interface between the lumen and surrounding tissues; this arrangement is found only within the sinusoids of the liver (see Fig. 15.12).
- **The presence of arteriovenous shunts.** These provide direct connections between the arterial and venous systems.
- **The abundance of the capillary network.** This depends on the functional requirements of the tissue. For example, the dense collagenous tissue of tendons has a sparse capillary network; in contrast, cardiac muscle has an extensive capillary network which pervades the interstices between the muscle fibres.

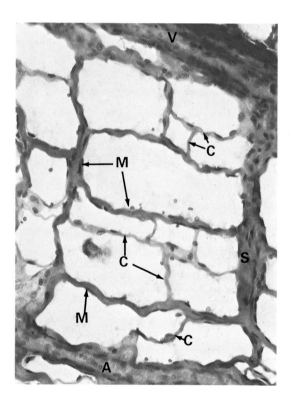

Fig. 8.11 **The microcirculation**
Mesenteric spread, H & E × 120

This micrograph demonstrates an anastomosing network of capillaries between an arteriole **A** and a venule **V**. The capillary network comprises small diameter capillaries **C**, consisting of only a single layer of endothelial cells, and larger diameter capillaries known as *metarterioles* **M**, characterised by a discontinuous outer layer of smooth muscle cells.

Note that small capillaries arise from both arterioles and metarterioles. At the origin of each capillary there is a sphincter mechanism, the precapillary sphincter, which is involved in regulation of capillary blood flow. Note also a direct wide-diameter communication between the arteriole and venule, an *arteriovenous shunt* **S**. Metarterioles also form direct communications between arterioles and venules. Contraction of the smooth muscle of the shunts and metarterioles directs blood through the network of small capillaries. Thus regulation of blood flow in the microcirculation is mediated by arterioles, metarterioles, precapillary sphincters and arteriovenous shunts. The smooth muscle activity of these vessels is modulated by the autonomic nervous system and circulating hormones, e.g. adrenal catecholamines. In addition, the concentration of oxygen and metabolites, such as lactic acid, regulate the local flow of blood within tissues; this process is called *autoregulation*.

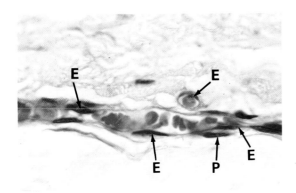

Fig. 8.12 Capillaries H & E × 800

The vessels seen here in longitudinal section and transverse section illustrate the characteristic features of capillaries.

A single layer of flattened endothelial cells **E** lines the capillary lumen. The thin layer of cytoplasm is difficult to resolve by light microscopy. The flattened endothelial cell nuclei bulge into the capillary lumen; in longitudinal section the nuclei appear elongated whereas in transverse section they appear more rounded in shape. Muscular and adventitial layers are absent. Occasional flattened cells called *pericytes* **P** embrace the capillary endothelial cells and may have a contractile function. Note that the diameter of capillaries is similar to that of the red blood cells contained within them.

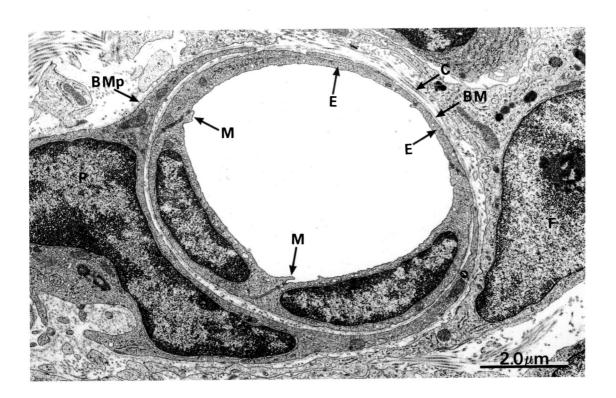

Fig. 8.13 Capillary: continuous endothelium type EM × 12 000

This electron micrograph illustrates the ultrastructure of capillaries of the continuous endothelium type, the type found in most tissues.

Four endothelial cells **E** are seen to encircle the capillary lumen, their plasma membranes approximating one another very closely and bound together by scattered tight junctions of the fascia occludens type (see Fig. 5.12). Small cytoplasmic flaps called *marginal folds* **M** extend across the intercellular junctions at the luminal surface. The capillary endothelium is supported by a thin basement membrane **BM** and adjacent collagen fibrils **C**. A pericyte **P** embraces the capillary. The pericyte is supported by its own basement membrane **BMp**. In the adjacent supporting tissue, note a fibroblast **F** and larger diameter collagen fibrils cut in transverse and longitudinal section.

Exchange between the lumen of the continuous-type capillary and the surrounding tissues is believed to occur in three ways. Passive diffusion through the endothelial cell cytoplasm mediates exchange of gases, ions and low molecular weight metabolites. Proteins and some lipids are transported by pinocytotic vesicles. White blood cells pass through the intercellular space between the endothelial cells in some way negotiating the endothelial intercellular junctions. Some workers maintain that the intercellular spaces also permit molecular transport. In capillaries of the continuous endothelial type, the basement membrane is thought to present little barrier to exchange between capillaries and surrounding tissues.

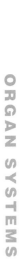

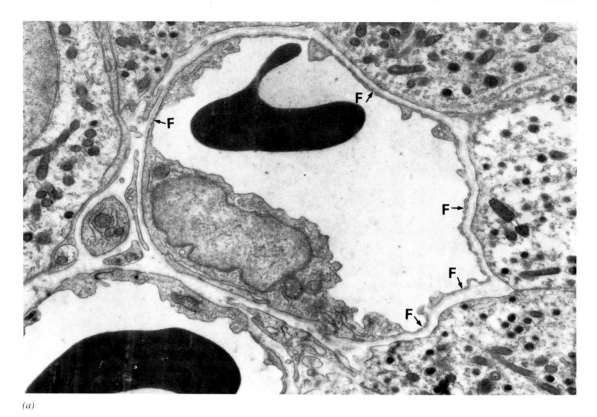

(a)

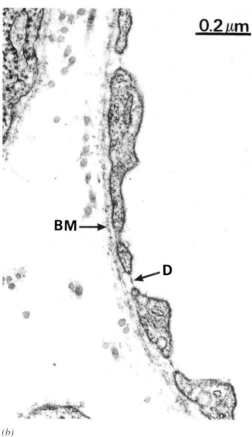

(b)

0.2 μm

Fig. 8.14   Fenestrated capillary
(a) EM × 13 000 (b) EM × 60 000

Fenestrated capillaries are found in some tissues where there is extensive molecular exchange with the blood; such tissues include the small intestine, endocrine glands and the kidney.

At low magnification (a), fenestrations **F** appear as pores through attenuated areas of the endothelial cytoplasm; however, only a small proportion of these areas are fenestrated. At high magnification (b), the fenestrations appear to be traversed by a thin electron-dense line **D** which may constitute a diaphragm; the biochemical and functional nature of this is not understood. A diaphragm is not seen across the fenestrations of the glomerular capillaries of the kidney (see Fig. 16.14).

The permeability of fenestrated capillaries is much greater than that of continuous endothelium-type capillaries and molecular labelling techniques have demonstrated that fenestrations permit the rapid passage of macromolecules smaller than plasma proteins from the lamina of fenestrated capillaries into surrounding tissues.

Like continuous endothelium-type capillaries, all fenestrated capillaries are supported by a basement membrane **BM** which is continuous across the fenestrations. Pericytes are rarely found in association with fenestrated capillaries.

Fig. 8.15 The endothelial cell

Endothelial cells are flat polygonal cells which are connected to their neighbours by junctional complexes. They have numerous pinocytotic vesicles and also contain specialised membrane-bound organelles called Weibel–Palade bodies which store von Willebrand factor (factor VIII in the coagulation cascade). Endothelial cells have many metabolic functions which are summarised in the table opposite. Many of the products synthesized and secreted by endothelial cells are associated with the fine control of blood coagulation and thrombosis, and with local control of blood vessel constriction/dilatation and vessel wall permeability. Abnormalities of endothelial cell function lead to loss of this fine local control and may lead to thrombosis or haemorrhage, or exudation of some of the components of blood into the extravascular tissues.

Summary of functions of endothelial cells
• Act as a permeability barrier
• Synthesize collagen and proteoglycans for basement membrane maintenance
• Synthesize and secrete molecules which promote protective thrombus formation, e.g. von Willebrand factor (Factor VIII)
• Synthesize and secrete molecules which minimise pathological thrombus formation, e.g. prostacyclin, thrombomodulin, nitrous oxide (which inhibits platelet adhesion and aggregation)
• Secrete vasoactive factors controlling blood flow, e.g. nitrous oxide, prostacyclin, vasoactive peptides such as endothelin.
• Produce molecules which mediate the acute inflammatory reaction, e.g. interleukins 1, 6 and 8, cell adhesion molecules
• Produce some growth factors, e.g. fibroblast growth factor, platelet-derived growth factor, blood cell colony stimulating factor

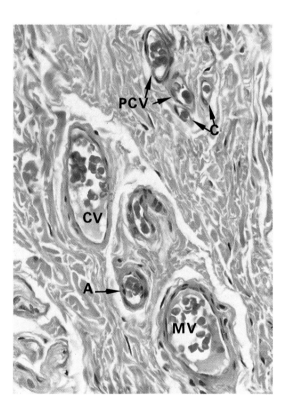

Fig. 8.16 Postcapillary and collecting venules
H & E × 480

The capillary beds are drained by a series of thin-walled vessels which form the first part of the venous system. Examples of each type of vessel are seen in micrograph (a).

Postcapillary venules **PCV** are the smallest of these vessels and are formed by the union of several capillaries **C** to produce a vessel similar in structure but of a wider diameter. Blood flow in postcapillary venules is sluggish and these vessels appear to be the main point at which white blood cells enter and leave the circulation. Postcapillary venules drain into *collecting venules* **CV** which are characterised by their large diameter and a greater number of enveloping pericytes. Collecting venules drain into vessels of progressively greater diameter, the walls of which contain a recognisable layer of smooth muscle and which are therefore known as *muscular venules* **MV**. This micrograph also shows a very small arteriole **A** with only a single layer of smooth muscle cells in its wall.

The venous system

With the exception of the venous components of the microcirculation, the venous system merely functions as a low pressure collecting system for the return of blood from the capillary networks to the heart. Blood flow in veins occurs passively down a pressure gradient towards the heart. With each inspiratory cycle, a negative pressure is created within the chest and hence within the right atrium of the heart. Venous return from the limbs is aided by the contraction of skeletal muscles which compress the veins contained within them. During expiration, the pressure gradients are reversed and blood tends to flow in the opposite direction. This is prevented by the presence of valves in veins of medium size. The valves also overcome the problem of reverse flow due to the effects of gravity especially in the lower limbs. Valve failure is the basis for the development of varicose veins.

The structure of the venous system conforms to the general three-layered arrangement elsewhere in the circulatory system, but the elastic and muscular components are much less prominent features. A major part of the total blood volume is contained within the venous system. Variations in relative blood volume, due for example to dilation of capillary beds or haemorrhage, may be compensated by changes in the capacity of the venous system. These changes are mediated by smooth muscle in the tunica media which controls the luminal diameter of muscular venules and veins.

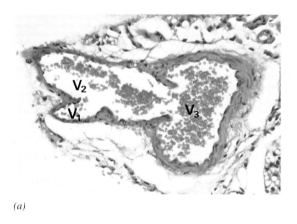

(a)

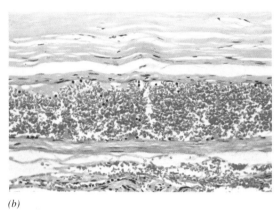

(b)

Fig. 8.17 **Muscular venules and small veins** (a) H & E × 128 (b) H & E × 128

Micrograph (a) illustrates the confluence of a small muscular venule **V₁** with a larger muscular venule **V₂** which then joins a small vein **V₃** cut in transverse section. Note the valve at the junction of the large venule and vein. Muscular venules are characterised by a clearly defined intimal layer devoid of elastic fibres and a tunica media consisting of one or two layers of smooth muscle fibres. Veins are characterised by a thicker muscular wall

and a poorly developed internal elastic lamina. Note that the tunica adventitia of these vessels is continuous with the surrounding collagenous supporting tissue.

Micrograph (b) shows a small vein cut in longitudinal section and fixed whilst still distended with blood. The wall of the vein consists of two to three layers of smooth muscle fibres. Note the wide diameter of the lumen relative to the thickness of the wall.

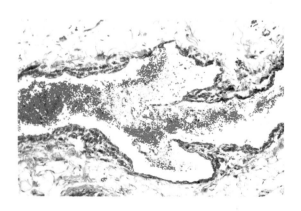

Fig. 8.18 **Vein with valve**
Masson's trichrome × 128

This micrograph demonstrates a valve in a small vein. The valve consists of delicate semilunar projections of the tunica intima of the vein wall; the projections are composed of fibroelastic tissue lined on both sides by endothelium. Each valve usually consists of two leaflets, the free edges of which project in the direction of blood flow. Valves only occur in veins of more than 2 mm in diameter, particularly those draining the extremities.

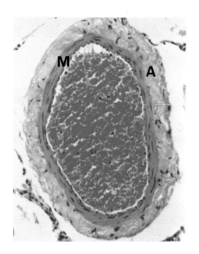

Fig. 8.19 Vein H & E × 128

Small and medium-sized veins are characterised by the following features demonstrated in this micrograph of a medium-sized vein. The tunica intima consists of little more than the endothelial lining; in veins that are not distended with blood the endothelium may be thrown up into small folds. The tunica media **M** is thin compared with that of arteries and consists of two or more layers of circularly arranged smooth muscle fibres. The tunica adventitia **A** is the broadest layer of the vessel wall and is composed of longitudinally arranged thick collagen fibres which merge with the surrounding collagenous tissue.

Note that the wall of the vein is thin relative to the diameter of the lumen. In contrast, in most arteries, the thickness of the wall approximates the diameter of the lumen.

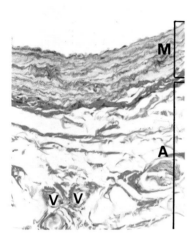

Fig. 8.20 Large muscular vein Elastic van Gieson × 128

Large veins such as the femoral and renal veins have a relatively thick muscular wall **M** consisting of several layers of smooth muscle (stained yellow in this specimen) separated by layers of collagenous connective tissue (stained red). The tunica media and tunica intima also contain a few elastic fibres (stained black in this preparation) but there is no distinct internal elastic lamina as in arteries of comparable size.

The tunica adventitia **A** is broad and contains numerous vasa vasorum **V** reflecting the need for arterial blood by the tissues of the vein wall. Vasa vasorum as well as lymphatics also penetrate the whole thickness of the muscular wall and are much more numerous than in arterial vessels of similar size.

The largest vessels of the venous system, the *venae cavae*, have a structure similar to that just described except that the smooth muscle is disposed longitudinally rather than in a circular fashion. This arrangement may reflect the need for elongation and shortening to accommodate chest expansion and contraction during the respiratory cycle.

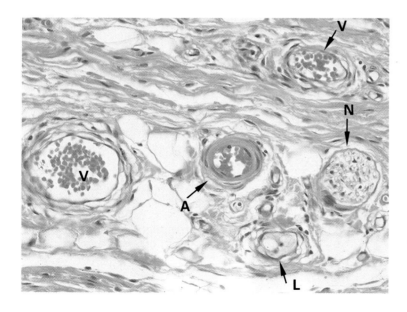

Fig. 8.21 Small neurovascular bundle H & E × 150

The vessels supplying and draining a particular area of tissue tend to pass together, frequently accompanied by a peripheral nerve and invested by a condensation of the surrounding collagenous tissue which forms an ill-defined protective sheath. This micrograph shows such a small neurovascular bundle containing a small arteriole **A**, venules **V**, a lymphatic **L** and a nerve **N**.

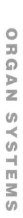

The lymph vascular system

The lymph vascular system drains excess fluid, the *lymph*, from extracellular spaces and returns it to the blood vascular system. Lymph is formed in the following manner. At the arterial end of blood capillaries, the hydrostatic pressure of blood exceeds the colloidal osmotic pressure exerted by plasma proteins. Water and electrolytes therefore pass out of capillaries into the extracellular space; some plasma proteins also leak out through the endothelial wall. At the venous end of blood capillaries, the pressure relationships are reversed and fluid tends to be drawn back into the blood vascular system. In this way, about 2% of plasma passing through the capillary bed is exchanged with the extracellular tissue fluid. The rate of tissue fluid formation at the arterial end of capillaries generally exceeds the re-uptake of fluid at the venous end. The excess fluid, lymph, is drained by a system of lymph capillaries which converge to form progressively larger diameter lymphatic vessels. Lymph enters the venous system by a single vessel on each side of the body, namely the thoracic duct (on the left) and the right lymphatic duct. Movement of lymph in the lymph vascular system is similar to movement of blood in the venous system but valves are more numerous in lymphatic vessels.

Along the course of the larger lymphatic vessels are aggregations of lymphoid tissues called lymph nodes where lymph is sampled for the presence of foreign material (antigen) and where activated cells of the immune system and antibodies join the general circulation (see Ch. 11). Lymphatic vessels are found in all tissues except the central nervous system, cartilage, bone, bone marrow, thymus, placenta, cornea and teeth. The structure of lymphatic vessels conforms closely to that of vessels of similar diameter in the venous system. Lymphatic vessels may be distinguished from venous vessels by the absence of erythrocytes and the presence of small numbers of leucocytes, mainly lymphocytes. Lymphatic capillaries differ from blood capillaries in several respects which reflect the greater permeability of lymphatic capillaries. In particular, the endothelial cell cytoplasm of lymphatics is extremely thin, the basement membrane is rudimentary or absent and there are no pericytes. Fine collagenous filaments known as **anchoring filaments** link the endothelium to the surrounding supporting tissue preventing collapse of the lymphatic lumen.

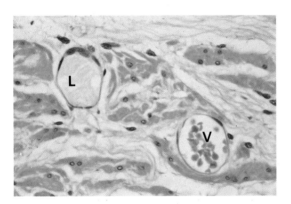

Fig. 8.22   Small lymphatic vessel H & E × 320

This micrograph illustrates the characteristic histological differences between a small lymphatic **L** and a venule **V**. Lymphatics do not contain erythrocytes but often contain a few lymphocytes. The stained amorphous material seen in this lymphatic is the protein of lymph which becomes precipitated during tissue processing. The presence of such material is often a distinguishing feature of lymphatics in histological preparations.

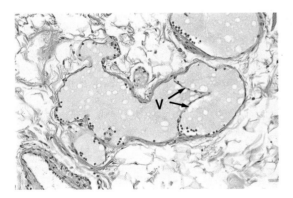

Fig. 8.23   Valve of a lymphatic vessel
H & E × 40

A characteristic feature of the lymphatic system is the numerous delicate valves in small and medium-sized vessels. The structure of these valves **V** is similar to that of valves in the venous system, but the supporting tissue core consists merely of reticulin fibres and a little ground substance. Note the presence of lymphocytes at the periphery of the lumina.

9. Skin

Introduction

The skin has four major functions:

- **Protection.** The skin provides protection against ultraviolet light and mechanical, chemical and thermal insults; its relatively impermeable surface prevents dehydration and acts as a physical barrier to invasion by microorganisms.
- **Sensation.** The skin is the largest sensory organ in the body and contains a variety of receptors for touch, pressure, pain and temperature. These are described and illustrated in Chapter 7.
- **Thermoregulation.** In humans, skin is a major organ of thermoregulation. The body is insulated against heat loss by the presence of hairs and subcutaneous adipose tissue. Heat loss is facilitated by evaporation of sweat from the skin surface and increased blood flow through the rich vascular network of the dermis.
- **Metabolic functions.** Subcutaneous adipose tissue constitutes a major store of energy, mainly in the form of triglycerides. Vitamin D is synthesised in the epidermis and supplements that derived from dietary sources.

The skin has three main layers:

- an outer keratinising stratified squamous epithelium which is self-regenerating – the *epidermis*
- an underlying tough supporting and nourishing layer of fibroelastic tissue – the *dermis*
- a variable deep layer, mainly adipose tissue – the *hypodermis* or *subcutis*.

In addition there are specialised epithelial appendages such as sweat glands, hair follicles and sebaceous glands, which arise as downgrowths into the dermis from the epidermis during embryological development. Within this basic pattern there are variations in structure at different sites on the body surface according to the major function of the skin at that site; for example, the soles of the feet have a very thick protective keratin layer and an epidermis with a complex interdigitation with the underlying dermis to resist the strong shearing frictional forces in walking.

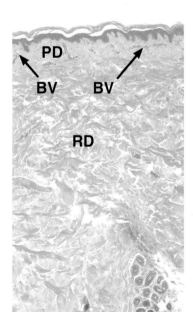

Fig. 9.1 Normal human skin (thin) H & E × 16

This micrograph shows the general structure of thin human skin from the middle of the back. The top layer is the thin epidermis with an overlying layer of loose keratin. The external surface of the epidermis is fairly smooth and flat, but the junction between epidermis and thick dermis is marked by downward folds of epidermis (*rete ridges*) which offer resistance to separation of the epidermal surface due to shearing. The dermis comprises two layers: the *papillary dermis* PD just beneath the epidermis which contains fine collagen and elastic fibres and small blood vessels arising from the vascular plexus BV; and the thicker, stronger *reticular dermis* RD which contains large compact collagen fibres and thick elastin fibres. Within the dermis also reside the skin appendages and their ducts (an eccrine gland is seen at bottom right) and larger blood vessels, nerves and some nerve endings. Beneath the reticular dermis is the adipose subcutis (hypodermis), which is not shown here.

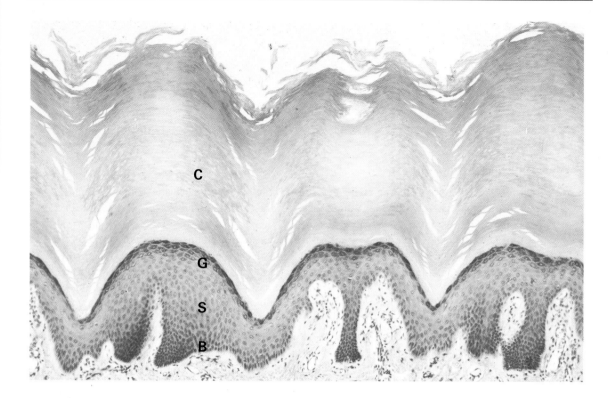

Fig. 9.2 **Epidermis (thick skin)** H & E × 104

The layers of the epidermis are best seen in thick skin, e.g. sole. Cells produced by mitosis in the germinal basal layer adjacent to the dermis undergo maturational changes concerned with the production of keratin. The outer keratinised layer is shed continuously and is replaced by the progressive movement and maturation of cells from the germinal layer; thus all of the cells of this lineage are often described as *keratinocytes*. The rate of mitosis in the germinal layer generally equals the rate of desquamation of keratin from the outer surface; in humans, the process of maturation of a basal cell through to desquamation takes from 25 to 50 days, being more rapid in areas exposed to heavy frictional forces.

The phases of this dynamic process are represented in four morphological layers:

- The *stratum basale* or basal layer **B** is the germinal layer of the epidermis. Mitotic activity in this layer provides a constant supply of new keratinocytes to replace those lost by normal wear and tear.
- The *stratum spinosum* or *prickle cell layer* **S**, so named for the 'prickly' appearance of the cells at high magnification (see Fig. 9.4), contains cells which are in the process of growth and early keratin synthesis.
- The *stratum granulosum* or *granular layer* **G** is characterised by intracellular granules which contribute to the process of keratinisation.
- The *stratum corneum* or *cornified layer* **C** consists of flattened, fused cell remnants composed mainly of the fibrous protein, keratin.

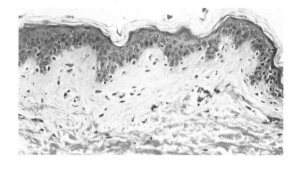

Fig. 9.3 **Thin skin** H & E × 128

In this preparation of thin skin from the abdomen, the individual cellular layers are more difficult to discern. In comparison with thick skin, the stratum corneum is thin and the combined thickness of the other layers is reduced to a lesser extent. The rete (epidermal) ridge system is much less prominent, reflecting the relatively lower shearing forces to which such thin skin is subjected.

Fig. 9.4 Epidermis
(a) Masson's trichrome × 600 (b) H & E × 1000
(c) Epoxy resin section, toluidine blue × 1200

Micrograph (a) shows the cells of the full thickness of the epidermis, (b) shows the low columnar basal cells (stratum basale), and (c) shows the keratinocytes of the stratum spinosum.

Stratum basale B. The cells of this layer are cuboidal or low columnar and form a single layer separated from the dermis **D** by a basement membrane. The basal aspect of each germinal cell is highly irregular and bound to the basement membrane by numerous hemidesmosomes. Like the cells of the adjacent stratum spinosum, small cytoplasmic projections extend across the intercellular spaces to abut upon those of adjacent cells; desmosomes bind these contact points. Mitotic figures are most frequently observed in this layer but cell division also occurs to a lesser extent in the stratum spinosum.

Stratum spinosum S. The so-called 'prickle cells' of this zone are relatively large and polyhedral in shape and have numerous cytoplasmic 'prickles' bound by desmosomes to adjacent cells. Prominent nucleoli and cytoplasmic basophilia indicate active protein synthesis. A fibrillar protein *cytokeratin*, the predominant synthetic product of these cells, aggregates to form intracellular fibrils known as *tonofibrils* which converge upon the desmosomes of the cytoplasmic 'prickles' clearly seen in (c); tonofibrils become more prominent towards the stratum granulosum. Tonofibrils are also found in small numbers in the cells of the stratum basale.

Stratum granulosum G. The cells of this layer are characterised by numerous, dense basophilic granules which crowd the cytoplasm and tend to obscure the tonofibrils. The chemical nature of these *keratohyalin granules* is distinct from that of the fibrous protein of the tonofibrils. The process of keratinisation is thought to involve the combination of tonofibril and keratohyalin elements to form the mature keratin complex. In the outermost aspect of the stratum granulosum, cell death occurs due to rupture of lysosomal membranes; released lysosomal enzymes may play an important role in the final process of keratinisation.

Stratum corneum C. The dead and dying cells of this surface layer are flattened, devoid of nuclei and other organelles and filled with mature keratin. In the deeper aspect of this layer, the cornified cells retain their desmosomal junctions and the intracellular keratin has an ordered pattern. Towards the surface, the desmosomes and internal structure of the cells become completely disrupted, a process which precedes desquamation.

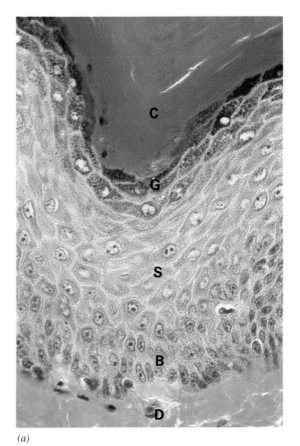

(a)

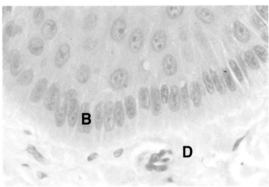

(b)

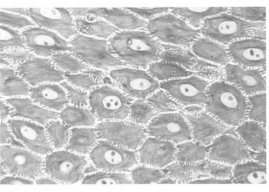

(c)

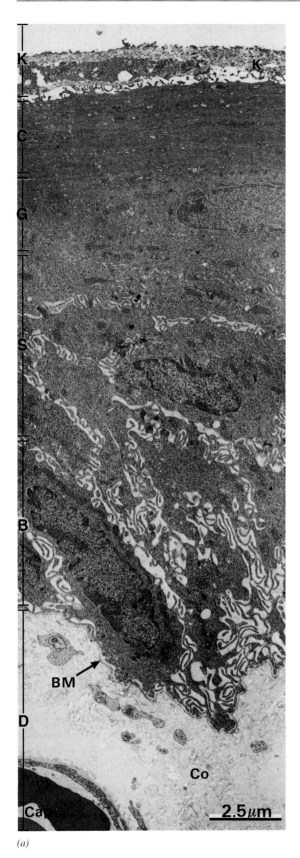

(a)

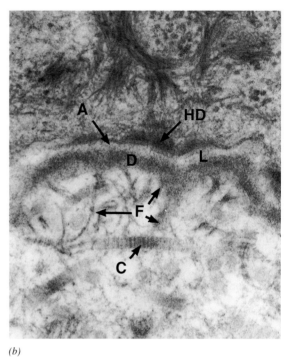

(b)

Fig. 9.5 Ultrastructure of epidermis
(a) Rat, EM × 8000 (b) Human, EM × 24 000

Micrograph (a) is a strip through the epidermis of an albino rat, showing dermis **D** (containing collagen fibres **Co** and capillaries **Cap**), basement membrane **BM**, cells of the basal layer **B**, stratum spinosum **S**, granular layer **G**, stratum corneum **C** and a superficial desquamating flake of keratin **K**. Micrograph (b) shows the detail of the dermo-epidermal *basement membrane*. The basement membrane has two distinct components, a *lamina lucida* **L** and a *lamina densa* **D**. The basal cells sit on the lamina lucida but are tethered to the lamina densa by anchoring proteins **A** arising from a hemidesmosome **HD**. There is a third ill-defined zone (the *fibroreticular lamina*) which contains fibrils **F** connecting the lamina densa to collagen fibres **Co** and elastin in the dermis.

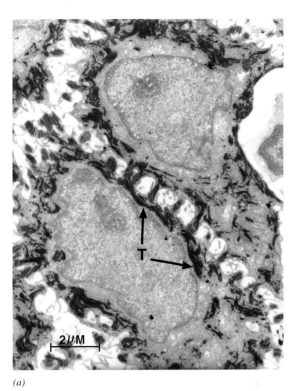

(a)

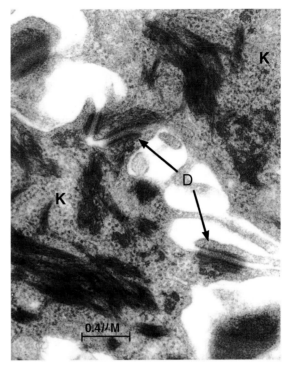

(b)

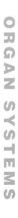

(c)

Fig. 9.6 Ultrastructure of epidermis
(a) EM × 5000 (b) EM × 25 000 (c) EM × 5000

The keratinocytes of the stratum spinosum shown in micrograph (a) contain many tonofilaments **T** of keratin which are particularly concentrated at the periphery of the cytoplasm and in the projections that terminate in desmosomal junctions which link neighbouring keratinocytes. The spaces between adjacent keratinocytes may contain the fine cytoplasmic processes of melanocytes and Langerhans cells.

Electron micrograph (b) shows details of the desmosomal junctions **D** between two keratinocytes **K**. Tonofilaments of keratin terminate in the desmosome but do not pass from one cell to the other.

Electron micrograph (c) shows keratinocytes of the granular layer **G** and the base of the stratum corneum **C**. Granular layer keratinocytes contain round *keratohyaline granules* **K** which contain sulphur-rich amino acids such as cysteine and small oval lamellated bodies (*Odland bodies* or *keratinosomes* – too small to be seen here) which contain a mixture of water-repellent lipids. The stratum corneum contains a mixture of keratohyaline granules and keratin tonofilaments, coated by non-wettable lipids released from the Odland bodies (*keratinosomes*).

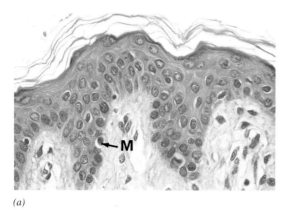

(a)

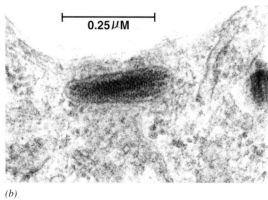

0.25 μM

(b)

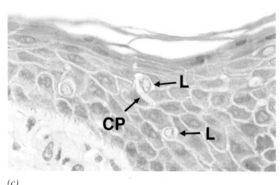

(c)

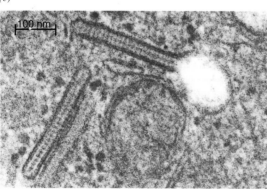

(d)

Fig. 9.7 Other cells in the epidermis
(a) Melanocyte, H & E × 320 (b) Premelanosome, EM × 100 000 (c) Langerhans cells, H & E × 700 (d) Birbeck granule, EM × 100 000

Melanocytes **M** as seen in micrograph (a) are responsible for the synthesis and release of the brown pigment *melanin* which is largely responsible for skin coloration. They are located in the basal layer of the epidermis and appear as round cells with pale-staining cytoplasm scattered infrequently between the low columnar basal cells. From this cell body there are numerous long cytoplasmic processes which run in the spaces between the keratinocytes of the stratum spinosum. Melanocyte cytoplasm contains specialised membrane-bound oval granules called *premelanosomes* and *melanosomes* which synthesise the pigment melanin. Tyrosine is converted into dihydroxyphenylalanine (DOPA) which is then polymerised into melanin; the melanin pigment binds to protein, and the melanoprotein is transferred along cytoplasmic processes to be transferred into the cytoplasm of basal and stratum spinosum keratinocytes, the highest concentration being in basal cells. The amount of melanin deposited varies from race to race, but racially white-skinned individuals can increase the amount of melanin synthesised and deposited by increasing skin exposure to UV light.

The premelanosome which synthesises melanin is oval to boat-shaped, membrane-bound and contains characteristic transverse striations (micrograph (b)). After a period of melanin synthesis this striated pattern is obscured by the melanin (melanosomes).

Micrograph (c) illustrates *Langerhans cells* **L** which are present in all layers of the epidermis, but are most easily seen in the stratum spinosum; they also occur around blood vessels in the papillary dermis. They have an oval, reniform or irregular pale nucleus surrounded by pale-staining cytoplasm which extends as cytoplasmic processes **CP** between the keratinocytes.

Ultrastructurally, Langerhans cell cytoplasm contains characteristic *Birbeck granules*, seen in micrograph (d), which are rod-like structures with regular cross-striations, one end of which frequently distends in a vesicle so that they resemble a tennis racket. These are antigen-presenting cells and are an important component of the immune defence mechanism (see Ch. 11).

Merkel cells (not shown here) are specialised touch receptors scattered very sparsely among the cells of the basal layer. By light microscopy they are difficult to distinguish from melanocytes. They contain round neuroendocrine vesicles at their base and have a synaptic junction with a fine nerve ending in the papillary dermis.

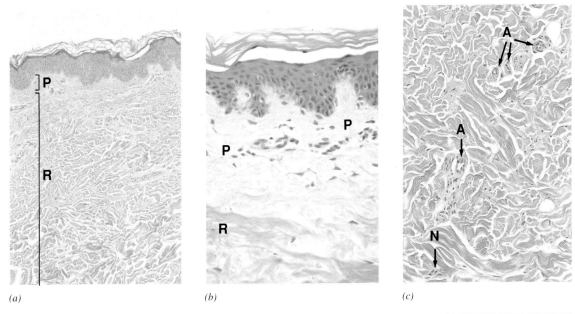

(a)   (b)   (c)

Fig. 9.8 **Dermis** (a) H & E × 60 (b) H & E × 200 (c) H & E × 100 (d) Elastic van Gieson × 150

The dermal layer of the skin provides a flexible but robust base for the epidermis and contains a generous vascular supply for the metabolic support of the avascular epidermis and for thermoregulation.

Micrograph (a) shows the full extent of the dermis which is divided into two zones, a superficial thin *papillary dermis* **P** and the more extensive deeper *reticular dermis* **R**. Micrograph (b) shows the papillary dermis **P** which is loose and contains very fine interlacing collagen fibres. It contains venules, arterioles and capillary loops, as well as lymphatics and fine nerve twigs from the sensory nerve endings, Meissner's corpuscles (see Fig. 7.28).

Micrograph (c) shows the reticular dermis which consists of coarse irregularly situated bundles of collagen within which are the blood vessels that join the plexus of vessels in the papillary dermis with the larger deeper vessels at the junction between dermis and subcutis. Some arterioles **A** and a small nerve twig **N** can be seen.

Elastin is an important constituent of both layers of the dermis and in micrograph (d) it shows black against the red stained collagen. In the reticular layer **R** the elastic fibres are long and thick and follow the course of the collagen bundles. In the papillary dermis **P** the elastic fibres are very fine, scanty and scarcely stained by this method. The cellular component of the dermis is mainly the fibroblasts which are responsible for the production of collagen and elastin, but lymphocytes, mast cells and tissue macrophages involved in non-specific defence and immune surveillance are also present.

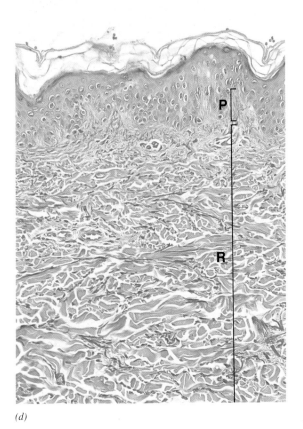

(d)

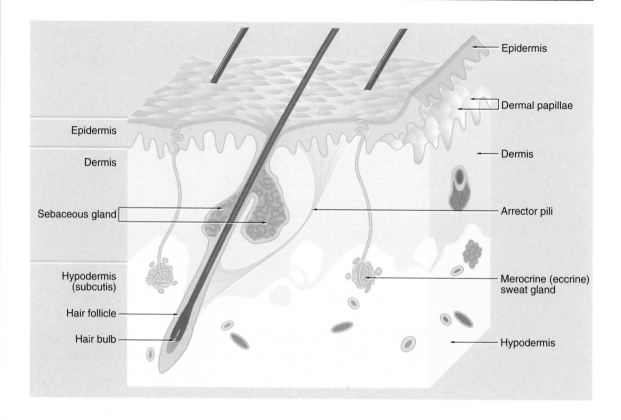

Epidermis

Dermal papillae

Dermis

Arrector pili

Merocrine (eccrine) sweat gland

Hypodermis

Epidermis

Dermis

Sebaceous gland

Hypodermis (subcutis)

Hair follicle

Hair bulb

Fig. 9.9 **Skin appendages**

Skin has a variety of appendages, principally hairs, sebaceous glands and sweat glands, which are derived embryonically from the surface epithelium (epidermis). The distribution, arrangement and detailed structure of the appendages vary from one part of the skin to another but nevertheless the general structure conforms to a basic pattern. The three-dimensional arrangement shown in this diagram has been deduced from studies of serial sections of skin; individual sections of skin rarely demonstrate all these features.

Hairs. Hairs are highly modified keratinised structures produced by *hair follicles* which are essentially cylindrical downgrowths of the surface epithelium ensheathed by collagenous tissue. Hair growth takes place within a terminal expansion of the follicle, the *hair bulb*, which consists of actively dividing epithelial cells surrounding a papilla of vascular tissue, the *dermal papilla*.

A bundle of smooth muscle cells, the *arrector pili* muscle, is attached to the follicular sheath and is inserted into the dermal papillary zone. Contraction of the arrector pili causes the hair to become erect and pulls down its point of insertion, producing the effect known as 'goose-flesh'.

The arrector pili muscles are innervated by the sympathetic nervous system and pilo-erection is activated by cold or fear. In furry animals, hair erection traps a thicker layer of air over the skin surface thus increasing insulation against heat loss; hair erection also makes the animal appear larger and is thus a protective mechanism in dangerous circumstances. These functions are probably of little physiological significance in humans. However, contraction of the arrector pili may play some part in expulsion of sebum from sebaceous glands.

Sebaceous glands. One or more sebaceous glands are associated with each hair follicle; these glands secrete an oily substance called *sebum* onto the hair surface in the upper part of the follicle. Sebum acts as a waterproofing and moisturising agent for the hair and skin surface. In regions of transition from the skin to the body tracts such as the lips, eyelids, glans penis, labia minora and nipples, sebaceous glands are found independent of hair follicles and secrete directly on to the skin surface.

Sweat glands. In most areas of the skin, sweat glands are simple, coiled tubular glands which secrete a watery fluid onto the skin surface by the process of merocrine secretion (see Ch. 5). The coiled, secretory portions of these glands are an important component of the thermoregulatory mechanism in humans. When the body requires to lose heat, skin blood flow and sweat production are increased; evaporation of sweat causes cooling of the skin surface and loss of heat from the underlying vascular bed. Merocrine (eccrine) sweat glands are innervated by cholinergic fibres of the sympathetic nervous system; sweating is stimulated not only by excessive body heat but also by fear-provoking stimuli.

A different type of sweat gland is found in the skin of the axilla and genital regions of humans. In contrast to the merocrine sweat glands, these glands are believed to secrete by the apocrine process (see Ch. 5) and are thus called *apocrine sweat glands*. They also differ in that they produce a viscid secretion which is discharged into hair follicles rather than directly onto the surface. Apocrine sweat glands are innervated by adrenergic fibres of the sympathetic nervous system.

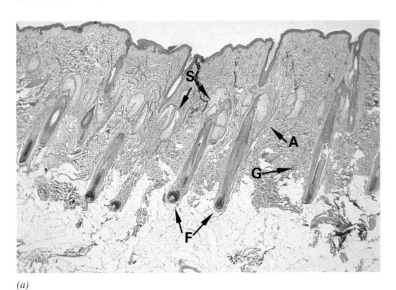

(a)

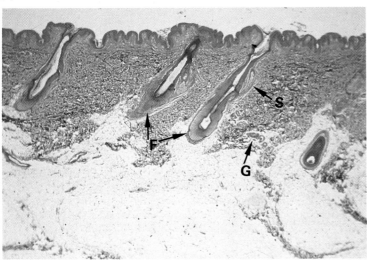

(b)

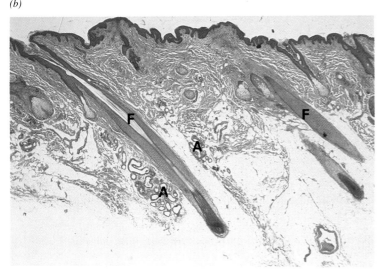

(c)

Fig. 9.10 Regional variations of skin structure (a) Scalp skin, Masson's (green) trichrome × 12 (b) Abdominal skin (male), Masson's (blue) trichrome × 12 (c) Pubic skin, H & E × 12

The structure of the skin differs considerably from one part of the body to another, the principal differences being in epidermal thickness, the size, density and state of activity of the hair follicles, and the nature and density of sweat glands and sensory receptors. These micrographs illustrate three extremes of structure in hairy skin.

As seen in micrograph (a), the skin of the scalp is robust due to a thick, densely collagenous dermis (stained blue-green in this preparation), and the hair follicles **F** are numerous and closely packed. In fair-haired people, the follicles are fewer in number and somewhat smaller in size, producing finer hair. The follicles of the scalp are particularly long and have more numerous sebaceous glands **S** than those of other areas. Note the arrector pili muscles **A** extending from the base of the follicles towards the upper dermis. Merocrine sweat glands **G** are numerous though less prominent than in the skin of the trunk and limbs due to the profusion of other appendages.

Micrograph (b) illustrates the typical histological appearance of the skin which covers most of the body. The hair follicles **F** and associated sebaceous glands **S** are sparse and merocrine sweat glands **G** are relatively shorter; the hairs produced are finer.

The skin of the axillae and pubic region, shown in micrograph (c), exhibits a moderate density of hair follicles **F** which, unlike those of the scalp, tend to be oriented obliquely to the skin surface and are often curved rather than straight causing the hairs to be curled. Apocrine sweat glands **A** are a common feature of this type of skin and are seen typically associated with hair follicles into which they discharge their secretions.

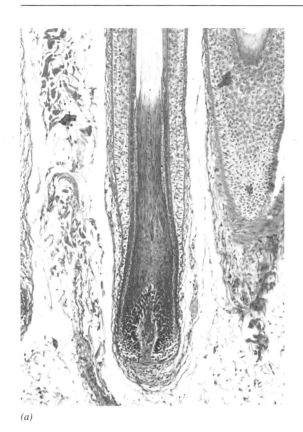

(a)

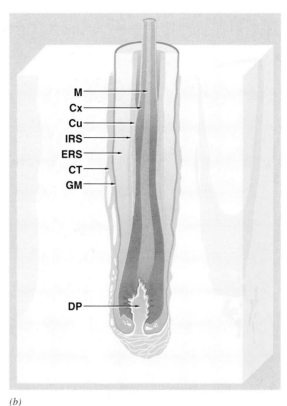

(b)

Fig. 9.11   Hair follicle (a) H & E × 120 (b) Explanatory diagram

The hair follicle is a tubular structure consisting of five concentric layers of epithelial cells. At the base, there is a bulbous expansion, the hair bulb, enclosing the dermal papilla **DP**. As they are pushed towards the skin surface from the hair bulb, the inner three epithelial layers undergo keratinisation to form the hair shaft whilst the outer two layers form an epithelial sheath. At the hair bulb, all the layers merge to become indistinguishable from one another; the mass of cells destined to form the hair is known as the *hair matrix*.

During active hair growth, the epithelial cells surrounding the dermal papilla proliferate to form the four inner layers of the follicle whilst the outermost layer merely represents a downward continuation of the stratum germinativum of the surface epithelium. The whole epithelial mass surrounding the dermal papilla constitutes the *hair root*.

The cells of the innermost layer of the follicle undergo moderate keratinisation to form the *medulla* **M** or core of the hair shaft; the medullary layer is often not distinguishable in fine hairs. The medulla is surrounded by a broad, highly keratinised layer, the *cortex* **Cx**, which forms the bulk of the hair. The third cell layer of the follicle undergoes keratinisation to form a hard, thin *cuticle* **Cu** on the surface of the hair. The cuticle consists of overlapping keratin plates, an arrangement which is said to prevent matting of the hair.

The fourth layer of the follicle constitutes the *internal root sheath* **IRS**; the cells of this layer become only lightly keratinised and disintegrate at the level of the sebaceous gland ducts leaving a space into which sebum

is secreted around the maturing hair. The outermost layer, the *external root sheath* **ERS**, does not take part in hair formation; this layer is separated from the sheath of connective tissue **CT** surrounding the follicle by a thick, specialised basement membrane known as the *glassy membrane* **GM**.

In the growing follicle, large active melanocytes (see Fig. 9.7a) are scattered amongst the proliferating cells with melanin being incorporated in the cortex of the hair shaft. Black, brown and yellow forms of melanin are produced in various combinations to determine final hair colour. In infancy, childhood and females, body hair is fine and soft and known as *vellus* in contrast to the coarser hair of the scalp which is known as *terminal hair*. Male sex hormone production at puberty is responsible for the development of further terminal pubic and axillary hair in both sexes and for the replacement of vellus hair with terminal hair on the mature male body.

The cross-sectional shape of hairs also varies between races. The straight hair of the Mongol races is round in cross-section, the wavy hair characteristic of Europeans is oval and the curly hair of black skinned peoples is more kidney-shaped.

In addition, the structure of hair follicles depends on the type of hair being produced. For example, the follicles of the scalp and other terminal hairs tend to be long and straight, whereas those of the body, which produce fine, downy hair (vellus), are relatively short and plump; curly hair may be produced by curved follicles or follicles in which the hair bulb lies at an angle to the hair shaft.

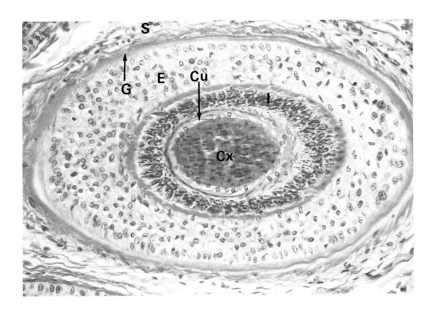

Fig. 9.12 Hair follicle
H & E × 198

This is a slightly oblique, transverse section through the lower part of a hair follicle. The broad external root sheath **E** is separated from the collagenous root sheath **S** by the glassy membrane **G**. Passing inwards, the internal root sheath **I** is recognised by its content of eosinophilic (keratohyalin) granules; the outermost cells of the internal root sheath have a more homogeneous appearance. Deep to the internal root sheath is the thin, pale stained cuticle layer **Cu** which surrounds the strongly stained cortex **Cx**. A medulla is not present in this specimen.

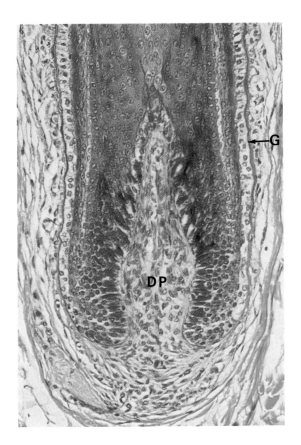

Fig. 9.13 Hair bulb Masson's trichrome × 198

This staining method permits clear delineation of the epithelial and collagenous elements of the hair follicle. The dermal papilla **DP** is highly vascular and is separated from the epithelial cells by a basement membrane which is continuous with the glassy membrane **G** surrounding the follicle externally. The sheath of the follicle is also rich in blood vessels and contains a delicate plexus of sensory nerve endings which are receptive to minute movements of the hair follicle and thus act as highly sensitive touch receptors.

Note the five cell layers of the hair follicle merging with the proliferating cells of the hair root. Note also the large amount of pigment in the basal layer extending up into the cortical layer and produced by melanocytes scattered along the basement membrane of the hair root.

Individual hair follicles undergo cycles of growth and quiescence and this is reflected in changes in their structure. In the ***growing phase***, follicles penetrate deeply into the hypodermis and the hair bulb is prominent, whereas during the ***resting phase***, follicles are shorter and the hair bulb is smaller and lacking in a dermal papilla; quiescent follicles are known as ***club hairs***.

This cyclical growth pattern is the factor which determines the limits of length reached by hairs in different parts of the body. For example, the growth phase of head hairs is of the order of 2 years or more, each hair being shed during a follicular resting phase lasting a matter of months. Only a small proportion of follicles are normally in the resting phase at any one time, thus maintaining a continuous crop of hair. In contrast, body hairs, eyebrows, eyelashes, etc. have a relatively short growth phase and longer resting phase preventing inappropriate overgrowth. This explains why pubic hair does not reach the knees!

ORGAN SYSTEMS

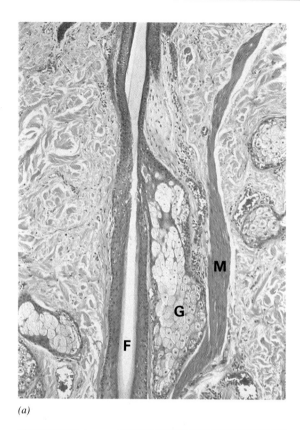

(a)

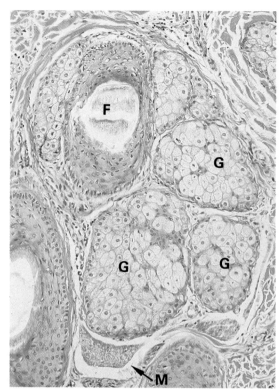

(b)

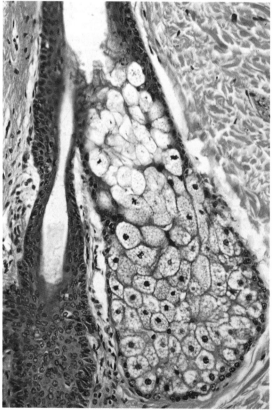

(c)

Fig. 9.14 **Sebaceous glands**
(a) H & E × 33 (b) H & E × 150 (c) H & E × 198

Micrograph (a) illustrates the relationship of a sebaceous gland **G** and an arrector pili muscle **M** to a hair follicle **F**. At a point about one-third of its length from the surface, each hair follicle is surrounded by one or more sebaceous glands which discharge their secretions onto the hair shaft and thence onto the skin surface. As seen in micrograph (b), sebaceous glands lie within the sheath surrounding the hair follicle and the glandular epithelium represents an outgrowth of the external root sheath.

The arrector pili muscle of each follicle consists of a bundle of smooth muscle fibres. The muscle inserts at one end into the sheath of the follicle at a point below the sebaceous glands, and at the other end into the dermal papillary area beneath the epidermis. Each hair follicle and its associated arrector pili muscle and sebaceous glands is known as a *pilosebaceous unit*. Note that the bulk of the sebaceous glands and the arrector pili muscle lie on that aspect of the hair to which the hair follicle inclines.

More detail of sebaceous gland structure can be seen in micrograph (c). Each sebaceous gland has a branched acinar form, the acini converging upon a short duct which empties into the hair follicle beside the maturing hair. Each acinus consists of a mass of rounded cells which are packed with lipid-filled vacuoles; during tissue preparation the lipid is largely removed leaving the cytoplasm of these cells poorly stained. Towards the duct, the lipid content of the acinar cells increases greatly and the distended cells degenerate, so releasing their contents, sebum, into the duct by the process known as holocrine secretion (see Ch. 5). Cells lost by holocrine secretion are replaced by mitosis in the basal layer of the acinus.

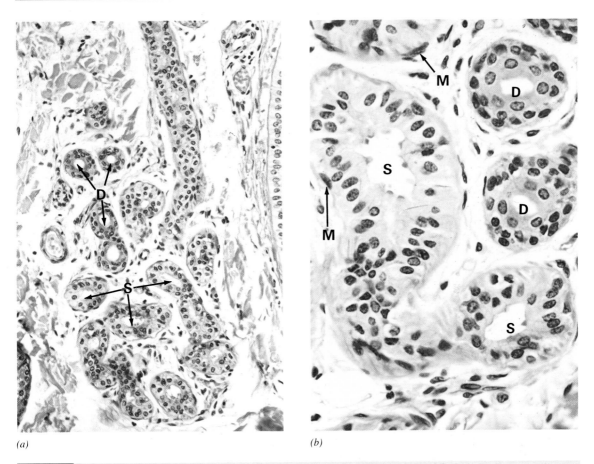

(a)   *(b)*

Fig. 9.15 **Merocrine (eccrine) sweat glands** (a) H & E × 198 (b) H & E × 480

Merocrine sweat glands are distributed in the skin of most parts of the body with the exception of areas such as the margins of the lip and the glans penis. Merocrine sweat glands secrete a watery fluid, hypotonic with respect to plasma, the evaporation of which plays an important role in thermoregulation. Sweat contains significant quantities of sodium and chloride ions, some other ions, urea and small molecular weight metabolites; thus sweating may be considered as a minor mode of excretion.

Merocrine sweat glands are unbranched tubular glands, the secretory portion forming a compact coil in the more superficial part of the fatty hypodermis. In histological section, the glands appear as a mass of tubules cut in various planes; secretory portions are interspersed with sections of the first part of the excretory duct. The secretory portion **S** consists of a single layer of large cuboidal or columnar cells, whereas the excretory duct **D** is lined by two layers of smaller cuboidal cells. The surrounding dermis contains a rich capillary plexus.

At higher magnification, the secretory portions **S** of merocrine sweat glands are seen to be mainly composed of pale stained, pyramidal cells which rest on a prominent basement membrane. These cells are believed to pump sodium ions into the gland lumen; this is followed by passive diffusion of water. A second less numerous, darkly stained cell type, which is difficult to identify with light microscopy, has ultrastructural features typical of protein-secreting cells. The dark cells are believed to secrete a glycoprotein; nevertheless the content of such in sweat is very low. Myoepithelial cells **M** form a discontinuous layer between the secretory cells and the basement membrane; contraction of these cells expels sweat into the excretory ducts.

Sections of the excretory duct **D** are readily distinguishable from sections of the secretory portion. The excretory duct has a narrower lumen, a double layer of small cuboidal cells, no underlying myoepithelial cells and a characteristically eosinophilic luminal aspect which may result from adsorption of the glycoprotein product of the dark secretory cells. The duct epithelium is thought to reabsorb sodium ions from the basic secretion, thus making it hypotonic with respect to plasma. When seen at low magnification, the ducts pursue a helical course through the dermis to discharge at the skin surface via a *sweat pore* located on an epidermal ridge.

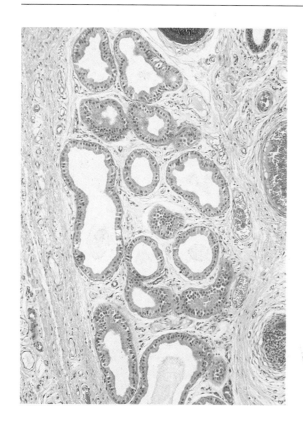

Fig. 9.16   Apocrine sweat glands H & E × 128

Apocrine sweat glands are mainly confined to the areolae of the breasts, axillae and genital regions where they produce a viscid, milky secretion which becomes malodorous after the action of skin commensal bacteria.

Apocrine sweat glands are large glands which always secrete into an adjacent hair follicle via a duct which is histologically similar to that of merocrine sweat glands. The secretory portion of the gland is of the coiled, tubular type with a widely dilated lumen. The secretory cells are usually low cuboidal and have an eosinophilic cytoplasm. The budding appearance of the apical cytoplasm of some cells gave rise to the belief that the mode of secretion was of the apocrine type, but recent evidence suggests that this appearance may be due to a fixation artefact and that the original interpretations were erroneous. Like merocrine sweat glands, apocrine glands have a discontinuous layer of myoepithelial cells between the base of the secretory cells and the prominent basement membrane.

Apocrine sweat glands do not become functional until puberty and in women undergo cyclical changes under the influence of the hormones of the menstrual cycle.

Apocrine glands are analogous to the odiferous glands of many mammals but their biological significance in humans is unknown.

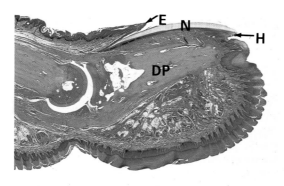

(a)

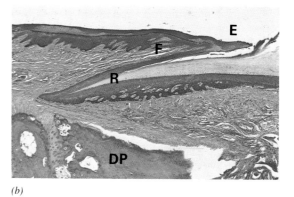

(b)

Fig. 9.17   Fingernail (monkey) (a) H & E × 5 (b) H & E × 20

The dorsal skin surface of the tip of each finger and toe forms a highly specialised appendage, the nail **N**, consisting of a dense keratinised plate, the *nail plate*, which rests on a stratified squamous epithelium called the *nail bed*. The proximal end of the nail, the *nail root* **R**, and the underlying nail bed extend deeply into the dermis to lie in close apposition to the distal interphalangeal joint, and the dermis beneath the nail plate is firmly attached to the periosteum of the distal phalanx **DP**.

Nail growth occurs by proliferation and differentiation of the epithelium underlying the nail root (known as the

nail matrix), and the nail plate slides distally over the rest of the nail bed which does not actively contribute to nail growth. Reflecting its proliferative activity, the nail matrix is thicker than that of the rest of the nail bed and exhibits pronounced epidermal ridges as seen in micrograph (b); on the surface, the distal part of the nail matrix is marked by the white crescent-shaped *lunular* at the base of the nail.

The skin overlying the root of the nail is known as the *nail fold* **F** and its highly keratinised free edge is known as the *eponychium* **E**. The skin beneath the free end of the nail is known as the *hyponychium* **H**.

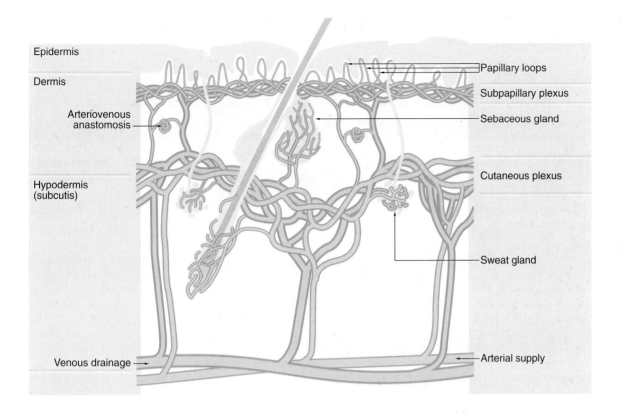

Epidermis

Dermis

Arteriovenous anastomosis

Hypodermis (subcutis)

Venous drainage →

Papillary loops
Subpapillary plexus
Sebaceous gland
Cutaneous plexus
Sweat gland
← **Arterial supply**

Fig. 9.18 **The skin circulation**

The circulation of the skin has an unusual arrangement which accommodates several different, sometimes conflicting, functional requirements: nutrition of the skin and appendages, increased blood flow to facilitate heat loss in hot conditions, and decreased blood flow to minimise heat loss in cold conditions whilst nevertheless maintaining adequate nutritional flow.

The arteries supplying the skin are located deep in the hypodermis from which they give rise to branches passing upwards to form two plexuses of anastomosing vessels. The deeper plexus lies at the junction of the hypodermis and dermis and is known as the ***cutaneous plexus***; the more superficial plexus lies just beneath the dermal papillae and is known as the ***subpapillary plexus***. Branches of the cutaneous plexus supply the fatty tissue of the hypodermis, the deeper aspect of the dermis and

capillary networks which envelop the hair follicles and deep sebaceous glands and sweat glands. The subpapillary plexus supplies the upper aspect of the dermis and the capillary networks around the superficial appendages. The subpapillary plexus also gives rise to a capillary loop in each dermal papilla. The venous drainage of the skin is arranged into plexuses broadly corresponding to the arterial supply.

Numerous shunts provide direct arteriovenous communications which play an important role in thermoregulation by controlling blood flow to the appropriate part of the dermis.

The skin has a rich lymphatic drainage which forms plexuses corresponding to those of the blood vascular system.

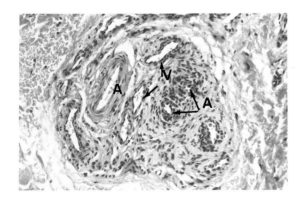

Fig. 9.19 **Glomus body** H & E × 128

In the dermis of the fingertips, and other odd peripheral sites prone to excessive cold such as the external ear, the flow in arteriovenous shunts is controlled by structures called ***glomus bodies***. The glomus consists of a highly convoluted segment of an arteriovenous shunt enveloped by condensed collagenous tissue. In histological section, one or more convolutions of the arterial **A** and venous **V** elements of the shunt are usually seen. Just before the arteriovenous junction, the wall of the artery becomes greatly thickened and its smooth muscle cells assume an epithelioid appearance.

10. Skeletal tissues

Introduction

The skeletal system is composed of a variety of specialised forms of supporting/connective tissue. Bone provides a rigid protective and supporting framework for most of the soft tissues of the body, whereas cartilage provides semi-rigid support in limited sites such as the respiratory tree and external ear. Cartilage formation is also a precursor in the processes of bone formation by either the membranous or endochondral ossification processes. Joints are composite structures which join the bones of the skeleton and, depending on the function and structure of individual joints, permit varying degrees of movement. Ligaments are robust but flexible bands of collagenous tissue which contribute to the stability of joints. Tendons provide strong, pliable connections between muscles and their points of insertion into bones.

The functional differences between the various tissues of the skeletal system relate principally to the different nature and proportion of the ground substance and fibrous elements of the extracellular matrix. The cells of all the skeletal tissues, like the cells of the less specialised supporting/connective tissues, have close structural and functional relationships and a common origin from primitive mesenchymal cells (see Ch. 4).

Cartilage

Cartilage is a semi-rigid form of supporting tissue, the characteristics of which mainly stem from the nature and predominance of ground substance in the extracellular matrix. Proteoglycans (see Ch. 4), disposed in *proteoglycan aggregates* of 100 or more molecules, make up the ground substance and account for the solid, yet flexible, consistency of cartilage. Sulphated glycosaminoglycans (chondroitin sulphate and keratan sulphate) predominate in the proteoglycan aggregates with molecules of the non-sulphated GAG, hyaluronic acid, forming the central backbone of the complex.

Within the ground substance are embedded varying proportions of collagen and elastic fibres giving rise to three main types of cartilage: *hyaline cartilage, fibrocartilage* and *elastic cartilage*.

Cartilage formation commences with the differentiation of stellate-shaped, primitive mesenchymal cells (see Fig. 4.2) to form rounded cartilage precursor cells called *chondroblasts*. Subsequent mitotic divisions give rise to aggregations of closely packed chondroblasts which grow and begin synthesis of ground substance and fibrous extracellular material. Secretion of extracellular material traps each chondroblast within the cartilaginous matrix thereby separating the chondroblasts from one another. Each chondroblast then undergoes one or two further mitotic divisions to form a small cluster of mature cells separated by a small amount of extracellular material. Mature cartilage cells, known as *chondrocytes*, maintain the integrity of the cartilage matrix. This differentiation and maturation sequence is most advanced in the centre of a mass of growing cartilage. Towards the periphery of the cartilage, chondroblasts at progressively earlier stages of differentiation merge with the surrounding loose supporting tissue. On completion of growth, the cartilage mass consists of chondrocytes embedded in a large amount of extracellular matrix. At the periphery of mature cartilage is a zone of condensed supporting tissue called *perichondrium* containing chondroblasts with cartilage-forming potential. Growth of cartilage occurs by *interstitial growth* from within and *appositional growth* at the periphery.

Most cartilage is devoid of blood vessels and consequently the exchange of metabolites between chondrocytes and surrounding tissues depends on diffusion through the water of solvation of the ground substance. This limits the thickness to which cartilage may develop whilst maintaining viability of the innermost cells; in sites where cartilage is particularly thick (e.g. costal cartilage), *cartilage canals* convey small vessels into the centre of the cartilage mass.

In mature mammals, cartilage has a limited distribution, whereas in immature mammals cartilage forms a template for most of the developing bony skeleton.

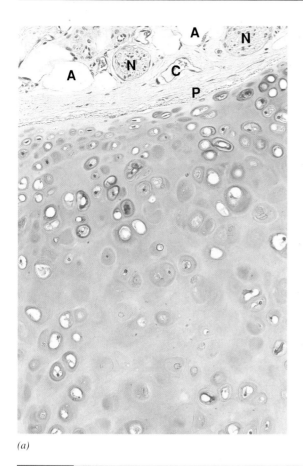

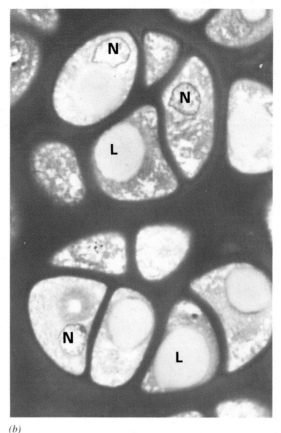

(a)   (b)

Fig. 10.1 **Hyaline cartilage (a) H & E × 150 (b) Thin section, toluidine blue × 1200**

Hyaline cartilage is the most common type of cartilage and is found in the nasal septum, larynx, tracheal rings, most articular surfaces and the sternal ends of the ribs. It also forms the precursor of bone in the developing skeleton. Mature hyaline cartilage is characterised by small aggregations of chondrocytes embedded in an amorphous matrix of ground substance reinforced by collagen fibres.

In the preparation of mature hyaline cartilage shown in micrograph (a), two zones are evident: an inner, strongly basophilic zone and a narrow, pale stained peripheral zone which merges with adjacent supporting tissue containing adipocytes **A**, capillaries **C** and small nerves **N**. The chondrocytes of the inner zone are arranged in characteristic clusters usually consisting of two or four fully differentiated cells. The clusters are separated by a large mass of amorphous cartilage matrix whilst the cells of each cluster are separated by only a thin layer of matrix. In standard histological preparations, considerable shrinkage distorts the cellular detail of the chondrocytes so that they may appear not to fully occupy their spaces within the matrix.

Extending from the inner zone towards the outer surface of the cartilage, the chondrocytes are progressively less differentiated so that the cells of the *perichondrium* **P** at the surface resemble mature fibroblasts. Note that the cells of the peripheral cartilage have not divided to form clusters. The morphological gradation of cartilage cells from the perichondrium to the most mature chondrocytes of the inner zone represents the progressive changes that occur during the development of cartilage. In adult cartilage, cell differentiation in the perichondrium and cartilage periphery is suspended

unless growth is stimulated. When growth is stimulated, isolated chondrocytes divide to form clusters thereby promoting interstitial growth whilst, at the same time, chondroblasts of the perichondrium differentiate into chondrocytes resulting in appositional growth.

The matrix of hyaline cartilage appears fairly amorphous since the ground substance and collagen have similar refractive properties. With the exception of articular cartilage, the collagen of hyaline cartilage, designated as collagen type II (see Ch. 4), is not cross-banded and is arranged in an interlacing network of fine fibrils; this collagen cannot be demonstrated by light microscopy. The variable staining intensity of the cartilage matrix reflects the concentration of acidic, sulphated proteoglycans which is greatest around the clusters of fully differentiated cells and least in the perichondrium.

With the technique employed in micrograph (b), the cellular detail of chondrocytes is preserved. Note that the chondrocytes fully occupy the spaces in the matrix, each space containing a single chondrocyte. Mature chondrocytes are characterised by small nuclei with dispersed chromatin and basophilic, granular cytoplasm reflecting a well developed rough endoplasmic reticulum. Lipid droplets **L**, often larger than the nuclei **N**, are a prominent feature of larger chondrocytes; the cytoplasm is also rich in glycogen. These characteristics reflect the active role of chondrocytes in synthesis of both the ground substance and fibrous elements of the cartilage matrix. In fully formed cartilage, the constituents of the extracellular matrix are continuously turned over, the integrity of the matrix being thus absolutely dependent on the viability of the chondrocytes.

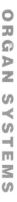

ORGAN SYSTEMS

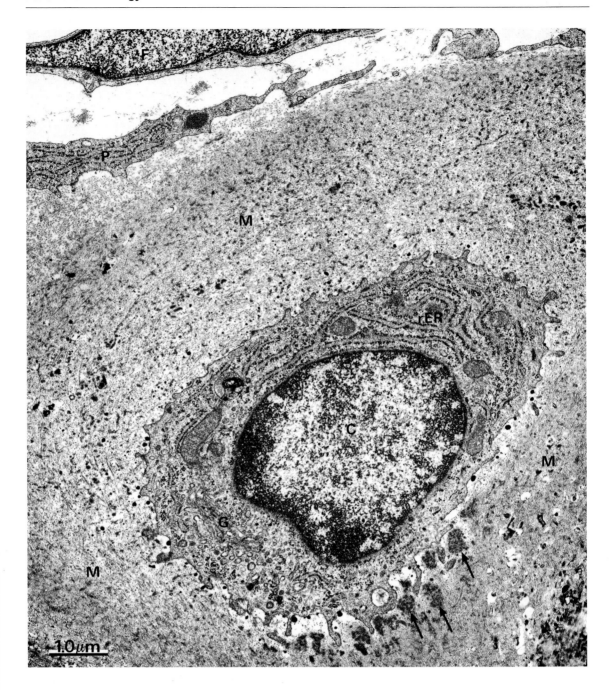

Fig. 10.2 Chondrocytes EM × 16 000

This micrograph illustrates a chondrocyte **C** lying within its lacuna and surrounded by cartilage matrix **M**. At the surface, part of the cytoplasm of a flattened perichondrial chondrocyte **P** can also be seen. Beyond this lies the nucleus and surrounding cytoplasm of a fibroblast **F** in the adjacent supporting tissue. Typical of cells active in protein synthesis (in this case matrix turnover), chondrocytes have prominent rough endoplasmic reticulum **rER** which is distended with secretory material. By contrast, note the absence of rER in the fibroblast in this micrograph. A well developed Golgi apparatus **G** is present. Glycogen granules are scattered in the cytoplasm. Note that the chondrocyte completely fills its lacuna within the matrix. Small cytoplasmic extensions mediate the constant interaction between chondrocytes and matrix. At this magnification, the fibrous elements of the matrix can just be discerned. The electron-dense material adjacent to the deep aspect of the cell (arrowed) represents recently secreted matrix material.

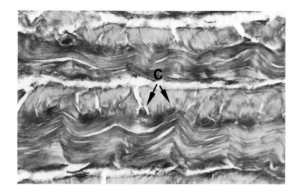

Fig. 10.3 Fibrocartilage H & E/Alcian blue × 320

Fibrocartilage, which has features intermediate between cartilage and dense fibrous supporting tissue, is found in the intervertebral discs, some articular cartilages, the pubic symphysis, and in association with dense collagenous tissue in joint capsules, ligaments and the connections of some tendons to bone. Fibrocartilage consists of alternating layers of hyaline cartilage matrix and thick layers of dense collagen fibres oriented in the direction of the functional stresses.

This micrograph is taken from the same specimen of intervertebral disc illustrated in Fig. 10.30. Pink stained collagen characteristically permeates the blue stained cartilage ground substance. Chondrocytes **C** are typically arranged in rows between the dense collagen layers within lacunae in the glycoprotein matrix.

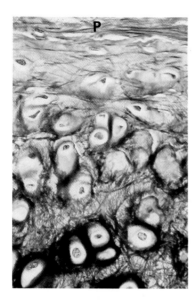

Fig. 10.4 Elastic cartilage Elastic van Gieson × 128

Elastic cartilage occurs in the external ear and external auditory canal, the epiglottis, parts of the laryngeal cartilages and the walls of the Eustachian tubes.

The histological structure of elastic cartilage is similar to that of hyaline cartilage, its elasticity, however, being derived from the presence of numerous bundles of branching elastic fibres in the cartilage matrix; this network of elastic fibres (stained black in this preparation) is particularly dense in the immediate vicinity of the chondrocytes. Collagen (stained red) is also a major constituent of the cartilage matrix and makes up the bulk of the perichondrium **P** intermingled with a few elastic fibres.

Development and growth of elastic cartilage occurs by both interstitial and appositional growth in the same manner as for hyaline cartilage.

Bone

Bone is composed of cells and a predominantly collagenous extracellular matrix (type I collagen) called *osteoid* which becomes mineralised by the deposition of calcium hydroxyapatite, thus giving the bone considerable rigidity and strength.

The cells of bone are:

- *osteoblasts*—which synthesize osteoid and mediate its mineralisation; they are found lined up along bone surfaces
- *osteocytes*—which represent largely inactive osteoblasts trapped within formed bone; they may assist in nutrition of bone
- *osteoclasts*—phagocytic cells which are capable of eroding bone and which are important, along with osteoblasts, in the constant turnover and refashioning of bone.

Osteoblasts and osteocytes are derived from a primitive mesenchymal cell called the *osteoprogenitor cell*. Osteoclasts are multinucleate phagocytic cells derived from the macrophage–monocyte cell line.

Bone forms the strong and rigid endoskeleton to which skeletal muscles are attached to permit movement. It is also acts as a calcium reservoir and is important in calcium homeostasis. Bone is heavy and its architecture is optimally arranged to provide maximum strength for the least weight. Most bones have a dense rigid outer shell of compact bone, the cortex, and a central medullary or cancellous zone of thin interconnecting narrow bone trabeculae. The number, thickness and orientation of these bone trabeculae are dependent upon the stresses to which the particular bone is exposed; for example, there are many thick intersecting trabeculae in the constantly weight-bearing vertebrae, but very few in the centre of the ribs which are not subjected to constant stress. The spaces in the medullary bone between trabeculae is occupied by haemopoietic bone marrow (see Fig. 3.12).

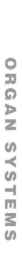

ORGAN SYSTEMS

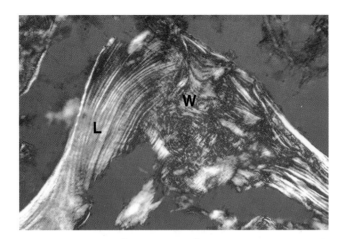

Fig. 10.5 **Woven and lamellar bone**
Eosin × 120

Bone exists in two main forms, woven bone **W** and lamellar bone **L**. Woven bone is an immature form with randomly arranged collagen fibres in the osteoid. Lamellar bone is composed of regular parallel bands of collagen arranged in sheets. Woven bone is produced when osteoblasts produce osteoid rapidly, as in fetal bone development and in adults when there is pathological rapid new bone formation, e.g. healing fracture and Paget's disease. The rapidly formed woven bone is eventually remodelled to form lamellar bone which is physically stronger and more resilient. Virtually all bone in a healthy adult is lamellar.

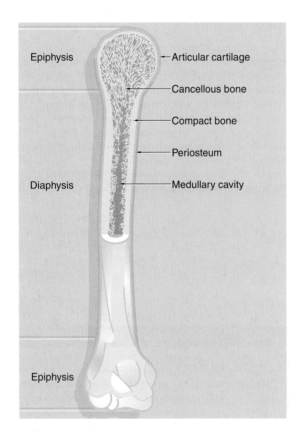

Fig. 10.6 **Long bone**

This diagram illustrates the general structure of long bones in the mature skeleton and the gross morphological appearance of the two types of lamellar bone found in the mature skeleton, i.e. compact (cortical) bone and cancellous (medullary) bone.

Compact bone forms the dense walls of the shaft or *diaphysis* while cancellous bone occupies part of the large central *medullary cavity*. Cancellous bone consists of a network of fine, irregular plates called *trabeculae* separated by intercommunicating spaces. In immature animals, the medullary cavities of most bones contain active (red) marrow which is responsible for the production of the cellular elements of blood. In the adult, active marrow is restricted to a few sites (see Ch. 3); the medullary cavities of other bones are filled with inactive (yellow) marrow which is largely composed of adipose tissue.

The articular (joint) surfaces of the expanded ends, or *epiphyses*, of long bones are protected by a layer of specialised hyaline cartilage called *articular cartilage*. The external surface of the bone is invested in a dense fibrous layer called the *periosteum* into which are inserted muscles, tendons and ligaments. The inner surfaces of the bone, including the trabeculae of cancellous bone, are invested by a delicate layer called the *endosteum*. The endosteum and periosteum contain cells of the osteogenic series which are responsible for growth, continuous remodelling and repair of bone fractures.

Prior to the attainment of skeletal maturity, the long bones grow in length by the process of endochondral ossification which occurs at a *growth* or *epiphysial plate* situated at each end of the bone at the junction of the diaphysis (shaft) and epiphysis. The *metaphysis* (not illustrated) is defined as the junction of the shaft with the growth plate.

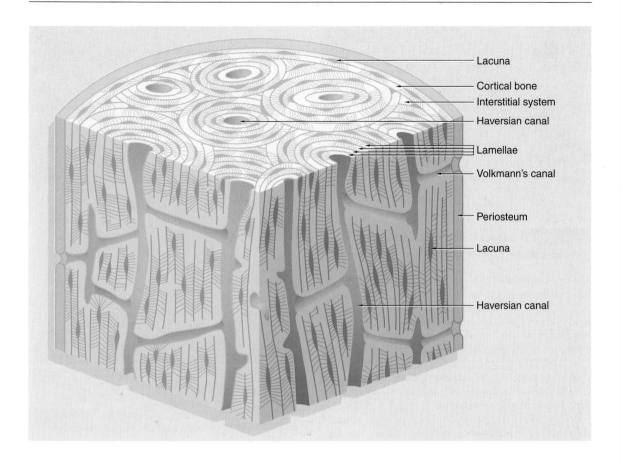

Lacuna
Cortical bone
Interstitial system
Haversian canal
Lamellae
Volkmann's canal
Periosteum
Lacuna
Haversian canal

Fig. 10.7 Compact bone

Compact bone is made up of parallel bony columns which, in long bones, are disposed parallel to the long axis, i.e. in the line of stress exerted on the bone. Each column is made up of concentric bony layers or *lamellae* disposed around a central channel containing blood vessels, lymphatics and nerves. These neurovascular channels are known as *canals of Havers* or *Haversian canals*, and with their concentric lamellae form *Haversian systems*. The neurovascular bundles interconnect with one another, and with the endosteum and periosteum, via *Volkmann's canals* which pierce the columns at right angles (or obliquely) to the Haversian canals.

Each Haversian system begins as a broad channel, at the periphery of which osteoblasts lay down lamellae of bone. With the deposition of successive lamellae, the diameter of the Haversian canal decreases and osteoblasts are trapped as osteocytes in spaces called *lacunae* in the matrix. The osteocytes are thus arranged in concentric rings within the lamellae. Between adjacent lacunae and the central canal are numerous minute interconnecting canals called *canaliculi* which contain fine cytoplasmic extensions of the osteocytes.

As a result of the continuous resorption and redeposition of bone, complete newly formed Haversian systems are disposed between partly resorbed systems formed earlier. The remnants of lamellae no longer surrounding Haversian canals form irregular *interstitial systems* between intact Haversian systems.

At the outermost aspect of compact bone, Haversian systems give way to concentric lamellae of dense *cortical bone* laid down at the bone surface by osteoblasts of the periosteum. At the inner medullary aspect, similar but irregular circumferential lamellae merge with trabeculae of cancellous bone (not illustrated).

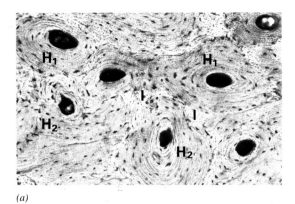

(a)

Fig. 10.8 Compact bone (ground sections, unstained) (a) TS × 80 (b) TS × 600 (c) LS × 150

These ground sections illustrate many of the features described in the preceding figure. In micrograph (a), the bone has been cut transversely thereby demonstrating newly formed Haversian systems H_1 and older, partly resorbed Haversian systems H_2; irregular interstitial systems **I**, representing the remnants of former Haversian systems, fill the spaces between the Haversian systems. Concentric rings of flattened lacunae can be seen to surround the central Haversian canals which appear as very dark areas in this preparation.

Micrograph (b) focuses on a single Haversian system, the central canal being surrounded by concentric lamellae of bone matrix containing empty lacunae **L**. Fine canaliculi **C** radiate from each lacuna to anastomose with those of adjacent lacunae. In life, the osteocytes do not completely fill the lacunae, the remaining narrow space being filled with extracellular bone fluid. Fine cytoplasmic processes of the osteocytes pass in the canaliculi to communicate via gap junctions with the processes of osteocytes in adjacent lamellae. The canaliculi provide passages for circulation of extracellular fluid and diffusion of metabolites between the lacunae and vessels of the Haversian canals.

Osteocytes maintain the structural integrity of the mineralised matrix and mediate short-term release or deposition of calcium for the purpose of calcium homeostasis in the body as a whole. The activity of osteocytes in calcium regulation is controlled directly by plasma calcium concentration and indirectly by the hormones parathormone and calcitonin secreted by the parathyroid and thyroid glands, respectively (see Ch. 17). Osteoblasts and osteocytes also appear to respond to minute piezo-electric currents induced by bone deformation, increasing or decreasing local bone formation as appropriate and inducing complementary activity in local osteoclasts via the secretion of local humoral factors. In this fashion bone is remodelled to adapt to mechanical stresses imposed on it.

Micrograph (c) shows compact bone cut in longitudinal section, the plane of section including some Haversian canals **HC**. These appear dark in colour as in micrograph (a) due to an optical artefact related to air trapped in the section. For the same reason, the tiny osteocyte lacunae appear as brown specks elongated in shape and arranged in concentric layers around the Haversian canals.

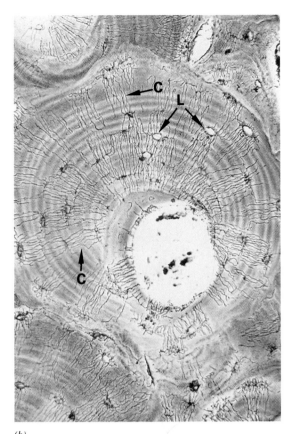

(b)

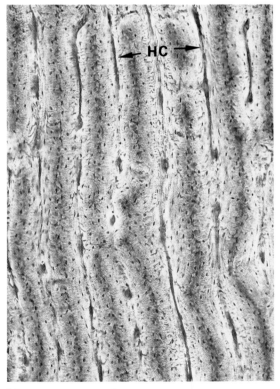

(c)

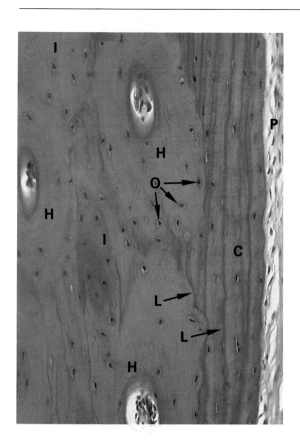

Fig. 10.9 | Compact bone TS, H & E × 198

The morphology of the cells and organic components of bone may be studied in standard decalcified preparations, as in this micrograph. Several Haversian systems **H** are seen in transverse section separated by irregular interstitial systems **I**. The matrix of decalcified mature bone is strongly eosinophilic because of its high content of collagen. The collagen of the lamellae is disposed in a helical manner around the long axes of the Haversian systems.

At its outer aspect, the Haversian bone gives way to lamellae of cortical bone **C** which provides a more dense, protective outer surface to most bones. Where the Haversian systems and cortical lamellae abut one another, fine basophilic cement lines **L** are seen, rich in proteoglycan ground substance. Note the fibrous periosteum **P** investing the surface of the cortical bone.

Osteocytes **O** have densely stained, irregular nuclei and pale, basophilic cytoplasm which undergoes considerable shrinkage in routine preparations such as this. Unlike the chondrocytes of cartilage, osteocytes do not usually completely occupy their lacunae in the bone matrix but rather they and their cytoplasmic processes are surrounded by a narrow space filled with extracellular fluid. Recent evidence suggests that this *bone fluid* may be of different composition to that of extracellular fluid of other tissues, the surface osteocytes and osteoblasts forming some form of 'bone membrane' separating the bone fluid from other extracellular fluid. Canaliculi, containing the fine cytoplasmic processes of osteocytes, are not usually visible in this type of preparation. Within the Haversian canals, note the presence of small blood vessels and nuclei representing endosteal osteoblasts.

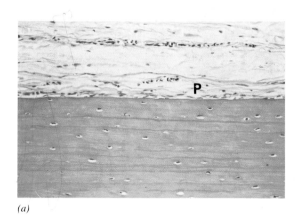

(a)

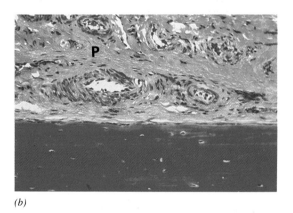

(b)

Fig. 10.10 | Mature periosteum (a) H & E × 128 (b) Masson's trichrome × 200

The outer surface of most bone is invested by a layer of condensed fibrous tissue, the periosteum **P**, which contains numerous osteoprogenitor cells which are practically indistinguishable from fibroblasts. During bone growth or repair, the osteoprogenitor cells differentiate into osteoblasts which are responsible for the deposition of concentric lamellae of cortical bone by appositional growth. The periosteum is bound to the underlying bone by bundles of collagen fibres called *Sharpey's fibres* which may penetrate the whole thickness of the cortical

bone; collagen is stained blue-green in micrograph (b). The periosteum is richly supplied with blood vessels from adjacent tissues.

Periosteum is not present on the articular surfaces of bone, the sites of insertion of tendons and ligaments, and at several other discrete sites such as the subcapsular area of the neck of the femur. The periosteum plays an important role in the repair of bone fractures and its absence may lead to delay or failure of healing, particularly of subcapsular fractures of the femoral neck.

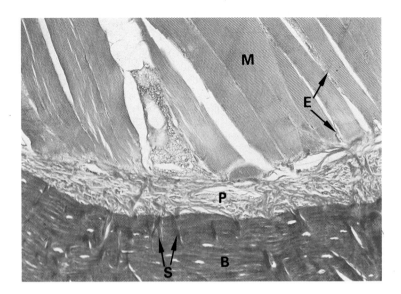

Fig. 10.11 | **Muscular insertion into bone** Phosphotungstic acid/ haematoxylin × 480

Muscle may be attached directly to bone, in which case the area of attachment is relatively extensive, or alternatively, the muscle may be inserted into a tendon which is attached to bone over a more localised area.

This micrograph shows the direct attachment of skeletal muscle **M** to bone **B**. The ends of the muscle fibres abut onto the periosteum **P**, the collagenous fibres of which extend between the muscle fibres to mingle with the collagen of the endomysium **E**; collagen stains red with this staining method. In areas of muscle attachment, the surface of the cortical bone tends to be roughened and the periosteal Sharpey's fibres **S** are robust and extend deeply into the bony cortex.

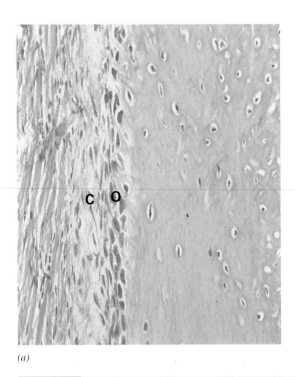

(a)

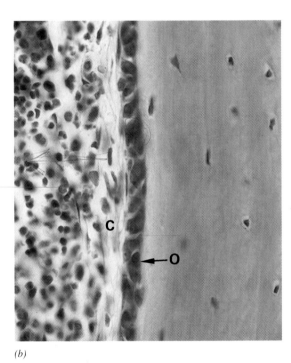

(b)

Fig. 10.12 | **Active periosteum** (a) H & E × 200 (b) H & E × 480

These micrographs illustrate highly active periosteum from a developing fetal long bone. The periosteum consists of plump, basophilic osteoblasts **O**, two to three cells deep on the surface of the developing bone, and a thin layer of immature, loose collagenous tissue **C**. The cytoplasmic basophilia of active osteoblasts reflects their large content of rough endoplasmic reticulum involved in synthesising the collagen, ground substance and other organic constituents of bone matrix. When appositional bone growth at the periosteal surface is complete, osteoblasts revert to quiescent, osteoprogenitor cells which closely resemble fibroblasts. Note that the bone of the developing shaft is of the woven type; the process of remodelling, to form lamellar bone, occurs at a later stage (see Fig. 10.22).

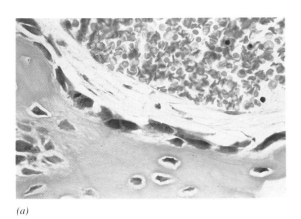

(a)

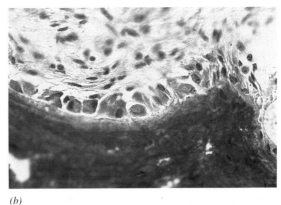

(b)

Fig. 10.13 Osteoblasts and osteoid (a) H & E × 320 (b) Undecalcified section, Goldner's trichrome × 320

These micrographs illustrate active osteoblasts in the process of laying down the organic components of bone matrix; before mineralisation occurs, the organic matrix is known as *osteoid*. In comparison with mature osteocytes, osteoblasts are large cells with abundant basophilic cytoplasm, a large Golgi apparatus and a pale stained nucleus with a prominent nucleolus. These features reflect a high rate of protein and proteoglycan synthesis.

In normally developing bone, as seen in micrograph (a), osteoid becomes calcified soon after deposition. Under conditions in which adequate calcium and phosphate ions are not available (e.g. rickets, chronic renal failure), there is a lag in mineralisation of osteoid; under such circumstances osteoid tissue accumulates. Osteoid is readily demonstrated in undecalcified sections as shown in micrograph (b), a biopsy specimen from a man with chronic renal failure. With this staining method, osteoid appears as a red stained zone between a layer of active osteoblasts and the mineralised bone (stained blue). In normal subjects the amount of unmineralised matrix is minimal.

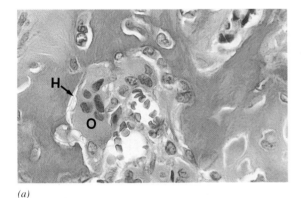

(a)

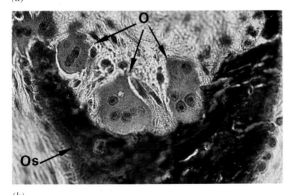

(b)

Fig. 10.14 Osteoclasts (a) H & E × 400
(b) Undecalcified section, Goldner's trichrome × 320

Resorption of bone is performed by large multinucleate cells called osteoclasts **O** which are often seen lying in depressions resorbed from the bone surface called *Howship's lacunae* **H**. The aspect of the osteoclast in apposition to bone is characterised by fine microvilli which form a *ruffled border* that is readily visible with the electron microscope. The ruffled border secretes several organic acids which dissolve the mineral component whilst lysosomal proteolytic enzymes are employed to destroy the organic matrix.

In decalcified preparations as in micrograph (a), osteoclasts tend to shrink and become detached from the bone surface; the intimate relationship of osteoclasts with bone is seen better in micrograph (b).

Osteoclastic resorption contributes to bone remodelling in response to growth or changing mechanical stresses upon the skeleton. Osteoclasts also participate in the long-term maintenance of blood calcium homeostasis by their response to parathyroid hormone and calcitonin (see Ch. 17). Parathyroid hormone stimulates osteoclastic resorption and the release of calcium ions from bone, whereas calcitonin inhibits osteoclastic activity.

The specimen shown in micrograph (b) is from a woman with a low serum calcium level. This condition stimulates release of parathyroid hormone which promotes excessive osteoclastic resorption in an attempt to restore serum calcium levels. In addition, under these circumstances there is a lag in mineralisation of newly deposited bone matrix which is manifest by the presence of osteoid **Os**.

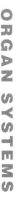

ORGAN SYSTEMS

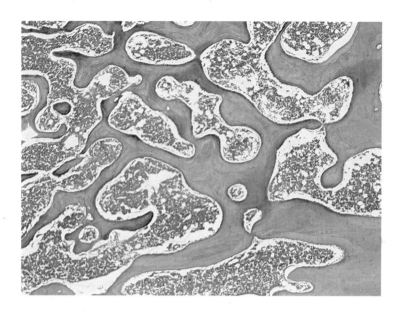

Fig. 10.15 Cancellous bone
H & E × 50

Cancellous (spongy) bone is composed of a network of bony trabeculae separated by a labyrinth of interconnecting spaces containing bone marrow (see Ch. 3). The trabeculae are thin and composed of irregular lamellae of bone with lacunae containing osteocytes (not seen at this magnification). Spongy bone does not usually contain Haversian systems and the osteocytes exchange metabolites via canaliculi with blood sinusoids in the marrow. The trabeculae are lined by a delicate layer of tissue called endosteum which contains osteoprogenitor cells, osteoblasts and osteoclasts.

Bone matrix and mineralisation

Mature compact bone is made up of about 70% inorganic salts and 30% organic matrix by weight. Collagen makes up over 90% of the organic component, the remainder being ground substance proteoglycans and a group of non-collagen molecules which appear to be involved in regulation of bone mineralisation.

The collagen of bone represents about half of the total body collagen and is almost exclusively in the form of type I fibres, a polymer of numerous elongated overlapping tropocollagen subunits (see Ch. 4). Spaces within this three-dimensional structure, often referred to as *hole zones*, are the initial site of mineral deposition.

Ground substance proteoglycans contribute a much smaller proportion of the matrix than in cartilage and mainly consist of chondroitin sulphate and hyaluronic acid in the form of proteoglycan aggregates. As well as controlling the water content of bones, ground substance is probably involved in regulating formation of collagen fibres in a form appropriate for subsequent matrix mineralisation. The remaining non-collagen organic material includes *osteocalcin (Gla protein)*, involved in binding calcium during the mineralisation process, *osteonectin* which may serve some bridging function between collagen and the mineral component, *sialoproteins* (rich in sialic acid) and certain proteins which appear to be concentrated from plasma.

The mineral component of bone mainly consists of calcium and phosphate in the form of hydroxyapatite crystals. These are conjugated to a small proportion of magnesium carbonate, sodium and potassium ions but also have affinity for heavy metal and radioactive environmental pollutants.

Collagen and the other organic matrix constituents are synthesised by the rough endoplasmic reticulum of osteoblasts, packaged by the Golgi and secreted from the cell surface resulting in the production of osteoid. After a maturation phase lasting several days, amorphous (non-crystalline) calcium phosphate salts begin to precipitate in the 'hole zones' of the collagen. These mineralisation foci expand and coalesce into hydroxyapatite crystals by further remodelling. Nevertheless, 20% or more of the mineral component remains in the amorphous form providing a readily available buffer in whole body calcium homeostasis.

The concentration of calcium and phosphate ions in bony extracellular fluid is greater than required for spontaneous deposition of calcium salts, and a variety of inhibitors including *pyrophosphate* play a crucial role in controlling bone mineralisation. The deposition of calcium appears to be associated with membrane-bound vesicles derived from osteoblast plasma membrane called *matrix vesicles*; these contain *alkaline phosphatase* and other phosphatases which may play a role in neutralising the inhibitory effect of pyrophosphate.

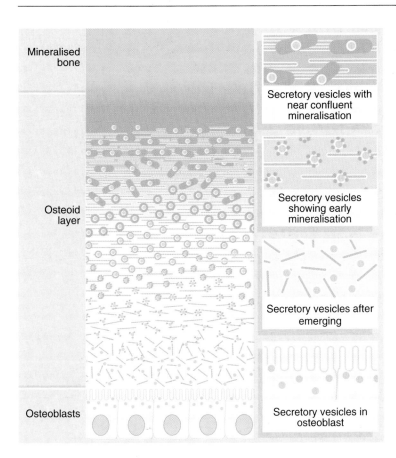

Mineralised bone

Osteoid layer

Osteoblasts

Secretory vesicles with near confluent mineralisation

Secretory vesicles showing early mineralisation

Secretory vesicles after emerging

Secretory vesicles in osteoblast

Fig. 10.16 **Mineralisation of bone**

This diagram shows the events believed to occur in the mineralisation of osteoid to form mineralised bone. The active cuboidal osteoblasts secrete osteoid collagen (red) but also matrix vesicles (yellow). The matrix vesicles are the focus for deposition of hydroxyapatite crystals (green), the first step in mineralisation. Continued accretion of mineral on these early foci leads eventually to confluent mineralisation of the osteoid collagen and supporting glycosaminoglycan matrix.

The matrix vesicles are rich in the enzymes alkaline phosphatase and pyrophosphatase which can both produce phosphate ions from a range of molecules. The phosphate ions accumulate in the matrix vesicles with calcium ions and form the raw material for the production of hydroxyapatite.

Bone development and growth

The fetal development of bone occurs in two ways, both of which involve replacement of primitive collagenous supporting tissue by bone. The resulting woven bone is then extensively remodelled by resorption and appositional growth to form the mature adult skeleton which is made up of lamellar bone. Thereafter, resorption and deposition of bone occur at a much reduced rate to accommodate changing functional stresses and to effect calcium homeostasis. The long bones, vertebrae, pelvis and bones of the base of the skull are preceded by the formation of a continuously growing cartilage model which is progressively replaced by bone; this process is called *endochondral ossification* and the bones so formed are called *cartilage bones*. In contrast, the bones of the vault of the skull, the maxilla and most of the mandible are formed by the deposition of bone within primitive mesenchymal tissue; this process of direct replacement of mesenchyme by bone is known as *intramembranous ossification* and the bones so formed are called *membrane bones*. Bone development is controlled by growth hormone, thyroid hormone and the sex hormones.

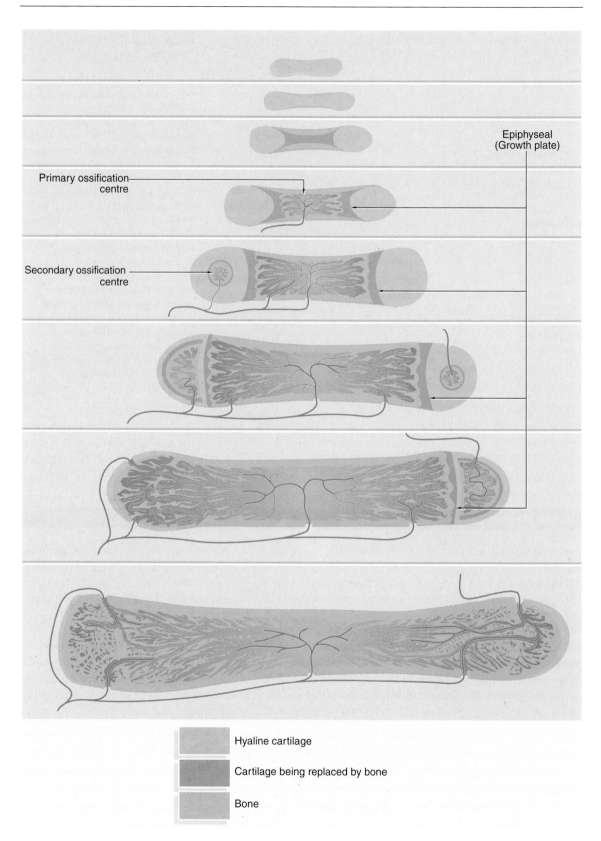

Epiphyseal
(Growth plate)

Primary ossification
centre

Secondary ossification
centre

Hyaline cartilage

Cartilage being replaced by bone

Bone

Fig. 10.17 Endochondral ossification *(illustration opposite)*

Endochondral ossification is a method of bone formation which permits functional stresses to be sustained during skeletal growth. It is well demonstrated in the development of the long bones.

A small model of the long bone is first formed in solid hyaline cartilage. This undergoes mainly appositional growth to form an elongated, dumb-bell shaped mass of cartilage consisting of a shaft (diaphysis) and future articular portions (epiphyses) surrounded by perichondrium.

Within the shaft of the cartilage model the chondrocytes enlarge greatly, resorbing the surrounding cartilage so as to leave only slender perforated trabeculae of cartilage matrix. This cartilage matrix then becomes calcified and the chondrocytes degenerate leaving large, interconnecting spaces. During this period, the perichondrium of the shaft develops osteogenic potential and assumes the role of periosteum. The periosteum then lays down a thin layer of bone around the surface of the shaft. At the same time, primitive mesenchymal cells and blood vessels invade the spaces left within the shaft after degeneration of the chondrocytes. The primitive mesenchymal cells differentiate into osteoblasts and blood-forming cells of the bone marrow. The osteoblasts form a layer of cells on the surface of the calcified remnants of the cartilage matrix and commence the formation of irregular, woven bone.

The ends of the original cartilage model have by now become separated by a large site of *primary ossification* in the shaft. The cartilaginous ends of the model, however, continue to grow in diameter. Meanwhile, the cartilage at the ends of the shaft continues to undergo regressive changes followed by ossification so that the developing bone now consists of an elongated, bony diaphysial shaft with a semilunar cartilage epiphysis at each end. The interface between the shaft and each epiphysis constitutes a *growth* or *epiphysial plate*. Within the growth plate, the cartilage proliferates continuously, resulting in progressive elongation of the bone. At the diaphysial aspect of each growth plate, the chondrocytes mature and then die, the degenerating zone of cartilage being replaced by bone. Thus the bony diaphysis lengthens and the growth plates are pushed further and further apart. On reaching maturity, hormonal changes inhibit further cartilage proliferation and the growth plates are replaced by bone, causing fusion of the diaphysis and epiphyses.

In the meantime, in the centre of the mass of cartilage of each developing epiphysis, regressive changes and bone formation similar to that in the diaphysial cartilage occur along with appositional growth of cartilage over the whole external surface of the epiphysis. This conversion of central epiphysial cartilage to bone is known as *secondary ossification*. A thin zone of hyaline cartilage always remains at the surface as the articular cartilage.

Under the influence of functional stresses, the calcified cartilage remnants and the surrounding irregular woven bone are completely remodelled so that the bone ultimately consists of a compact outer layer with a medulla of cancellous bone. By maturity, the medullary bone is almost completely resorbed to leave a large medullary space filled with bone marrow.

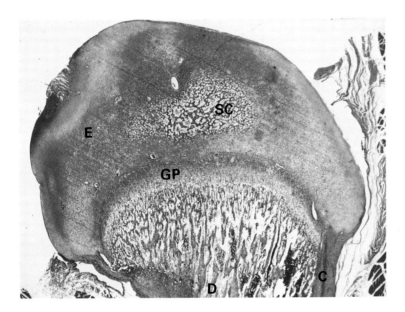

Fig. 10.18 Epiphysis
H & E/Alcian blue × 12

This micrograph illustrates the head of a kitten femur at an advanced stage of development.

The cartilaginous epiphysis **E** is separated from the diaphysis **D** by the epiphysial growth plate **GP**. Note the thickening compact bone **C** at the outer aspect of the diaphysis and the trabeculae of bone in the medulla. Note also the centre of secondary ossification **SC** in the epiphysial cartilage.

Epiphysial growth plates provide for growth in length of long bones whilst accommodating functional stresses in the growing skeleton. The next three micrographs focus, at higher magnification, on particular areas of the epiphysial plate.

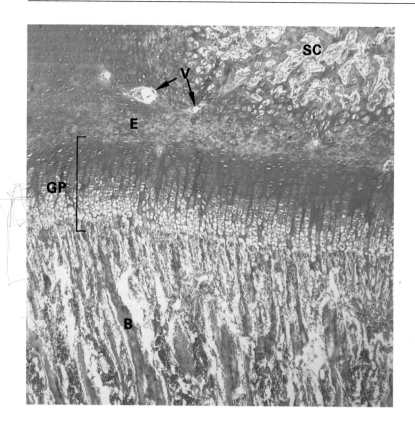

Fig. 10.19 Epiphysial growth plate H & E/Alcian blue × 40

At higher magnification, the epiphysial growth plate **GP** shows a progression of morphological changes between the epiphysial cartilage **E** and the newly forming bone **B** of the diaphysis. Similar, but less stratified, morphological changes are seen between the epiphysial cartilage and the centre of secondary ossification **SC** within the epiphysis although this does not represent a growth plate. The Alcian blue counter-stain has been employed as it has particular affinity for the ground substance of cartilage. Note blood vessels **V**, cut in transverse section, passing into the secondary ossification centre via cartilage canals.

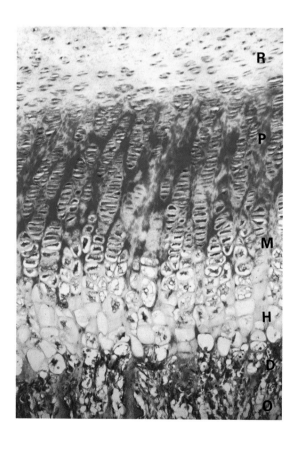

Fig. 10.20 Epiphysial growth plate H & E/Alcian blue × 120

The dynamic process of endochondral ossification is summarised in this micrograph of the epiphysial growth plate at high magnification. The transition between epiphysial cartilage and new bone occurs in six functional and morphological stages:

- *Zone of reserve cartilage* **R**: this consists of typical hyaline cartilage (see Fig. 10.1) with the chondrocytes arranged in small clusters surrounded by a large amount of moderately stained matrix.
- *Zone of proliferation* **P**: the clusters of cartilage cells undergo successive mitotic divisions to form columns of chondrocytes separated by strongly stained matrix rich in proteoglycans.
- *Zone of maturation* **M**: cell division has ceased and the chondrocytes increase in size.
- *Zone of hypertrophy and calcification* **H**: the chondrocytes become greatly enlarged and vacuolated and the matrix becomes calcified.
- *Zone of cartilage degeneration* **D**: the chondrocytes degenerate and the lacunae of the calcified matrix are invaded by osteogenic cells and capillaries from the marrow cavity of the diaphysis.
- *Osteogenic zone* **O**: the osteogenic cells differentiate into osteoblasts which congregate on the surface of the spicules of calcified cartilage matrix where they commence bone formation. This transitional zone is known as the *metaphysis*.

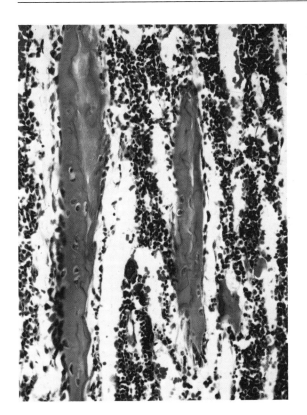

Fig. 10.21 Endochondral ossification:
metaphysis H & E/Alcian blue × 198

In the metaphysis seen in this preparation, the blue stained
spicules of calcified cartilage matrix are surrounded by
osteoblasts and newly formed woven bone which is
stained pink. Further growth of metaphysial woven bone
is followed by extensive remodelling to produce mature
compact and spongy bone.

At physical maturity the process of endochondral
ossification ceases. This stage is recognised by the fusion
of the diaphysis with the epiphysis, resulting in the
obliteration of the growth plates. From this point onwards
no further endochondral ossification is possible. Although
endochondral ossification is the means of growth in
length of a long bone, growth in diameter of the shaft
occurs by appositional growth at the periosteal surface
and complementary osteoclastic resorption at the
endosteal (medullary) aspect.

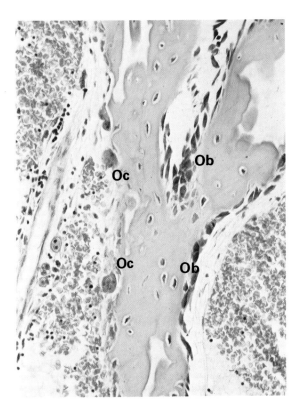

Fig. 10.22 Bone remodelling and repair
H & E × 480

This micrograph illustrates an irregular spicule of woven
bone from a fetus. Some of the surfaces of the spicule
exhibit osteoblastic proliferation and activity **Ob** whereas
other surfaces are in the process of being resorbed by
osteoclasts **Oc**.

Woven bone is not only the first type of bone to be
formed during skeletal development but is also the first
bone to be laid down during the repair of a fracture.
At the fracture site, a blood clot initially forms, later
being replaced by highly vascular collagenous tissue
(*granulation tissue*) which becomes progressively more
fibrous. Mesenchymal cells then differentiate into
chondroblasts and progressively replace this *fibrous
granulation tissue* with hyaline cartilage. This firm but
still flexible bridge is known as the *provisional callus*.
The provisional callus is then strengthened by deposition
of calcium salts within the cartilage matrix. Meanwhile,
osteoprogenitor cells in the endosteum and periosteum are
activated and lay down a meshwork of woven bone within
and around the provisional callus; the provisional callus
thus becomes transformed into the *bony callus. Bony
union* is achieved when the fracture site is completely
bridged by woven bone. Under the influence of functional
stresses, the bony callus is then slowly remodelled to
form mature lamellar bone.

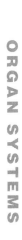

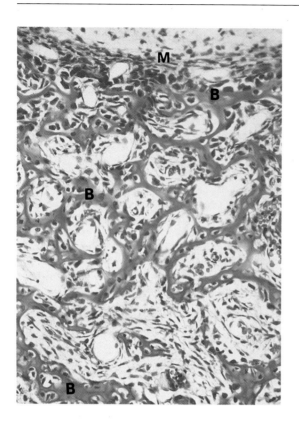

Fig. 10.23 Intramembranous ossification
H & E × 75

Intramembranous bone formation occurs within 'membranes' of condensed, primitive mesenchymal tissue. Mesenchymal cells differentiate into osteoblasts which begin synthesis and secretion of osteoid at multiple *centres of ossification*; mineralisation of osteoid follows closely. As osteoid is laid down, osteoblasts are trapped in lacunae to become osteocytes and their fine cytoplasmic extensions shrink to form the fine processes contained within the canaliculi. Osteoprogenitor cells at the surface of the centres of ossification undergo mitotic division to produce further osteoblasts which lay down more bone. Progressive bone formation results in the fusion of adjacent ossification centres to form bone which is spongy in gross appearance.

The collagen fibres of developing bone are randomly arranged in interlacing bundles, giving rise to the term woven bone. The woven bone then undergoes progressive remodelling into lamellar bone by osteoclastic resorption and osteoblastic deposition to form mature compact or spongy bone. The primitive mesenchyme remaining in the network of developing bone differentiates into bone marrow.

This preparation from the developing skull vault of a cat fetus illustrates spicules of woven bone **B**, separated by primitive mesenchymal tissue. Note the condensed primitive mesenchyme **M** which delineates the outer margin of the developing bone.

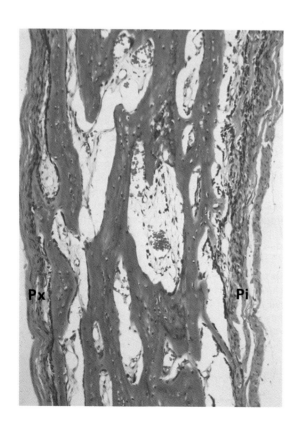

Fig. 10.24 Skull (cat) H & E × 30

This micrograph shows a full thickness view of the skull vault of a mature cat which, as in humans, is formed by the process of intramembranous ossification. The skull vault consists of cancellous bone which is condensed at its internal and external aspects to form continuous, relatively smooth surfaces. The external surface of the skull is invested by periosteum **Px** which merges with the deep layers of the overlying scalp. The internal surface of the skull is also lined by periosteum **Pi**; this layer also constitutes the outermost membranous covering of the brain, the dura mater.

During skeletal growth, the skull vault expands in response to the pressure of the growing brain within. The developing skull bones, which are bound together by *sutures* of periosteum, are pushed outwards and new membrane bone is laid down at the sutural margins. At the same time, periosteal deposition of new bone on the outer surfaces, and corresponding osteoclastic resorption at the inner surfaces, provides for the necessary recontouring of the skull bones which become progressively flatter. At skeletal maturity the sutures between the skull bones become almost closed and filled with dense fibrous tissue which represents the periosteal layers of opposing bones. With advancing age the sutures tend to ossify.

Joints

Joints may be classified into two main functional groups, *synovial* and *non-synovial*, both of which may show wide morphological variations.

Synovial joints

In this type of joint there is extensive movement of the bones upon one another at the articular surfaces. The articular surfaces are maintained in apposition by a fibrous capsule and ligaments, and the surfaces are lubricated by *synovial fluid*. Synovial joints are known as *diarthroses*. In some diarthroses such as the temporomandibular and knee joints, plates of fibrocartilage may be completely or partially interposed between the articular surfaces but remain unattached to the articular surfaces.

Non-synovial joints

These joints have limited movement, the articulating bones having no free articular surfaces, instead being joined by dense collagenous tissue. This may be of three types:

- **Dense fibrous tissue**. This forms the sutures between the bones of the skull and permits moulding of the fetal skull during its passage through the birth canal. The sutures are progressively replaced by bone with advancing age. Such fibrous tissue joints are called *syndesmoses*, and when replaced by bone are called *synostoses*.
- **Hyaline cartilage**. This type of joint, called a *synchondrosis* or *primary cartilagenous joint*, unites the first rib with the sternum and is the only synchondrosis found in the human adult.
- **Fibrocartilage**. The opposing surfaces of some bones are covered by hyaline cartilage but, instead of a synovial space, are directly connected to each other by a plate of fibrocartilage. Such fibrocartilaginous joints are called *symphyses* or *secondary cartilaginous joints* and occur in the pubic symphysis and at the intervertebral discs. The fibrocartilage disc of the pubic symphysis develops a central cavity and the intervertebral discs have a fluid-filled central cavity.

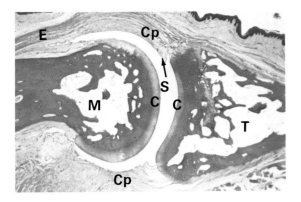

Fig. 10.25 **Synovial joint (monkey)** H & E × 12

This micrograph illustrates a typical synovial joint, in this case the distal interphalangeal joint of the finger. The articular surfaces of the terminal phalanx **T** and the middle phalanx **M** are covered by hyaline cartilage **C**. The joint space is artefactually widened. In vivo, the articular surfaces are maintained in close contact by a fibrous capsule **Cp** which is inserted into the articulating bones at some distance beyond the articular cartilages. The *synovium* **S** is a specialised layer of collagenous tissue which lines the inner aspect of the capsule. Note the extensor tendon **E** which inserts into the base of terminal phalanx.

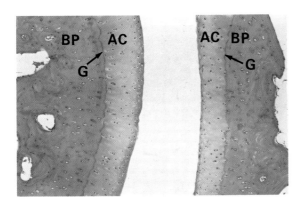

Fig. 10.26 **Articular cartilage** H & E × 20

This micrograph focuses on the opposing articular cartilages **AC** of the synovial joint shown in the previous micrograph.

Each articular cartilage is bonded to its long bone at a region called the *bony end plate* **BP**; this region is composed of an unusual type of bone which lacks Haversian systems and canaliculi and in which osteocytes occupy particularly large lacunae. The articular cartilage is sharply demarcated from the underlying bony end plate by a thick layer of glycoprotein-rich substance **G** which resembles the cement lines of Haversian bone.

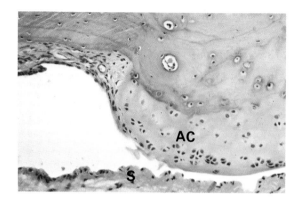

Fig. 10.27 Articular cartilage H & E × 128

This micrograph shows the lower rim of the articular cartilage **AC** of the middle phalanx of the joint shown in Fig. 10.25. Articular cartilage differs from other hyaline cartilage in two respects. Firstly, the articular surface is not covered by perichondrium. Secondly, the collagen fibres of the articular cartilage matrix are of type I, exhibiting the characteristic cross-banding of the collagen fibres typical of supporting tissue and bone. In contrast, the collagen fibres of hyaline cartilage elsewhere (type III collagen) are not cross-banded (see Ch. 4).

Articular cartilage, like other hyaline cartilage, is avascular; it is nourished by diffusion from the synovial fluid of the joint cavity. Note part of the synovial layer **S** of the joint capsule.

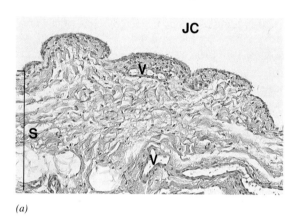

(a)

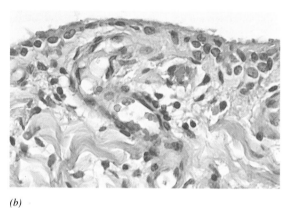

(b)

Fig. 10.28 Synovium (a) H & E × 100 (b) H & E × 400

The inner surface of the capsule of synovial joints and tendon sheaths is lined by a specialised collagenous tissue, the synovium, which is responsible for the elaboration of the synovial fluid which lubricates the movement of articular surfaces. Depending on the location, the bulk of the synovial tissue may be of loose collagenous type (*areolar synovium*), of more dense collagenous type (*fibrous synovium*) or predominantly composed of fat (*adipose synovium*) as in the case of intra-articular fat pads.

As seen in micrograph (a), the surface of the synovium **S** is thrown up into folds and smaller villi which may extend for some distance into the joint cavity **JC**. The synovial tissue contains numerous blood vessels **V**, lymphatics and nerves.

As seen in micrograph (b), the free surface of the synovium is characterised by a discontinuous layer of cells up to four cells deep. These *synovial cells* are not connected by junctional complexes and do not rest on a basement membrane, and the synovial surface therefore does not constitute an epithelium. The synovial cells are of mesenchymal origin. The majority are plump with an extensive Golgi complex and numerous lysosomes, features suggestive of macrophages (*type A synovocytes*). The remainder have profuse rough endoplasmic reticulum and represent fibroblasts (*type B synovocytes*). Also in this micrograph, note the rich network of capillaries and the thick strands of collagen which would define this as fibrous synovium.

In the normal joint, the synovial fluid is little more than a thin film covering the articular surfaces. In that the articular space is not demarcated from the synovium by an epithelium, the synovial fluid represents a highly specialised fluid form of synovial extracellular matrix rather than a secretion in the usual sense. Its major constituents are hyaluronic acid and associated glycoproteins secreted by the type B synovocytes and its fluid component is a transudate from synovial capillaries. This arrangement facilitates the continuous exchange of oxygen, carbon dioxide and metabolites between blood and synovial fluid which is the major source of metabolic support for articular cartilage. Normal synovial fluid also contains a small number of leucocytes (less than 100/mm^3), predominantly monocytes.

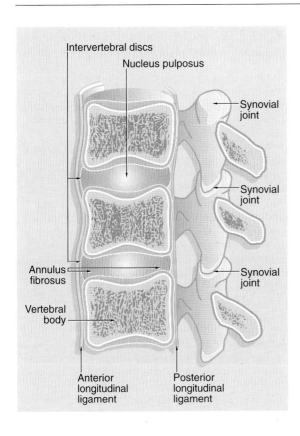

Intervertebral discs
Nucleus pulposus
Synovial joint
Synovial joint
Synovial joint
Annulus fibrosus
Vertebral body
Anterior longitudinal ligament
Posterior longitudinal ligament

Fig. 10.29 **The intervertebral joints**

The vertebrae articulate by means of two different types of joints:

- The vertebral bodies are united by symphysial joints, the *intervertebral discs*, which permit movement between the vertebral bodies whilst maintaining a union of great strength. The fibrocartilage of each intervertebral disc is arranged in concentric rings forming the *annulus fibrosus*. Within the disc, there is a central cavity containing a viscous fluid, the *nucleus pulposus*, which acts as a shock absorber. The annulus fibrosus is reinforced peripherally by circumferential ligaments. A thick ligament extending down the anterior aspect of the spinal column merges with and further reinforces the annulus fibrosus and a similar, but thinner, ligament reinforces the posterior aspect.
- The vertebral arches articulate with each other by pairs of synovial joints known as facet or zygoapophyseal joints. Strong elastic ligaments connecting the bony processes of the vertebral arches contribute to the stability of the spinal column.

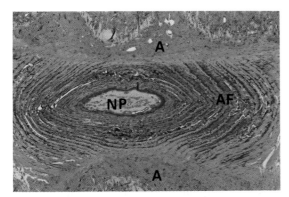

(a)

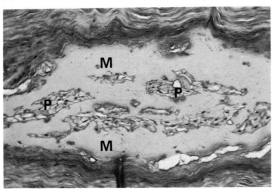

(b)

Fig. 10.30 **Intervertebral disc (rat)**
(a) H & E/Alcian blue × 20
(b) H & E/Alcian blue × 128

An intervertebral disc is shown in these micrographs of the tail of an immature rat; this has been chosen since the much larger intervertebral discs of mature mammals and humans would not be amenable to sectioning and photomicroscopy in this manner.

The intervertebral disc lies between the articular surfaces **A** of adjacent vertebral bodies. The disc consists of concentric layers of fibrocartilage, constituting the annulus fibrosus **AF**, which surrounds the central nucleus pulposus **NP**. This staining method distinguishes the collagen component of the fibrocartilage, which is stained pink, from the ground substance component, which is stained blue.

At high magnification, the nucleus pulposus is seen to consist of an unusual fluid form of supporting tissue; this is the only remnant of the embryonic notochord persisting in adult mammals. The cells of the nucleus pulposus, called *physaliphorous cells* **P**, are scattered in irregular clumps throughout an extracellular matrix **M** which consists of ground substance only.

The intervertebral disc functions in the manner of a hydraulic shock absorber, the nucleus pulposus acting as hydraulic fluid. With advancing age, the fibrocartilage of the annulus fibrosus becomes thinned and weakened and the nucleus pulposus tends to be extruded, particularly at the postero-lateral aspect where the disc is least reinforced by surrounding ligaments. This gives rise to the inappropriately named condition, 'slipped disc'.

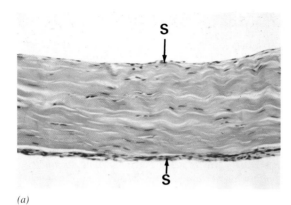

(a)

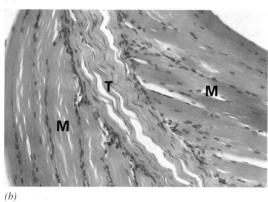

(b)

Fig. 10.31 Tendon
(a) H & E × 128 (b) H & E × 128

Tendons are tough inextensible but flexible straps which connect certain muscles to various skeletal structures allowing the muscular forces to be exerted at some distance from the body of the muscle itself and, in some cases, in a different direction.

Tendon is the densest form of collagenous supporting tissue, consisting of bundles of coarse collagen fibres among which are scattered rows of fibroblasts with elongated nuclei. Each tendon is composed of small bundles of this dense tissue bound together by a small amount of looser collagenous supporting tissue which contains the scanty blood supply and tiny nerve fibres from the tendon stretch receptors. The tendon surface is smooth and condensed with minimal connections with the surrounding tissue so as to allow relatively unimpeded movement of the tendon.

In some sites, as shown in micrograph (a), tendons are invested in a fibrous sheath lined by synovium **S**, movement of the tendon within the sheath being lubricated by synovial fluid.

Micrograph (b) shows the insertion of two masses of skeletal muscle **M** into a common tendon **T**; in this case, the tendon will exert the muscular force in a direction different from the direction of pull of the individual skeletal muscles attached to it.

Ligaments are dense bands of fibrous tissue which reinforce joint capsules and maintain bones in the correct anatomical arrangement. Ligaments are histologically similar to tendons but have a less ordered arrangement of the collagen fibres and a variable content of elastic fibres.

11. Immune system

Introduction

All living tissues are subject to the constant threat of invasion by disease-producing foreign agents and micro-organisms (pathogens), i.e. bacteria, viruses, fungi, protozoa and multicellular parasites. These organisms may invade the body, multiply and destroy functional tissue. Three main lines of defence have consequently evolved:

- protective surface mechanisms
- non-specific tissue defence
- specific immune responses.

Protective surface mechanisms

In humans, these provide the first line of defence. Pathogens may enter the body via breaches in the skin or linings of the gut, respiratory and genitourinary tracts. The skin constitutes a relatively impenetrable barrier to most microorganisms unless breached by injury such as abrasion or burning. The seromucous surfaces of the body, such as the conjunctivae and oral cavity, are protected by a variety of antibacterial substances including the enzyme *lysozyme* which is secreted in tears and saliva. The respiratory tract is protected by a layer of surface mucus which is continuously removed by ciliary action and replaced by goblet cell activity. Maintenance of an acidic environment in the stomach, vagina and, to a lesser extent, the skin, inhibits the growth of pathogens in these sites. When such defences fail, the two other main types of defence mechanism are activated.

Non-specific tissue defences

Damage to tissues usually excites a non-specific response called *inflammation* (which may be *acute* or *chronic*), which is aimed at removal of any dead tissue and foreign matter, replacement of lost tissue by scar formation and in some cases regeneration of normal tissue. Acute inflammation is characterised by vascular changes, including dilatation and enhanced permeability of capillaries and increased blood flow, resulting in the production of a fibrin-rich *inflammatory exudate*. Neutrophils, and later macrophages, migrate into the damaged tissues, and phagocytose and kill pathogens. Tissue debris is removed by phagocytosis. Destruction of organisms by phagocytosis is often greatly enhanced by involvement of immunological mechanisms as described below. Destroyed tissue is initially replaced by proliferation of capillary-rich *granulation tissue*, which is then slowly replaced by fibroblast proliferation and collagen deposition with the eventual formation of a relatively avascular and acellular fibrous *scar*. Some tissues, such as liver, skin and epithelial linings, are able to regenerate to a greater or lesser degree.

Complement is a series of plasma proteins constituting an enzyme cascade analogous to the clotting system. The cascade can be activated via either the *classical pathway* (usually involving antigen–antibody complexes, see below) or the *alternative pathway* (direct activation by certain organisms). The various peptides and proteins thus generated mediate a diverse range of processes including vascular changes (dilatation and increased permeability), cell lysis, *opsonisation* (coating of organisms with complement which enhances phagocytosis by leucocytes), and leucocyte activation and attraction (*chemotaxis*). The alternative pathway probably evolved first as a non-specific defence system, with the classical pathway evolving later as an effector mechanism linked to the immune response.

The immune system

This highly specific system depends upon the recognition of exogenous materials as being foreign to the body, any particular foreign substance so recognised being known as an *antigen*. This results in the activation of the immune system with the purpose of neutralising or destroying the antigen. Some normal body components may also act as antigens in *autoimmune reactions*, a pathological situation resulting from failure of *self-tolerance*. Lymphocytes play the central role in the immune response but rely on the phagocytic cells of the monocyte–macrophage system for *presentation of antigen* to T lymphocytes. Components of the non-specific defence system (i.e. complement, neutrophils, macrophages) are frequently employed and amplified in the final destruction of antigen. As any one microorganism is usually made up of many different antigens (i.e. peptides, proteins, polysaccharides), the immunological response may involve a combination of mechanisms.

The cells of the immune system, particularly lymphocytes, are distributed throughout the body as single cells, as non-encapsulated aggregations in the gastrointestinal, respiratory and other tracts (***mucosa-associated lymphoid tissue, MALT***), or within the lymphoid organs, namely the ***thymus, lymph nodes*** and ***spleen***. This chapter begins with an overview of the function of the immune system, which is an essential prerequisite for understanding the structure and function of the different lymphoid tissues.

The immune system is traditionally divided into two branches, namely ***cell-mediated immunity*** and ***humoral immunity***, corresponding to two types of lymphocytes identified by early immunological research. ***B lymphocytes (B cells)*** are responsible for antibody production and mediate the humoral response. In cell-mediated immunity, ***T lymphocytes (T cells)*** function as cytotoxic cells, directly killing abnormal cells. More recent research has revealed a system of interrelationships and controls making this classification a gross oversimplification. Lymphocyte subtypes such as ***T helper*** and ***T suppressor*** cells control B and T cell responses.

Antigen presenting cells (APCs) of various types, including macrophages and B lymphocytes, control the activation of T cells. The entire system forms an exquisitely balanced mechanism which can be switched on and off in response to antigen challenge and which can respond with a varied armamentarium to different pathogens.

The specificity of the immune system is entirely attributable to the remarkable chemical structure of antigen receptors on lymphocytes, namely ***surface immunoglobulin (sIg)*** on B cells and the ***T cell receptor (TCR)*** on T cells. The ability of this system to respond to the huge variety of antigens confronting it depends on rearrangement of the genes for these receptors by DNA splicing to generate an enormous diversity of receptor structures in a random manner.

Lymphocytes

Lymphocytes comprise some 20–50% of leucocytes in the circulation, their numbers increasing in response to viral infections. Most circulating lymphocytes measure 6–9 μm (i.e. about the same size as erythrocytes) and are called ***small lymphocytes***. About 3% are ***large lymphocytes***, measuring 9–15 μm.

The light and electron microscopic appearance of circulating lymphocytes has been illustrated in Chapter 3. Lymphocyte nuclei are ovoid or kidney-shaped with the dense chromatin typical of cells with relatively little biosynthetic activity. Nucleoli are not visible with the usual Romanowsky stains of light microscopy, but can be demonstrated using the methyl green/pyronin method.

In small lymphocytes, the nucleus occupies about 90% of cell volume, the cytoplasm forming only a narrow rim. The cytoplasm exhibits pale basophilia (i.e. stains light blue) due to a considerable number of free ribosomes; rough endoplasmic reticulum is minimal. With the electron microscope, the Golgi apparatus appears rudimentary and a few lysosomes can be seen. The glycogen content is variable. The plasma membrane exhibits small cytoplasmic projections which, with the scanning electron microscope, appear as short microvilli; these are much more numerous on B lymphocytes. With phase contrast microscopy, lymphocytes exhibit slow amoeboid movement without the cytoplasmic spreading seen in monocytes.

Large lymphocytes have a greater amount of cytoplasm. The majority of large lymphocytes seen in blood represent activated B lymphocytes en route to the tissues where they will become antibody-secreting ***plasma cells*** (see Fig. 11.2). Some circulating large lymphocytes are ***natural killer (NK) cells***. NK cells are able to kill virus-infected cells by inducing apoptosis by a mechanism which is not antigen-specific. Granules containing ***granzymes*** and ***perforin*** are found in the cytoplasm of NK cells, which are thus sometimes described as ***large granular lymphocytes (LGL)***. NK cells have some but not all features of T lymphocytes and may constitute a separate lymphocyte subset in addition to T and B lymphocytes.

The role of T lymphocytes

T cells have a number of effector and regulatory functions. Both T and B cells are derived from stem cells in the bone marrow. Immature T lymphocytes migrate from the bone marrow to the thymus where they develop into mature T (thymus-dependent) lymphocytes. The process of maturation includes proliferation, rearrangement of TCR genes to produce a huge range of antigen specificities, and acquisition of the ***surface markers*** of the mature T cell (see Fig. 11.4). At this stage, T cells with the ability to react with 'self-antigens' (normal body components) are removed by apoptosis, creating a state of ***self-tolerance***. Mature T cells then populate the peripheral lymphoid tissues (lymph nodes, mucosa-associated lymphoid tissues and spleen) and from here continuously circulate via the bloodstream in a constant quest for antigen. On encountering antigen, T lymphocytes effect antigen destruction either directly by cytotoxic activity or indirectly by activation of B lymphocytes or macrophages.

T lymphocytes are divided into several functional subsets known as *T helper cells, cytotoxic T cells* and *suppressor T cells*. These subsets can be identified by the presence of different surface markers.

- **T helper cells** (T_H cells). These T lymphocytes 'help' other lymphocytes to perform their effector functions by secreting a variety of locally acting mediators known as *cytokines*. Such functions include activation of B cells to produce antibody, regulation of cytotoxic T cell function and activation of macrophages to mount a granulomatous inflammatory response (*delayed-type hypersensitivity*). T_H cells are characterised by the presence of the surface marker CD4 as well as the *pan-T cell markers* (CD2, CD3 and the TCR) which are present on all mature T cells (see Fig. 11.4).
- **Cytotoxic T cells** (T_C cells). These lymphocytes function in the killing of virus-infected and malignant cells. Most carry the surface marker CD8 as well as the pan-T cell markers. They require interaction with T_H cells to become activated and proliferate to form clones of effector cells.
- **Suppressor T cells** (T_S cells). The existence of this functional subset is still controversial, although suppressor function can be demonstrated by CD8-bearing lymphocytes in experimental animals. These cells are thought to be responsible for switching off the immune response when the initiating stimulus is removed and possibly for suppressing immune responsiveness to self-antigens. However, other mechanisms are known which can carry out at least some of these functions and the exact role of suppressor cells in vivo is thus unknown. Because they carry the CD8 marker, suppressor cells are often lumped together with T_C cells in one subgroup designated *suppressor/cytotoxic T cells*.

The role of B lymphocytes

B lymphocytes are derived from precursors in the bone marrow and also mature there. B cell maturation was first studied in birds in an organ called the *Bursa of Fabricius*; this is the origin of the designation 'B' lymphocyte.

B lymphocytes are characterised by their ability to mature into plasma cells which synthesise *antibodies (immunoglobulins)*, which bind to specific antigens. Immunoglobulins, which fall into five different structural classes, namely IgG, IgA, IgD, IgM and IgE, are secreted and circulate in the blood. They are also found bound to the surface of B cells where they behave as antigen receptors, activating the B cell when the appropriate antigen binds with the surface antibody. As a general rule, activation of B cells requires the 'help' of a T helper cell (see above) responding to the same antigen.

Once activated, the B cell undergoes mitotic division to produce a clone of cells, able to synthesise immunoglobulin of the same antigen specificity. Most of the B cells of such a clone mature into plasma cells which are capable of synthesis and secretion of large quantities of immunoglobulin. When an antigen is encountered for the first time, this is described as the *primary immune response*. A few cells from the same clone mature to become memory cells, small long-lived circulating lymphocytes which are able to respond quickly to any subsequent challenge with the same antigen. Antibody production during this *secondary immune response* occurs much more rapidly, is of much greater magnitude and produces IgG rather than IgM. This phenomenon explains the lifetime immunity which follows many common infections; it is also the general principle on which vaccination is based.

Antibodies neutralise or destroy invading organisms by a number of methods, all of which involve binding of antibody to one or more antigens associated with the organism; further details are given in Figure 11.1.

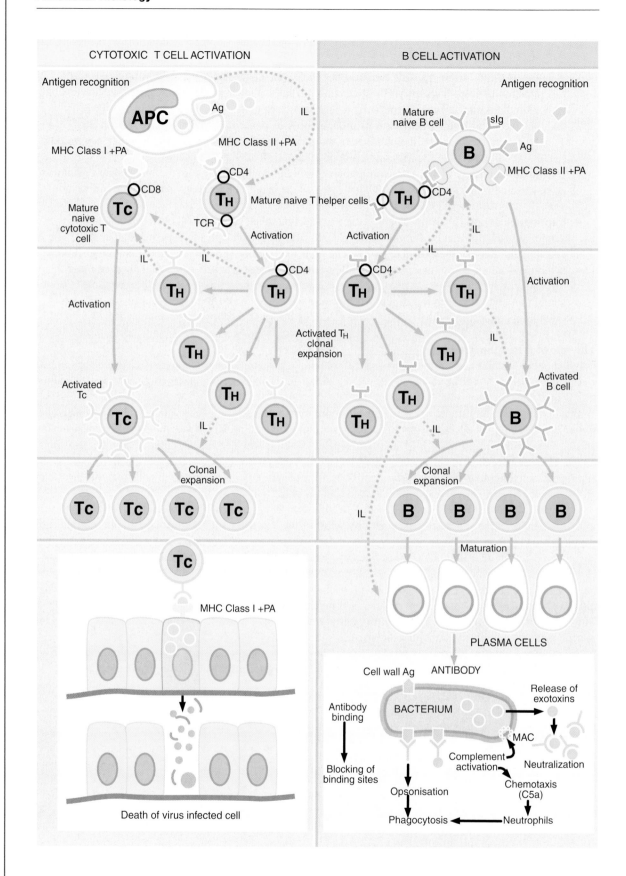

Fig. 11.1 **Essential immunological processes** (*illustration opposite*)

The essential processes in the development of an immunological response are summarised below and the better understood pathways are illustrated in simplified form in the diagram.

Activation of the immune system

Initiation of an immune response first requires contact between antigen **Ag** and mature lymphocytes; in the case of T cells, this requires an antigen presenting cell **APC**. There are several mechanisms of immunological activation:

1. Interaction of a B cell with a protein or polysaccharide antigen which has a repeating chemical structure (e.g. the polysaccharide coat of bacteria such as **Pneumococcus**). Few naturally occurring antigens are of this type (not illustrated). Such antigens are often known as T-independent antigens.

2. Antigen is taken up by an antigen presenting cell **APC** (e.g. macrophage, B lymphocyte **B** via binding to surface immunoglobulin **sIg**, Langerhans cells of skin) and processed (see Fig. 11.2). Processed antigen **PA** is then bound to a major histocompatibility complex protein **MHC** and the MHC–peptide complex is incorporated into the cell membrane such that part of the molecule, including the bound antigenic peptide, is exposed to the outside milieu. If the antigen in that form comes into contact with a mature T lymphocyte which bears a T cell receptor **TCR** with appropriate specificity, it will activate an immune response. The nature of the response depends on whether the peptide is presented bound to MHC class I or II (see Fig. 11.3) as these only interact with CD8- or CD4-bearing T lymphocytes, respectively. Antigenic peptides bound to class II MHC molecules thus induce a T helper cell T_H response, which is then available to 'help' B cells to respond to the same antigen with the production of immunoglobulins. T_H cells secrete a variety of interleukins **IL** which mediate activation, clonal expansion and maturation of the B cell response. The architecture of lymph nodes and other lymphoid tissues and the routes of circulation of T lymphocytes are designed to bring as many lymphocytes as possible into contact with each antigen.

3. Antigen synthesised within a body cell (e.g. tumour cell, virus-infected cell) is incorporated in the cell membrane (bound to a class I MHC protein) where it is available for recognition by CD8-bearing cytotoxic T lymphocytes T_C. T_H activation is also required for a T_C response to be mounted. Activation of both T_C and T_H requires the antigen presentation by an APC.

4. Cells that bear different MHC proteins on their cell surfaces (i.e. transplanted tissues) are able to excite an immune response which involves at least T helper cells and either cytotoxic T cells or macrophages (not illustrated).

During activation of the immune response, the surface antigens on the lymphocytes alter, for simplicity, only essential markers are included in this diagram (see Fig. 11.3).

Generation of the means of antigen destruction

1. **Production of antibodies** by plasma cells. Mechanisms of antibody-mediated antigen elimination are as follows:

   - Antibody blocks the entry of organisms (such as viruses) into cells by binding to viral surface antigens.
   - Antigen-antibody complexes (**immune complexes**) activate complement to produce (among other factors) the **membrane attack complex** **MAC** which makes a hole in the outer membrane of the attacking organism.
   - Bound antibody with or without complement **opsonises** organisms, which facilitates phagocytosis by neutrophils and macrophages.
   - Antibody is essential for **antibody-dependent cell cytotoxicity** (ADCC) (see below).
   - Antibody bound to toxins inactivates them and facilitates their removal by phagocytic cells.

2. **Cell-mediated cytotoxicity** is the destruction of altered or abnormal cells by cytotoxic cells, which may be classical cytotoxic T cells **Tc**, natural killer 'NK' cells or cytotoxic cells which require specific antibody to carry out their cytotoxic function (ADCC).

3. Certain types of antigens (e.g. of mycobacteria) interact with T lymphocytes promoting the secretion of certain lymphokines; such lymphokines activate macrophages to kill organisms which they have previously ingested but which they are otherwise unable to destroy; this is the mechanism of **chronic granulomatous inflammation** (not illustrated).

Termination of the immune response

There are a number of mechanisms for switching off the immune response when the need for it has been removed; these include the idiotype-antiidiotype antibody networks, cross-linking of surface immunoglobulins to Fc receptors by antigens, down-regulation by immune complexes, suppressor T cells and factors they may produce, and neuroendocrine interactions.

Immunological memory

When activated lymphocytes undergo clonal expansion during an immune response, some of the cells generated mature to become memory T and B cells. These lymphocytes have a similar appearance to naive lymphocytes but are able to produce a faster and more effective response to a smaller quantity of antigen encountered at a later date. This is known as a secondary immune response.

ORGAN SYSTEMS

Fig. 11.2 Lymphocytes and antigen presenting cell (a) Schematic diagram (b) EM × 18 000 *(opposite)*

Antigen presenting cells **APC** are vital in the activation of lymphocytes to produce an immune response. They include macrophage–monocyte type cells and other bone-marrow derived cells, *dendritic cells*, which are found in lymphoid tissue. When antigen (e.g. bacteria) breaches a surface barrier to enter the tissues it is taken up by phagocytosis by tissue APCs. These then migrate via the lymph to organised lymphoid tissue such as the regional lymph nodes to present the antigen to lymphocytes. The steps in the process are shown diagrammatically in (a). Antigen taken up by APCs is first found in the cytoplasm within an early endosome **EE** (see Ch. 1). The antigen is broken down into small peptide fragments by enzymatic hydrolysis and the late endosome formed **LE** fuses with a transport vesicle containing *major histocompatibility complex class II (MHCII)* molecules (see Fig. 11.1). Peptide and MHCII form a complex which is then transported to the plasma membrane. When the plasma membrane and transport vesicle **TV** fuse, the MHCII–peptide complex is found on the cell surface where it may come into contact with passing T_H lymphocytes. If the T_H cell is able to bind, via its T cell receptor **TCR**, to that particular MHCII–peptide complex, it will become activated and the specific immune response will proceed. Obviously a bacterium, after processing, will generate many different antigenic peptides, but only one peptide and one T_H cell is shown in this diagram for simplicity. In general T_H cells are able to recognise peptide bound to MHC class II and T_C cells recognise antigen bound to MHC class I.

Micrograph (b) illustrates several lymphocytes and an APC in a lymph node. Lymphocytes and antigen presenting cells exhibit similar features in other lymphoid tissues. The lymphocytes **L** are relatively small with round nuclei and condensed chromatin which tends to be clumped around the periphery. Cell outlines are fairly

regular with occasional surface projections. The scanty cytoplasm is homogeneous and contains plentiful free ribosomes and modest numbers of mitochondria but little rough or smooth endoplasmic reticulum and few lysosomes or secretory granules.

The centre of the field is occupied by the large cell body of an antigen presenting cell **APC**, in this case an *interdigitating dendritic cell*. These have numerous long branched cytoplasmic extensions **CE** reaching out between the surrounding lymphocytes so that a single APC can be in contact with many different lymphocytes. Its nucleus is deeply indented with dispersed chromatin; in this example, the plane of section has resulted in a small nuclear extension appearing to be separate from the main part of the nucleus. Typically, the APC cytoplasm is very heterogeneous, containing numerous small lysosomal granules **G**, larger phagosomes **P** and scattered profiles of rough endoplasmic reticulum and microtubules.

APCs found in different lymphoid tissues include *interdigitating dendritic cells* in the paracortical area of lymph nodes and *interdigitating cells* of the thymus. *Follicular dendritic cells* in the germinal centres of lymph nodes are similar cells which are able to bind antibody–antigen complexes to their surface without prior processing where they are accessible to B cells. Most APCs are mobile, such as the *Langerhans cells* of the skin, which migrate from their site of antigen uptake in the skin to regional lymph nodes where they mature into paracortical interdigitating dendritic cells.

Antigen presentation is not exclusively the function of cells derived from the macrophage–monocyte system. B lymphocytes and, in certain circumstances, a variety of other cells, including vascular endothelial cells, dermal fibroblasts, thyroid epithelial cells and brain astrocytes, may present antigen to T lymphocytes.

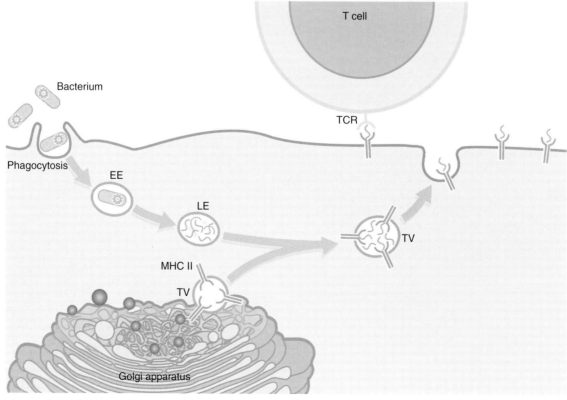

(a)

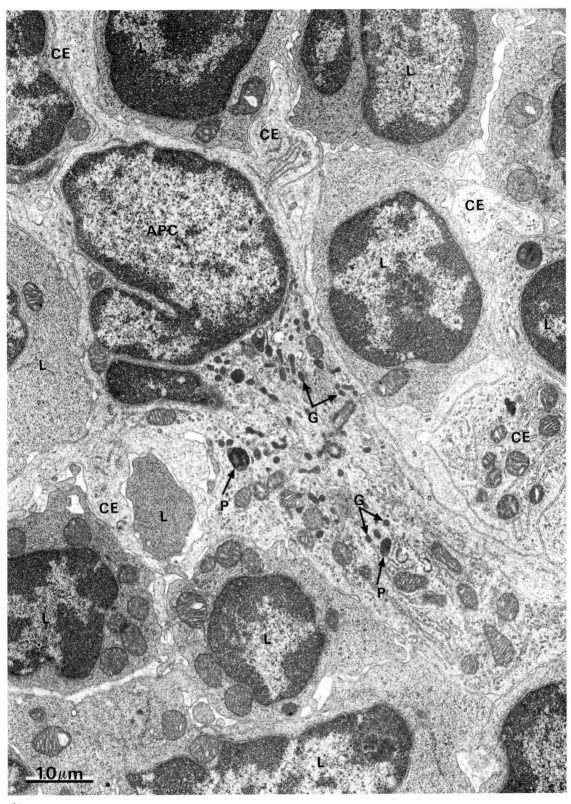

(b)

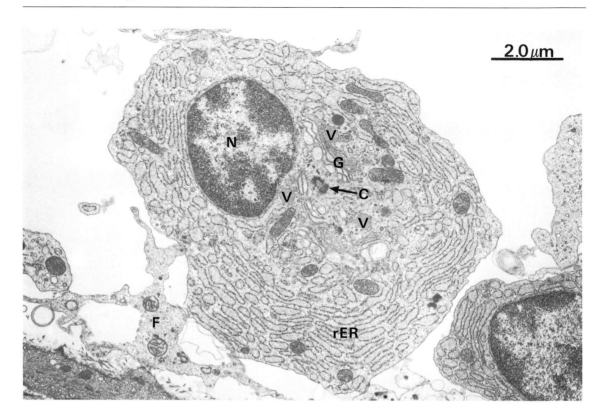

Fig. 11.3 Plasma cell EM × 10 000

When B lymphocytes are stimulated by antigen, they differentiate to form plasma cells which produce large quantities of antibody. Plasma cells are not usually found in the circulation but function in the tissues, in particular the medullary cords of lymph nodes, the white pulp of the spleen, the supporting tissues of mucosal surfaces (e.g. lamina propria of intestine) and the bone marrow. Antibody production involves the synthesis of the immunoglobulin polypeptide chains by rough endoplasmic reticulum. The basic antibody unit is made up of two identical light chains and two identical heavy chains. These are then transferred to the Golgi apparatus where synthesis is completed and the immunoglobulin is packaged into small vesicles before secretion into the extracellular space by exocytosis.

Maturation of a B lymphocyte into an antibody-secreting plasma cell involves three steps: activation, proliferation and maturation. Two types of antigen can activate B cell responses: T cell-dependent and T cell independent. The former require T cell help mediated by activated T_H cells. The latter are usually large molecular weight polymers with simple repeating structures which induce cross-linking of cell surface receptors. T cell-dependent antigens are by far the most important in physiological terms.

Several cell divisions are involved in the process of transformation from resting small lymphocyte to *plasmablast* and thence to mature plasma cells, which can undergo successive cycles of mitosis in the medullary cords of lymph nodes to enlarge the clone of cells still further.

Each stage of this process requires several signals, including recognition of appropriate antigen by the surface immunoglobulins (sIg) of resting B cells and secretion by activated T_H cells of soluble factors including interleukins 4, 5 and 6 (lymphokines). Interleukin release by T_H cells is dependent on simultaneous activation and clonal expansion of T_H cells, which must therefore also recognise and be activated by the antigen.

Morphology

Plasma cells are large with an eccentric round or oval nucleus **N** the chromatin of which is coarsely clumped in a characteristic 'cartwheel' or 'clock face' pattern. By light microscopy, the cytoplasm is amphophilic (purple) due to its large content of ribosomal RNA and protein which stains with both acidophilic and basophilic dyes (see Fig. 1.9c). With electron microscopy, the ribosomes are seen to be associated with an extensive rough endoplasmic reticulum **rER**. A well developed Golgi apparatus **G** displaces the nucleus to one side of the cell and with light microscopy is represented by a perinuclear halo. The light and heavy chains of immunoglobulin are synthesised in the rER and the carbohydrate element added by the Golgi. Secretory vesicles **V** then convey the antibody to the surface where it is secreted into the extracellular fluid. Plasma cells do not express surface immunoglobulin (sIg). In the centre of the cell and surrounded by the Golgi complex is the centrosome **C** from which radiate the microtubules of the cytoskeleton. Note the fine cytoplasmic extensions of fibroblasts **F** in the surrounding tissues.

Function	T cell	B cell
Antigen receptor	TCR	sIg
Accessory binding molecules	CD4 (T$_H$) CD8 (T$_c$) CD2 CD28	CD19 CD40
Signal transduction	CD3	sIg
Other	CD25	CR2

Fig. 11.4 Lymphocyte surface markers

Lymphocytes carry on their surface membranes a wide range of transmembrane glycoproteins which are often known as *surface markers* or *surface antigens*. This name has arisen because they are routinely detected by antibodies for both diagnostic and research purposes (see Fig 11.14). These molecules have a wide range of functions in controlling the activation of the immune response and are the means by which lymphocytes interact with their environment. Known functions of these molecules include acting as receptors for antigen, acting as cobinding/costimulatory molecules whose function is to enhance the activation of lymphocytes, and signal transmission through the plasma membrane to the inside of the cell. Many of these surface markers are named according to the *CD (cluster of differentiation) system*, an internationally agreed system which may seem confusing to the immunologically naïve reader but which is infinitely better than the previous haphazard free-for-all that preceded it. There are well over 100 known CD molecules now. Fortunately, for the purposes of this text, only a few need to be touched on here.

Antigen receptors

Lymphocytes are constantly being produced in the bone marrow, each cell subsequently acquiring the ability to recognise a single particular chemical configuration, i.e. a particular antigen to which it might be exposed at some time in the future. This occurs by the random rearrangement of segments of the genes which code for the binding site of the receptor. B cells produce small amounts of immunoglobulin which are inserted into the plasma membrane (business end out) and act as the antigen receptor. When this *surface immunoglobulin* **sIg** binds to antigen, the process of activation of the B cell is initiated, resulting in the production of clones of plasma cells which secrete large amounts of immunoglobulin specific for that antigen.

T cells have a structurally similar antigen receptor, known as the *T cell receptor* **TCR**, which serves the same triggering function when bound to antigen. During T cell development the TCR genes are rearranged in a manner similar to immunoglobulin genes, in order to produce T cells with a wide range of possible antigen specificities.

Accessory binding/costimulatory molecules

Binding of the TCR to antigenic peptide is insufficient to trigger T cell activation. Activation requires binding between accessory molecules on the surface of the T cell and their counterparts on the APC. T$_H$ cells are recognised by the CD4 surface marker which binds to *major histocompatibility complex class II molecules* on the surface of APCs, thereby providing increased binding affinity and an additional signal to the T cell. CD8 on the surface of the cytotoxic/suppressor type of T cells binds in a similar fashion to MHCI on APCs. Thus, T$_H$ cells are said to be *MHC class II restricted* and T$_c$ cells *MHC class I restricted*.

MHC molecules are the major antigens that differentiate tissues of one individual from another and were first discovered in the context of organ transplant rejection; in humans, the system is called *HLA (human leucocyte antigen)*. The MHC antigens are of three different classes, designated class I, class II and class III. Class I MHC antigens are present on the surfaces of virtually all cells in the body, with the important exception of erythrocytes. Class II MHC antigens are normally present only on APCs and B lymphocytes, the cells which present antigen to T cells.

Other surface molecules which have cobinding/costimulatory activity include CD28 and CD2 on T cells and CD19 and CD40 on B cells.

Signal transduction molecules

CD3 on T cells is a protein complex closely associated with the TCR. When the TCR binds antigen and CD4/8-MHC binding occurs, CD3 passes the message to the inside of the cell to trigger the intracellular events leading to cell activation. On B cells, sIg seems to perform the same function

Other surface markers

These include a diverse range of transmembrane proteins such as complement receptors **CR2**, interleukin receptors **CD25** and various others.

Thymus

The thymus is a flattened lymphoid organ located in the upper anterior mediastinum and lower part of the neck. The thymus is most active during childhood, reaching a weight of about 30–40 g at puberty, after which it undergoes slow involution so that in the middle-aged or older adult it may be difficult to differentiate from adipose tissue macroscopically.

In the embryo, the thymus originates from epithelial outgrowths of the ventral wing of the third pharyngeal pouch on each side. These merge in the midline, forming a single organ subdivided into numerous fine lobules. The epithelium develops into a sponge-like structure containing a labyrinth of interconnecting spaces which become colonised by immature T lymphocytes derived from haemopoietic tissue elsewhere in the developing embryo. Towards the centre of the organ, the epithelial framework has a coarser structure with smaller interstices and a much smaller lymphocyte population, so that, on microscopic examination, the gland has a highly cellular outer *cortex* and a less cellular central *medulla* which is continuous throughout the gland.

The epithelial cells of the thymus provide a mechanical supporting framework for the lymphocyte population. Cortical epithelial cells, known as *nurse cells*, envelop multiple lymphocytes promoting T cell differentiation and proliferation. Furthermore, the epithelial cells secrete at least four different hormones which regulate T cell maturation and proliferation within the thymus and in other lymphoid organs and tissues.

Functions of the thymus

The prime functions of the thymus include:

- Development of immunocompetent T lymphocytes from T cell precursors derived from bone marrow to produce mature T_H and T_C cells.
- Proliferation of clones of mature naïve T cells to supply the circulating lymphocyte pool and peripheral tissues.
- Development of immunological self-tolerance.
- Secretion of hormones and other soluble factors which regulate T cell maturation, proliferation and function within the thymus and peripheral tissues. There are at least four polypeptides with hormonal characteristics, namely *thymulin*, *thymopoietin* and α_1 and β_4 *thymosin*.

Fig. 11.5 Thymus (a) H & E × 15 (b) H & E × 15 (c) H & E × 75 (d) Immunoperoxidase × 100

The infant thymus (a) is a lobulated organ invested by a loose collagenous capsule **C** from which short interlobular septa **S** containing blood vessels radiate into the substance of the organ. The thymic tissue is divided into two distinct zones, a deeply basophilic outer cortex **Cx** and an inner eosinophilic medulla **M**; distinction between the two is most marked in early childhood, as in this specimen.

In the middle-aged adult, the thymus (b) is already well into the process of involution, which involves two distinct processes, fatty infiltration and lymphocyte depletion. Adipocytes first begin to appear at birth, their numbers slowly rising until puberty when the rate of fatty infiltration increases markedly. Fatty infiltration of the interlobular septa occurs first, spreading out into the cortex and later the medulla. Thus islands of lymphoid tissue **L** are separated by areas of adipose tissue **A** in the mature thymus.

Lymphocyte numbers begin to fall from about 1 year of age, the process continuing thereafter at a constant rate. Despite this, the thymus continues to provide a supply of mature T lymphocytes to the circulating pool and peripheral tissues. Lymphocyte depletion results in collapse of the epithelial framework. However, cords of epithelial cells persist and continue to secrete thymic hormones throughout life.

The normal process of slow thymic involution associated with ageing should be distinguished from *acute thymic involution*, which may occur in response to severe disease and metabolic stress associated with pregnancy, lactation, infection, surgery, malnutrition, malignancy and other systemic insults. Stress involution is characterised by greatly increased lymphocyte death and is probably mediated by high levels of corticosteroids; thus the size and activity of the adult thymus are often underestimated if examined after prolonged illness.

Micrograph (c) shows part of a pubertal thymus at higher magnification. The cortex **Cx** is packed with lymphocytes accounting for its basophilia, whereas the medulla **M** contains fewer lymphocytes and has a coarser epithelial framework. In the centre of the medulla, eosinophilic structures known as *Hassal's corpuscles* **H** are found (see Fig. 11.7). The epithelial framework of the cortex is more delicate and finely branched than that of the medulla, and is sometimes described as 'reticular'; there is, however, no evidence that the cells are phagocytic or represent part of the reticuloendothelial system (see Ch. 4). At an ultrastructural level, the epithelial cells have typical desmosomes at their points of contact and the cytoplasm contains bundles of keratin intermediate filaments. Note the collagenous capsule **C** which is continuous with an interlobular septum **S** terminating at the corticomedullary junction.

Sympathetic and parasympathetic fibres derived respectively from the sympathetic chain and phrenic nerves accompany the blood vessels into the thymus.

In micrograph (d) the epithelial cells of the thymus are highlighted using the immunoperoxidase technique. These cells are not easily identified using the standard H & E sections. An antibody to keratin, the intermediate filament typical of epithelial cells was used here, and individual epithelial cells **E**, as well as Hassal's corpusules **H**, are stained brown.

The inner surfaces of the thymic capsule and septa are invested by a continuous layer of thymic epithelial cells resting on a basement membrane (not seen at this magnification). The epithelium also forms sheaths around the blood vessels, creating a barrier to the entry of antigenic material into the system of spaces within the epithelial framework. This is known as the *blood–thymus barrier*.

Numerous small branches of the internal thoracic and inferior thyroid arteries enter the thymus via the interlobular septa, branching at the corticomedullary junction to supply the cortex and medulla. Postcapillary venules in the corticomedullary region have a specialised cuboidal endothelium similar to that of the high endothelial venules of the lymph node (see Fig. 11.15), which allows passage of lymphocytes into and out of the thymus. The venous and lymphatic drainage follows the course of the arterial supply; there are no afferent lymphatics.

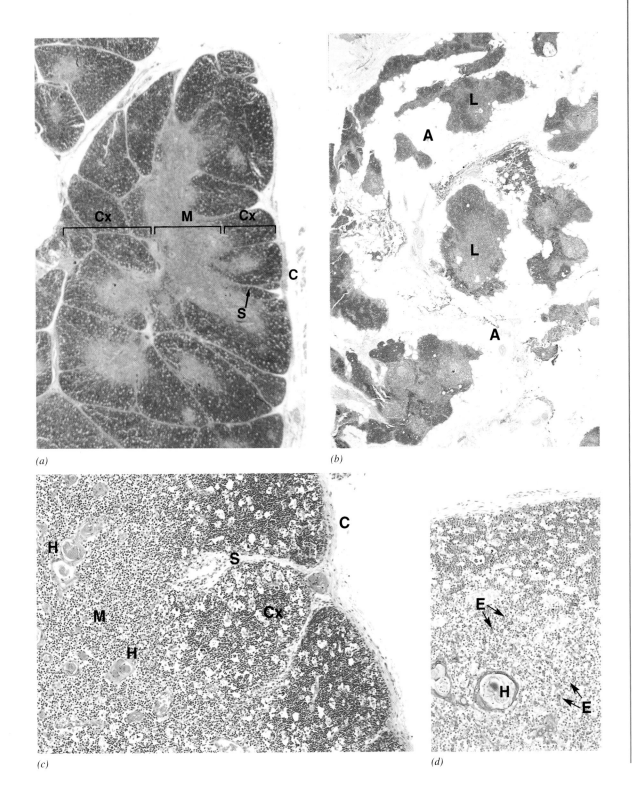

(a)

(b)

(c)

(d)

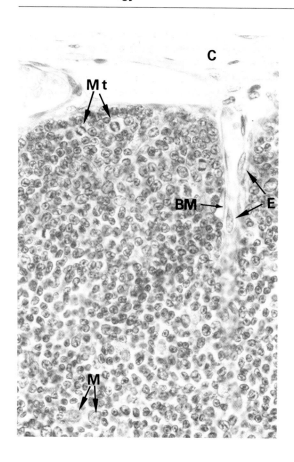

Fig. 11.6 Thymic cortex H & E × 480

The thymic cortex is packed with immature and maturing T cells, often called *thymocytes*. In the outer cortex, large lymphocytes (*lymphoblasts*) divide by mitosis to produce clones of smaller mature T cells. These undergo further maturation as they move deeper into the cortex towards the medulla. It is during this process that the TCR genes are rearranged and the cells acquire the surface markers (*phenotype*) of mature helper and cytotoxic T cells. Several mitotic figures **Mt** can be seen in the outer cortex in this micrograph. Cells failing to make these adjustments successfully, die by apoptosis and are taken up by pale-stained macrophages **M** at the corticomedullary junction. This is often picturesquely known as a *starry sky appearance* and is easily seen in Figure 11.5 (c).

Note also in this micrograph, a small capillary lined by flattened endothelial cells **E** entering the cortex from the capsule **C**. Around the capillary the basement membrane **BM** of epithelial cells can be discerned at the interface between the thymic framework and supporting tissue elements. The cells of the cortical epithelial framework stain poorly and cannot be distinguished, being obscured by the mass of lymphocytes.

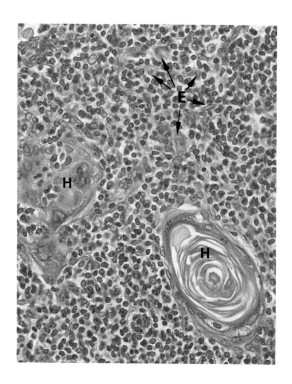

Fig. 11.7 Thymic medulla H & E × 480

The dominant feature of the thymic medulla is the robust epithelial component **E**, the cells having large pale-stained nuclei, eosinophilic cytoplasm and prominent basement membranes. A particular feature are the concentrically lamellated *Hassall's corpuscles* **H** which first appear in fetal life and increase in number and size thereafter. These are formed from groups of keratinised epithelial cells and probably represent a degenerative phenomenon.

Also found in the medulla is a type of APC, known as a *thymic interdigitating cell*, which expresses high levels of both class I and II MHC proteins. It appears that these cells present normal self-components, *self-antigens*, to maturing T-cells. Any self-reactive T cells which identify themselves by becoming activated are obliterated by apoptosis, a process known as *clonal deletion* or *negative selection*. Thus the thymus is the organ where self-reactive T cells are removed, preventing the development of autoimmunity.

At the end of their journey through the thymus, the mature T cells enter the blood vessels and lymphatics to join the pool of circulating T lymphocytes and populate the T lymphocyte domains of other lymphoid organs.

Although the thymus is usually considered a specifically T cell organ, occasional mature B lymphocytes, B cell germinal centres and, rarely, plasma cells can be found in the thymus, particularly in children. Ultrastructural studies have shown that these lie outside the epithelial enclosure and within the perivascular spaces of the medulla, corticomedullary junction and septa; this has led to a concept of two functional compartments of the thymus, namely an intraepithelial compartment and an extraepithelial (perivascular) compartment.

Lymph nodes

Mature lymphocytes are distributed throughout the body, where they are arranged in aggregations which exhibit various degrees of structural organisation. Isolated lymphocytes are found in most loose supporting tissues and amongst epithelial cells, particularly the epithelium of the gastrointestinal and respiratory tracts; in addition, large non-encapsulated aggregations of lymphocytes are found in the walls of these tracts. These include the palatine tonsils and the Peyer's patches of the small intestine. Many lymphocytes are, however, located in encapsulated, highly organised structures called *lymph nodes*, which are interposed along the larger regional vessels of the lymph vascular system. Lymph nodes tend to occur in groups, particularly in areas where the lymphatics converge to form larger trunks as in the neck, axillae, groins, lung hila and para-aortic areas.

Four interrelated functions occur within lymph nodes:

- Non-specific filtration of particulate matter and microorganisms from lymph by the phagocytic activity of macrophages, thus preventing exogenous material from reaching the general circulation.
- Interaction of circulating lymphocytes with antigen-containing lymph as it is filtered through the narrow confines of the node; initiation of an immune response usually requires antigen presenting cells.
- Activation and proliferation of B lymphocytes; in response to appropriate antigenic stimulation, this leads to plasma cell formation and antibody production.
- Aggregation, activation and proliferation of T lymphocytes to produce activated T_H and T_C lymphocytes.

Cell types in the lymph node

The cells of the lymph node can be divided into three functional types:

- **Lymphoid cells**, including small, medium and large lymphocytes and plasma cells. All originate from bone marrow but T cells have passed through a maturation phase in the thymus (see above) before reaching the lymph node. Lymphocytes enter the node in the lymph via the afferent lymphatics and from the blood via the postcapillary venules in the paracortex.
- **Immunological accessory cells**. These include a variety of antigen presenting cells. These cells originate in the bone marrow and pass to the peripheral tissues before reaching the lymph node in lymph. They include the macrophages found in the lymph node sinuses, the follicular dendritic cells and the interdigitating dendritic cells of the paracortex.
- **Stromal cells**. These include lymphatic and vascular endothelial cells and fibroblasts responsible for elaboration of the lymph node supporting framework.

Recirculation of lymphocytes

Mature resting (naïve) lymphocytes constantly traffic between the periphery and organised lymphoid tissue via the blood and lymph circulation. Lymphocytes enter the lymph node from the blood or via the afferent lymphatics. In the node, the lymphocytes come into close contact with the dendritic cells of the follicles and paracortex. Lymphocytes unable to respond to antigen exhibited within the node move on via the efferent lymph to the next lymph node in the chain and eventually return to the blood by way of the thoracic duct to repeat the process over and over in their endless quest for antigen. Lymphocytes which are able to bind displayed antigen in the node via their surface receptors (sIg on B cells and TCR on T cells) are trapped in the node to undergo clonal expansion before returning to the general circulation. The lymphoblasts and memory cells produced by this process are able to home to sites of tissue inflammation and perform their effector functions.

Lymph nodes are small, bean-shaped organs situated in the course of lymphatic vessels such that lymph draining back to the bloodstream passes through one or more lymph nodes. Inactive nodes are only a few millimetres long but may increase greatly in size when mounting an active immunological response. Most lymph nodes in the body show some degree of reactive change in response to the constant barrage of antigen they are exposed to. The outer part of the lymph node is highly cellular and is known as the *cortex*, whilst the central area, the *medulla*, is less cellular.

The lymph node is surrounded by a collagenous *capsule* from which *trabeculae* extend for a variable distance into the substance of the node. *Afferent lymphatic vessels* divide into several branches outside the node, then pierce the capsule to drain into a narrow space called the *subcapsular sinus* which encircles the node beneath the capsule. From here, a labyrinth of channels called *cortical sinuses* passes towards the medulla through the cortical cell mass; sinuses adjacent to the trabeculae pursue a more direct course towards the medulla, but nevertheless form part of the cortical sinus system. The dominant feature of the medulla is the network of broad interconnected lymphatic channels called *medullary sinuses* which coverge upon the hilum in the concavity of the node. Lymph drains from the hilum into one or more *efferent lymphatic vessels*, which in turn drain into more proximal nodes before eventually joining the bloodstream via the *thoracic duct* or *right lymphatic duct*.

The parenchyma of the lymph node consists of an open meshwork of reticulin fibres which provides support for an ever-changing population of lymphocytes. The cortex consists of densely-packed lymphocytes. Cellular *medullary cords* project into the medulla between the medullary sinuses. In the outer cortex, lymphocytes form a variable number of densely packed *lymphoid follicles,* many of which show less dense *germinal centres*. The deep cortex (*paracortical zone*) is devoid of lymphoid follicles.

The blood supply of the lymph node is derived from one or more small arteries which enter at the hilum and branch in the medulla, giving rise to extensive capillary networks corresponding to the cortical follicles, paracortical zone and medullary cords. Lymphocytes enter lymph nodes mainly via the arterial system, gaining access by migrating across the walls of specialised postcapillary venules (*high endothelial venules, HEV*) as described later. The HEV drain into small veins which leave the node via the *hilum*.

The micrograph illustrates the main histological features of a lymph node. The node is made up of an outer, densely staining cell-rich cortex **Cx** and a pale-stained inner medulla **M** which is continuous with the hilum **H**. The superficial cortex contains a number of dense cellular aggregations, the follicles **F**, many of which have a pale-stained germinal centre. The deeper cortex or paracortical zone **P** is also densely cellular but has a more homogeneous staining appearance. At the left of the field, some lymphoid follicles appear to be located deep in the paracortex; this is not the case but is a product of the plane of section, which passes at that point through the superficial cortex. Extensions of the cortical cell mass extend into the medulla as medullary cords **MC**. The superficial cortex, the paracortex, the medulla and the sinuses represent the four different zones of immunological activity in the lymph node, containing mainly B lymphocytes, T lymphocytes, plasma cells and macrophages, respectively.

Several trabeculae **T** extend from the capsule **C** into the substance of the node. The subcapsular sinus **S** is found immediately beneath the capsule and is continuous with the trabecular sinuses. The cortical sinuses are generally difficult to visualise because of their highly convoluted shape and numerous fine extensions which penetrate the cellular mass of the cortex. Antigens are phagocytosed by various types of antigen presenting cells exposed to the lymph, processed and then passed to their cytoplasmic extensions to be presented to lymphocytes. Lymphocytes entering the node in afferent lymph constitute less than 10% of all lymphocytes entering the node, except in mesenteric nodes where they may constitute up to 30%.

The vascular system provides the main route of entry of lymphocytes into the node as well as supplying its metabolic requirements. Within the paracortex, the postcapillary high endothelial venules have a cuboidal endothelium specialised for the exit of lymphocytes. Recognition by lymphocytes of these exit sites appears to involve the presence of specific complementary *adhesion molecules* on the surface of the endothelial cells and lymphocytes. Different groups of lymphocytes home to different tissues. Thus lymphocytes from the mucosa of the gut home to mesenteric lymph nodes and then migrate to the spleen, the resulting blasts homing back to mucosal tissues. Lymphocytes from the skin home to their regional lymph nodes and return, perhaps via the spleen, to peripheral tissue. This is made possible by the different adhesion molecules or *vascular addressins* in the HEV of the different lymph node groups and the corresponding binding molecules on the lymphocytes. The vessels of the superficial cortex and medullary cords are not thought to be specialised and do not appear to allow exit of lymphocytes.

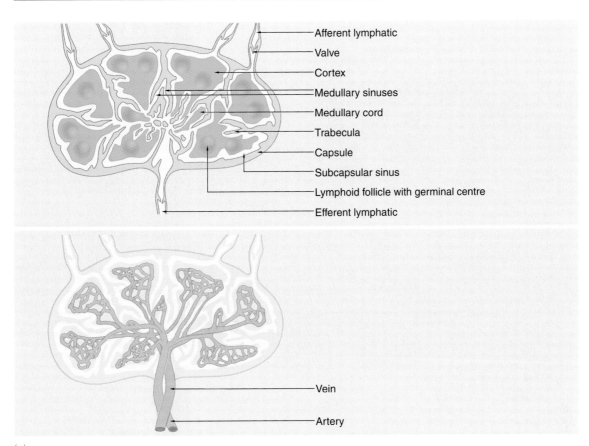

Afferent lymphatic
Valve
Cortex
Medullary sinuses
Medullary cord
Trabecula
Capsule
Subcapsular sinus
Lymphoid follicle with germinal centre
Efferent lymphatic

Vein

Artery

(a)

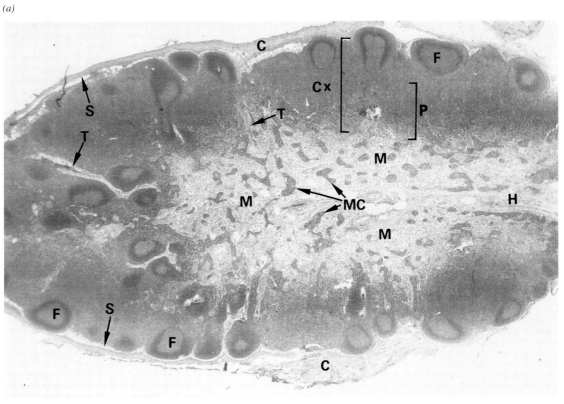

(b)

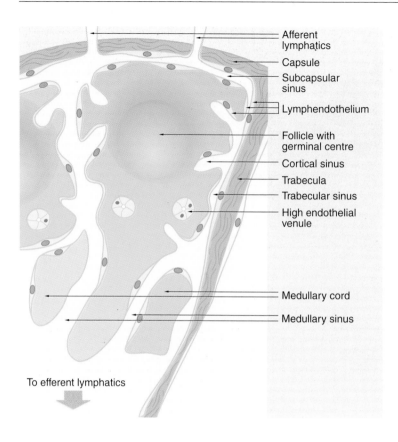

Afferent lymphatics
Capsule
Subcapsular sinus
Lymphendothelium
Follicle with germinal centre
Cortical sinus
Trabecula
Trabecular sinus
High endothelial venule
Medullary cord
Medullary sinus

To efferent lymphatics

Fig. 11.9 Functional compartments of the lymph node

This diagram illustrates the three functional compartments within the lymph node:

- **A network of lymphatic sinuses** lined by a mixture of lymphatic endothelial cells and macrophages and continuous with the lumen of the afferent and efferent lymphatic vessels. These contain macrophages, which enter the node in the lymph and carry a load of phagocytosed antigen.
- **The blood vascular compartment** represented by the microvascular network of the node; its specialised *high endothelial venules* are the major site of entry of circulating lymphocytes into the node.
- **The interstitial compartment**, into which pass circulating lymphocytes in the quest for antigen; lymphocytes which do not recognise antigen leave the node within a few hours via the lymphatic compartment and efferent lymph to rejoin the general circulation.

The lymphatic and vascular endothelia thus define the boundaries of the three compartments and control passage of cells and molecules between the different compartments.

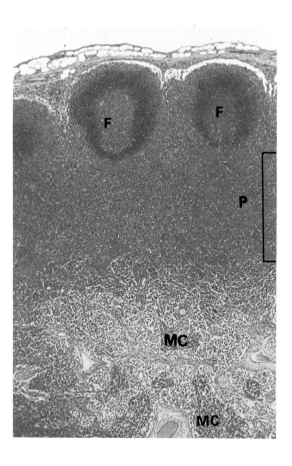

Fig. 11.10 Lymphocyte domains in the lymph node **H & E × 30**

The interstitial compartment of the lymph node has three functional domains; each populated by different types of lymphocytes.

The lymphocytes of the superficial cortex are mainly arranged in spheroidal lymphoid follicles **F** and these are the major sites in which B lymphocytes localise and proliferate. Lymphoid follicles are classified as *primary follicles* if a central pale area is absent and as *secondary follicles* if the pale area, the *germinal centre*, is present. Germinal centres are the site of B lymphocyte proliferation and are paler because the nuclear chromatin of the cells is not condensed as it is in the small lymphocytes which make up the primary follicles and the rim or *mantle zone* of secondary follicles.

The deep cortical zone or paracortex **P** consists mainly of T lymphocytes which are never arranged as follicles.

The medullary cords **MC** mainly contain B lymphocytes and plasma cells involved in immunoglobulin synthesis.

The number of cortical lymphoid follicles and the depth of the paracortex vary greatly according to the immunological state of the particular lymph node and the individual as a whole. A predominantly T cell response is associated with paracortical expansion whereas a predominantly humoral response is characterised by many secondary follicles.

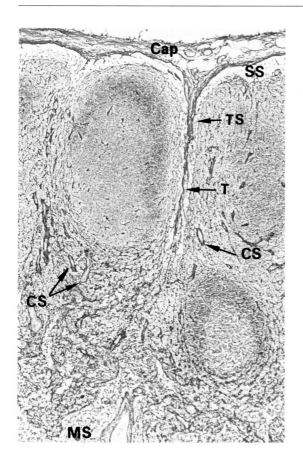

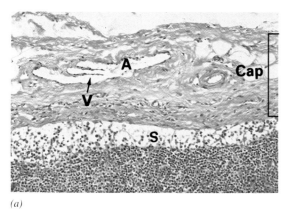

(a)

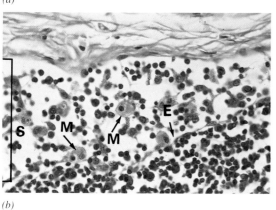

(b)

Fig. 11.11 Supporting tissue of the lymph node Reticulin method × 30

This technique shows the fine reticular architecture of the lymph node; reticulin fibres are stained blackish-brown and lymphocyte nuclei appear lighter brown.

The main structural support for the lymph node is derived from the collagenous capsule **Cap** and trabeculae **T**, which extend into the node. From these, a fine meshwork of reticulin fibres extends throughout the node, providing a supporting framework for the mass of lymphocytes and accessory cells within the cortex and medullary cords. The reticular network is particularly dense in the cortex, except for the follicular areas where it is relatively sparse. The subcapsular sinus **SS**, trabecular sinuses **TS**, other cortical sinuses **CS** and medullary sinuses **MS** are kept patent by a fine skeleton of reticulin fibres which traverse the sinuses.

The reticulin framework and collagen of the capsule and trabeculae are laid down by fibroblasts as in other supporting tissues, and a few fibroblast-like cells are found on the reticulin network. Numerous macrophages are draped over the whole reticular meshwork, their long dendritic cytoplasmic processes providing a large surface area for the clearance of particles, organisms and soluble antigens from the afferent lymph.

Fig. 11.12 Capsule and subcapsular sinus (a) H & E × 128 (b) H & E × 320

As seen in micrograph (a), the fibrous capsule **Cap** of the lymph node is pierced by branches of afferent lymphatic vessels **A** with valves **V** to ensure one-way flow. Beneath the capsule is the subcapsular sinus **S** which drains via the cortical sinuses towards the medulla.

Micrograph (b) focuses on the subcapsular sinus **S** at high magnification. A fine eosinophilic line **E** can been seen representing the sinus lining, consisting of a mixture of endothelial cells and macrophages. The lymph node sinuses are traversed by fine reticulin strands, which are very difficult to identify with ordinary light microscopic methods. The reticulin strands provide support for large eosinophilic *sinus macrophages* **M**. These macrophages may carry antigen which was phagocytosed elsewhere or may engulf particles, soluble antigens and other debris from afferent lymph. The macrophages are then able to process antigen and present it to lymphocytes within the node as shown in Figure 11.2(a). Some antigen may be released from macrophages and taken up by other APCs. Cortical lymphocytes and dendritic cells may also sample antigen directly as it percolates through the node.

Langerhans cells in the skin may also be found in the subcapsular sinus. These cells have a highly folded surface membrane and for this reason are sometimes known as *veiled cells*. They are probably the precursors of the dendritic interdigitating cells of the paracortex (see Fig. 11.15).

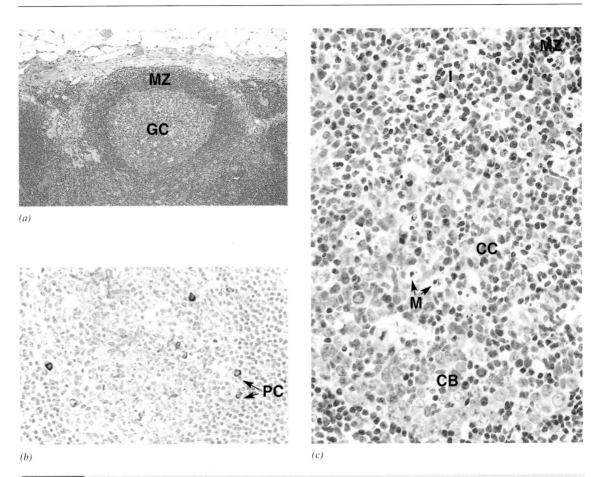

(a)

(b)

(c)

Fig. 11.13 Lymphoid follicle and germinal centre
(a) H & E × 50 (b) Immunoperoxidase × 200 (c) H & E × 300

Micrograph (a) shows a lymphoid follicle with a pale *germinal centre* **GC** and a darker stained *mantle zone* **MZ** surrounding it. The periphery of the mantle zone is somewhat paler than the inner part and is sometimes called the *marginal zone*, as in the lymphoid follicles of the spleen (see Fig. 11.24b), although it is much less distinct than in the spleen. The mantle zone is made up of small resting B cells, the condensed nuclear chromatin giving the dark blue colour. It is usually asymmetric, with the side nearest the capsule being broader than the side towards the medulla. Intermixed with the B cells is a scattering of T_H cells, follicular dendritic cells and macrophages. Primary follicles which are unstimulated consist entirely of the same cell types as the mantle zone.

The cells of the germinal centre of secondary follicles (c) are also mainly B cells, often called *follicle centre cells*. The germinal centre is not uniform in colour but is darker towards the medullary end and paler towards the capsule end, reflecting the organisation of the different cell types within it. Resting B cells enter the lymph node via the high endothelial venules and, if they encounter an antigen with which they can react, enter the cycle of blast transformation to produce clones of plasma cells and B memory cells. The first step is activation to give rise to *centroblasts* **CB**, large, mitotically active cells with round nuclei which are found at the darker medullary end of the germinal centre. These differentiate into *centrocytes* **CC**, which are found in the pale midzone of the germinal centre. These cells are of variable size and have folded, irregular nuclear membranes and are therefore often known as *cleaved cells*. Mitotic figures are absent in this area but there are many *tingible body macrophages* **M**,

due to the high rate of apoptosis in these cells. Centrocytes migrate towards the paler capsular end of the germinal centre where they go through further cycles of division to produce either *immunoblasts* **I** or memory B cells. Immunoblasts migrate to the medullary cords where they complete their differentiation into plasma cells capable of secreting large amounts of antibody. Memory cells, which resemble small lymphocytes, may take up residence in the mantle zone **MZ** of the follicle or may join the recirculating pool of small lymphocytes.

Other cells found in the germinal centres include:

• *Follicular dendritic cells*, the major antigen presenting cells of the follicles. These are difficult to see in routine H & E stains but their dendritic processes can be demonstrated (stained brown) as in micrograph (b) using an antibody to IgM which is trapped on the plasma membrane. These cells are found in all areas of the germinal centre and also form a meshwork in the mantle zone and in primary follicles. They can retain antigen on their surface for many months and may have a role in maintaining the activity of memory cells as well as stimulating a primary immune response. Occasional plasma cells **PC** are also stained by virtue of their cytoplasmic IgM.

• The interestingly named *tingible body macrophages* **M** are easily seen in routine sections in active germinal centres. They contain within their cytoplasm numerous apoptotic bodies derived from B lymphocytes which have not survived the process of blast transformation, presumably due to some error in DNA replication during the frenzy of mitosis which goes on in the germinal centre.

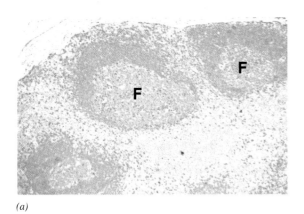 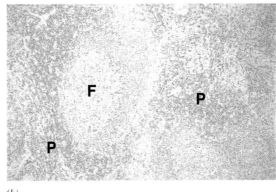

(a)   *(b)*

| **Fig. 11.14** | **Cortical distribution of T and B lymphocytes** |

Immunoperoxidase method: (a) B cells × 50 (b) T cells × 50

Micrograph (a) employs an immunoperoxidase method for a B lymphocyte surface marker, which stains the plasma membrane brown. Nuclei are counterstained blue with haematoxylin. The follicles **F** are composed mainly of B cells.

Micrograph (b) employs the same method, in this case utilising a T cell marker. T lymphocytes make up the majority of the cells in the paracortex **P**, but scattered T cells are also present in the follicles **F**. These are mainly T_H cells which must also recognise antigen to provide help for B cell stimulation.

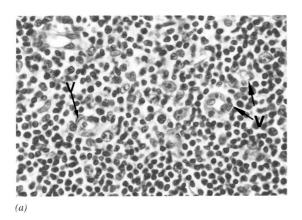 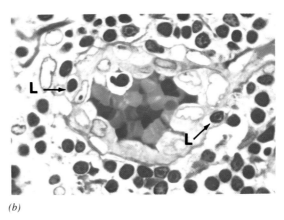

(a)   *(b)*

| **Fig. 11.15** | **Paracortical zone** (a) H & E × 320 (b) Thin section: toluidine blue × 800 |

T lymphocytes are the main cell type in the paracortical zone.

Circulating T lymphocytes of both helper and cytotoxic/suppressor subsets enter the lymph node in arterial blood and then migrate through the walls of high endothelial venules **V** into the paracortical zone; they rejoin the circulation some 6–16 hours later, passing out of the lymph node in efferent lymph.

When activated, T lymphocytes enlarge to form immunoblasts, histologically similar to their B cell counterparts, before mitotic proliferation to produce expanded clones of activated T lymphocytes. Indeed, in a T cell-dominated immunological response, the paracortical zone may be greatly expanded, a pattern known as the *paracortical reaction*. Activated T cells are then disseminated via the circulation to peripheral sites where much of their activity occurs.

The main antigen presenting cell in the paracortex is the *interdigitating dendritic cell*. These are named for their numerous cytoplasmic processes which form a meshwork in the paracortex and are in close contact

with the naïve T cells which circulate through this zone. It is now believed that the veiled cells of the subcapsular sinuses may represent the precursors of interdigitating dendritic cells. Veiled cells are probably derived from the Langerhans cells of the skin. Another type of accessory cell found in the paracortex are macrophages with their cytoplasm packed with lipid (possibly engulfed cellular membrane) and nuclear debris.

Postcapillary venules of the paracortex have an unusual structure which facilitates the passage of T lymphocytes from the blood circulation into the lymph node. Micrograph (b) illustrates a high endothelial venule which is lined by tall cuboidal rather than the usual squamous endothelial cells. These endothelial cells express on their surface specific lymphocyte binding molecules known as *addressins*, which allow lymphocytes to bind to the endothelium as the first step of migration across it into the tissue. Several lymphocytes **L** can be seen in various stages of progress through the wall between the high endothelial cells.

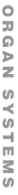

ORGAN SYSTEMS

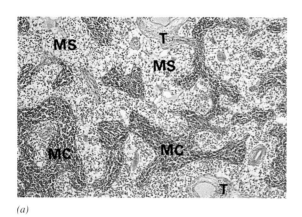

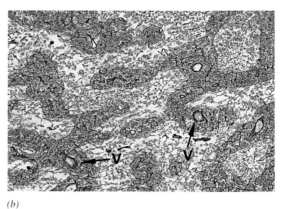

(a)   *(b)*

Fig. 11.16 Medullary cords and sinuses (a) H & E × 20 (b) Reticulin method/neutral red × 20

Micrograph (a) illustrates the structure of the lymph node medulla with branching medullary cords **MC** separated by irregular medullary sinuses **MS**. Throughout the medulla are trabeculae **T** extending from the collagenous supporting tissue of the capsule and hilum and conveying afferent and efferent blood vessels.

The medullary cords largely contain plasma cells and their precursors as well as small lymphocytes (memory cells, T_H cells) and macrophages. The cells of the medullary cords are supported by a reticulin framework as seen in micrograph (b), the black-staining reticulin being condensed around trabecular blood vessels **V**.

As in the subcapsular and trabecular sinuses, fine reticular strands traverse the medullary sinuses providing support for highly active sinus macrophages.

The dominant cell population of the medullary cord comprises plasma cells and their precursors, *immunoblasts*, which have migrated from the germinal centres of the cortex to the medullary cords. Here, the final stages of maturation to form plasma cells take place. Plasma cells synthesise antibody which is carried from the node to the general circulation via efferent lymph; some mature plasma cells probably also migrate from the node in a similar manner.

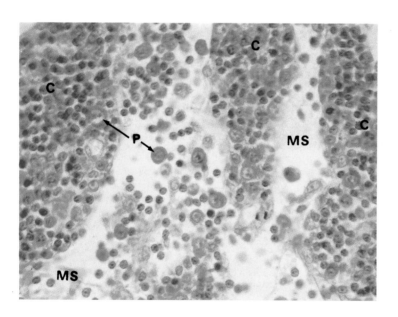

Fig. 11.17 Medullary cords and sinuses Methyl green/pyronin × 480

This preparation, taken from a lymph node undergoing an intense B cell response, has been stained by a technique to demonstrate plasma cells. The plasma cells **P** are large with an extensive, red-stained cytoplasm and a pale-stained nucleus with a prominent nucleolus. The red dye, pyronin, has a marked affinity for ribosomal RNA and hence stains the plasma cell cytoplasm strongly, since it is packed with ribosomes involved in antibody synthesis. Note the presence of numerous plasma cells in both the medullary cords **C** and sinuses **MS**.

The main accessory cells in the medulla are macrophages which are located predominantly in the sinuses.

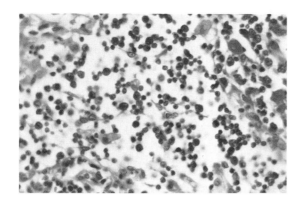

Fig. 11.18 Efferent lymph H & E × 320

This micrograph shows efferent lymph in a medullary sinus. Efferent lymph differs from afferent lymph in several important respects. Afferent lymph contains particulate matter (often including microorganisms), soluble antigens, relatively few lymphocytes and some antigen presenting cells migrating from peripheral tissues. In contrast, efferent lymph contains little particulate matter or soluble antigens but contains large numbers of recirculating T lymphocytes and a variable number of B lymphocytes and plasma cells. Antibody is also carried in efferent lymph to the general circulation and thence to the site of antigenic stimulation.

Mucosa-associated lymphoid tissue (MALT)

Lymphoid tissue is distributed throughout the gastrointestinal tract either as a diffuse population or as large, discrete non-encapsulated aggregations, such as in the tonsils and intestinal *Peyer's patches*. In the large aggregations, follicles may form with germinal centres similar to those of lymph nodes. Smaller follicular aggregations and diffuse populations of lymphocytes are also seen in the tracheobronchial tree (see Fig. 12.9) and genitourinary tract.

The total mass of lymphoid tissue in the gastrointestinal, respiratory and genitourinary tracts is enormous, but until recently its function was unknown and largely discounted. This mass of lymphoid tissue is now considered to be a lymphoid organ in its own right and is collectively known as *mucosa-associated lymphoid tissue (MALT)*. The larger aggregations function in a manner analogous to lymph nodes, sampling antigenic material entering the tracts and mounting both antibody-mediated and cytotoxic immune responses where appropriate; they contain discrete B and T cell zones as well as antigen-processing accessory cells.

The diffusely scattered lymphocytes seen in the lamina propria of the gut and respiratory tree are mainly T lymphocytes. Smaller numbers of B cells are also present, as well as plasma cells. All classes of antibody are produced, with IgA predominating.

IgA is secreted into the lumen bound to a carbohydrate moiety, *secretory piece*, which is synthesised in the epithelium and renders IgA resistant to proteolytic enzymes. This *secretory IgA* protects against pathogens in the gut lumen before they breach the tissues. IgA also reaches the gut in bile, being taken up from blood and secreted into bile in a similar fashion.

IgG and IgM are also secreted into the lamina propria to deal with organisms that elude the surface protective mechanisms. IgE is also produced and mediates release of histamine from mast cells which are present in large numbers in the lamina propria.

Considerable numbers of lymphocytes are found within the epithelium of the small and large intestines and are present in particularly large numbers in the epithelium overlying Peyer's patches. These lymphocytes are almost exclusively T cells and the majority are of the suppressor/cytotoxic subset, with most of the rest being NK cells.

The epithelium overlying all MALT aggregations is specialised for the sampling of luminal contents for antigen and acts as the equivalent of the afferent lymphatics of the lymph node. The lymphatics associated with MALT are all efferent, passing to regional lymph nodes (e.g. tonsillar, mesenteric, hilar), along with the lymphatics of the surrounding tract wall.

MALT is formed during fetal life, but germinal centres do not develop until after exposure to antigen at birth. The amount of MALT is maximal during childhood, undergoing progressive atrophy in adulthood.

MALT appears to act as an integrated unit with separate but parallel routes of lymphocyte recirculation. When antigen is encountered, it is carried to local MALT tissue. Stimulated lymphocytes migrate to regional lymph nodes where clonal expansion takes place. Effector cells then pass via the thoracic duct and general circulation to the gastrointestinal and respiratory mucosae. MALT lymphocytes carry surface binding molecules which attach to the addressins on HEVs in MALT tissue but not in peripheral tissue.

The lymphoid aggregates of the respiratory tract are similar to, though generally smaller than, those of the gut and are covered by similar antigen sampling and transport cells. As in the gut, there are no afferent lymphatics but efferent lymphatics drain lymph to the regional nodes and activated lymphocytes derived from the respiratory tract aggregations home specifically to the respiratory and other mucosal tissues.

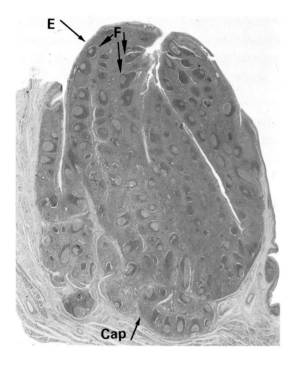

Fig. 11.19 Palatine tonsil H & E × 6

The palatine tonsils are large non-encapsulated masses of lymphoid tissue which, along with the lingual, pharyngeal and tubal tonsils (adenoids), form *Waldeyer's ring*.

The luminal surface is covered by stratified squamous epithelium **E** which deeply invaginates the tonsil, forming blind-ended tonsillar crypts. The base of the tonsil is separated from underlying muscle by a dense collagenous hemicapsule **Cap**. The tonsillar parenchyma contains numerous lymphoid follicles **F** dispersed just beneath the epithelium of the crypts and incorporating germinal centres broadly similar to those found in lymph nodes. Tracer studies have demonstrated that particulate matter entering the crypts from the oropharynx is passed to the follicles, a process that may involve phagocytosis by the epithelial cells of the crypt lining. Likewise, bacteria applied to the tonsils of germ-free animals have been shown to enter the follicle in a similar manner, inducing the formation of germinal centres. An immune response is initiated in a similar manner to that in Peyer's patches. Efferent lymphatics pass to the deep cervical chain of nodes and lymphoblasts migrate to the lamina propria of the oral mucosa and nasopharynx and other mucosae.

Antigen uptake occurs in a similar manner in the lingual, pharyngeal and tubal tonsils, the latter being covered with respiratory-type epithelium rather than stratified squamous epithelium.

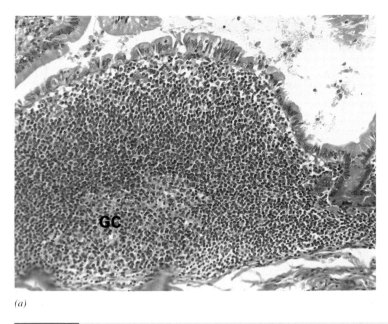

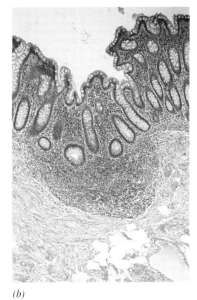

(a) *(b)*

Fig. 11.20 **Peyer's patches and colonic lymphoid aggregations** (a) H & E × 150 (b) H & E × 64

Peyer's patches are groups of lymphoid follicles found scattered in the small intestinal mucosa where they bulge dome-like into the gut lumen. They are least numerous in the duodenum and most prominent in the terminal ileum. Micrograph (a) illustrates part of a Peyer's patch in the ileum, showing a single lymphoid follicle. The follicle is similar to those in lymph nodes, consisting of a germinal centre **GC** composed of large proliferating B cells (centroblasts and centrocytes) surrounded by a mantle of small resting lymphocytes. Immediately beneath the epithelium is a zone of mixed lymphocytes and macrophages. The area between follicles is occupied by T lymphocytes and, like its lymph node equivalent, the paracortex, contains high endothelial venules.

The mucosa overlying these *dome areas* is specialised for antigen uptake and contains large numbers of intraepithelial lymphocytes. The epithelial cells are cuboidal, rather than the usual tall columnar form; goblet cells are scanty. Scattered among the cuboidal epithelial cells are *M cells*, modified epithelial cells which exhibit numerous surface microfolds instead of the usual microvilli. These cells take up antigen from the lumen of the gut by phagocytosis and transport it into the underlying Peyer's patch.

Antigen entering the patch via the M cells is taken up by macrophages and presented to T lymphocytes, thus initiating the immune response. Peyer's patches are not a site of significant IgA secretion and it appears that IgA-committed B cell precursors and memory cells are stimulated in the Peyer's patches passing to mesenteric lymph nodes via efferent lymphatics where the

immunological response is greatly amplified. *Immunoblasts* enter the circulation via the thoracic duct, and home to the lamina propria of the gut where they undergo final maturation into plasma cells. Unlike the Peyer's patches, the lamina propria does not contain high endothelial venules and the mechanism by which Peyer's patch-derived lymphoblasts recognise and home in upon the gut lamina propria is unknown. During lactation, Peyer's patch-derived B lymphocytes also migrate to the breast where they mature into plasma cells and secrete IgA into the milk; thus the newborn is protected from the same ingested pathogens to which the mother is exposed. T_H cells in Peyer's patches control the differentiation of IgA-committed B cell precursors and thus, ultimately, IgA secretion.

Micrograph (b) illustrates a primary lymphoid follicle in the wall of the colon. It does not contain a germinal centre (although secondary follicles are sometimes seen) and the distribution of lymphoid cells is more diffuse, spreading out into the lamina propria between the colonic glands. The epithelium overlying colonic lymphoid tissue is similar to that overlying Peyer's patches and contains M cells and intraepithelial lymphocytes.

Lymph nodes draining the skin receive little of their lymphocyte traffic via afferent lymphatics; however, the mesenteric lymph nodes receive 30–50% of lymphocytes via lymphatics or lacteals draining the gut wall. The mesenteric node thus appears to be a meeting place for lymphocytes from Peyer's patches and the gut lamina propria with recirculating lymphocytes entering the node from the bloodstream.

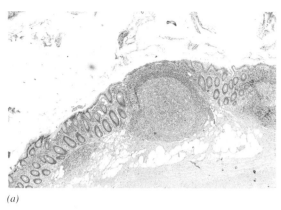

(a)

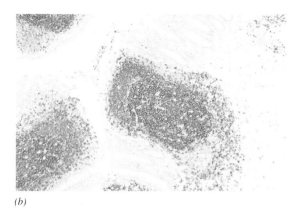

(b)

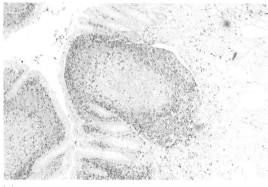

(c)

Fig. 11.21 Appendix

(a) H & E × 20 (b) Immunoperoxidase method for B lymphocytes × 40 (c) Immunoperoxidase method for T lymphocytes × 40

The appendix is a blind-ended tubular sac attached to the caecum with its general structure conforming to that of the large intestine. In children the lymphoid tissue of the appendix is more prominent than in adults, sometimes forming a continuous layer in the lamina propria.

Micrograph (a) shows the typical appearance of a lymphoid follicle in the appendix, which is similar in form to Peyer's patches. Micrographs (b) and (c) use markers for T and B cells, respectively, showing that the follicle is dominated by B lymphocytes with only a small proportion of T cells mainly at the follicular periphery and beneath the overlying epithelium. In micrograph (b) the B cells are stained brown; in (c) the T cells are brown.

Spleen

The spleen is a large lymphoid organ situated in the left upper part of the abdomen. It receives a rich blood supply via a single artery, the *splenic artery*, and is drained by the *splenic vein* into the hepatic portal system.

In humans, the spleen has two main functions:

- production of immunological responses against blood-borne antigens
- removal of particulate matter and aged or defective blood cells, particularly erythrocytes, from the circulation.

In dogs and horses, the spleen also acts as a reservoir of blood which can be mobilised by contraction of the organ. In the human fetus, the spleen is an important site of haemopoiesis and this function may be resumed in adulthood in certain disease states.

Removal of the spleen in childhood or adolescence renders the individual susceptible to infection by certain pyogenic bacteria. This effect is not seen in mature adults in whom splenectomy appears to have few deleterious effects; presumably they have been naturally immunised against these organisms.

The manner in which the spleen performs its function and many of its ultrastructural details are still widely disputed; in many respects, however, the spleen may be considered analogous to a lymph node in which the lymphatic circulation is replaced by a blood circulation. The structure of the spleen allows intimate contacts to be made between blood and lymphocytes, just as the structure of the lymph node facilitates the interaction of afferent lymph and lymphoid cells. Although it is well established that the spleen is involved in removal of aged or defective blood cells from the circulation, it is still not clear whether this is a purely mechanical process or whether immunological recognition plays an important role.

Accounts of the histology of the spleen vary according to the animal models used, all being somewhat different from the human spleen and thus imposing certain inconsistencies in terminology; for example, there are no marginal sinuses in the human spleen. This description is specific to the human spleen. There is considerable variation in the normal between individuals and in the same individual under different physiological and immunological circumstances.

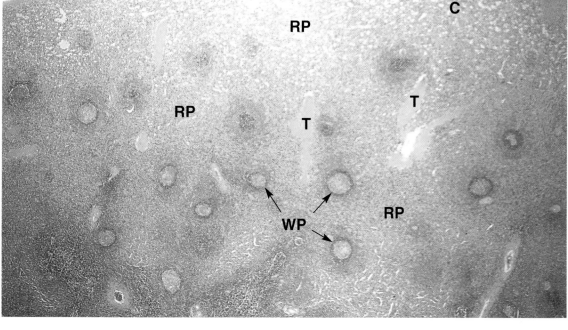

Fig. 11.22 Spleen H & E × 12

On macroscopic examination of the cut surface, the spleen appears to consist of discrete 0.5–1 mm white nodules, called the *white pulp*, embedded in a red matrix called the *red pulp*. Microscopically, as seen in micrograph (a), the white pulp **WP** is seen to consist of lymphoid aggregations and the red pulp **RP**, making up the bulk of the organ, to be a highly vascular tissue.

The spleen has a thin but dense fibroelastic outer capsule **C** from which short trabeculae **T** extend into the parenchyma. The capsule is thickened at the hilum and is continuous with supporting tissues that sheath the larger blood vessels entering and leaving the organ. In some mammals, these supporting tissues contain smooth muscle which exerts a rhythmic pumping action, clearing the spleen of blood and allowing it to act as a reservoir. In humans, only a few smooth muscle cells persist.

The splenic artery divides into several major branches, which enter the splenic hilum and branch to form numerous arterioles which ramify into the splenic parenchyma.

In the white pulp, the T cell areas surround the central arteries, forming what is known as the *periarteriolar lymphoid sheath: (PALS)*. In humans, this lymphoid tissue is less well organised than in other animals, but the term PALS persists in the literature.

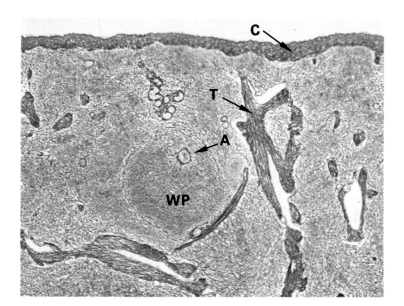

Fig. 11.23 Splenic supporting tissue Reticulin method/neutral red × 42

This staining technique demonstrates the reticular architecture of the spleen. The capsule **C** and perivascular supporting tissue sheaths **T** provide a robust framework which supports a fine reticulin meshwork ramifying throughout the organ in the red pulp. The reticular skeleton is almost absent in the centre of the white pulp nodules **WP** but is well developed at their margins and around the central arteriole **A**.

An overview of the splenic circulation is shown in diagram (a) and a more detailed view of the red pulp in diagram (b). Blood enters the spleen in the splenic artery **SA** which branches repeatedly within the parenchyma (only a few branches are shown for simplicity). The larger arteries are surrounded by a fibrocollagenous sheath which disappears in the smaller branches. These vessels, known as *central arteries* **C**, are so named because they have a cylindrical cuff of lymphoid tissue around them. This lymphoid tissue, known as the *periarteriolar lymphoid sheath* **PALS**, consists mainly of T cells, predominantly T_H cells. The central artery gives off a number of short branches at right angles, which are called *penicillary arteries* **PA**, and these terminate in two to three *sheathed capillaries* **SC** (only one is shown for each penicillary artery). These unique vessels are small blind-ending capillaries which have no endothelial lining but are surrounded instead by an aggregate of macrophages. Thus the blood arriving in a sheathed capillary must traverse this wall of macrophages before entering the red pulp **RP**. The sheathed capillaries therefore form the first part of the filtering mechanism of the spleen.

Splenic red pulp

The splenic parenchyma is permeated by an interconnected network of sinuses **S** which drain into larger sinuses, which in turn drain into tributaries of the splenic vein **SV** and thence the hepatic portal vein. The sinuses are lined by flattened endothelial cells resting upon a basement membrane which is interrupted by numerous narrow slits. The reticulin fibres of the sinusoidal basement membrane are arranged in a circular fashion and are continuous with the reticulin meshwork within the parenchyma (see Fig. 11.25b).

Blood cells entering the parenchyma from the sheathed capillaries squeeze through the walls of the sinuses to drain out of the organ via the splenic vein, an arrangement known as the *open circulation*. The rate of flow in this system approximates the rate through capillaries elsewhere in the body.

Most of the red pulp parenchyma (micrograph b) consists of loose tissue supported by reticulin fibres permeated by capillaries **C** terminating as sheathed capillaries **SC**. The parenchyma removes particulate matter and aged or abnormal erythrocytes from the bloodstream, the defective cells being less deformable and thus unable to negotiate the narrow slits in the sinusoidal basement membrane. Trapped cells are removed by the macrophages of the sheathed capillaries and the parenchyma. The mechanism of recognition of effete red cells is probably based on diminished deformability, but immunological mechanisms may also be involved.

Numerous small patches of the red pulp parenchyma (comprising in total a volume comparable to that of the white pulp) are devoid of capillaries and contain mainly T and B lymphocytes and macrophages. Adjacent sinuses are blind-ended and bulb-shaped and their endothelial lining cells have been shown to have characteristics similar to high endothelial venules of lymph nodes. Lymphocytes probably exit these sinuses to enter these non-filtering areas of the red pulp parenchyma **NFA**, and these areas should be considered as a functional part of the splenic lymphoid tissue.

Perilymphoid (perifollicular) zones

The zone of red pulp immediately surrounding the white pulp differs from the rest of the red pulp, being devoid of sinuses, having only a sparse reticulin meshwork and containing a large number of red and white blood cells in the same proportion as that of blood. About 10% of blood entering the spleen is believed to pass into this perilymphoid parenchyma, from which it passes much more slowly into the surrounding, more widely spaced sinuses than in the rest of the red pulp. The function of these *perilymphoid (perifollicular) zones* is unclear, but the sluggish blood flow may be a means of enhancing the interaction of blood cells, antigens and antibodies.

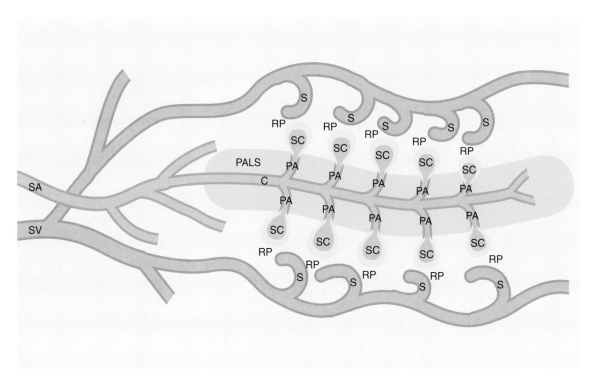

(a)

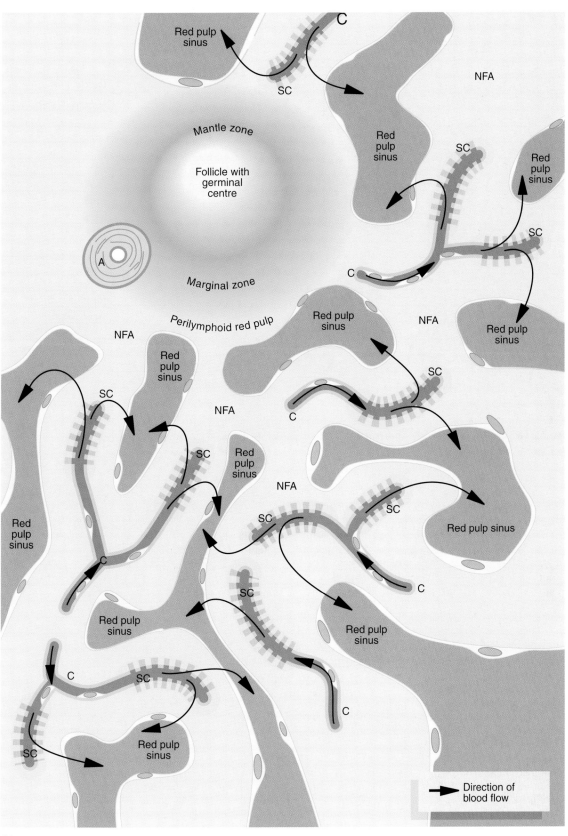

(b)

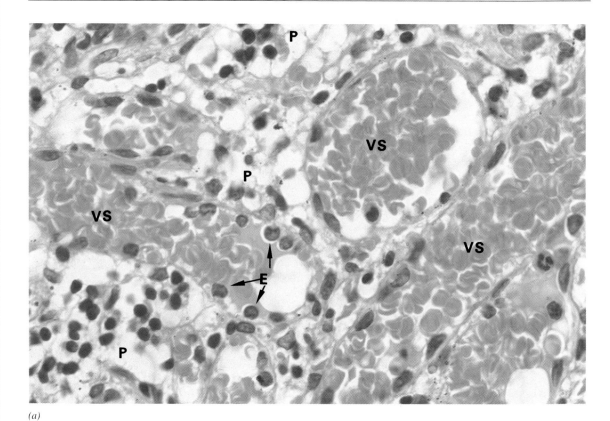

(a)

Fig. 11.25 **Red pulp (a) H & E × 800**
(b) Reticulin method × 200

Micrograph (a) illustrates the red pulp, its major constituent being the parenchyma **P** which is permeated by broad interconnected venous sinuses **VS**. Seen in section, the parenchymal tissue between the sinusoids is considerably thinner than the diameter of the sinusoids, and the area occupied by sinuses is greater than that of the parenchyma; in three-dimensional terms, however, the parenchyma makes up 70% of the volume and the sinuses only 30%. The two-dimensional view gave rise to the misleading term *cords (of Bilroth)* to describe the parenchymal tissue. Together, the sinuses and intervening parenchyma make up the red pulp, its three dimensional structure being analogous to a Swiss cheese, the holes representing the sinuses and the cheese representing the parenchyma.

The parenchyma is composed of the macrophages of sheathed capillaries, other macrophages and blood cells which have left the capillaries and not yet crossed into the sinuses. Non-filtering areas are devoid of sheathed capillaries and contain a greater proportion of lymphocytes. The phagocytic cells are responsible for destruction of aged or damaged blood cells. The different nucleated cell types of the parenchyma cannot be reliably distinguished in this type of preparation.

The venous sinuses are lined by elongated, spindle-shaped endothelial cells **E** which lie parallel to the long axes of the sinuses. The venous sinuses have thus been likened to all wooden barrels with both ends open, with the epithelial cells represented by the wooden staves and hence described as *stave cells*. Slits occur between the endothelial cells, the endothelial basement membrane

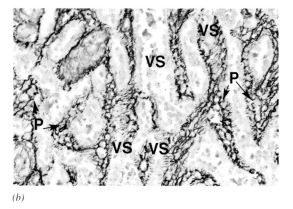

(b)

being discontinuous over the slits. Blood cells, particularly viable erythrocytes, squeeze between the stave cells to reach the venous sinuses; these drain into progressively larger vessels which converge to form the splenic vein.

Micrograph (b) shows red pulp stained by the reticulin method to demonstrate the supporting framework of the parenchyma **P**. The basement membranes of the venous sinuses **VS** show the greatest concentration of reticulin fibres, which encircle the endothelium in a manner reminiscent of the steel bands holding together a wooden barrel. Fine reticular strands traverse the parenchyma, linking the whole structure together and providing support for parenchymal macrophages and a small number of fibroblasts responsible for elaboration of the reticulin. In some sinuses, the plane of section is such that the parallel bands of reticulin can be seen encircling the sinuses. Other sinuses are cut in such a way that only the erythrocytes in the lamina are visible.

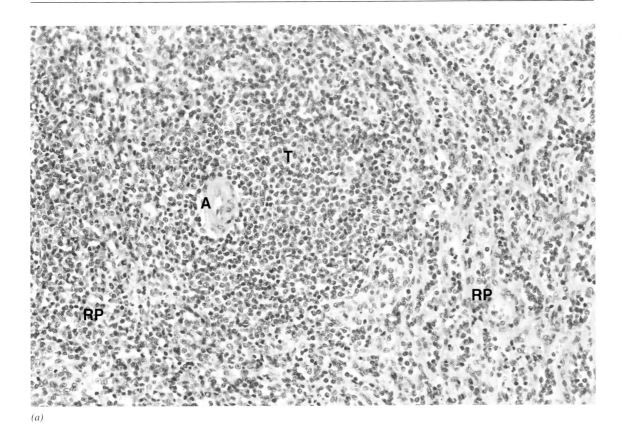

(a)

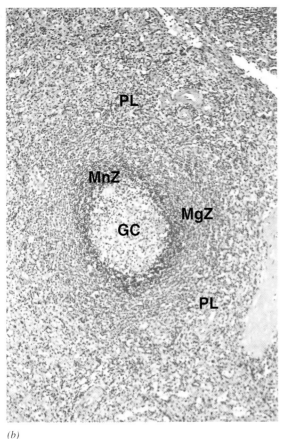

(b)

Fig. 11.26 Splenic lymphoid tissue
(a) H & E × 225 (b) H & E × 150

The splenic white pulp is of two types, T cell and B cell, together making up 5–20% of the total mass of the spleen. The functions of these areas appear to be similar to those of the paracortex and superficial cortex of lymph nodes, respectively. The non-filtering areas of red pulp parenchyma (see Fig. 11.24) should probably be considered part of the splenic lymphoid tissue mass also, but its immunological function remains to be elucidated.

Micrograph (a) shows a T cell area typically forming an eccentric cylindrical sheath **T** around a central arteriole **A** and containing small lymphocytes mainly of the T helper subset. This is equivalent to the periarteriolar lymphoid sheath in animals. Note the way the T cell mass merges with the surrounding red pulp parenchyma **RP.** Small lymphatics arise in the T lymphocyte areas, forming a network around the arterioles and then continuing with the larger arteries to the hilum to drain into a group of adjacent lymph nodes.

B cells form follicles usually located in the vicinity of an arteriole, as illustrated in micrograph (b). In young people, many of the follicles exhibit germinal centres **GC** similar to those of the lymph node, although the proportion of follicles with germinal centres diminishes with age. At the follicle periphery is a narrow zone of small lymphocytes called the *mantle zone* **MnZ** beyond which is a broader *marginal zone* **MgZ** of less densely packed medium-sized lymphocytes supported by a framework of reticulin fibres. The red pulp around the marginal zone, the perilymphoid red pulp **PL**, also contains lymphocytes which may simply be migrating from the sinuses to the white pulp.

12. Respiratory system

Introduction

Respiration is a term used to describe two different but interrelated processes: **cellular respiration** and **mechanical respiration**. Cellular respiration is the process by which cells produce energy by metabolism of organic molecules (see Ch. 1). Mechanical respiration is the process by which oxygen required for cellular respiration is absorbed from the atmosphere into the blood vascular system and carbon dioxide is excreted into the atmosphere. Mechanical respiration is the function of the respiratory system.

The respiratory system has two functional components: a conducting system for transport of inspired and expired gases into and out of the lungs and an interface for passive exchange of gases between the atmosphere and blood. The conducting system begins essentially as a single tube, which divides repeatedly to form airways of ever decreasing diameter. The terminal branches of the conducting system open into blind-ended sacs called *alveoli* which are the sites of gas exchange. The alveoli, which constitute the bulk of the lung tissue, are thin-walled structures enveloped by a rich network of capillaries, the *pulmonary capillaries*. This arrangement provides a huge area where blood and air are separated by a very thin barrier allowing gas exchange. The continuous process of gaseous diffusion requires appropriate gaseous pressure gradients to be maintained across the alveolar wall. This is achieved by rapid and continuous perfusion of the pulmonary capillaries by deoxygenated venous blood from the right side of the heart and regular replacement of alveolar gases through the process of breathing.

The respiratory system is divided anatomically into two parts, the *upper* and *lower respiratory tracts*, which are separated by the *pharynx*. The pharynx is best considered functionally and histologically as part of the gastrointestinal tract despite its important role as an airway.

Upper respiratory tract

The upper respiratory tract comprises a system of interconnected spaces, the *nasal cavity*, *paranasal sinuses* and the *nasopharynx*, and is principally involved in filtering, humidifying and adjusting the temperature of inspired air. In addition, the nasal cavity contains receptors for the sense of smell (see Ch. 21), whilst the paranasal sinuses act as resonance chambers for speech, as well as reducing the bony mass of the facial skeleton. The nasopharynx is connected via the *auditory (Eustachian) tubes* (see Fig. 21.23) to the middle ear cavities, an arrangement which permits equilibration of air pressure in the middle ear with that of the external environment.

The upper respiratory tract is lined by pseudostratified columnar epithelium with numerous goblet cells (respiratory epithelium, see Fig. 5.5). The epithelium is supported by a loose collagenous layer, the *lamina propria*. Collectively, the epithelium and lamina propria are known as *respiratory mucous membrane* or *respiratory mucosa*. The terms mucous membrane and mucosa are also used for the moist linings of other tracts, such as the gastrointestinal tract, and always refer to both the epithelium and its supporting lamina propria. A further supporting tissue layer called the *submucosa* separates the mucosa from underlying structures.

Lower respiratory tract

The lower respiratory tract begins at the *larynx* and then continues into the thorax as the *trachea*, before repeatedly dividing into smaller and smaller airways to reach the alveoli; there are about 20 orders of branches in humans. The vocal cords of the larynx protect the lower respiratory tract against the entry of foreign bodies, in addition to performing a vital function in speech. The vocal cords are lined by stratified squamous epithelium, which is better adapted than respiratory epithelium to withstand frictional stress.

The trachea first divides into left and right *primary* or *main bronchi* which supply the lungs. Each primary bronchus gives rise to *secondary* or *lobar bronchi* supplying the lobes of the lungs before dividing again to form *tertiary* or *segmental bronchi* which supply the segments of each lobe. The tertiary bronchi then ramify into numerous orders of progressively smaller airways called *bronchioles*, the smallest of which are called *terminal bronchioles* and mark the end of the purely conducting portion of the tract. The terminal bronchioles branch further into a series of transitional airways, the *respiratory bronchioles* and *alveolar ducts*, which become increasingly involved in gaseous exchange. These passages finally terminate in dilated spaces called *alveolar sacs*, which open into the alveoli. The unit of lung structure consisting of a terminal bronchiole and its respiratory bronchioles and alveoli is sometimes called the *acinus*.

Each type of airway has its own characteristic structural features, but there is a gradual, rather than abrupt, transition from one type of airway to the next along the whole length of the tract. In general terms, the airways are pliable tubes lined by respiratory mucosa and containing variable amounts of muscle plus cartilage in the larger airways. The principal structural features of the lower respiratory tract are as follows:

- The respiratory epithelium undergoes progressive transition from a tall, pseudostratified columnar, ciliated form in the larynx and trachea to a simple, cuboidal, non-ciliated form in the smallest airways. Goblet cells are numerous in the trachea but decrease in number and are absent from the distal terminal bronchioles. Scattered throughout the respiratory tract epithelium are cells which contain electron-dense, secretory granules. These cells are known as *Kulchitsky* or *K cells* and constitute part of the diffuse neuroendocrine system (see Ch. 17); serotonin, bombesin and calcitonin are among the secretory products so far identified.
- The lamina propria consists of fibroelastic tissue which contains lymphoid aggregates of variable size; these form part of the mucosa-associated lymphoid tissue (see Ch. 11). One of the functions of this immunological tissue is the production of secretory IgA, which is secreted onto the mucosal surface as a defence against invading microorganisms.
- A layer of smooth muscle lies deep to the mucosa (except in the trachea) and becomes increasingly prominent as the airway diameter decreases. Smooth muscle tone controls the diameter of the conducting passages and thus controls resistance to air flow within the respiratory tree. Smooth muscle tone is modulated by the autonomic nervous system, adrenal medullary hormones and local factors. Sympathetic activity causes smooth muscle relaxation and thus dilatation of the airways, which is a desirable response in the 'fight or flight' situation. Parasympathetic activity, on the other hand, causes airway constriction; the functional significance of this may be to reduce 'dead space' on expiration.
- The submucosal layer underlying the smooth muscle layer contains serous and mucous glands which become progressively less numerous in the narrower airways and are not present beyond the tertiary bronchi.
- Cartilage provides a supporting skeleton for the larynx, trachea and bronchi and prevents the collapse of these airways during respiration. The cartilage lies outside the submucosa, diminishing as the calibre of the airway decreases to be completely absent beyond the tertiary bronchi.
- The outermost layer of cartilage or smooth muscle, as the case may be, is surrounded by fibroelastic tissue called the *adventitia* which merges with the surrounding lung parenchyma.

Blood supply of the lungs

The lungs have a dual blood supply, the *pulmonary system* and the *bronchial system*. The pulmonary supply carries deoxygenated blood from the right side of the heart via a large pulmonary artery to each lung.

The *pulmonary arteries* enter the roots or *hila* of the lungs with the main bronchi and then divide and course in parallel with the branching airways to supply the pulmonary capillaries surrounding the alveoli. The pulmonary arterial system is structurally unusual in two respects. Firstly, the pulmonary arterial vessels are relatively thin-walled and of large calibre, their diameter approximating that of the accompanying airway. The arterial blood pressure in the pulmonary system is thus much lower than systemic blood pressure. Secondly, the pulmonary arteries have the histological characteristics of elastic arteries rather than of muscular arteries. Elastic expansion and recoil of the vessels maintain the pulmonary arterial pressure at a relatively constant level throughout the cardiac cycle.

The bronchial arterial system constitutes the systemic circulation of the lower respiratory tract. It arises as small branches of the aorta and supplies oxygenated blood to the tissues of the airway walls and to the *pleura*, the layer which invests the outer surface of each lung. The bronchial vessels are of the usual type found in the rest of the systemic circulation.

A common venous system returns most of the blood to the left side of the heart via the *pulmonary veins*, which are thin-walled vessels of wide diameter. A small proportion of blood from the bronchial system drains to the right side of the heart via the *azygous venous system*.

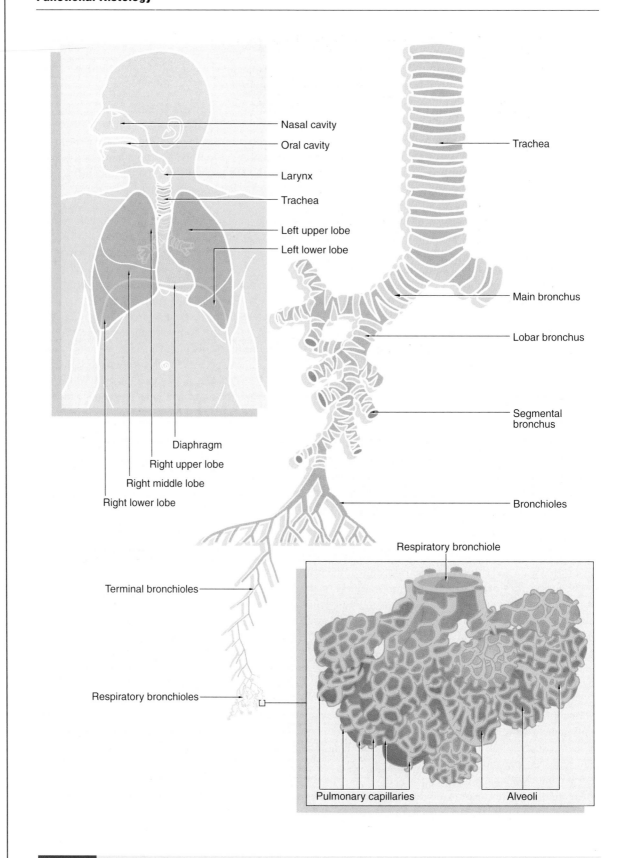

Nasal cavity

Oral cavity

Larynx

Trachea

Left upper lobe

Left lower lobe

Diaphragm

Right upper lobe

Right middle lobe

Right lower lobe

Trachea

Main bronchus

Lobar bronchus

Segmental
bronchus

Bronchioles

Terminal bronchioles

Respiratory bronchioles

Respiratory bronchiole

Pulmonary capillaries

Alveoli

Fig. 12.1 Structure of the respiratory system

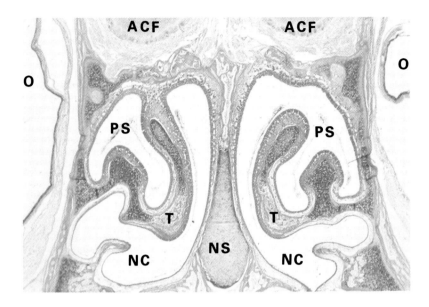

Fig. 12.2 Nasal cavity – kitten (coronal section) H & E/Alcian blue × 12

The nose is subdivided into two nasal cavities **NC** by the cartilaginous *nasal septum* **NS**; cartilage is stained blue in this preparation.

The nasal cavities and paranasal sinuses **PS** are lined by respiratory mucosa, the major function of which is to adjust the temperature and humidity of inspired air. Particulate matter entering the nares is usually trapped by the hairs at that site but some smaller particles are caught on the respiratory mucosa. These functions are enhanced by a large surface area provided by the turbinate system of bones **T** which project into the nasal cavities.

Part of the nasal mucosa, the *olfactory mucosa*, contains receptors for the sense of smell (see Fig. 21.2). Although the olfactory mucosa is extensive in lower mammals, in man it is confined to a relatively small area in the roof of the nasal cavities.

Note the close proximity of the nasal cavities to the orbital cavities **O** and the anterior cranial fossa **ACF**.

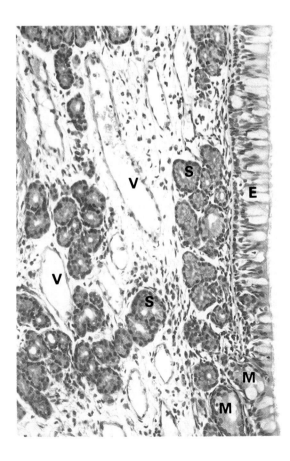

Fig. 12.3 Nasal mucosa H & E × 200

The nasal mucosa consists of a pseudostratified columnar ciliated epithelium **E** with numerous goblet cells, *respiratory epithelium*, supported by a richly vascular lamina propria containing serous and mucous glands. These features reflect the functions of the nasal mucosa, to warm and humidify the incoming air, which are common to the conducting parts of the respiratory system.

The entrance to each nasal cavity, the *nasal vestibule*, is lined by skin with short, coarse hairs called *vibrissae* which trap the largest particles in inspired air before they reach the nasal mucosa.

Small particles in inspired air are trapped in a thin layer of surface mucus secreted by the goblet cells and the mucous glands **M** of the respiratory passages. Coordinated, wave-like beating of cilia propels mucus with trapped particles towards the pharynx where it is swallowed. Any pathogenic organisms so trapped are inactivated in the stomach by gastric acid.

The temperature of inspired air is adjusted to that of the body by heat exchange between the air and blood flowing in a rich plexus of thin-walled venules **V** in the lamina propria. Inspired air is humidified by the watery secretions of serous glands **S**, also located in the lamina propria.

A mucosa similar to that of the nasal cavities also lines the nasopharynx, paranasal sinuses and auditory tubes.

ORGAN SYSTEMS

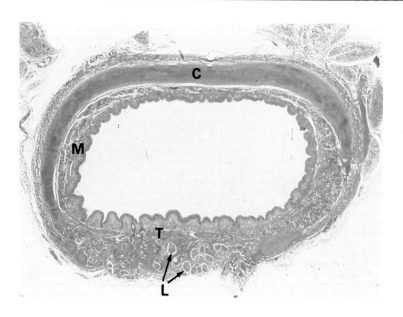

Fig. 12.4 **Trachea**

H & E/Alcian blue × 9

This specimen from a newborn child shows the general structure of the trachea. This is a flexible tube of fibroelastic tissue and cartilage which permits expansion in diameter and extension in length during inspiration, and passive recoil during expiration.

A series of C-shaped rings of hyaline cartilage **C** (stained blue) support the tracheal mucosa **M** and prevent its collapse during inspiration.

Bands of smooth muscle, called the *trachealis muscle* **T**, join the free ends of the rings posteriorly; contraction of the trachealis reduces tracheal diameter and thereby assists in raising intrathoracic pressure during coughing. A few strands of longitudinal muscle **L** can be seen disposed behind the trachealis muscle.

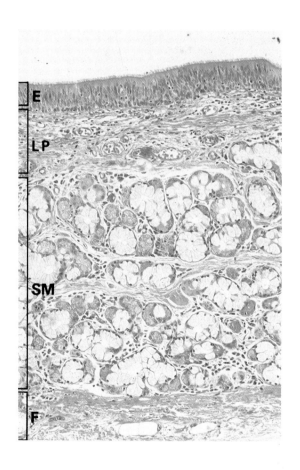

Fig. 12.5 **Trachea** H & E × 198

The layers of the tracheal wall are shown in this specimen from a young adult. The respiratory epithelium **E** of the trachea is similar to the rest of the bronchial tree and nasal epithelium. The epithelium of the respiratory system is supported by an unusually thick basement membrane. A variety of cell types are found in the epithelium, including:

- tall pseudostratified columnar cells with cilia
- goblet cells
- serous cells identical to the cells of the submucosal serous glands
- Kulchitsky cells which are part of the diffuse neuroendocrine system
- stem or reserve cells which are able to divide and differentiate to replace other cell types.

The various cell types are present in different proportions in different parts of the trachea, with ciliated columnar cells relatively more plentiful in the lower trachea, and goblet and basal cells more common in the upper trachea. Beneath the basement membrane, the lamina propria **LP** consists of loose, highly vascular supporting tissue which becomes more condensed at its deeper aspect to form a band of fibroelastic tissue.

Underlying the lamina propria is the loose submucosa **SM** containing numerous mixed seromucinous glands which decrease in number in the lower parts of the trachea; the serous cells stain strongly with H & E whilst the mucous cells remain poorly stained. The submucosa merges with the perichondrium of the underlying hyaline cartilage rings (not seen in this field) or, as here, with the dense fibroelastic tissue **F** between the cartilage rings.

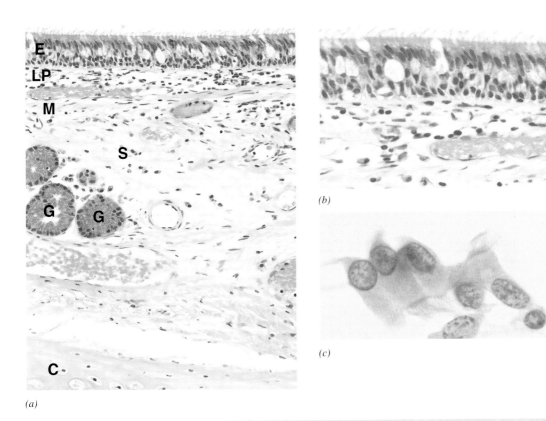

(a)

(b)

(c)

Fig. 12.6 **Primary bronchus** **(a) H & E × 150 (b) H & E × 300 (c) Cytology: H & E × 900**

The basic structure of the bronchi is similar to that of the trachea, but differs in several details, as follows:

- The respiratory epithelium **E** is less tall and contains fewer goblet cells; the goblet cells have darkly stained, granular cytoplasm with the staining method used in micrograph (a).
- The lamina propria **LP** is more dense with a large quantity of elastin in its more superficial layers.
- The lamina propria is separated from the submucosa **S** by a discontinuous layer of smooth muscle **M** which becomes progressively more prominent in smaller airways.
- The submucosal layer contains fewer seromucinous glands **G**.

- The cartilage framework **C** is arranged into flattened, interconnected plates rather than discrete C-shaped rings as in the trachea.

In micrograph (b), which shows the bronchial epithelium at high power, the mixture of tall columnar ciliated cells and goblet cells can be appreciated. Some of the basal nuclei in the micrograph represent the nuclei of Kulchitsky cells and reserve cells which do not extend to the luminal surface of the epithelium. Micrograph (c) is a cytology specimen obtained by bronchial brushing during bronchoscopic examination for suspected bronchogenic cancer. It illustrates the normal tapered shape of the tall columnar ciliated epithelial cells with the nuclei located towards the base.

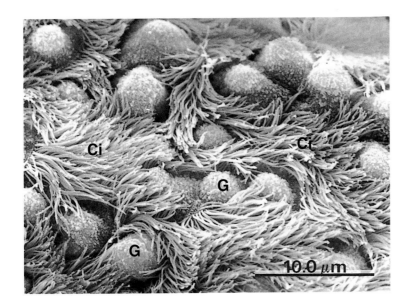

Fig. 12.7 **Primary bronchus epithelium SEM × 2000**

This micrograph illustrates the surface of a primary bronchus at high magnification; the film of surface mucus has been removed before fixation and processing. The ciliated epithelial cells **Ci** have an appearance reminiscent of clumps of seaweed, the cilia being several microns in length. Goblet cells **G**, recognisable by their bulbous surface outline, lack of cilia and the presence of small surface projections associated with mucus secretion, are scattered amongst ciliated cells.

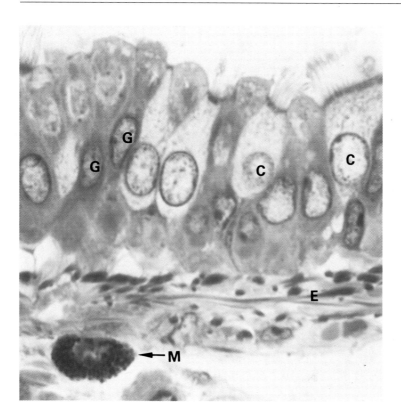

Fig. 12.8 Bronchial epithelium – rat
Thin section: toluidine blue × 800

This micrograph illustrates the structure of the bronchial epithelium at the limit of resolution of the light microscope. The epithelium is pseudostratified, the bases of all the cells extending down to the basement membrane, although not all the cells reach the luminal surface. The ciliated cells **C** have large nuclei and stain very poorly with this method. The goblet cells **G** stain most strongly due to their content of mucus.

The underlying lamina propria contains a considerable amount of elastin **E** and mast cells **M**, the latter having numerous darkly stained granules which contain histamine and the glycoprotein heparin. It is the heparin which is responsible for the intense staining with this method (see also Fig. 4.14). The role of mast cells in normal function is unclear; however, when antigen–antibody complexes are formed on their cell membranes, they release large quantities of histamine, causing smooth muscle constriction and vasodilatation leading to mucosal swelling. In the bronchioles, these phenomena are partly responsible for the clinical condition of asthma.

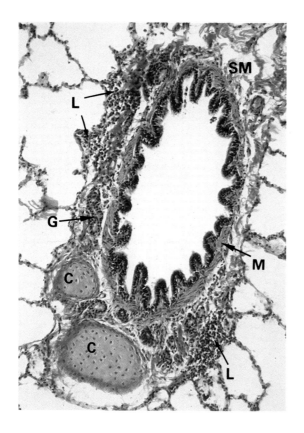

Fig. 12.9 Tertiary (segmental) bronchus
Elastic van Gieson × 75

As the bronchi diminish in diameter, the structure progressively changes to resemble more closely that of large bronchioles. The respiratory epithelium, which cannot be seen at this magnification, is now tall and columnar with little pseudostratification, and goblet cell numbers are greatly diminished.

The lamina propria is thin, elastic and completely encircled by smooth muscle **M** which is disposed in a spiral manner. This arrangement of smooth muscle permits contraction of the bronchi in both length and diameter during expiration. Seromucinous glands **G** are sparse in the submucosa; they are rarely found in smaller airways.

The cartilage framework **C** is reduced to a few irregular plates; cartilage does not usually extend beyond the tertiary bronchi. Note that the submucosa **SM** merges with the surrounding adventitia and thence with the lung parenchyma. Small aggregations of lymphocytes **L**, part of the mucosa-associated lymphoid tissue (MALT), are seen in the adventitia.

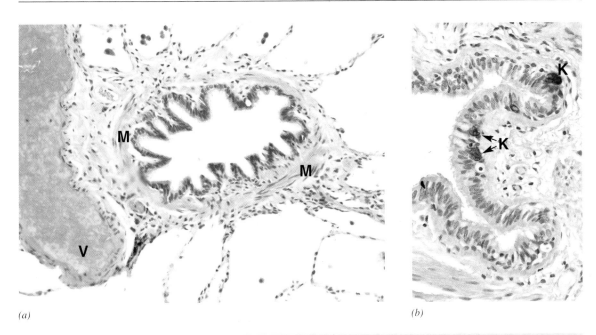

(a)

(b)

Fig. 12.10 Bronchiole (a) H & E × 150 (b) Immunoperoxidase × 200

Bronchioles, as in micrograph (a), are airways of less than 1 mm in diameter and have neither cartilage support nor submucosal glands. The respiratory epithelium is composed of ciliated columnar cells and contains few goblet cells. In the terminal and respiratory bronchioles, goblet cells are entirely replaced by *Clara cells*, tall columnar non-ciliated cells which contain apical secretory granules. Clara cells are thought to secrete one of the components of surfactant and also to act as reserve cells.

The smooth muscle layer **M** is disposed in discrete bundles arranged in various orientations. The total cross-sectional area of all bronchioles combined is far greater than that of the rest of the conducting passages combined,

and thus the tone of the bronchiolar smooth muscle effectively controls resistance to air flow within the lungs.

A vein **V** can be seen accompanying the bronchiole in this micrograph.

Micrograph (b) employs the immunoperoxidase technique to demonstrate *Kulchitsky cells* **K**. These are part of the diffuse neuroendocrine system and contain dense core granules in common with other neuroendocrine cells. The antibody used in this preparation reacts with *chromogranin A*, a protein found in the dense core granules of all neuroendocrine cells. The granules contain a variety of peptide hormones such as serotonin, bombesin, calcitonin and leu-enkephalin, which are thought to regulate muscle tone in bronchi and vessel walls.

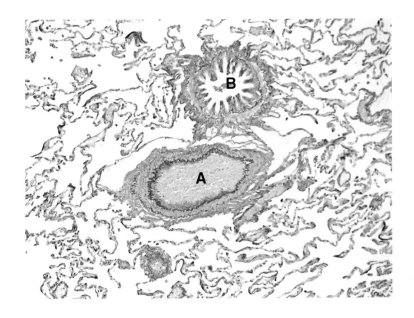

Fig. 12.11 Pulmonary artery
Elastic van Gieson × 75

This micrograph shows a branch of the pulmonary artery **A** adjacent to a bronchiole **B**. The airway can be identified as such by the absence of cartilage and submucosal glands, and the relatively thin muscular layer.

The pulmonary arterial vessels are described as elastic arteries (see Fig. 8.7) and contain relatively little smooth muscle; in this preparation, elastin is stained black and smooth muscle tan.

The walls of the pulmonary arteries are relatively thin in relation to their diameter, the pressures being much lower than that in the systemic circulation. Note the red-stained collagen in the supporting tissue of the vessel and airway.

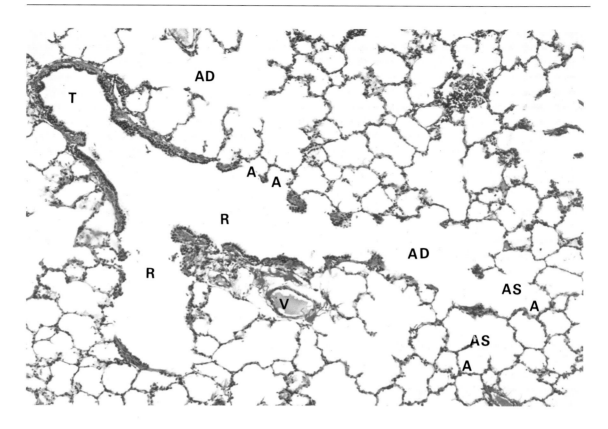

Fig. 12.12 Terminal portion of the respiratory tree Elastic van Gieson × 40

Terminal bronchioles **T** are the smallest diameter passages of the purely conducting portion of the respiratory tree; beyond this, further branches become increasingly involved in gaseous exchange.

Each terminal bronchiole divides to form short, thinner-walled branches called *respiratory bronchioles* **R** which contain a small number of single alveoli **A** in their walls. The epithelium of the respiratory bronchioles is devoid of goblet cells and largely consists of ciliated cuboidal cells and smaller numbers of non-ciliated cells called *Clara cells*. In the most distal part of the respiratory bronchioles, Clara cells become the predominant cell type. Clara cells have three functions:

- They produce one of the components of *surfactant*.
- They act as reserve cells, i.e. they are able to divide, differentiate and replace other damaged cell types.
- They contain enzyme systems which can detoxify noxious substances.

Each respiratory bronchiole divides further into several *alveolar ducts* **AD** which have numerous alveoli **A** opening along their length. The alveolar ducts end in an *alveolar sac* **AS**, which in turn opens into several alveoli. In histological sections, all that can be seen of the walls of the alveolar ducts are small aggregations of smooth

muscle cells, collagen and elastic fibres which form rings surrounding the alveolar ducts and the openings of the alveolar sacs and alveoli. The smooth muscle of the respiratory bronchioles and alveolar ducts regulates alveolar air movements.

Each alveolus consists of a pocket, open at one side and lined by flattened epithelial cells. Surrounding each alveolus is a rich network of pulmonary capillaries supplied by pulmonary vessels **V** which follow the general course of the airways. The wall or *alveolar septum* between adjacent alveoli forms a sandwich of:

- the two layers of alveolar epithelium with their basement membranes (the bread)
- plentiful capillaries enmeshed in elastin and fine collagen fibres (the filling).

The collagen and elastin fibres condense around the opening of each alveolus and merge with those around the openings of adjacent alveoli to form a fine, three-dimensional supporting meshwork for the whole lung parenchyma. The alveolar septa contain small openings about 8 μm in diameter, called *alveolar pores*, which allow equalisation of pressure between alveoli and provide a collateral air circulation should a bronchiole become obstructed.

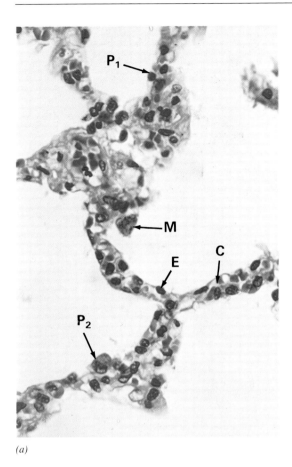

(a)

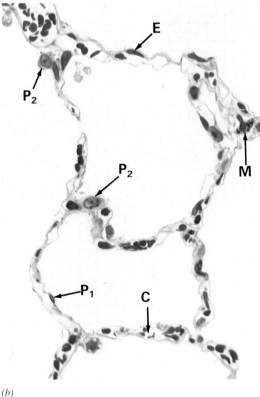

(b)

Fig. 12.13 Alveoli (a) H & E × 480
(b) Thin section: toluidine blue × 480

The conventional method of studying the structure of the alveolar wall in light microscopy has been to use relatively thick (5–8 μm) paraffin-embedded sections, stained by routine methods as in micrograph (a); however, the resolution obtained by such methods is limited. In contrast, thin resin sections, as shown in micrograph (b), reveal much greater structural detail since they permit better resolution.

In general terms, the alveolar wall consists of three tissue components: *surface epithelium*, *supporting tissue* and *blood vessels*.

Epithelium provides a continuous lining to each alveolus and consists of cells of two types. Most of the alveolar surface area is covered by large, squamous cells called *type I pneumocytes (alveolar lining cells)*; since the cytoplasm of these cells covers such an extensive area, the characteristic densely stained nuclei of type I pneumocytes P_1 are relatively infrequently seen in histological section. A second epithelial cell type, known as the *type II pneumocyte*, represents some 60% of cells in the lining epithelium; these cells are rounded in shape and thus occupy a much smaller proportion (about 5%) of the alveolar surface area. Type II pneumocytes P_2 have large, rounded nuclei with a prominent nucleolus and vacuolated cytoplasm. Type I pneumocytes constitute part of the extremely thin gaseous diffusion barrier, whereas type II pneumocytes secrete a surface-active material called *surfactant* which reduces surface tension within the alveoli, preventing alveolar collapse during expiration. Clara cells of the respiratory bronchioles probably synthesise other components of surfactant. Type II pneumocytes retain the capacity for cell division and can differentiate into type I pneumocytes in response to damage to the alveolar lining.

Supporting tissue forms an attenuated layer beneath the epithelium and surrounding the blood vessels of the alveolar wall. This layer consists of fine reticular, collagenous and elastic fibres and occasional fibroblasts.

Blood vessels, mainly capillaries **C** (7–10 μm in diameter), form an extensive plexus around each alveolus. In most of the alveolar wall, the basement membrane which supports the capillary endothelium is directly applied to the basement membrane supporting the surface epithelium; in such sites the two basement membranes are fused and the supporting tissue layer is absent. This arrangement provides an interface of minimal thickness between alveolar air and blood. Note in these micrographs the nuclei of capillary endothelial cells **E** and the close proximity of the densely stained erythrocytes within these capillaries to the alveolar air spaces.

Although the defence mechanisms of the conducting passages filter most particulate matter from inspired air, small particles such as carbon reach the alveoli and are engulfed by large phagocytic cells (macrophages) found in the alveolar wall or free in the alveolar space. These *alveolar macrophages* **M** are derived from circulating blood monocytes and are usually recognisable by their content of engulfed, particulate material.

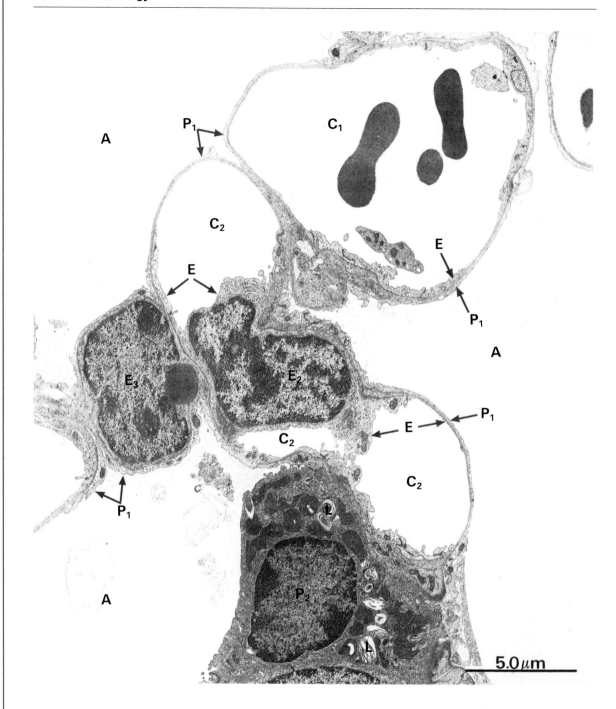

Fig. 12.14 Alveolar wall **EM × 6000**

This micrograph shows the alveolar wall between three alveoli **A** at low magnification. Capillaries make up the bulk of the alveolar wall, branching and anastomosing to create a basket-like arrangement around each alveolus. This field shows parts of several capillaries, the uppermost C_1 containing erythrocytes and a platelet. The plane of section has cut the lumen of a second capillary C_2 in three places and includes the nucleus of one of its lining endothelial cells E_2. The nucleus of an endothelial cell E_3 of another capillary is also included in this section. The cytoplasm of type I pneumocytes P_1, which cover most of the alveolar surface, and capillary endothelial cells **E** are both extremely attenuated and distinction between them is best made by tracing their basement membranes. Alveolar lining cells lie on the convex side of the basement membrane, whilst endothelial cells are on the concave side and adjacent to any erthrocytes within the capillary.

A type II pneumocyte P_2 is also seen, typically located at a branching point of the alveolar septum; the cytoplasm is filled with vesicles containing phospholipid in the form of *lamellar bodies* **L**. These bodies are discharged into the alveolar air space where they contribute to a surfactant layer at the epithelium/air interface.

Fig. 12.15 **Alveolar septum**
EM × 34 000

This micrograph shows, at high magnification, the components of the diffusion barrier between blood and alveolar air. This consists of the attenuated cytoplasm of a type I pneumocyte **P₁**, the fused basement membrane **BM** and the thin cytoplasm of a capillary endothelial cell **E**. Note the erythrocyte **Er** in the capillary lumen.

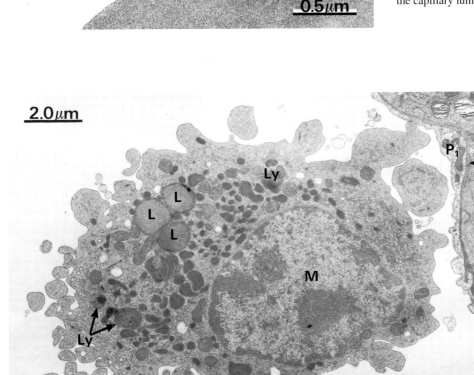

Fig. 12.16 Alveolar macrophage EM × 8000

Macrophages are an important component of the defence system of the lungs, being responsible for phagocytosis of microorganisms and other particulate matter evading the airway defences and reaching the alveoli. The macrophage population is essentially derived from circulating blood monocytes, although some appear to arise from mitotic division of macrophages already resident in the lungs. Alveolar macrophages can be found on the surface of alveolar lining cells as well as in the supporting tissue of the alveolar septa. After engulfment of exogenous material, the majority appear to migrate into the airways where they are carried up on the mucociliary escalator and disposed of by coughing and swallowing. Others appear to be sequestered in the septa and account for the black discoloration (often called *anthracotic pigment*) of the lung parenchyma in individuals chronically inhaling contaminated air, e.g. cigarette smokers.

The macrophage **M** in this micrograph lies within an alveolus adjacent to a septal capillary **C** and a type II pneumocyte (surfactant cell) **P₂** between which is an alveolar pore **AP**. The aspect of the surfactant cell seen here is typically invested by the thin cytoplasm of a type I pneumocyte (alveolar lining cell) **P₁**, the two being separated by a common basement membrane **BM** (see Fig. 12.17). The alveolar macrophage exhibits the typical features of macrophages elsewhere in the body (see Fig. 4.16), but in particular contains numerous secondary lysosomes **Ly** and lipid droplets **L**.

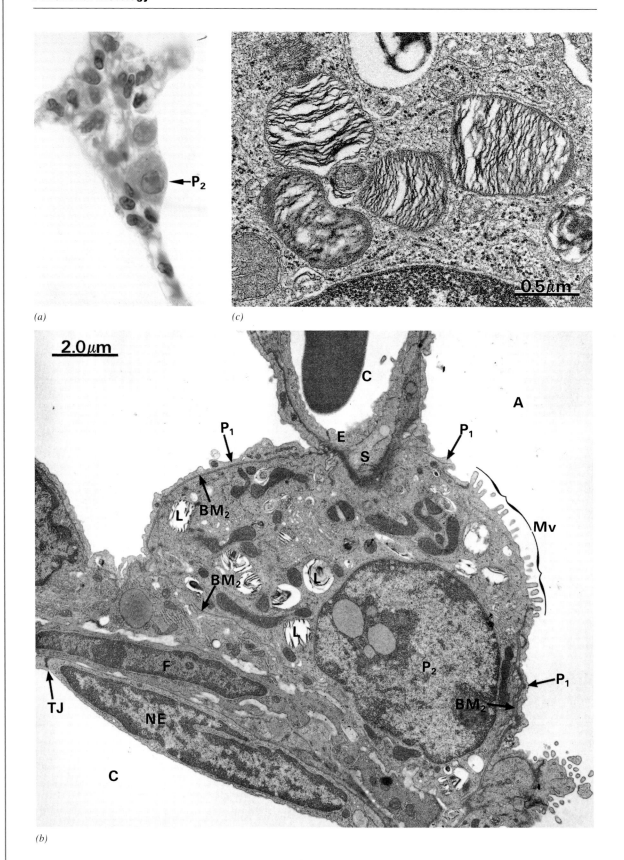

(a)

(c)

0.5μm

2.0μm

(b)

Fig. 12.17 Type II pneumocytes *(illustrations opposite)* (a) H & E × 400 (b) EM × 9000 (c) EM × 35 000

Micrograph (a) shows the light microscope appearance of type II pneumocytes P_2 or *surfactant cells*, which are responsible for surfactant production; their nuclei are large and plump with dispersed chromatin and prominent nucleoli. The plentiful eosinophilic cytoplasm is filled with fine unstained vacuoles representing lamellar bodies, the phospholipid of which is dissolved out during tissue preparation. In comparison, the nuclei of type I pneumocytes (alveolar lining cells) and capillary endothelial cells are small, dense and flattened.

Micrograph (b) shows a branching point in an alveolar wall typically containing a type II pneumocyte P_2, recognisable by its lamellar bodies **L**. Most of the type II pneumocyte is surrounded by basement membrane BM_2 and only a small proportion of its surface is exposed directly to the alveolar space **A**, where it exhibits numerous small microvilli **Mv** associated with surfactant secretion. Elsewhere, the alveolar aspect of the type II pneumocyte is invested by a thin layer of cytoplasm of type I pneumocytes P_1 but separated by a common basement membrane. At the top of the field, the type II pneumocyte abuts a capillary **C**, its cytoplasm being separated from that of the capillary endothelium **E** by the basement membranes of each cell and a little intervening

supporting tissue **S**. At the lower left of the field, the type II cell rests upon a thin layer of septal supporting tissue containing a fibroblast **F**. Beyond this lies the flattened nucleus of a capillary endothelial cell **NE**, its attenuated cytoplasm spreading out to line the capillary lumen **C**. A tight junction **TJ** is seen where this endothelial cell abuts an adjacent cell. Basement membranes can be traced on both aspects of this alveolar supporting tissue. The surfactant cell contains rough ER, free ribosomes and moderate numbers of elongated mitochondria.

Micrograph (c) shows lamellar bodies at high magnification. These are membrane-bound and the lamellae within them are composed mainly of phospholipids, particularly palmitoyl phosphatidylcholine. Phospholipid is released by exocytosis, spreading out over the alveolar surface where it combines with other carbohydrate- and protein-containing secretory products (some of which are derived from Clara cells) to form a tubular lattice of lipoprotein described as *tubular myelin*. In the event of two alveolar surfaces coming together, this overcomes the effects of surface tension which would otherwise cause them to adhere. This allows for normal inflation of the alveoli at birth and for the reinflation of alveoli which collapse after airway obstruction.

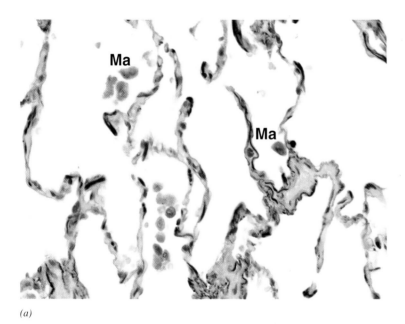

(a)

(b)

Fig. 12.18 Pulmonary elastic tissue (a) Elastic van Gieson × 130 (b) EM × 26 000

The staining method used in micrograph (a) demonstrates the large amount of elastin (stained black) in the alveolar walls. At the margins of the openings into the alveoli, the elastin is condensed to form a supporting ring. The elastin and septal collagen of the alveolar wall are continuous with those of adjacent alveoli, forming a fibroelastic supporting framework for the lung parenchyma as a whole. Occasional alveolar macrophages **Ma** can be seen within the lumen of the alveoli.

Micrograph (b) shows part of an alveolar septum containing elements of the elastin meshwork. The septum consists of the thin cytoplasmic layers of a type I pneumocyte P_1 and two capillary endothelial cells **En** separated by a common basement membrane **BM**; note the marginal fold **M** of one endothelial cell overlapping the other, creating a seal and reinforced by a tight junction **J**.

The elastin **E** is an amorphous, moderately electron-dense mass insinuated between the two epithelial layers. This space also contains a fine cytoplasmic extension of a fibroblast **F**.

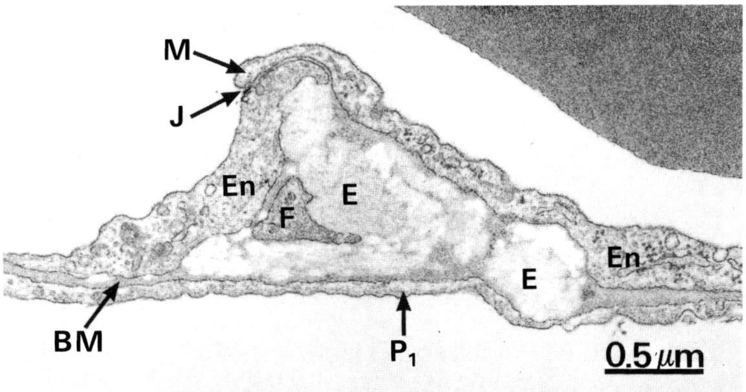

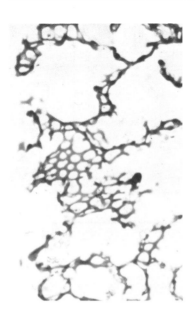

Fig. 12.19 **Pulmonary capillaries** Dye-perfused preparation × 420

The pulmonary arterial system terminates at the alveolar ducts where arterioles ramify to form a widely interconnected capillary basket surrounding each alveolus; the capillaries are of relatively large diameter (7–10 μm). Control of blood flow in the pulmonary capillary bed is predominantly effected by the partial pressure of gases within the alveoli. In poorly ventilated alveoli, the partial pressure of oxygen is low and that of carbon dioxide high; this causes local vasoconstriction, thus directing blood away from the poorly ventilated alveoli.

The lung tissue illustrated in this micrograph was prepared by perfusion of the pulmonary vasculature with a blue dye. This procedure outlines the pulmonary capillary bed; no other histological detail can be seen. In the centre of the field, the richly anastomosing capillary network of part of an alveolar wall is included in the plane of section (see also Fig. 12.1). This type of technique, in combination with the study of very thick histological sections, provided early microscopists with valuable information about the structure, function and vascular system of the lungs.

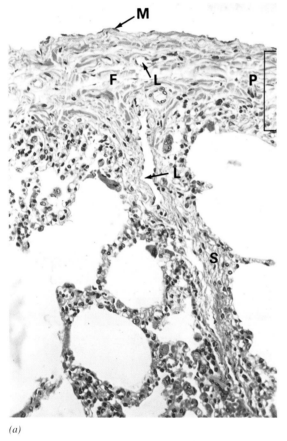

(a)

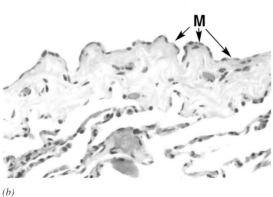

(b)

Fig. 12.20 **Visceral pleura**
(a) H & E × 100 (b) H & E × 200

The cavities containing the lungs, the *pleural cavities*, are lined by a thin, flattened epithelium (mesothelium) called the *pleura*, which is similar in structure to the pericardium and the peritoneum. The pleura lining the thoracic wall, the *parietal pleura*, is reflected at the hilum of the lung so as to invest the outer surface of the lung, the *visceral pleura*. The visceral and parietal pleura are directly applied to one another but separated by a potential space (the *pleural space*) containing a minute amount of serous fluid. The two pleural layers adhere to one another by surface tension so that movements of the thoracic wall during ventilation result in corresponding expansion and contraction of the lungs.

Micrograph (a) illustrates visceral pleura **P.** The outer surface is lined by a layer of flattened mesothelium **M** which is supported by a thin basement membrane. The underlying fibrous supporting tissue **F** consists primarily of collagen and elastin fibres. The fibrous layer of visceral pleura extends into the lung as fibrous septa **S** which are continuous with the fibroelastic framework of the lung parenchyma.

The visceral pleura contains a superficial plexus of lymph vessels which drain via the septa into a deep plexus surrounding the pulmonary blood vessels and airways. Lymph from the deep plexuses drains into the thoracic duct via lymph nodes in the hilar region. Lymph capillaries are not found in alveolar walls, but they are present in the walls of respiratory bronchioles and all larger airways. Several lymph vessels **L** can be seen in the pleura in this micrograph. The visceral pleura also contains numerous small blood vessels and capillaries.

Micrograph (b) is a higher power view of the pleura showing the flattened cuboidal mesothelial cells **M.** These cells stretch to accommodate the movement of the lungs so that the height of the cells varies from flattened to columnar. Ultrastructurally, mesothelial cells have plentiful long surface microvilli which serve to trap hyaluronic acid, thus enhancing the lubrication of the two pleural surfaces. Like other epithelia, mesothelial cells contain prekeratin intermediate filaments.

13. Oral tissues

Introduction

The digestive process commences in the oral cavity with the ingestion, fragmentation and moistening of food, but in addition to its digestive role, the oral cavity is involved in speech, facial expression, sensory reception and breathing. The major structures of the oral cavity, the *lips, teeth, tongue, oral mucosa* and the associated *salivary glands*, participate in all these functions.

Mastication or chewing is the process by which ingested food is made suitable for swallowing. Chewing involves not only coordinated movements of the mandible and the cutting and grinding action of the teeth, but also activity of the lips and tongue, which continually redirect food between the *occlusal surfaces* of the teeth. The watery component of saliva moistens and lubricates the masticatory process, whilst salivary mucus helps to bind the food bolus ready for swallowing.

The entire oral cavity is lined by a protective mucous membrane, the *oral mucosa*, which contains many sensory receptors, including the taste receptors of the tongue. The epithelium of the oral mucosa is of the stratified squamous type which tends to be keratinised in areas subject to considerable friction such as the palate. The oral epithelium is supported by dense collagenous tissue, the *lamina propria*. In highly mobile areas such as the soft palate and floor of the mouth, the lamina propria is connected to the underlying muscle by loose submucosal supporting tissue. In contrast, in areas where the oral mucosa overlies bone, such as the hard palate and tooth-bearing ridges, the lamina propria is tightly bound to the periosteum by a relatively dense fibrous submucosa. Throughout the oral mucosa, numerous small accessory salivary glands of both serous and mucous types are distributed in the submucosa.

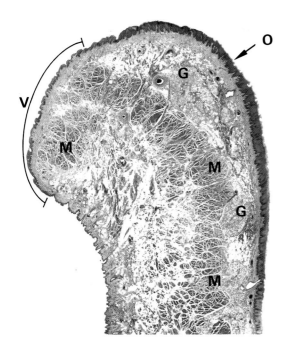

Fig. 13.1 Lip H & E × 6

This micrograph illustrates a midline section through a human lower lip, the bulk of which is made up of bundles of circumoral skeletal muscle **M** seen in transverse section.

The external surface of the lip is covered by hairy skin which passes through a transition zone to merge with the oral mucosa **O** of the inner surface. The transition zone constitutes the free *vermilion border* of the lip **V**, and derives its colour from the richly vascular dermis, which here has only a thin, lightly keratinised epidermal covering. The free border is highly sensitive due to its rich sensory innervation. Since the vermilion border is devoid of sweat and sebaceous glands, it requires continuous moistening by saliva to prevent cracking.

The oral mucosa covering the inner surface of the lip has a thick stratified squamous epithelium and the underlying submucosa contains numerous accessory salivary glands **G** of serous, mucous and mixed seromucous types.

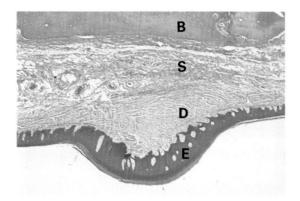

Fig. 13.2 **Palatal mucosa** H & E × 28

Like the rest of the mouth, the palate is covered by a thick stratified squamous epithelium **E** supported by a tough, densely collagenous lamina propria **D**. To assist mastication, the palatal mucosa is thrown up into transverse folds or *rugae*, one of which is shown in this micrograph.

The mucosa of the hard palate is bound down to the underlying bone **B** by relatively dense submucosal tissue **S** containing a few accessary salivary glands.

In rodents and many other mammals with a coarse diet, the surface epithelium of particularly exposed areas is keratinised for extra protection, as in this specimen taken from a monkey.

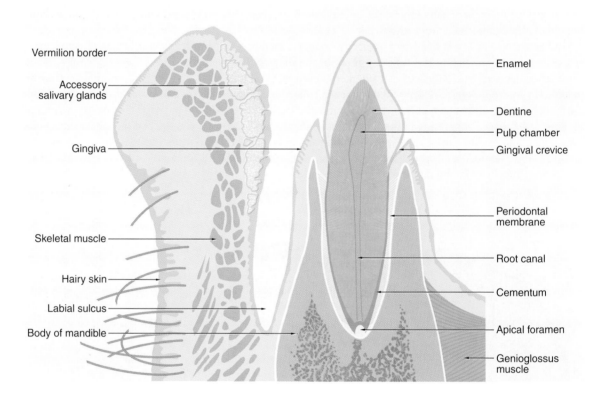

Fig. 13.3 **Lip and tooth**

This drawing of a section through the lower jaw near the midline illustrates the general arrangement of the lip and a tooth with its supporting structures.

Each tooth may be grossly divided into two segments, the *crown* and the *root*; the crown is that portion which projects into the oral cavity and is protected by a layer of highly mineralised *enamel* which covers it entirely. The bulk of the tooth is made up of *dentine*, a mineralised tissue which has a similar chemical composition to bone. The dentine has a central pulp cavity containing the *dental pulp* which consists of specialised supporting tissue containing many sensory nerve fibres. The tooth root is embedded in a bony ridge in the jaw called the *alveolar ridge*; the tooth socket is known as the *alveolus*.

At the lip or cheek (*buccal*) aspect of the alveolus, the bony plate is generally thinner than at the tongue (*palatal*) aspect. The root of the tooth is invested by a thin layer of *cementum* which is connected to the bone of the socket by a thin fibrous layer called the *periodontal ligament* or *periodontal membrane*.

The oral mucosa covering the upper part of the alveolar ridge is called the *gingiva*, and at the junction of the crown and root of the tooth (the *neck of the tooth*) the gingiva forms a tight protective cuff around the tooth. The potential space between the gingival cuff and the enamel of the crown is called the *gingival crevice*. All of the tissues which surround and support the tooth are collectively known as the *periodontium*.

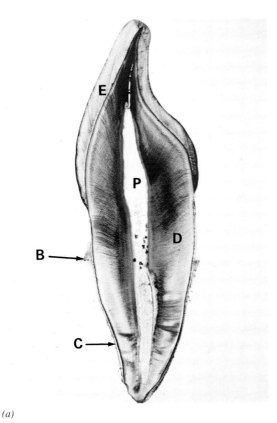

(a)

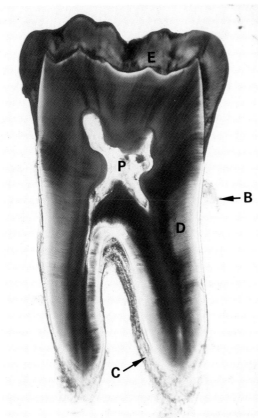

(b)

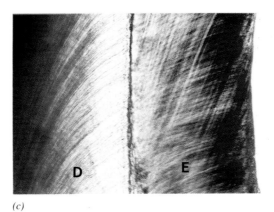

(c)

Fig. 13.4 **Tooth structure** **Undecalcified sections, unstained: (a) × 5 (b) × 5 (c) × 50**

These undecalcified sections cut with a diamond wheel demonstrate the arrangement of the calcified tissues of an upper central incisor tooth micrograph (a) and a lower molar tooth micrograph (b). Micrograph (c) demonstrates the tissues of the crown at high magnification.

The dentine **D**, which forms the bulk of the crown and root, is composed of a calcified organic matrix similar to that of bone. The inorganic component constitutes a somewhat larger proportion of the matrix of dentine than that of bone and exists mainly in the form of hydroxyapatite crystals. Teeth are thus harder than bone. From the pulp cavity **P**, minute parallel tubules, called *dentine tubules*, radiate to the periphery of the dentine; in longitudinal sections of teeth, the tubules appear to follow an S-shaped course.

The crown of the tooth is covered by enamel **E**, an extremely hard, translucent substance composed of parallel *enamel rods* or *prisms* of highly calcified material cemented together by an almost equally calcified *interprismatic material*.

The root is invested by a thin layer of *cementum* **C** which is generally thicker towards the apex of the root. The cementum is an amorphous calcified tissue into which the fibres of the periodontal membrane are anchored. Fragments of alveolar bone **B** have remained attached to the roots after extraction of these specimens.

The morphological form of the tooth crown and roots varies considerably in different parts of the mouth; nevertheless, the basic arrangement of the dental tissues is the same in all teeth.

In humans, the *primary (deciduous) dentition* consists of 20 teeth, comprising two *incisors*, one *canine* and two *molars* in each quadrant. These begin to be formed at the age of 6 weeks during fetal development and erupt between the ages of 6 and 30 months after birth. Between the ages of 6 and 12 years, the deciduous teeth are succeeded by permanent teeth, namely two incisors, one canine and two *premolars* in each quadrant. Distal to these will develop three *permanent molars* which have no primary precursors; the first permanent molar erupts at age 6, the second at age 12 and the third (wisdom tooth) at age 17–21 years. The sharp points found on the posterior teeth are known as *cusps*.

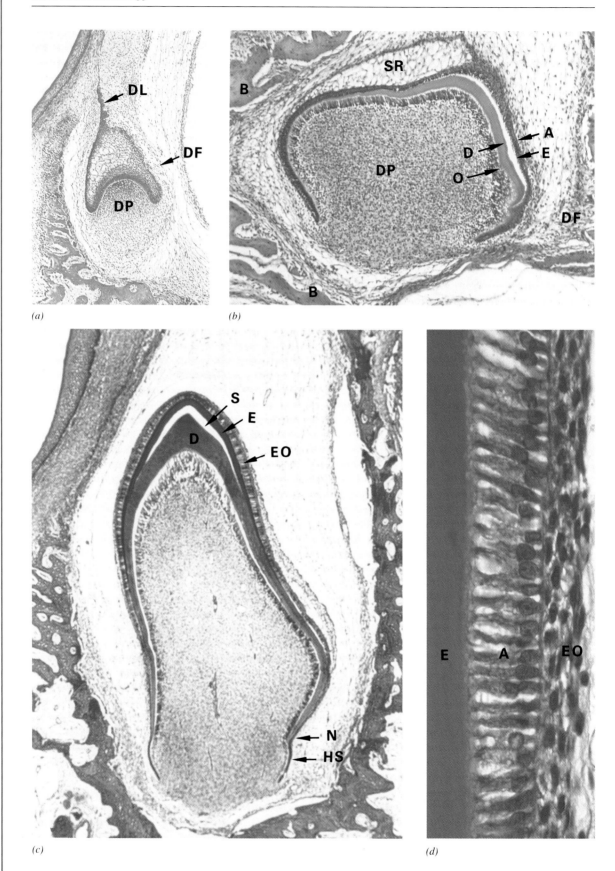

Fig. 13.5 **Tooth development** (*illustrations opposite*) **(a) H & E: cap stage** × 28 **(b) H & E: bell stage** × 96 **(c) H & E: onset of root development** × 45 **(d) H & E: ameloblasts** × 640

This series of micrographs illustrates the important stages of tooth development.

The tissues of the teeth are derived from two embryological sources. The enamel is of epithelial (ectodermal) origin, whilst the dentine, cementum, pulp and periodontal ligament are of mesenchymal (mesodermal) origin. The first evidence of tooth development in humans occurs at 6 weeks of fetal life with the proliferation of a horseshoe-shaped epithelial ridge from the basal layer of the primitive oral epithelium into the underlying mesoderm in the position of the future jaws; this is known as the *dental lamina*. In each quadrant of the mouth, the lamina then develops four globular swellings which will become the *enamel organs* of the future deciduous central and lateral incisors, canines and first molar teeth. Subsequently, the dental lamina proliferates backwards in each arch, successively giving rise to the enamel organs of the future second deciduous molar and the three permanent molars. The permanent successors of the deciduous teeth will later develop from enamel organs which bud off from the inner aspect of the enamel organs of their deciduous predecessors.

The primitive mesenchyme immediately subjacent to the developing enamel organ proliferates to form a cellular mass, the *dental papilla* **DP**. At the same time, the enamel organ becomes progressively cap-shaped, as seen in micrograph (a), enveloping the dental papilla. During the cap stage, the cells lining the concave face of the enamel organ in contact with the dental papilla begin to differentiate into tall columnar cells, *ameloblasts*, which will be responsible for the production of enamel. This, in turn, induces the differentiation of a layer of columnar *odontoblasts*, the future dentine-producing cells, in the apical region of the dental papilla. The interface between the differentiating ameloblast and odontoblast layers marks the position and shape of the future junction between enamel and dentine.

As the enamel organ develops further, it assumes a characteristic bell shape as seen in micrograph (b), the free edge of the 'bell' proliferating so as to determine the eventual shape of the tooth crown.

Meanwhile, the cells of the main bulk of the enamel organ become large and star-shaped, forming the *stellate reticulum* **SR**, the extracellular matrix of which is rich in glycosaminoglycans. Between the stellate reticulum and ameloblast layer, two or three layers of flattened cells form the *stratum intermedium*, whilst the outer surface of the enamel organ consists of a simple cuboidal epithelium called the *external enamel epithelium*. By the cap stage of development, the dental lamina **DL** connecting the enamel organ with the oral mucosa has become fragmented and, around the whole developing bud, a condensation of mesenchyme forms the *dental follicle* **DF** which will eventually become the periodontal ligament.

As ameloblasts and odontoblasts differentiate at the tip of the crown, a layer of dentine matrix is progressively laid down between the ameloblast and odontoblast layers. As the odontoblasts retreat, each leaves a long cytoplasmic extension, the *odontoblastic process*, embedded within the dentine matrix, thereby forming the dentine tubules. Dentine matrix has a similar biochemical composition to that of bone and undergoes calcification in a similar fashion. Deposition of dentine induces the production of enamel by the adjacent ameloblasts. Each retreating ameloblast lays down a column of enamel

matrix, which then undergoes mineralisation resulting in the formation of a dense prismatic structure as described below. With the deposition of dentine and enamel, the overlying stellate reticulum atrophies and the enamel organ is much reduced in thickness. These changes are well demonstrated in micrograph (b). A thin layer of dentine **D** has been laid down by the underlying odontoblastic layer **O** of the highly cellular dental papilla **DP**. The ameloblastic layer **A** is about to lay down enamel in the area of the artefactual space **E**; note that in this area, the stellate reticulum has disappeared. Note also the surrounding dental follicle **DF** and early formation of cancellous bone **B**.

By the time that dentine and enamel formation is well underway at the incisal edge or tips of the cusps (as the case may be), the enamel organ will have fully outlined the shape of the whole tooth crown. This is the case in micrograph (c), the neck of the tooth **N** marking the junction of crown and root. A thin, densely stained layer of poorly mineralised enamel **E** can be seen covered at its external surface by the now much thinner enamel organ **EO**. The unstained space **S** between this and the underlying dentine **D** represents fully mineralised enamel laid down earlier but dissolved away during tissue preparation. Although enamel production is confined to the crown, the rim of the 'bell' of the enamel organ nevertheless continues to proliferate, inducing dentine formation and thereby determining the shape of the tooth root. This part of the enamel organ, known as the *epithelial sheath of Hertwig* **HS** disintegrates once the outline of the root is completed. The cementum which later forms on the root surface is derived from the dental follicle. As the dentine of the crown and root are progressively laid down, the dental papilla shrinks and eventually becomes the dental pulp contained within the pulp chamber and root canals.

Growth of the tooth root is one of the principal mechanisms of tooth eruption, and root formation is not completed until some time after the crown has fully erupted into the oral cavity.

Micrograph (d) illustrates the characteristic appearance of ameloblasts. Active ameloblasts **A** are tall columnar epithelial cells which form a single layer apposed to the forming surface of the enamel **E**. Each ameloblast elaborates a column of organic enamel matrix which undergoes progressive mineralisation by the deposition of calcium phosphate mainly in the form of hydroxyapatite crystals. Fully formed enamel contains less than 1% organic material and is the hardest and most dense tissue in the body.

Mature enamel consists of highly calcified *enamel prisms* separated by *interprismatic enamel* consisting of similar crystals orientated in a different direction. Each prism extends from the dentino-enamel junction to the enamel surface. The prisms are made up of groups of long, thin, parallel crystallites of hydroxyapatite covered by a surface layer of organic material.

Underlying the ameloblast layer are several layers of cells, also of epithelial origin, which constitute the remainder of the enamel organ **EO**. As enamel formation progresses, the enamel organ becomes much reduced in thickness compared with earlier stages of its development. At tooth eruption, the enamel organ, including the ameloblasts, degenerates leaving the enamel exposed to the hostile oral environment, completely incapable of regeneration.

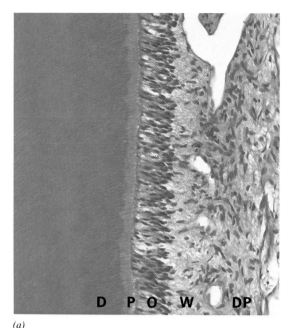

(a)

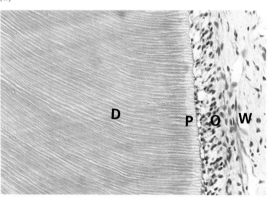

(b)

Fig. 13.6 Odontoblasts and dentine
Decalcified sections: (a) H & E × 200 (b) H & E × 128

Dentine, the dense calcified tissue which forms the bulk of the tooth, is broadly similar to bone in composition but is more highly mineralised and thus much harder than bone. The cells responsible for dentine formation, the *odontoblasts*, differentiate as a single layer of tall columnar cells on the surface of the dental papilla apposed to the *ameloblast* layer of the enamel organ. The odontoblasts initiate tooth formation by deposition of organic dentine matrix between the odontoblastic and ameloblastic layers; calcification of this dentine matrix then induces enamel formation by ameloblasts (see Fig. 13.5). Odontoblasts continue to produce dentine which subsequently calcifies. Unlike ameloblasts, each odontoblast leaves behind a slender cytoplasmic extension, the odontoblastic process, within a fine dentine tubule. When dentine formation is complete, the dentine is thus pervaded by parallel *odontoblastic processes* radiating from the odontoblast layer on the dentinal surface of the reduced dental papilla which now constitutes the dental pulp. After tooth formation is complete, a small amount of less organised *secondary dentine* continues to be laid down, resulting in the progressive obliteration of the pulp cavity with advancing age.

These micrographs illustrate active odontoblasts **O** forming a pseudostratified layer of columnar cells at the dentine surface. Parallel dentine tubules containing odontoblastic processes extend through a narrow pale-stained zone of uncalcified dentine matrix called *predentine* **P** into the mature dentine **D**; the dentine tubules are best seen in micrograph (b). Underlying the odontoblastic layer, a relatively acellular layer, called the *cell free zone of Weil* **W**, gives way to the highly cellular dental pulp **DP**.

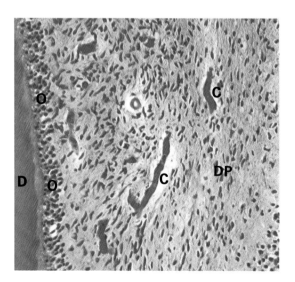

Fig. 13.7 Dental pulp
Decalcified section: H & E × 198

The dental pulp **DP** consists of a delicate supporting/connective tissue resembling primitive mesenchyme (see Fig. 4.3); it contains numerous stellate fibroblasts, reticulin fibres, fine collagen fibres and plentiful ground substance. The pulp contains a rich network of thin-walled capillaries **C** supplied by arterioles which enter the pulp canal from the periodontal membrane, usually via one foramen at each root apex. The pulp is also richly innervated by a plexus of myelinated nerve fibres from which fine, non-myelinated branches extend into the odontoblastic layer. Despite the acute sensitivity of dentine, nerve fibres are rarely demonstrable and the mechanism of sensory reception is unknown; it has been suggested that the odontoblastic processes may act as sensory receptors. Odontoblasts **O** and the edge of the dentine **D** can also be identified.

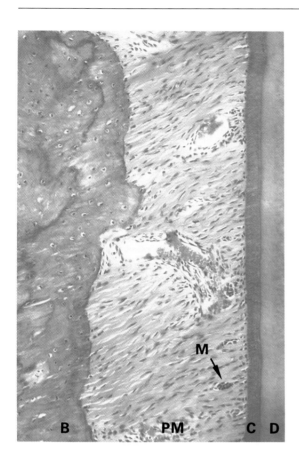

The periodontal membrane **PM** forms a thin fibrous
attachment between the tooth root and the alveolar bone.
The dentine **D**, comprising the root, is covered by a thin
layer of cementum **C** which is elaborated by cells called
cementocytes lying on the surface of the cementum.
Cementum consists of a dense, calcified organic material
similar to the matrix of bone, and is generally acellular.
Towards the root apex, the cementum layer becomes
progressively thicker and irregular and cementocytes are
often entrapped in lacunae within the cementum.

The periodontal membrane consists of dense
collagenous tissue. The collagen fibres, known as
Sharpey's fibres, run obliquely downwards from their
attachment in the alveolar bone **B** to their anchorage in
the cementum at a more apical position on the root
surface. The periodontal membrane thus acts as a sling for
the tooth within its socket, permitting slight movements
which cushion the impact of chewing. The points of
attachment of the collagen fibres in both cementum
and bone are in a constant state of reorganisation to
accommodate changing functional stresses upon the teeth.
Osteoclastic resorption is often seen at one aspect of a
tooth socket and complementary osteoblastic deposition
at the opposite side, thus indicating bodily movement of
the tooth through the bone; this is the mechanism which
permits tooth movement during orthodontic treatment.

The periodontal membrane is richly supplied by blood
vessels and nerves from the surrounding alveolar bone,
the apical region and the gingiva. Small clumps of
epithelial cells are often found scattered throughout the
periodontal membrane; these cells are remnants of
Hertwig's sheath (see Fig. 13.5) and are known as
epithelial rests of Malassez **M**.

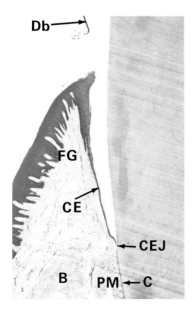

Fig. 13.9 Gingival attachment **Decalcified section: H & E × 320**

This micrograph shows the relationship of the gingiva (gum) to the neck of the
tooth. During tissue preparation the enamel has been completely dissolved
from the surface of the crown, but the extent of the outer surface of the enamel
can be visualised by shreds of remaining organic debris **Db** which had been
adherent to the tooth surface.

The gingiva may be divided into the *attached gingiva*, which provides a
protective covering to the upper alveolar bone **B**, and the *free gingiva* **FG**,
which forms a cuff around the enamel at the neck of the tooth. Between the
enamel and the free gingiva is a potential space, the *gingival crevice*, which
extends from the tip of the free gingiva to the cemento-enamel junction **CEJ**.

The thick stratified squamous epithelium, which constitutes the oral aspect
of the gingiva, undergoes abrupt transition at the tip of the free gingiva to form
a thin layer of epithelial cells, tapering to only two or three cells thick at the
base of the gingival crevice. This *crevicular epithelium* **CE** is easily breached
by pathogenic organisms, and the underlying supporting tissue is thus
frequently infiltrated by lymphocytes and plasma cells.

Collagen fibres of the periodontal membrane **PM** radiate from the cementum
C near the cemento-enamel junction into the dense supporting tissue of the free
gingiva; these fibres, together with circular fibres surrounding the neck of the
tooth, maintain the role of the gingiva as a protective cuff.

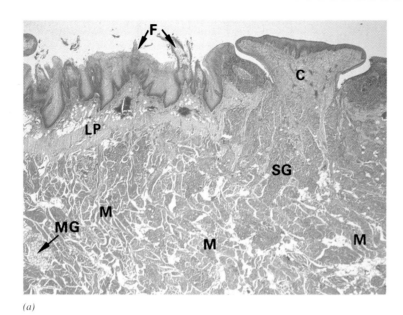

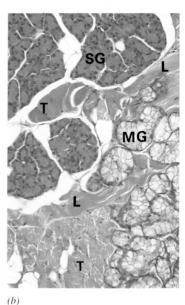

(a) *(b)*

Fig. 13.10 Tongue (a) H & E × 6 (b) H & E × 100

The tongue is a muscular organ covered by oral mucosa which is specialised for manipulating food, general sensory reception and the special sensory function of taste.

A V-shaped groove, the *sulcus terminalis*, demarcates the anterior two-thirds of the tongue from the posterior one-third. The mucosa of the anterior two-thirds is formed into papillae of three types. The most numerous, the *filiform papillae*, appear as short 'bristles' macroscopically. Among them are scattered the small red globular *fungiform papillae*. Six to 14 large *circumvallate papillae* form a row immediately anterior to the sulcus terminalis and these papillae contain most of the taste buds (see Figs 13.12 and 21.1); a circumvallate papilla **C** and numerous filiform papillae **F** are seen in micrograph (a). *Foliate papillae*, which are rudimentary in humans, are found in some animal species.

The body of the tongue consists of a mass of interlacing bundles of skeletal muscle fibres **M** which permit an extensive range of tongue movements. The mucous membrane covering the tongue is firmly bound to the underlying muscle by a dense, collagenous lamina propria **LP**, which is continuous with the epimysium of the tongue muscle.

Numerous small serous and mucous accessory salivary glands are scattered throughout the muscle and lamina propria of the tongue and are seen at higher magnification in micrograph (b); in these preparations the serous glands **SG** are stained strongly, whereas the mucous glands **MG** are poorly stained. Note bundles of skeletal muscle cut in both transverse **T** and longitudinal **L** sections.

Fig. 13.11 Filiform and fungiform papillae H & E × 30

This micrograph illustrates several filiform papillae **FL** and a fungiform papilla **Fg**. Filiform papillae are the most numerous type and consist of a dense supporting tissue core and a heavily keratinised surface projection. Fungiform papillae have a thin non-keratinised epithelium and a richly vascularised supporting tissue core, giving them a red appearance macroscopically amongst the much more numerous, whitish filiform papillae.

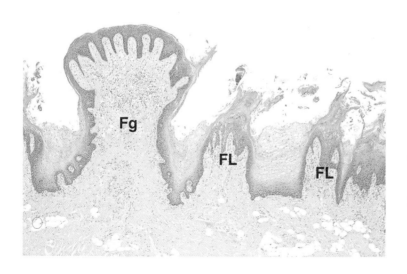

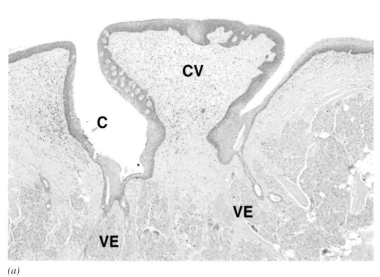

(a)

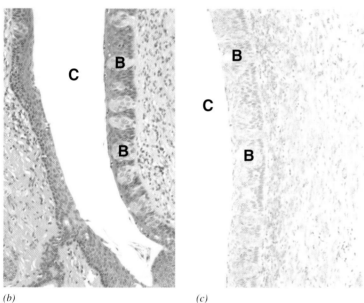

(b)   (c)

Fig. 13.12 **Circumvallate papillae (a) H & E × 15 (b) H & E × 100 (c) Immunoperoxidase × 100**

Circumvallate papillae **CV** are the largest and least common type of papillae on the tongue. They are set into the tongue surface and encircled by a deep cleft **C**. Aggregations of serous glands, called *von Ebner's glands* **VE**, open into the base of the circumvallate clefts (micrograph a), secreting a watery fluid which dissolves food constituents, thus facilitating taste reception. The stratified epithelium lining the papillary wall of the cleft contains numerous taste buds **B** as shown in micrograph (b) (see also Fig. 21.1).

Micrograph (c) is stained by the immunoperoxidase method for the enzyme neurone-specific enolase. This demonstrates the neural nature of the taste buds **B** and the meshwork of fine axons (stained brown) in the lamina propria underlying the taste buds which subserve taste sensation.

Fig. 13.13 **Lingual tonsil** **H & E × 15**

Apart from being of different embryological origin and having different sensory innervation to the anterior two thirds, the posterior one-third of the tongue has a distinctly different mucosal surface. The posterior surface has a relatively smooth stratified squamous epithelium **E** under which lies masses of lymphoid tissue **L** containing typical lymphoid follicles **F**. This mass of lymphoid tissue is known as the *lingual tonsil* and, with the palatine tonsils and adenoids, completes a ring of lymphoid tissue, *Waldeyer's ring*, guarding the entrance to the gastrointestinal and respiratory tracts. Like the palatine tonsils (see Fig. 11.19), the lingual lymphoid aggregations are penetrated by epithelial crypts **C** which function in a similar manner to those of the palatine tonsils. Some of the epithelial crypts in this micrograph do not appear to be connected to the surface, but this is due to the plane of section.

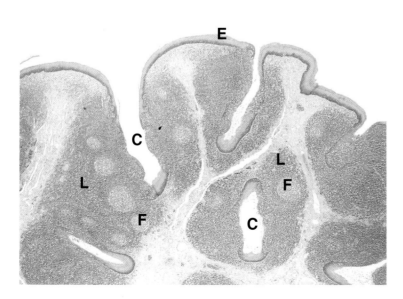

ORGAN SYSTEMS

Salivary glands

Saliva is produced by three pairs of major salivary glands, the ***parotid, submandibular*** and ***sublingual glands,*** and numerous minor ***accessory glands*** scattered throughout the oral mucosa. The minor salivary glands secrete continuously and are in general under local control, whereas the major glands mainly secrete in response to parasympathetic activity which is induced by physical, chemical and psychological stimuli. Daily saliva production in humans is 600–1500 ml.

Saliva is a hypotonic watery secretion containing variable amounts of mucus, enzymes (principally ***amylase*** and the antibacterial enzyme ***lysozyme***), antibodies and inorganic ions. Two types of secretory cells are found in the salivary glands: ***serous cells*** and ***mucous cells***. The parotid glands consist almost exclusively of serous cells and produce a thin watery secretion rich in enzymes and antibodies. The sublingual glands have predominantly mucous secretory cells and produce a viscid secretion. The submandibular glands contain both serous and mucous secretory cells and produce a secretion of intermediate consistency. The overall composition of saliva varies according to the degree of activity of each of the major gland types.

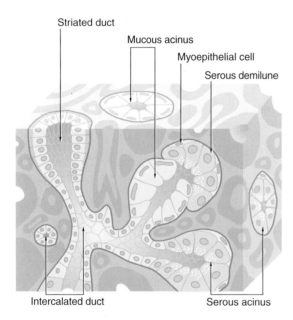

Striated duct
Mucous acinus
Myoepithelial cell
Serous demilune

Intercalated duct
Serous acinus

Fig. 13.14 Salivary secretory unit

The salivary secretory unit consists of a terminal branched tubulo-acinar structure composed exclusively of either serous or mucous secretory cells or a mixture of both types. In mixed secretory units where mucous cells predominate, serous cells often form semilunar caps called ***serous demilunes*** surrounding the terminal part of the mucous acini. Myoepithelial cells embrace the secretory units, their contraction helping to expel the secretory product.

The terminal secretory units merge to form small ***intercalated ducts*** which are also lined by secretory cells. They drain into larger ducts called ***striated ducts***, so named because of their striated appearance by light microscopy. The striations result from the presence of numerous interdigitations of the basal cytoplasmic processes of adjacent columnar lining cells.

The serous cells secrete a fluid isotonic with plasma. In the striated ducts ions are reabsorbed and secreted to produce hypotonic saliva containing less Na^+ and Cl^- and more K^+ and HCO_3^- than plasma. The mitochondria, which pack the basal processes, provide the energy for ion transport.

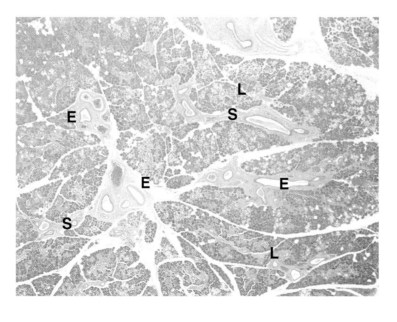

Fig. 13.15 Parotid gland
H & E × 15

The general architecture of the major salivary glands follows the pattern shown in this micrograph of the parotid gland. The gland is divided into numerous lobules **L**, each containing many secretory units. Supporting tissue septa **S** radiate between the lobules from an outer capsule and convey blood vessels, nerves and large excretory ducts **E**. The parotid gland consists mainly of serous secretory units which are darkly stained in this H & E preparation.

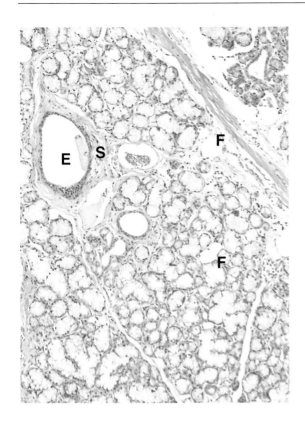

Fig. 13.16 Sublingual gland H & E × 75

Mucous acini predominate in the sublingual glands making them stain very poorly with H & E, in contrast to the serous units shown in the parotid in Figure 13.15. A large excretory duct **E**, lined by a stratified cuboidal epithelium, is also present in the fibrous tissue septum **S**. The duct is accompanied by blood vessels and nerves. As these ducts merge to form the major excretory duct, the epithelium gradually transforms into stratified squamous epithelium.

Note also that the gland contains occasional adipocytes **F**, a feature found in older individuals. The proportion of fat in the gland generally increases with increasing age.

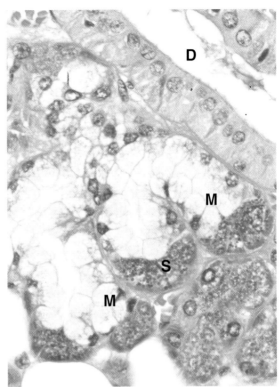

Fig. 13.17 Submandibular gland H & E × 450

The submandibular gland consists of a mixture of serous and mucous secretory units which are often found in the form of mixed seromucous secretory units as shown here. However, both pure serous and pure mucous secretory units are also found in the submandibular gland. The mixed secretory units consist of mucous acini **M** with serous demilunes **S**. In H & E stained preparations, *mucigen* granules within the mucous acini are poorly stained, whereas the enzyme-containing (*zymogen*) granules of serous acini are strongly stained. The nuclei of mucous cells are characteristically condensed and flattened against the basement membrane, whereas the nuclei of serous cells are rounded with dispersed chromatin and usually occupy a more central position within the cell.

Also running across the corner of the micrograph is a striated duct **D** cut in longitudinal section.

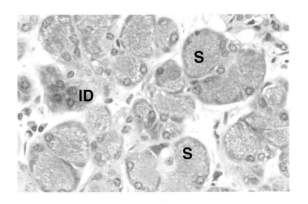

Fig. 13.18 Intercalated duct H & E × 300

This micrograph of serous secretory units is taken from the parotid gland. A small intercalated duct **ID** with several acini draining into it can be identified. Intercalated ducts have a lining of cuboidal secretory cells.

At this magnification, the serous secretory cells **S** have plentiful strongly stained apical cytoplasmic granules. The nucleus is pushed to the base of the cell. Adjacent to the nucleus, in EM sections (not illustrated), a large Golgi apparatus, prominent rough endoplasmic reticulum and mitochodria are found in common with other protein-secreting cells (see Fig. 15.15 of a pancreatic secretory cell, which is very similar ultrastructurally).

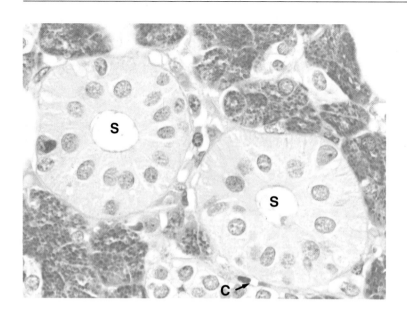

Fig. 13.19 Striated ducts
H & E × 600

The striated ducts **S** are lined by tall columnar cells with large nuclei located towards the apex of the cell. The basal cytoplasm appears striated, reflecting the presence of basal interdigitations of cytoplasmic processes of adjacent cells and associated columns of mitochondria. This feature greatly extends the area of membrane available for exchange of water and ions in a similar fashion to the proximal convoluted tubule of the kidney (see Fig 16.15). The duct epithelium also secretes lysozyme and IgA. In predominantly serous salivary glands, the striated ducts are larger than in predominantly mucous glands, a feature associated with the role of the striated duct in modifying isotonic basic saliva to produce hypotonic saliva. The sparse supporting tissue between the secretory acini contains a rich network of capillaries **C**.

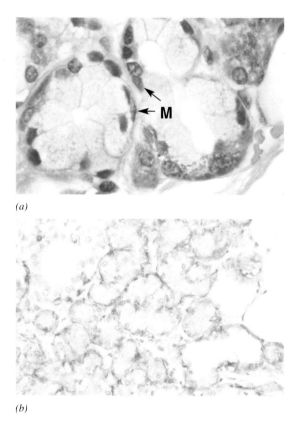

(a)

(b)

Fig. 13.20 Mucous acinus
(a) H & E × 300 (b) Immunoperoxidase × 200

Both serous and mucous acini are embraced by the processes of contractile cells called *myoepithelial cells* which, on contraction, force secretion from the acinar lumen into the duct system. Myoepithelial cells are located between the basal plasma membranes of secretory cells and the basement membrane. These cells are flattened and have long processes which extend around the secretory acinus, but in section they can only be recognised by their large flattened nuclei lying within the basement membrane surrounding the acinus. Micrograph (a) shows the typical appearance of myoepithelial cells **M** embracing mucous acini.

In micrograph (b), a similar section has been stained using the immunoperoxidase technique with an antibody specific for actin, an intermediate filament characteristic of muscle cells but not usually found in epithelial cells. The myoepithelial cells are stained brown, confirming the presence of cytoplasmic actin which is not seen in the luminal epithelial cells. However, these cells also show characteristics of epithelial differentiation, including cytoplasmic cytokeratin intermediate filaments. This technique demonstrates the large numbers of myoepithelial cells surrounding each of the secretory acini.

14. Gastrointestinal tract

Introduction

The gastrointestinal system is primarily involved in breaking down food for absorption into the body. This process occurs in five main phases: ingestion, fragmentation, digestion, absorption and elimination of waste products. The gastrointestinal system is essentially a muscular tube lined by a mucous membrane which exhibits regional variations reflecting the changing functions of the system from mouth to anus.

Ingestion and initial fragmentation of food occur in the oral cavity, resulting in the formation of a bolus of food; this is then conveyed to the *oesophagus* by the action of the tongue and pharyngeal muscles during swallowing (*deglutition*). Fragmentation and swallowing are facilitated by the secretion of saliva from three pairs of major *salivary glands* and numerous *minor salivary glands* (see Ch. 13).

The oesophagus conducts food from the oral cavity to the *stomach* where fragmentation is completed and digestion initiated. Digestion is the process by which food is enzymatically broken down into molecules which are small enough to be absorbed into the circulation; e.g. ingested proteins are first reduced to polypeptides and then further degraded to small peptides and amino acids which can then be absorbed. Initial digestion, accompanied by intense muscular action of the stomach wall, reduces the stomach contents to a semi-digested liquid called *chyme*. Chyme is squirted through a muscular sphincter, the *pylorus*, into the *duodenum*, the short first part of the *small intestine*. Digestive enzymes from a large exocrine gland, the *pancreas*, enter the duodenum together with bile from the liver via the *common bile duct*. Bile contains excretory products of liver metabolism, some of which act as emulsifying agents necessary for fat digestion. The duodenal contents pass onwards along the rest of the small intestine where the process of digestion is completed and the main absorptive phase occurs. The middle segment of the small intestine is called the *jejunum* and the distal segment the *ileum*. There is no distinct anatomical boundary between these two parts of the small bowel.

The liquid residue from the small intestine passes through a valve, the *ileocaecal valve*, into the *large intestine*. Here, water is absorbed from the liquid residue which becomes progressively more solid as it passes towards the anus. The capacious first part of the large intestine is called the *caecum*, from which projects a blind-ended sac, the *appendix*. The next part of the large intestine, the *colon*, is divided anatomically into *ascending*, *transverse*, *descending* and *sigmoid* segments, although histologically the segments are indistinguishable from one another. The terminal portion of the large intestine, the *rectum*, is a holding chamber for faeces prior to defaecation via the *anal canal*.

Food is propelled along the gastrointestinal tract by two main mechanisms: voluntary muscular action in the oral cavity, pharynx and upper third of the oesophagus is succeeded by involuntary waves of smooth muscle contraction called *peristalsis*. Peristalsis and the secretory activity of the entire gastrointestinal system are modulated by the autonomic nervous system and a variety of hormones, some of which are secreted by neuroendocrine cells located within the gastrointestinal tract itself. These cells constitute a diffuse neuro-endocrine system, with cells producing a variety of locally acting hormones found scattered along the whole length of the tract (see also Ch. 17). Autonomic regulation of certain glandular secretions and the smooth muscle of the gut and its blood vessels is mediated by the enteric nervous system, comprising postganglionic sympathetic fibres and ganglia and postganglionic fibres of the parasympathetic nervous system supplied by the vagus nerve.

Because of its continuity with the external environment, the gastrointestinal system is a potential portal of entry for pathogenic organisms. Thus the system incorporates a number of defence mechanisms, which include prominent aggregations of lymphoid tissue, known as the *gut-associated lymphoid system (GALT)*, distributed throughout the tract. GALT is part of MALT (see Ch. 11).

ORGAN SYSTEMS

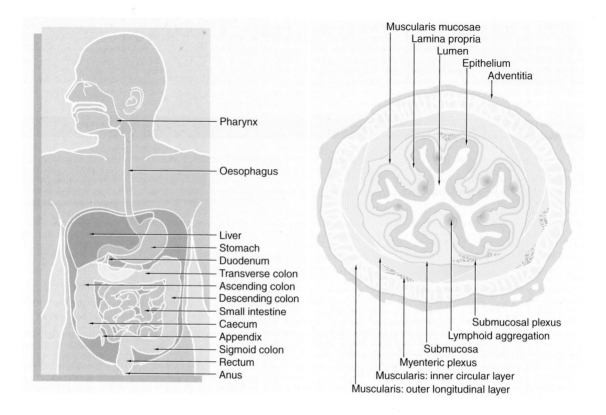

Labels (left diagram): Pharynx; Oesophagus; Liver; Stomach; Duodenum; Transverse colon; Ascending colon; Descending colon; Small intestine; Caecum; Appendix; Sigmoid colon; Rectum; Anus

Labels (right diagram): Muscularis mucosae; Lamina propria; Lumen; Epithelium; Adventitia; Submucosal plexus; Lymphoid aggregation; Submucosa; Myenteric plexus; Muscularis: inner circular layer; Muscularis: outer longitudinal layer

Fig. 14.1 Structure of the gastrointestinal tract

The structure of the gastrointestinal tract conforms to a general plan which is clearly evident from the oesophagus to the anus. The tract is essentially a muscular tube lined by a mucous membrane. The arrangement of the major muscular component remains relatively constant throughout the tract, whereas the mucosa shows marked variations in the different regions of the tract.

The gastrointestinal tract has four distinct functional layers: *mucosa, submucosa, muscularis propria* and *adventitia*.

- **Mucosa.** The mucosa is made up of three components: the *epithelium* a supporting *lamina propria* and a thin smooth muscle layer, the *muscularis mucosae*, which produces local movement and folding of the mucosa. At four points along the tract the mucosa undergoes abrupt transition from one form to another: the gastro-oesophageal junction, the gastroduodenal junction, the ileocaecal junction and the recto-anal junction.
- **Submucosa.** This layer of loose collagenous tissue supports the mucosa and contains the larger blood vessels, lymphatics and nerves.
- **Muscularis propria.** The muscular wall proper consists of smooth muscle which is usually arranged as an inner circular layer and an outer longitudinal layer. In the stomach only, there is an inner oblique layer of muscle. The action of the two layers, at right angles to one another, is the basis of peristaltic contraction.
- **Adventitia.** This outer layer of loose supporting tissue conducts the major vessels and nerves; in obese individuals it contains a large amount of adipose tissue. Where the gut lies within the abdominal cavity (peritoneal cavity), the adventitia is referred to as the *serosa (visceral peritoneum)* and is lined by a simple squamous epithelium (*mesothelium*). Elsewhere, the adventitial layer merges with retroperitoneal tissues.

The smooth muscle of the bowel has its own inherent rhythmicity which is modulated by the autonomic nervous system, in particular the parasympathetic nervous system. As in other organs of the body, parasympathetic efferent fibres synapse with effector neurones in small ganglia located in or close to the organ involved. In the gastrointestinal tract, parasympathetic ganglia are concentrated in plexuses in the wall of the tract. In the submucosa, isolated or small clusters of parasympathetic ganglion cells give rise to postganglionic fibres which supply the mucosal glands and the smooth muscle of the muscularis mucosae; this submucosal plexus, sometimes referred to as *Meissner's plexus*, also contains postganglionic sympathetic fibres arising from the superior mesenteric plexus. Larger clusters of parasympathetic ganglion cells are found between the two layers of the muscularis propria, the postganglionic fibres mainly supplying the surrounding smooth muscle. This plexus is known as the *myenteric plexus* or *Auerbach's plexus*.

Glands are found throughout the tract at various levels in its wall. In some parts of the tract (i.e. stomach, small and large intestine), the mucosa is arranged into glands which have a variety of secretory functions. In the lower oesophagus and duodenum, glands penetrate the muscularis mucosae to lie in the submucosa. The pancreas and liver are large glands draining into the gastrointestinal lumen but lying entirely outside the tract wall (see Ch. 15).

Lymphoid tissue is distributed throughout the gastrointestinal tract both as diffusely scattered cells, particularly in the lamina propria, and as dense aggregates which may form follicles; in toto, this mass of lymphoid tissue constitutes the gut component (GALT) of the mucosa-associated lymphoid tissue (MALT) described in Chapter 11.

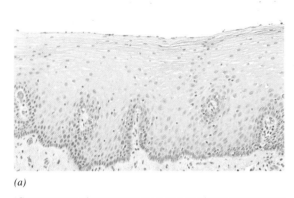

(a)

Fig. 14.2 **Basic mucosal forms in the gastrointestinal tract** H & E: (a) × 100 (b) × 100 (c) × 128 (d) × 128

There are four basic mucosal types found in the gastrointestinal tract, which can be classified according to their main function:

Protective. This type is found in the oral cavity, pharynx, oesophagus and anal canal. The surface epithelium is stratified squamous and may be keratinised in animals which have a coarse diet, e.g. rodents, herbivores.

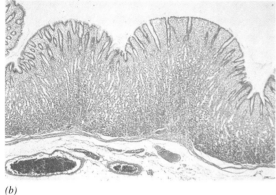

(b)

Secretory. This type occurs only in the stomach. The mucosa consists of long, closely packed tubular glands which are simple or branched depending on the region of the stomach.

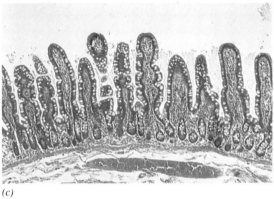

(c)

Absorptive. This mucosal form is typical of the entire small intestine. The mucosa is arranged into finger-like projections called villi (to increase surface area) with intervening short glands called crypts. In the duodenum, some crypts extend through the muscularis mucosae to form submucosal mucous glands called ***Brunner's glands***. This is the major histological feature which differentiates the duodenum from the jejunum and ileum.

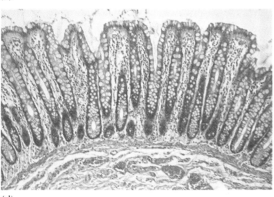

(d)

Absorptive/protective. This form lines the whole of the large intestine. The mucosa is arranged into closely packed, straight tubular glands consisting of cells specialised for water absorption and mucus-secreting goblet cells which lubricate the passage of faeces.

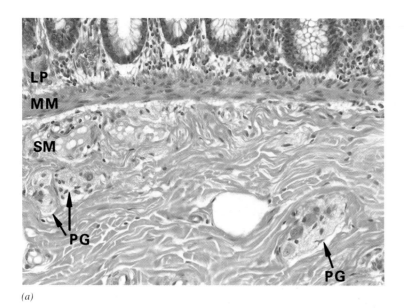

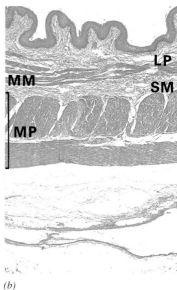

(a)

(b)

Fig. 14.3 Components of the wall of the gastrointestinal tract (a) H & E × 480 (b) H & E × 28 (c) H & E × 320

This series of micrographs illustrates the layers of the wall of the tract deep to the surface epithelium.

Micrograph (a) illustrates the deep part of the large bowel mucosa, the muscularis mucosae **MM** clearly demarcating the delicate lamina propria **LP** from the more robust underlying submucosa **SM**; this arrangement is typical of the whole of the gastrointestinal tract.

The *lamina propria* consists of loose areolar tissue which appears highly cellular due to the presence of considerable numbers of lymphocytes and plasma cells. At intervals in the oesophagus, small and large bowel and appendix, prominent aggregates of lymphocytes with lymphoid follicles are present. There are also smaller numbers of eosinophils and histocytes (see Fig. 4.17) which deal with any microorganisms breaching the intestinal epithelium until a specific immune response can be mounted. In contrast, the lamina propria of the normal stomach contains few white blood cells. The lamina propria is also typically rich in blood and lymphatic capillaries necessary to support the secretory and absorptive functions of the mucosa.

The *muscularis mucosae* consists of several layers of smooth muscle fibres, those in the deeper layers oriented parallel to the luminal surface. The more superficial fibres are oriented at right angles to the surface and extend up into the lamina propria between the glands; in the case of the small intestine, the fibres extend up into the villi, as seen in Figure 14.25. The activity of the muscularis mucosae keeps the mucosal surface and glands in a constant state of gentle agitation, which expels secretions from the deep glandular crypts, prevents clogging and enhances contact between epithelium and luminal contents for absorption.

The *submucosa* consists of loose supporting tissue which binds the mucosa to the main bulk of the muscular wall. The submucosa contains the larger blood vessels and lymphatics as well as the nerves supplying the mucosa. Tiny parasympathetic ganglia **PG** are scattered throughout the submucosa, forming the *submucosal*

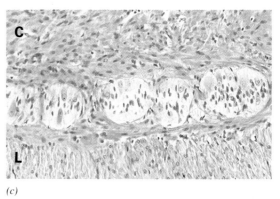

(c)

(Meissner's) plexus from which postganglionic fibres supply the muscularis mucosae.

The typical arrangement of the two layers of the muscular wall proper is seen in micrograph (b) which shows a longitudinal section of the oesophagus. The muscularis propria **MP** is made up of an outer longitudinal layer and a somewhat broader inner circular layer; there has been some artefactual separation of the layers making them easier to visualise. The submucosa **SM** is separated from the lamina propria **LP** by the muscularis mucosae **MM**. In the oesophagus, where the function of the mucosa is to protect against friction, the lamina propria is more collagenous than elsewhere and the muscularis mucosae is more prominent.

Micrograph (c) illustrates, at high magnification, the junction of outer longitudinal **L** and inner circular **C** layers of the muscularis propria in the large intestine; between the layers are clumps of parasympathetic ganglion cells of the *myenteric (Auerbach's) plexus*. The two layers of the muscularis propria undergo synchronised rhythmic contractions which pass in peristaltic waves down the tract, propelling the contents distally. Peristalsis is inherent in the smooth muscle itself but the level of activity is modulated by the autonomic nervous system, locally produced gastrointestinal tract hormones and other environmental factors. Parasympathetic activity enhances peristalsis whilst sympathetic activity slows gut motility.

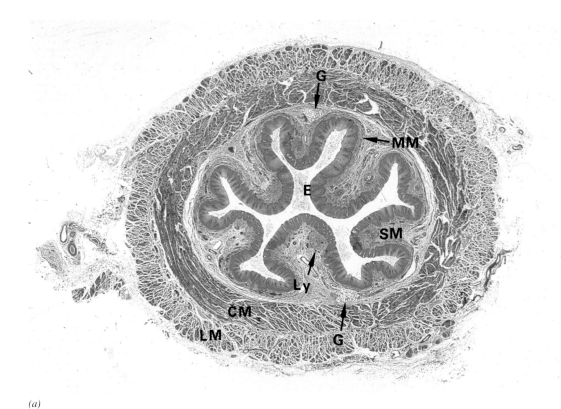

(a)

Fig. 14.4 **Oesophagus** (a) Masson's trichrome × 9 (b) Masson's trichrome × 320

The oesophagus is a strong muscular tube which conveys food from the oropharynx to the stomach. The initiation of swallowing is a voluntary act involving the skeletal musculature of the oropharynx which is then succeeded by a strong peristaltic reflex which conveys the bolus of food or fluid to the stomach. Food and fluid do not normally remain in the oesophagus for more than a few seconds and reflux and regurgitation are normally prevented by a physiological sphincter in the region of the gastro-oesophageal junction. Below the diaphragm, the oesophagus passes a centimetre or so into the abdominal cavity before joining the stomach at an acute angle. Sphincter control appears to involve four complementary factors: diaphragmatic contraction, greater intra-abdominal pressure than intragastric pressure being exerted upon the abdominal part of the oesophagus, unidirectional peristalsis and maintenance of correct anatomical arrangements of the structures.

Micrograph (a) shows the lower third of the oesophagus. In the relaxed state, the oesophageal mucosa is deeply folded, an arrangement which permits marked distension during the passage of a food bolus.

The lumen of the oesophagus is lined by a thick protective stratified squamous epithelium **E** (see Fig. 14.2). The underlying lamina propria is quite narrow and contains scattered lymphoid aggregates **Ly;** the underlying muscularis mucosae **MM** is barely visible at this magnification.

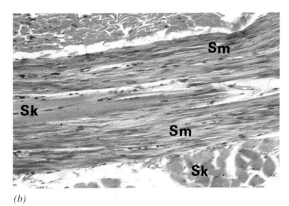

(b)

The submucosa **SM** is relatively loose with many elastic fibres, allowing for considerable distension during passage of a food bolus. The submucosa also contains small seromucous glands **G**, similar to salivary glands, which aid lubrication and are most prominent in the upper and lower thirds of the oesophagus.

The muscularis propria is thick, and inner circular **CM** and outer longitudinal **LM** layers of smooth muscle are clearly distinguishable. Since the first part of swallowing is under voluntary control, fasciculi of skeletal muscle predominate in the muscularis of the upper third of the oesophagus.

Micrograph (b) shows part of the muscularis propria of the upper oesophagus at high magnification in the area of transition from skeletal to smooth muscle fibres. A bundle of smooth muscle fibres **Sm** is seen, with two skeletal muscle fibres **Sk** in their midst. The collagen of the endomysial supporting tissue stains green with this method.

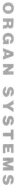

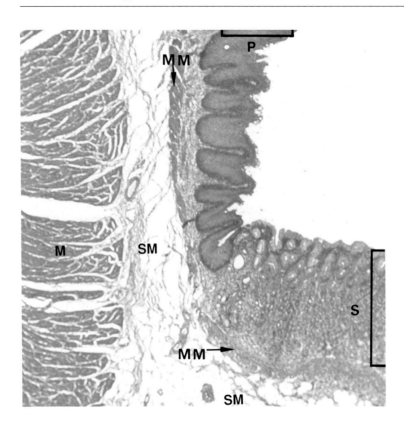

Fig. 14.5 Gastro-oesophageal junction H & E × 40

At the junction of the oesophagus with the stomach, the mucosa of the tract undergoes an abrupt transition from a protective stratified squamous epithelium **P** to a tightly packed glandular secretory mucosa **S**. The muscularis mucosae **MM** is continuous across the junction, although it is less easily seen in the stomach where it lies immediately beneath the base of the gastric glands. The underlying submucosa **SM** and muscularis propria **M** continue uninterrupted beneath the mucosal junction. The muscularis propria does not form a thick anatomical sphincter, but rather there is a physiological sphincter mechanism as described in Figure 14.4.

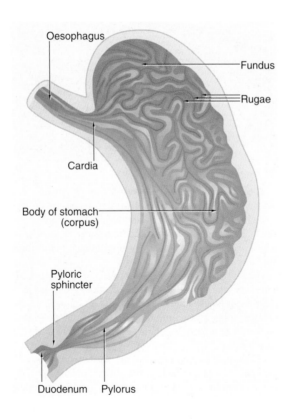

Fig. 14.6 Stomach

Food passes from the oesophagus into the stomach, a distensible organ, where it may be retained for 2 hours or more. In the stomach the food undergoes mechanical and chemical breakdown to form chyme. Solid foods are broken up by a strong muscular churning action, whilst chemical breakdown is produced by gastric juices secreted by the glands of the stomach mucosa. There is little absorption from the stomach, except for water, alcohol and some drugs. Once chyme formation is completed, the pyloric sphincter relaxes and allows the liquid chyme to be squirted into the duodenum.

In the non-distended state, the stomach mucosa is thrown into prominent longitudinal folds called *rugae* which permit great distension after eating. Anatomically the stomach is divided into four regions: the *cardia*, *fundus*, *body (corpus)* and *pylorus (pyloric antrum)*. The pylorus terminates in a strong muscular sphincter at the gastroduodenal junction.

The mucosa of the entire stomach has a tubular glandular form but there are three distinctly different histological zones:

- The cardia is a small area of predominantly mucus-secreting glands surrounding the entrance of the oesophagus (see Fig. 14.5).
- The mucosa of the fundus and the body forms the major histological region and consists of glands which secrete acid-peptic gastric juices as well as some protective mucus.
- The glands of the pylorus secrete mucus of two different types and associated endocrine cells secrete the hormone *gastrin*.

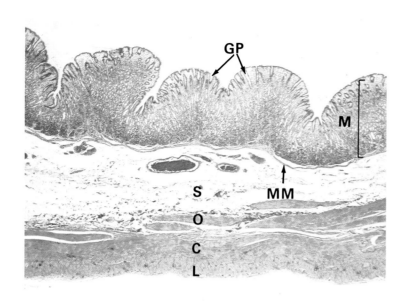

Fig. 14.7 **Body of the stomach** H & E × 12

This micrograph illustrates the body of the stomach in the non-distended state. The mucosa **M** is thrown into prominent folds or rugae and consists of *gastric glands* which extend from the level of the muscularis mucosae **MM** to open into the stomach lumen via *gastric pits* or *foveoli* **GP**.

The muscularis propria comprises the usual inner circular **C** and outer longitudinal **L** layers, but the inner circular layer is reinforced by a further inner oblique layer **O**. The submucosa **S** is relatively loose and distensible and contains the larger blood vessels. The serosal layer which covers the peritoneal surface is thin and barely visible at this magnification.

Fig. 14.8 **Body of stomach: structure of glands**

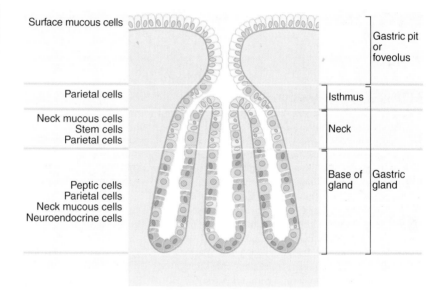

The mucosa of the fundus and body of the stomach consists of straight tubular glands which synthesise and secrete gastric juice. The gastric pits occupy about one-quarter of the thickness of the gastric mucosa and each has between one and seven gastric glands opening into it. Gastric juice is a watery secretion containing *hydrochloric acid* (pH 0.9–1.5) and the digestive enzyme *pepsin* which hydrolyses proteins into polypeptide fragments. The stomach mucosa is protected from self-digestion by a thick surface covering of mucus, which is maintained at a higher pH than the gastric juice by the secretion of bicarbonate ions by the gastric surface mucous cells.

The gastric glands contain a mixed population of cells:

- *Surface mucous cells* cover the luminal surface of the stomach and line the gastric pits. The cytoplasmic mucigen granules which pack these cells are stained poorly by H & E. These cells have short surface microvilli and secrete protective bicarbonate ions directly into the deeper layers of the surface mucous coat.
- *Neck mucous cells* are squeezed between the parietal cells in the neck and base of the gastric glands. These cells have larger secretory granules and more polyribosomes than surface mucous cells.
- *Parietal* or *oxyntic cells* are distributed along the length of the glands but tend to be most numerous in the *isthmus* of the glands. These large rounded cells have an extensive eosinophilic (oxyntic) cytoplasm and a centrally located nucleus. Parietal cells secrete gastric acid as well as *intrinsic factor* which is necessary for the absorption of vitamin B_{12} in the terminal ileum.
- *Chief*, *peptic* or *zymogenic cells* are located towards the bases of the gastric glands. Peptic cells are recognised by their condensed, basally located nuclei and strongly basophilic granular cytoplasm, which reflects their large content of ribosomes. These are the pepsin-secreting cells.
- *Neuroendocrine cells*, part of the diffuse neuroendocrine system, are also found in the base of the gastric glands. They secrete serotonin and other hormones (see also Fig. 14.13).
- *Stem cells* are found mainly in the neck of the gastric glands. These undifferentiated cells divide continuously to replace worn out epithelial cells of all other types. The maturing cells then migrate up or down as appropriate. These cells are not easily identified in sections of normal gastric mucosa but become very prominent with plentiful mitotic figures after damage to the mucosa has occurred, e.g. after gastritis.

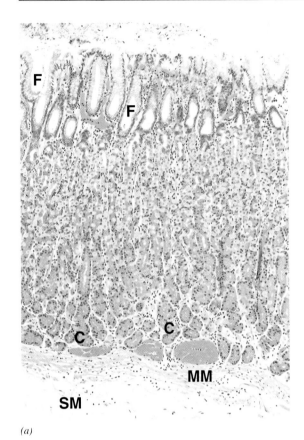

(a)

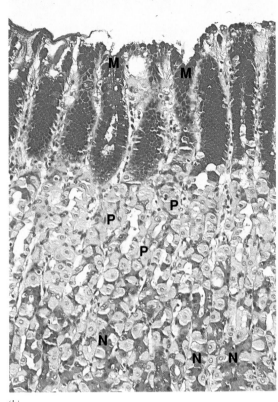

(b)

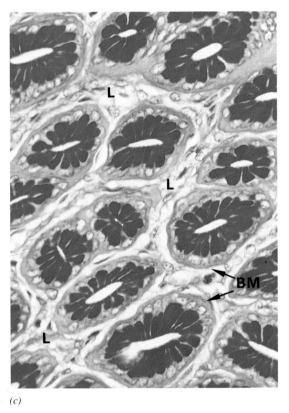

(c)

Fig. 14.9 **Gastric body mucosa**
(a) H & E × 75 (b) PAS/H & E × 150
(c) PAS/haematoxylin/orange G TS × 200

Micrograph (a) shows the full thickness of the gastric body mucosa and includes a small amount of submucosa **SM**. The gastric pits **F** lined by pale-stained surface mucous cells are easily identifiable. The isthmus and neck of the glands also appear pale due to the predominance of mucous neck cells and parietal cells. The base of the glands, where peptic (chief) cells **C** predominate, are stained darker in this H & E preparation. The glands extend down to the muscularis mucosae **MM**. Lymphoid follicles are not found in normal gastric mucosa.

A similar section stained by the PAS/H & E method (b) highlights the mucus-secreting cells of the gastric mucosa; mucus is PAS-positive because it is a polysaccharide. The stomach surface and gastric pits are lined by a single layer of tall columnar mucus-secreting cells **M** which are shed continuously and replaced by cells which migrate from the neck region of the gastric glands. The mucus-secreting cells of the stomach are not of the goblet form found in other parts of the body. The neck mucous cells **N**, which secrete a mucus of a slightly different chemical composition, are less intensely stained. Note that neck mucous cells are also found at the base of the gland. The mucus produced by these two types of mucous cells protects the epithelium from autodigestion.

The parietal cells **P** are recognised by their copious eosinophilic cytoplasm and central nucleus, which is often described as a 'fried egg appearance'.

In transverse section, as in micrograph (c), the tubular nature of the gastric pits is clearly evident. Between one and seven gastric glands may open into each gastric pit.

Note the loose vascular but scanty *lamina propria* **L** which supports the gastric pits and glands. The lightly PAS-positive basement membrane **BM** can be distinguished between the epithelium and lamina propria.

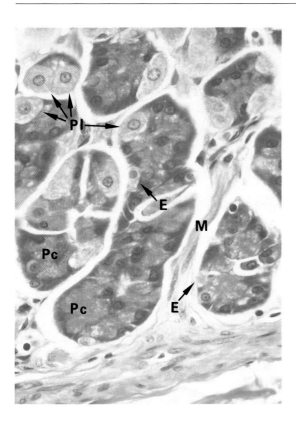

Fig. 14.10 Base of gastric gland H & E × 320

Peptic (chief) cells **Pc**, which synthesise and secrete the proteolytic enzyme *pepsin*, are the principal cell type in the basal third of the gastric glands, although some parietal cells **Pl** are also found at this level. Peptic cells have basally located nuclei and extensive granular cytoplasm packed with rough endoplasmic reticulum, the ribosomes accounting for the marked cytoplasmic basophilia. The inactive pepsin precursor, *pepsinogen*, is synthesised by the ribosomes and stored in numerous secretory granules located towards the luminal surface. Pepsinogen remains inactive until it reaches the lumen of the stomach where it is activated by the low pH of the gastric juices. Secretion of an inactive precursor molecule prevents autodigestion of the gastric glands.

The much larger parietal cells are round with large, centrally located nuclei and eosinophilic (pink-stained) cytoplasm due to the numerous mitochondria which are a feature of highly metabolically active cells.

The secretory activity of both parietal and peptic cells is controlled by the autonomic nervous system and the hormone *gastrin* secreted by neuroendocrine cells mainly located in the pyloric region. A variety of other neuroendocrine cells of the gastrointestinal endocrine system are also scattered in the gastric body mucosa and elsewhere in the gastrointestinal tract. Occasionally, the neuroendocrine cells **E** can be identified in sections fixed with chromium-containing fixatives, as in this example. Neuroendocrine cells in the pylorus are demonstrated in Figure 14.13c. Note a fine extension of the muscularis mucosae **M** extending up between the glands.

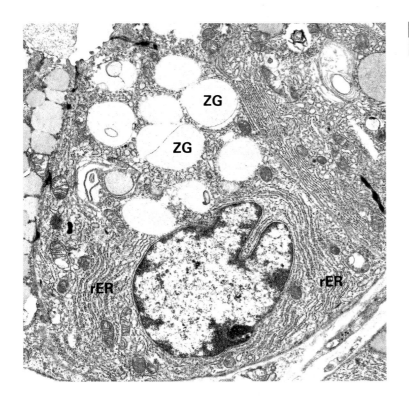

Fig. 14.11 Peptic cell – rat EM × 7200

This electron micrograph illustrates a peptic (chief) cell at the base of a gastric gland. The ultrastructural features of peptic cells are those of protein-secreting (zymogenic) cells in general; these features include an extensive rough endoplasmic reticulum **rER** and membrane-bound secretory vesicles (zymogen granules) **ZG** crowded in the apical cytoplasm, thus restricting the nucleus to the base of the cell. The extensive rough endoplasmic reticulum accounts for the intense basophilia of peptic cells in H & E sections.

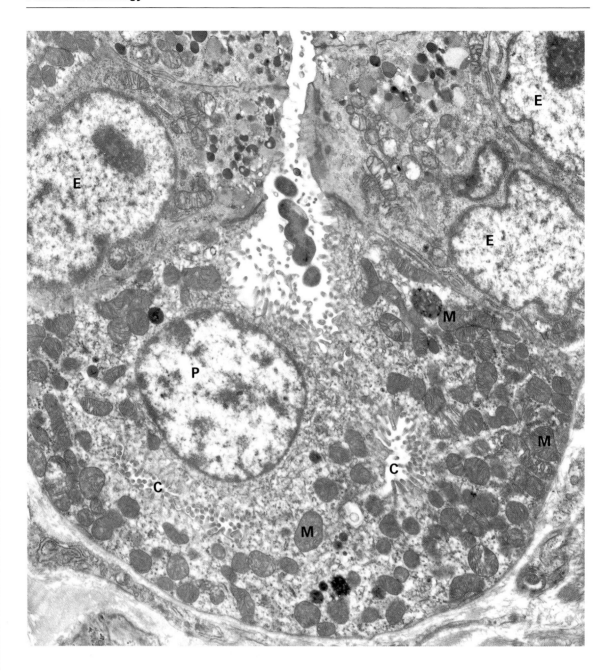

Fig. 14.12 Parietal cell – rat EM × 9600

This micrograph shows a parietal cell **P** within a gastric gland. The luminal plasma membrane of the parietal cell forms deep, branching canaliculi **C** which extend throughout the cytoplasm and between adjacent cells. Numerous short microvilli project into the lumina of the intracellular canaliculi, greatly increasing the surface area. The canaliculi are related to a tubulovesicular membrane complex (not well seen in this micrograph) and these two membrane systems secrete hydrochloric acid. In actively secreting cells, as in this case, the canalicular system is more prominent, whereas in resting parietal cells the canalicular system is inconspicuous and the tubulovesicular complex is prominent.

Secretion of hydrochloric acid begins with the production of carbonic acid which dissociates into hydrogen and bicarbonate ions. The hydrogen ions are actively transported into the lumen of the tubulovesicular

complex by the trans-membrane 'proton pump', a H^+/K^+ - ATPase. Chloride ions follow passively. The details of the next step are as yet unclear, but there may be fusion of the tubulovesicular complex vesicles with the canalicular system, so that the acid is now within the lumina of the canaliculi. This would explain the increase in the size of the canalicular system and decrease in the tubulovesicular complex that occurs in actively secreting cells. The end result is a hydrogen ion concentration in gastric juice about 1 million times that in plasma. This process is fueled by the many mitochondria **M** of the parietal cells.

Parietal cells also secrete a glycoprotein called *intrinsic factor* which is essential for the absorption of vitamin B_{12} in the terminal ileum. Also seen in this micrograph are several neuroendocrine cells **E**, recognised by their small electron-dense secretory granules (see Fig. 14.13).

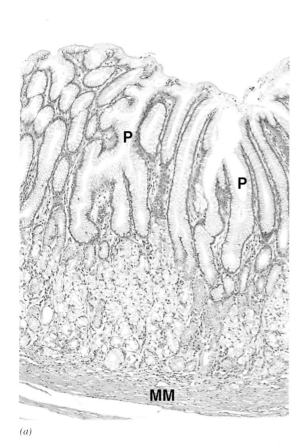

(a)

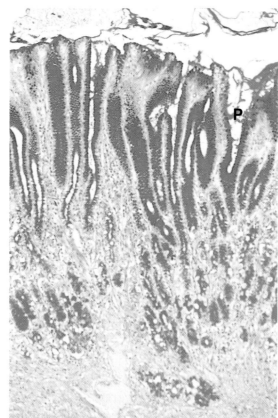

(b)

Fig. 14.13 Pyloric stomach
(a) H & E × 75 (b) PAS/H & E × 75
(c) Immunoperoxidase for gastrin × 150

In contrast to the simple tubular glands of the fundus and body, the pyloric glands are branched and coiled and the gastric pits **P** occupy about half the thickness of the pyloric mucosa (a). The glands are lined almost exclusively by mucus-secreting cells which are similar to the neck mucous cells of the gastric body and fundus. A small number of acid-secreting parietal cells are also scattered amongst the pyloric glands. Note the prominent muscularis mucosae **MM** separating the glands from underlying submucosa.

The PAS method which stains carbohydrates magenta has been used in specimen (b) to show better detail of the glandular structure. The glands open into deep, irregularly shaped pits **P**, giving the superficial mucosa a characteristic frond-like appearance in histological sections. The function of the mucus secreted by the pyloric glands is to protect the entrance to the duodenum from acid-pepsin attack and to lubricate the passage of chyme.

As in the body of the stomach, stem cells are found in the neck of the glands. Scattered amongst the pyloric mucous cells are neuroendocrine cells which secrete the peptide hormone *gastrin* and are thus called *G cells*. In micrograph (c) an antibody to gastrin has been used to highlight the G cells which contain gastrin in secretory granules in their cytoplasm. The G cells are stained brown **G** and are found mainly in the neck of the gland. Other neuroendocrine cells in the pylorus secrete products, including somatostatin, which is involved in the regulation of insulin, glucagon, gastrin and growth hormone secretion.

The presence of food in the stomach stimulates the secretion of gastrin into the bloodstream; gastrin then

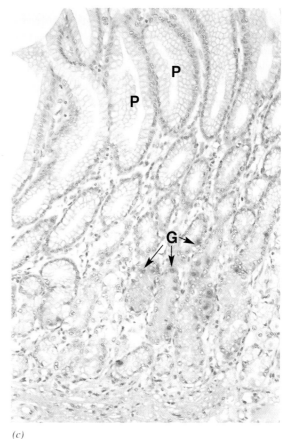

(c)

promotes secretion of pepsin and acid by the gastric glands of the fundus and body as well as enhancing gastric motility.

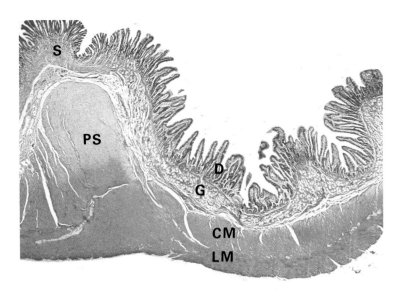

S

PS

D

G

CM

LM

Fig. 14.14 **Gastroduodenal junction – monkey** H & E × 12

The pyloric sphincter **PS** marks a sharp transition in the gastrointestinal mucosa from the glandular arrangement of the stomach **S** to the villous arrangement which characterises the duodenum **D** and the rest of the small intestine. In addition, the duodenum is distinguished from the rest of the small intestine by the presence of numerous mucus-secreting glands **G**. These glands, known as ***Brunner's glands***, are predominantly found in the submucosa but often extend into the mucosa.

The pyloric sphincter consists of a marked thickening of the circular layer of the muscularis at the gastroduodenal junction. Note the continuity of both the circular **CM** and longitudinal **LM** layers of the muscularis between the pylorus and duodenum. The inner oblique layer is found only in the body of the stomach.

Fig. 14.15 **Small intestine – monkey** *(illustrations opposite)* **(a) Duodenum H & E × 20 (b) Ileum H & E × 16**

The duodenum, seen in micrograph (a), represents the first part of the small intestine and receives partly digested food in the form of acidic chyme from the stomach via the pyloric canal. The main function of the duodenum is to neutralise gastric acid and pepsin and to intiate further digestive processes.

Micrograph (a) illustrates monkey duodenum, the wall of the human duodenum being too thick to be photographed in its entirety. The mucosa **M** has the characteristic villous form of the whole of the small intestine, with short glands known as ***crypts of Lieberkühn*** between the villi extending down to the muscularis mucosae **MM**. The feature unique to the duodenum is the extensive mass of coiled branched tubular glands **G** found mainly in the submucosa **SM**. The ducts of these ***Brunner's glands*** pass up through the muscularis mucosae to open into the crypts between the mucosal villi **V**. Beneath the mass of submucosal glands, the smooth muscle wall consists of an inner circular layer **CM** and an outer longitudinal layer **LM**, as in the rest of the small intestine.

The tall columnar cells of Brunner's glands have extensive, poorly stained mucigen-filled cytoplasm and basally located nuclei. The presence of chyme in the duodenum stimulates Brunner's glands to secrete a thin alkaline mucus which helps to neutralise the acidic chyme and to protect the duodenal mucosa from autodigestion. Other products of Brunner's glands include lysozyme and epidermal growth factor. Brunner's glands may also be involved in the secretion of IgA, produced by plasma cells of the lamina propria, into the lumen of the duodenum.

Chyme also stimulates the release of two peptide hormones, ***secretin*** and ***cholecystokinin-pancreozymin***

(***CCK***) from neuroendocrine cells scattered throughout the duodenal mucosa. Secretin and CCK promote pancreatic exocrine secretion into the duodenal lumen via the pancreatic duct; CCK also stimulates contraction of the gall bladder, thus propelling bile into the common bile duct. The pancreatic and common bile ducts merge to empty their contents into the duodenum via a single short duct which opens into the second part of the duodenum via the ***ampulla of Vater***.

Pancreatic juice is alkaline due to a high content of bicarbonate ions and thus helps to neutralise the acidic gastric contents entering the duodenum. The pancreas also secretes a variety of digestive enzymes, including the proteolytic enzymes ***trypsin*** and ***chymotrypsin***; like pepsin in the stomach, these are secreted in an inactive pro-enzyme form. On entering the duodenal lumen, trypsin is activated by the enzyme ***enterokinase*** secreted by the duodenal mucosa; activated trypsin in turn activates chymotrypsin. The pancreatic enzymes, which also include ***amylase*** and ***lipases***, initiate the processes of luminal digestion described in Figure 14.16. The biliary secretions contain ***bile acids***, which act as emulsifying agents and are particularly important in the absorption of lipids.

Micrograph (b) shows a section of ileum at very low magnification. The mucosa **M** is thrown into transverse folds, the ***plicae circulares*** **PC**, covered with villi **V**. The muscularis mucosae **MM** lies immediately beneath the basal crypts and is difficult to see at this magnification. The vascular submucosa **S** extends into the plicae circulares. Beneath it lie circular **CM** and longitudinal **LM** layers of the muscularis propria and the serosa **Sr**. Peyer's patches **P** dominate the mucosa at the left of the field.

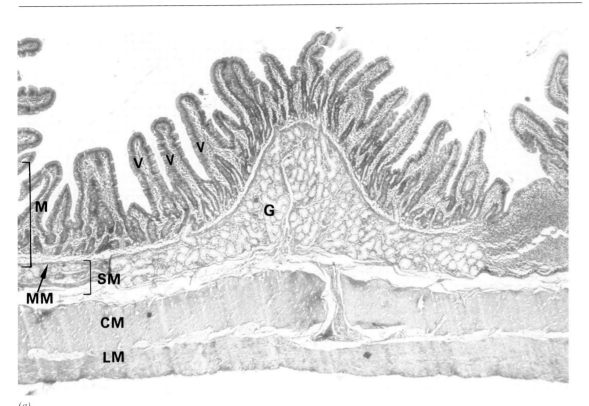

(a)

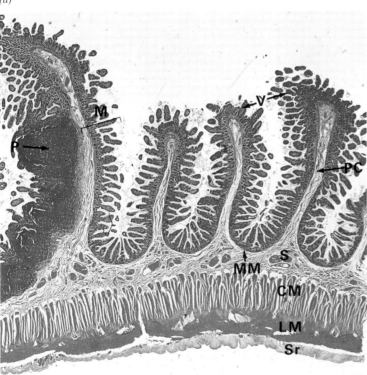

(b)

It is clear from these two micrographs that the small intestine has the same basic structure throughout. The major difference between the duodenum on the one hand, and the jejunum and ileum on the other, is the presence of Brunner's glands in the duodenum. Other qualitative differences include the following:

- The villi tend to be longest in the duodenum and become shorter towards the ileum.
- Lymphoid tissue becomes more prominent in the ileum and is relatively inconspicuous in the duodenum.
- The proportion of goblet cells in the epithelium increases distally.
- Plicae circulares are only found in the jejunum and ileum.

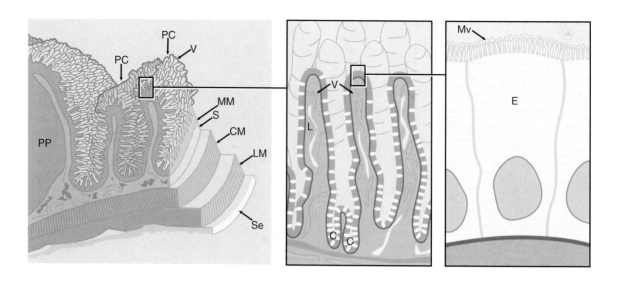

Fig. 14.16 Small intestine

The small intestine, comprising the duodenum, jejunum and ileum, is the principal site for absorption of digestion products from the gastrointestinal tract. Digestion begins in the stomach and is completed in the small intestine in association with the absorptive process. Four factors combine to provide an enormous surface area:

- The small intestine is extremely long (4–6 metres in humans).
- The mucosa and submucosa are thrown up into circularly arranged folds called *plicae circulares* **PC** or *valves of Kerkring* which are particularly numerous in the jejunum.
- The mucosal surface is made up of numerous finger-like projections called *villi* **V**, whilst the mucosa between the bases of the villi is formed into crypts, called *crypts of Lieberkühn* **C**.
- Plentiful *microvilli* **Mv** are present at the luminal surface of the *enterocytes* **E**, the columnar cells covering the villi and crypts; these cells are responsible for the processes of digestion and absorption.

The muscularis mucosae **MM** lies immediately beneath the mucosal crypts and separates the mucosa from the submucosa **S**. The vascular submucosa extends into, and forms the core of, the plicae circulares. Inner circular **CM** and outer longitudinal **LM** layers of the muscularis are responsible for continuous peristaltic activity of the small intestine. The peritoneal aspect of the muscularis is invested by the loose collagenous serosa **Se**, which is lined on its peritoneal surface by mesothelium identical in appearance to the mesothelial lining of the pleura (see Fig. 12.20).

A prominent feature of the small intestine are 200 or so lymphoid aggregations known as *Peyer's patches* **PP** within the lamina propria (see Fig. 11.20).

The mechanisms of digestion and absorption
Digestion occurs within the lumen or at the mucosal surface, the latter being linked with the process of absorption.

Luminal digestion involves the mixing of chyme with pancreatic enzymes, with subsequent molecular breakdown occurring within the intestinal lumen; the process is facilitated by adsorption of pancreatic enzymes onto the mucosal surface. *Membrane digestion* involves enzymes located in the luminal plasma membranes of the cells lining the small intestine. The principal means of digestion and absorption of the main food constituents are as follows:

- **Proteins** are initially denatured by the acidic gastric juice before being hydrolysed to polypeptide fragments by the enzyme pepsin. In the duodenum, pancreatic enzymes, including *trypsin, chymotrypsin, elastase* and *carboxypeptidases*, mediate further luminal digestion to small peptide fragments. Membrane-bound *peptide hydrolases* complete the process leading to amino acid absorption; this involves active transport with a different carrier system for each amino acid. In young infants, some proteins are absorbed without prior digestion by the process of endocytosis, colostrum having been shown to have some anti-digestive properties.
- **Carbohydrates** occur in the diet mainly in the form of starches and the disaccharides, sucrose and lactose. *Pancreatic amylase* hydrolyses starch to glucose and the disaccharide maltose in the small intestinal lumen. This process is commenced by *salivary amylase* in the mouth, although its contribution to digestion is probably insignificant. Membrane-bound disaccharidases and oligosaccharidases convert the sugars to monosaccharides, mainly glucose, galactose and fructose, which are absorbed by facilitated diffusion.
- **Lipids**, predominantly triglycerides, are converted by the mechanical action of the stomach into a coarse emulsion, which is converted to a fine emulsion in the duodenum by bile acids synthesised in the liver. Each triglyceride molecule is broken down into a monoglyceride and two free fatty acids by pancreatic *lipases*, although some glycerol and diglycerides are also produced. These smaller lipid molecules are then absorbed and resynthesised back into triglycerides within the enterocytes.

The products of protein and carbohydrate digestion, namely amino acids and monosaccharides, respectively, enter the intestinal capillaries and pass via the portal vein to the liver. In contrast, the reconstituted triglycerides pass into intestinal lymphatics known as *lacteals* **L**, and thence via the thoracic duct to the general circulation, bypassing the liver. For lymphatic transport, the triglycerides become coated with phospholipids and proteins to form fine globules known as *chylomicrons*. A minority of lipid digestion products, such as short-chain fatty acids and glycerol, pass in the portal system to the liver along with almost all the bile acids which are reabsorbed and recirculated.

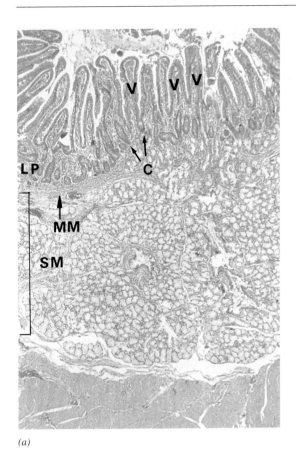

(a)

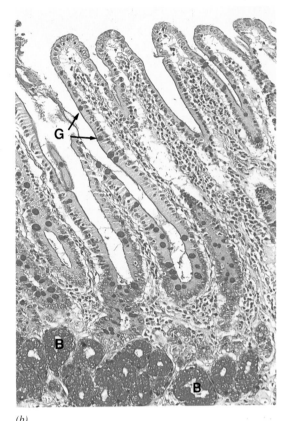

(b)

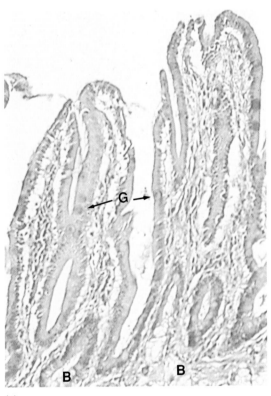

(c)

Fig. 14.17 **Duodenum (a) H & E × 15
(b) PAS/haematoxylin × 150 (c) Alcian blue × 150**

These micrographs of the human duodenum highlight the mucus-secreting cells. Micrograph (a) is stained by the standard H & E method which has little affinity for mucin. Nevertheless, the thickness of the Brunner's glands is evident, the main glandular mass lying in the submucosa **SM** deep to the muscularis mucosae **MM** with a small portion sometimes found in the lamina propria **LP**. The duodenal mucosa has the typical form found elsewhere in the small intestine, namely numerous elongated villi **V**, between the bases of which are shorter crypts **C**.

At higher magnification, micrograph (b) focuses on the duodenal mucosa stained by the PAS method; this stains most complex carbohydrates, including mucins, a strong magenta. Brunner's glands **B** are not the only mucus-secreting cells in the duodenum, mucus also being produced by goblet cells **G** scattered in the epithelium of the mucosal villi and crypts. The majority of the mucosal epithelial cells are not PAS-positive and are tall columnar absorptive cells (enterocytes).

Micrograph (c) shows a section from the same specimen stained by the Alcian blue method, which is specific for the acid mucin typical of goblet cells **G** but which leaves the alkaline mucus of Brunner's glands **B** unstained. All goblet cell mucus is Alcian blue-positive as in the respiratory tract and colon (see Fig. 14.28). Such differential staining provides a useful tool in histopathology for distinguishing mucus-secreting glandular tumours of gastric origin from those arising from the small and large intestines. In contrast, the mucin-producing cells of the stomach do not stain with the Alcian blue method.

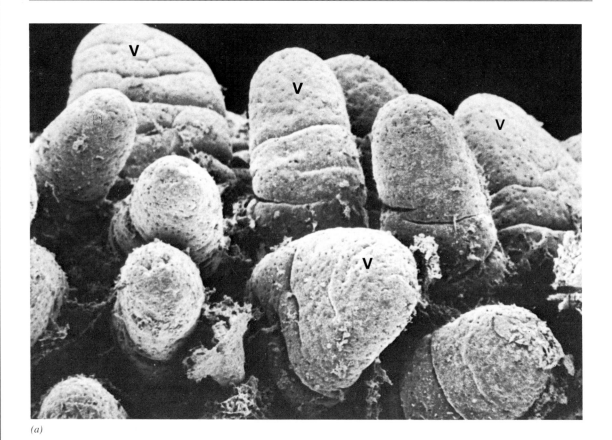

(a)

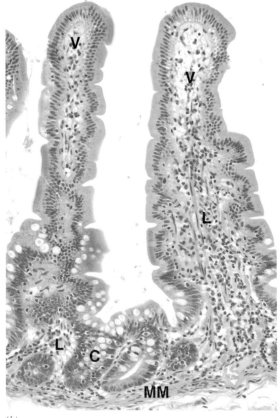

(b)

Fig. 14.18 Intestinal villi and crypts
(a) SEM × 100 (b) H & E × 150

This low power scanning electron micrograph (a) shows villi **V** along the crest of a plica circularis in the small intestine. Note the variability of the shape of the villi: some are finger-shaped, while others have a broader, leaf-like profile. Surface openings of scattered goblet cells stud the villous surface.

The intestinal villi **V** (micrograph (b)) are lined by a simple columnar epithelium which is continuous with that of the crypts **C**. As in other parts of the gastrointestinal tract, the epithelium includes a variety of cell types, each with its own specific function. Cell types in the small intestine epithelium include:

- *Enterocytes*, the most numerous cell type, are tall columnar cells with surface *microvilli* which are seen as a brush border in light micrographs. These cells are characteristic of the small intestine and are the main absorptive cells.
- *Goblet cells* are scattered among the enterocytes and produce mucin for lubrication of the intestinal contents and protection of the epithelium.
- *Paneth cells* are found at the base of the crypts and are distinguished by their prominent, eosinophilic apical granules. These cells have a defensive function.
- *Neuroendocrine cells* produce locally acting hormones which regulate gastrointestinal motility and secretion.
- *Stem cells*, found at the base of the crypts, divide continuously to replenish all of the above four cell types.
- *Intraepithelial lymphocytes*, which are mostly of T cell type, provide defence against invasive organisms.

The lamina propria **L** extends between the crypts and into the core of each villus and contains a rich vascular and lymphatic network into which digestive products are absorbed. The muscularis mucosae **MM** lies immediately beneath the base of the crypts.

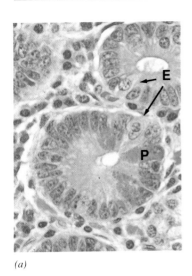

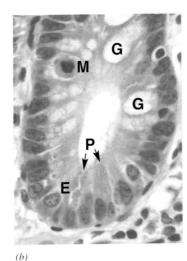

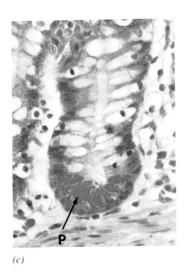

(a)   *(b)*   *(c)*

Fig. 14.19   **Crypts of Lieberkuhn (a) H & E, TS × 400 (b) H & E, LS × 300 (c) Phloxine-tartrazine × 320**

The majority of cells in the crypt bases are stem cells which replenish the epithelial cells of the villi; immature goblet cells **G** are readily seen in micrograph (b). A single mitotic figure **M** is identifiable. With H & E staining, Paneth cells **P** exhibit intensely eosinophilic apical cytoplasmic granules; these are even more clearly demonstrated by the phloxine-tartrazine method which stains the granules scarlet. The eosinophilic granules of Paneth cells contain various antimicrobial peptides known as *defensins*, as well as protective enzymes such as lysozyme and phospholipase A. These products, secreted into the lumen of the small bowel, provide the first line of

defence against any disease-producing microbes which survive passage through the stomach. The lumen of the small bowel is virtually sterile. Paneth cells are long-lived (weeks) in comparison to the short lifespan (2–3 days) of enterocytes and goblet cells.

Endocrine cells **E** also contain eosinophilic cytoplasmic granules which are found in a subnuclear position, in contrast to the granules of Paneth cells. Secretory products of such cells include secretin, somatostatin, enteroglucagon and serotonin. As a general rule, each endocrine cell produces only one hormone.

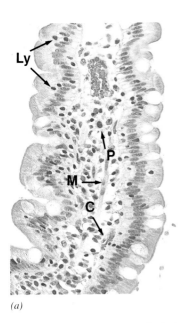

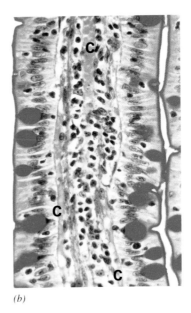

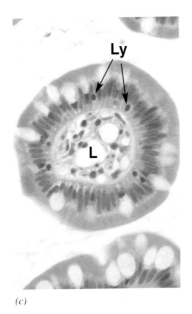

(a)   *(b)*   *(c)*

Fig. 14.20   **Intestinal villi (a) H & E, LS × 100 (b) PAS/iron haematoxylin/orange G × 320 (c) H & E, TS × 300**

These micrographs illustrate the tall columnar enterocytes which invest the intestinal villi, as well as the goblet cells scattered among them. The luminal surface of the enterocytes seen in micrograph (b) is strongly PAS-positive due to a particularly thick glycocalyx and a surface layer of goblet cell-derived mucus; both protect against autodigestion. The glycocalyx may also be the site for adsorption of pancreatic digestive enzymes.

T lymphocytes **Ly** are scattered among the enterocytes. Plasma cells **P** in the villous core secrete IgA into the intestinal lumen.

The cores of the villi are extensions of the lamina propria and consist of loose supporting tissue. Capillaries **C** lie immediately beneath the basement membrane and transport most digestive products to the hepatic portal vein. Tiny lymphatic vessels drain into a single larger vessel called a *lacteal* **L**, at the centre of the villus. The lacteals transport absorbed lipid into the circulatory system via the thoracic duct. Smooth muscle fibres **M** are seen in the long axis of the villous core in micrograph (a) and represent extensions of the muscularis mucosae.

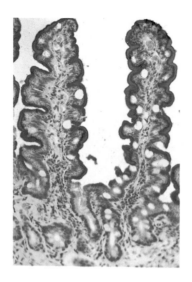

Fig. 14.21 **Intestinal villi**

Enzyme histochemical method for alkaline phosphatase × 128

This frozen section from an intestinal biopsy has been stained for the enzyme *alkaline phosphatase*, which is one of the many membrane-bound enzymes characteristic of enterocyte microvilli; enzyme activity is represented by a red deposit. Alkaline phosphatase is thought to be involved in the transport of calcium ions from the intestinal lumen. Other membrane enzymes are involved in the breakdown of peptides and disaccharides to amino acids and monosaccharides, respectively. The enzymes of the brush border are intrinsic membrane proteins and are synthesised by enterocytes, in contrast to those enzymes adsorbed on to the surface which are synthesised by the pancreas. Note that the relatively immature enterocytes in the intestinal crypts show little alkaline phosphatase activity.

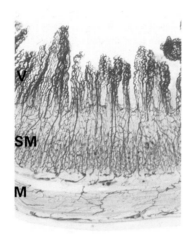

Fig. 14.22 **Intestinal villi** Carmine perfused × 10

This specimen of small intestine has been perfused before fixation with a red dye and demonstrates the blood supply of the mucosa. Long loops of branching capillaries, originating from a dense capillary network in the submucosa **SM**, extend up to the tips of the villi **V**. Note also the capillary network supplying the muscular wall **M**. Most of the absorbed food products, with the exception of triglycerides, enter the capillaries and pass via the portal vein to the liver.

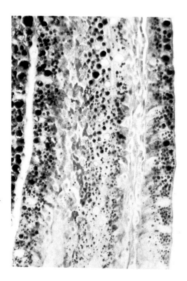

Fig. 14.23 **Intestinal villus** Sudan black × 320

This frozen section from the intestine of a rat fed with milk has been stained to demonstrate the presence of absorbed lipids. Ingested triglycerides are emulsified by bile and hydrolysed by the pancreatic enzyme, *lipase*; the degradation products, mainly free fatty acids and monoglycerides, are absorbed by enterocytes where they are resynthesised into triglycerides in the smooth endoplasmic reticulum. Here, the triglycerides are reconstituted into small globules and form a lipoprotein complex incorporating protein, cholesterol and phospholipids. Membrane-bound vesicles containing multiple droplets bud from the smooth endoplasmic reticulum and pass towards the base of the cell where they are released by exocytosis into the intercellular clefts; from here the small lipoprotein droplets, described as *chylomicrons*, pass into the lacteals and then into larger lymphatics, eventually entering the general circulation. Note the high concentration of black-stained lipid in the enterocyte cytoplasm and in the chylomicrons within the central lacteal.

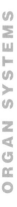

ORGAN SYSTEMS

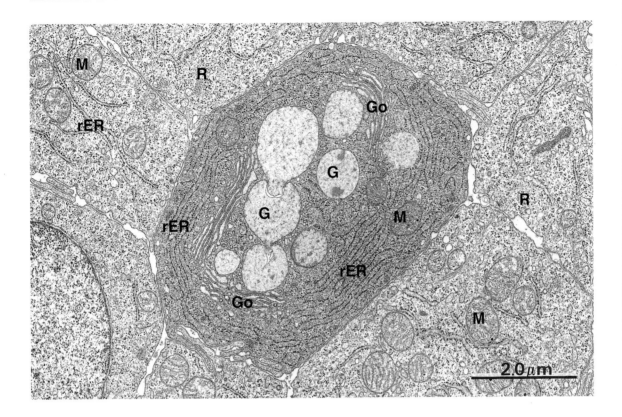

Fig. 14.24 Duodenal epithelium EM × 14 500

This low power electron micrograph of a horizontal section through the duodenal epithelium demonstrates several important features. In the central area there is a goblet cell containing several mucin-containing granules **G**. The goblet cell appearance by conventional light microscopy is actually an artefact of preparation whereby water is taken up by the granules which consequently expand and compress the surrounding cytoplasm.

Adjacent to the mucin granules are three Golgi apparatuses **Go** with plentiful rough endoplasmic reticulum **rER**, features typical of secretory cells. Occasional mitochondria **M** are also seen.

Surrounding the goblet cell are a number of enterocytes. These have much less prominent rER but contain large numbers of free ribosomes **R** and mitochondria **M**. (see Fig.14.27).

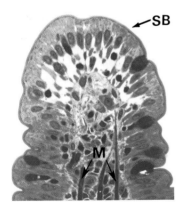

Fig. 14.25 Tip of intestinal villus Thin section, toluidine blue × 320

This method of tissue preparation demonstrates several features of the intestinal villus which are not as well seen in thicker conventional paraffin wax-embedded sections.

Firstly, degenerating enterocytes and goblet cells are seen about to be shed from the tip of the villus. Secondly, the striated or brush border **SB** is identifiable at the luminal surface of the enterocytes representing the microvilli seen with electron microscopy. Thirdly, smooth muscle fibres **M** are seen in the long axis of the villous core where they are disposed around the central lacteal; these muscle cells are extensions of the muscularis mucosae. Contraction of the smooth muscle strands enhances drainage of lymph from the lacteals and probably also keeps the villi in a constant motile state, reducing the prospect of clogging and enhancing contact of luminal contents with the villous surface.

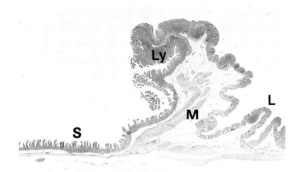

Fig. 14.26 Ileocaecal junction H & E × 5

Unabsorbed and indigestible food residues from the ileum are propelled by peristalsis into the distended first part of the large intestine, the caecum, through a simple cone-shaped valve which marks the ileocaecal junction. There is an abrupt transition in the lining of the valve from the villiform pattern in the small intestine **S** to the glandular form in the large intestine **L**.

The ileocaecal valve consists of a thickened extension of the muscularis propria **M** which provides robust support for the mucosa. Variable quantities of lymphoid tissue **Ly** are found in the mucosa.

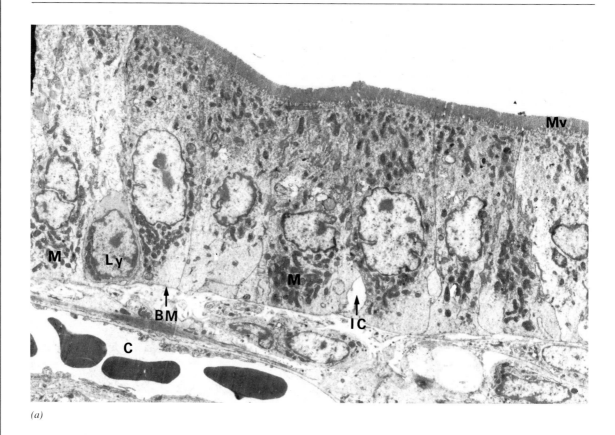

(a)

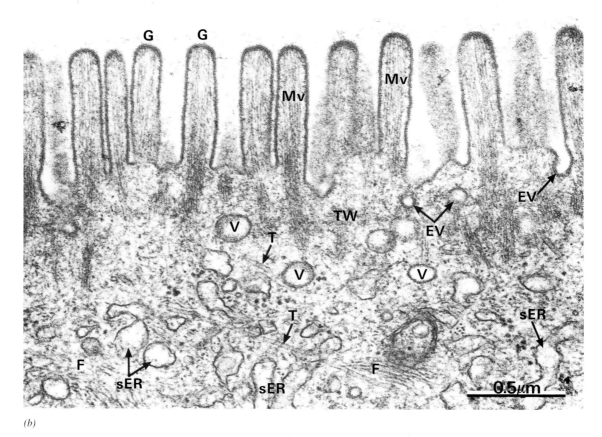

(b)

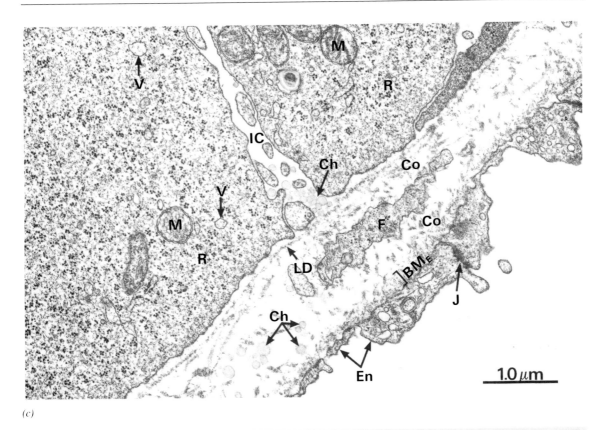

(c)

Fig. 14.27 **Enterocytes** (a) EM × 4540 (b) EM × 56 000 (c) EM × 22 000 *(illustrations (a) and (b) opposite)*

These micrographs illustrate the main ultrastructural features of enterocytes, the absorptive cells of the small intestine. Micrograph (a) shows the enormous number of *microvilli* **Mv** (up to 3000 per cell), which increase the surface area of the plasma membrane exposed to the lumen by some 30 times. The microvilli are of uniform length (approximately 1 μm) and constitute the ***brush border*** of light microscopy (see Fig. 14.20). Most absorption in the small intestine occurs by direct passage of low molecular weight digestion products across the luminal plasma membrane. Mitochondria **M** are particularly abundant within enterocytes, reflecting the high energy demands of such processes. Chylomicrons assembled in the enterocytes pass first into the ***intercellular clefts*** **IC**, then across the basement membrane **BM** into the core of the villus and then into the lacteal. Lymphocytes **Ly** are commonly found in the intercellular clefts between enterocytes where they play an important part in the immunological defence of the tract. Note the close proximity of a blood capillary **C** to the enterocyte basement membrane.

As seen in micrograph (b), the glycocalyx **G** of the enterocyte microvilli is unusually prominent. It provides protection against autodigestion and acts as the site for adsorption of pancreatic digestive enzymes. This micrograph also shows the filamentous cytoskeleton of the microvilli **MV** extending into the superficial cytoplasm. Here, in the terminal web **TW**, it becomes integrated into the cytoskeleton of the body of the cell. Deeper in the cell, filaments **F** and microtubules **T** are readily identified. Enterocytes are tightly bound near their luminal surface by junctional complexes (see Fig. 5.10) which prevent

direct access of luminal contents into the intercellular spaces as well as holding the epithelium together.

Endocytotic vesicles **EV** are often seen between the bases of microvilli, and endocytic vesicles **V** are common in the superficial cytoplasm. The importance of endocytosis as a mode of absorption in the small intestine is not well understood, although it may be a minor pathway of lipid and in some cases protein absorption. Smooth endoplasmic reticulum **sER** is seen deeper in the cytoplasm.

Micrograph (c) illustrates the basal aspect of two enterocytes separated by an intercellular cleft **IC**. Their basement membrane is thin, the lamina densa **LD** appearing to be discontinuous. Close beneath the base of the enterocytes is a tiny lymphatic tributary of the central lacteal, its endothelial lining **En** being thin and fenestrated; note the junctional complex **J** binding adjacent endothelial cells and the thin discontinuous endothelial basement membrane **BM**$_E$. The delicate supporting tissue between the basement membrane and lymphatic contains fibroblasts **F** and fine collagen fibrils **Co**.

The main feature of the basal enterocyte cytoplasm is numerous free ribosomes **R**, scattered mitochondria **M** and membranous vesicles **V** containing lipoprotein droplets en route for exocytosis into the intercellular cleft. The cleft contains numerous small chylomicrons **Ch** which cluster near the lamina densa as if temporarily held up in their passage towards the lymphatic. In the lamina propria, the chylomicrons are larger, probably due to fusion of smaller ones coursing through from the intercellular cleft. Note that the chylomicrons in the extracellular environment are not membrane-bound but have a fine electron-dense limiting layer of protein.

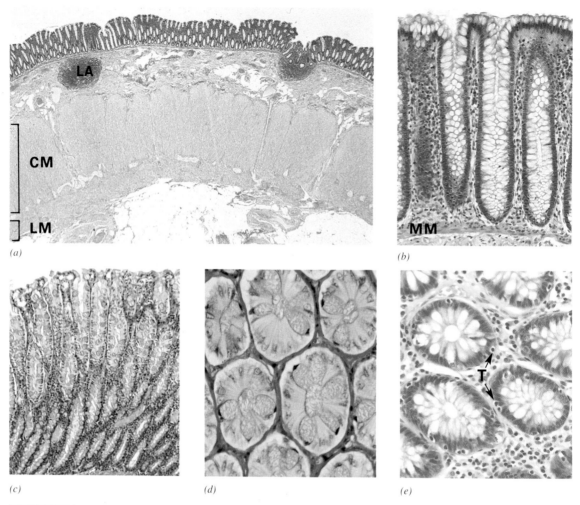

Fig. 14.28 Colon (a) H & E × 4 (b) H & E × 100 (c) LS, Alcian blue/van Gieson × 80
(d) TS, Alcian blue/van Gieson × 320 (e) TS, H & E × 200

The principal functions of the large intestine are the recovery of water and salt from the faeces and the propulsion of increasingly solid faeces to the rectum prior to defaecation.

As shown in micrograph (a), the muscular wall is consequently thick and capable of powerful peristaltic activity. As in the rest of the gastrointestinal tract, the muscularis propria of the large intestine consists of inner circular **CM** and outer longitudinal layers **LM** but, except in the rectum, the longitudinal layer forms three separate longitudinal bands called *teniae coli*.

The mucosa is folded in the non-distended state but it does not exhibit distinct plicae circulares like those of the small intestine. Immediately above the anal valves, the mucosa forms longitudinal folds called the *columns of Morgagni*. The muscularis mucosae is a prominent feature of the large intestinal mucosa; rhythmic contractions prevent clogging of the glands and enhance expulsion of mucus.

Consistent with its functions of water absorption and faecal lubrication, the mucosa consists of cells of two types: absorptive cells and mucus-secreting goblet cells. As seen in micrograph (b), these are arranged in closely packed straight tubular glands or crypts, which extend to the muscularis mucosa **MM**. As faeces pass along the large intestine and become progressively dehydrated, the mucus becomes increasingly important in protecting the mucosa from trauma. The Alcian blue method(micrograph c)

stains goblet cell mucus a greenish-blue colour whilst the absorptive cells remain poorly stained. Goblet cells predominate in the base of the glands, whereas the luminal surface is almost entirely lined by columnar absorptive cells.

Micrographs (d) and (e) show transverse sections through the upper part of large intestinal glands, highlighting the closely packed arrangement of the glands in the mucosa. The tall columnar absorptive cells have oval basal nuclei; in contrast, goblet cell nuclei are small and condensed. Stem cells at the base of the glands continually replace the epithelium. Intraepithelial T lymphocytes **T** are easily seen in (e). Lamina propria fills the space between the glands and contains numerous blood and lymphatic vessels into which water is absorbed by passive diffusion. The lamina propria also contains collagen (stained red in (c) and (d)) as well as lymphocytes and plasma cells. These form part of the defence mechanisms against invading pathogens along with intraepithelial lymphocyes and the lymphoid aggregates **LA**, which are smaller than Peyer's patches, found in the lamina propria and submucosa (a).

The large intestine is inhabited by a variety of commensal bacteria which further degrade food residues. Bacterial degradation is an important mechanism for the digestion of cellulose in ruminants, but in humans most cellulose is excreted. Small quantities of fat-soluble vitamins derived from bacterial activity are absorbed in the large intestine.

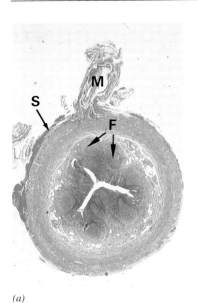

(a)

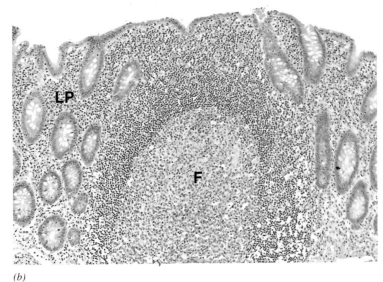

(b)

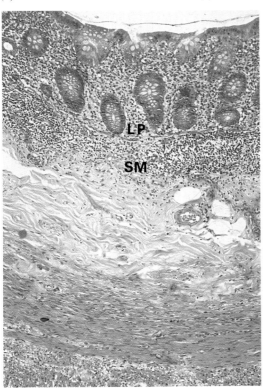

(c)

Fig. 14.29 Appendix (a) H & E × 5 (b) H & E × 75 (c) H & E × 42

The appendix is a small blind-ended tubular sac extending from the caecum just distal to the ileocaecal junction. The general structure of the appendix conforms to that of the rest of the large intestine. In some mammals, the appendix is capacious and involved in prolonged digestion of cellulose, but in humans its function is unknown.

Micrograph (a) illustrates the suspensory mesentery **M** in continuity with the outer serosal layer **S**. This contains extravasated blood resulting from haemorrhage during surgical removal. The mesenteries conduct blood vessels, lymphatics and nerves to and from the gastrointestinal tract.

The most characteristic feature of the appendix, particularly in the young, is the presence of masses of lymphoid tissue in the mucosa and submucosa. As seen in micrographs (b) and (c), the lamina propria **LP** and upper submucosa **SM** are diffusely infiltrated with lymphocytes. Note that the mucosal glands are much less closely packed than elsewhere in the large intestine. As seen in micrographs (a) and (b), the lymphoid tissue also forms follicles **F** often containing germinal centres (see also Fig. 11.21). These follicles bulge into the lumen and, like the follicles of Peyer's patches in the small intestine, are invested by a simple epithelium of M cells, which presumably facilitates sampling of antigen in the appendicular lumen.

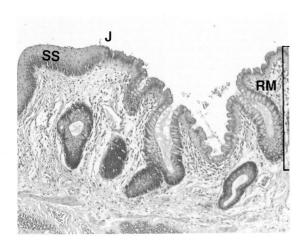

Fig. 14.30 Recto-anal junction H & E × 60

The rectum is the short dilated terminal portion of the large intestine. The rectal mucosa **RM** is similar to that of the rest of the large bowel except that it has even more numerous goblet cells. At the recto-anal junction **J**, it undergoes an abrupt transition to become stratified squamous epithelium **SS** in the anal canal. Branched tubular *circumanal glands* open at the recto-anal junction into small pits at the distal ends of the columns of Morgagni. The anal canal forms the last 2 or 3 cm of the gastrointestinal tract and is surrounded by voluntary muscle which forms the anal sphincter. Here, the stratified squamous epithelium undergoes a gradual transition to skin containing sebaceous glands and large apocrine sweat glands (see Fig. 9.16).

ORGAN SYSTEMS

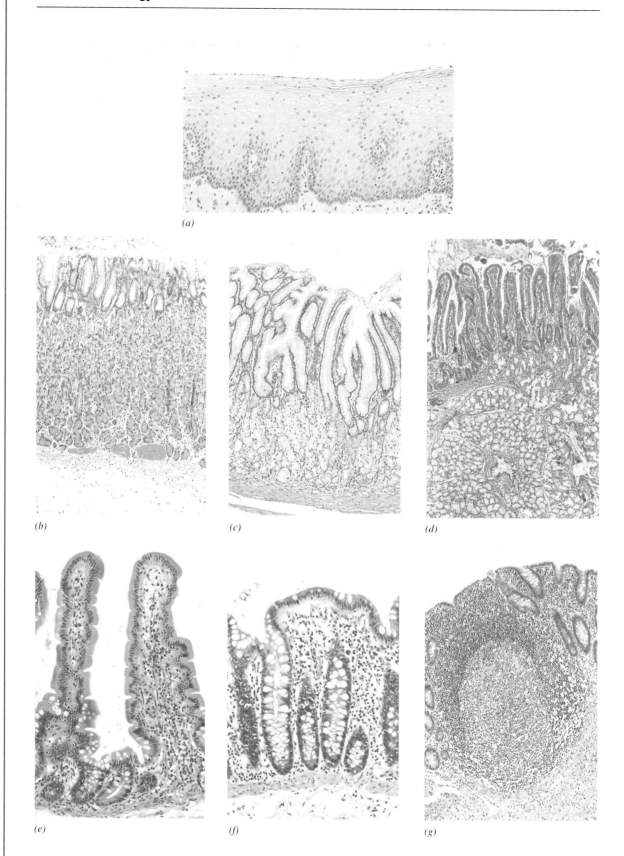

(a)

(b)

(c)

(d)

(e)

(f)

(g)

Fig. 14.31 Comparison of structure of parts of the gastrointestinal tract (a) H & E × 100 (b) H & E × 50 (c) H & E × 50 (d) H & E × 15 (e) H & E × 100 (f) H & E × 100 (g) H & E × 75 (h) H & E × 60 *(opposite and below)*

The table below outlines the main structural features of the different components of the gastrointestinal tract for easy reference and revision. Please note that the epithelium of all segments includes stem cells and neuroendocrine cells, which have not been included in the table for simplicity. Each line of the table refers to the correspondingly labelled micrograph opposite.

Part of gastrointestinal tract	Illustration	Type of epithelium	Main cell types of epithelium	Other distinctive features
Oesophagus	(a)	Stratified squamous	• Squamous cells	Submucosal glands
Body/fundus of stomach	(b)	Glandular – straight tubular	• Surface mucous cells • Neck mucous cells • Parietal cells • Chief (peptic) cells	Lymphoid cells very sparse No lymphoid aggregates
Pylorus	(c)	Glandular – coiled, branched tubular	• Mucous cells • Occasional parietal cells	Lymphoid cells very sparse No lymphoid aggregates
Duodenum	(d)	Glandular with villi and crypts of Lieberkühn	• Enterocytes with microvilli • Goblet cells • Paneth cells	Brunner's glands
Jejunum and ileum	(e)	Glandular with villi and crypts of Lieberkühn	• Enterocytes with microvilli • Goblet cells • Paneth cells	Peyer's patches become more prominent distally
Colon and rectum	(f)	Glandular – straight	• Goblet cells • Absorptive cells	Teniae coli
Appendix	(g)	Glandular – straight crypts	• Goblet cells • Tall columnar cells	Prominent lymphoid tissue
Anus	(h)	Glandular – straight Stratified squamous	• Absorptive and goblet cells • Squamous cells	Columns of Morgagni

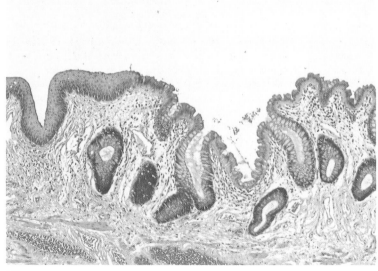

(h)

15. Liver and pancreas

Liver and biliary system

The liver, like the pancreas, develops embryologically as a glandular outgrowth of the primitive gut. The major functions of the liver may be summarised as follows:

- Detoxification of metabolic waste products, e.g. deamination of amino acids to produce urea.
- Destruction of spent red cells and reclamation of their constituents (in conjunction with the spleen).
- Synthesis and secretion of bile; bile contains many of the end products of the above processes and is thus an excretory product and an exocrine secretion.
- Synthesis of the plasma proteins, including albumin and clotting factors.
- Synthesis of plasma lipoproteins.
- Metabolic functions, e.g. glycogen synthesis, gluconeogenesis, storage of glycogen, some vitamins and lipid.
- Detoxification of various drugs and toxins, such as alcohol.

Many of these biosynthetic functions utilise the products of digestion. With the exception of most lipids, absorbed food products pass directly from the gut to the liver via the *hepatic portal vein*. Thus the liver is perfused by blood rich in amino acids, simple sugars and other products of digestion but relatively poor in oxygen. Oxygen required to support liver metabolism is supplied via the *hepatic artery*. The liver is thus unusual in having both arterial and venous blood supplies. Venous drainage of the liver occurs via the *hepatic vein*.

The structural components of the liver include plates of liver cells, called *hepatocytes*, separated by wide vascular channels known as *sinusoids*. Blood flow into the sinusoids comes from terminal branches of the portal vein and hepatic artery, bringing nutrient-rich blood from the gastrointestinal tract and oxygen-rich blood, respectively. The larger branches of these two vessels course side by side in fibrous tracts, known as *portal tracts*, along with *bile ductules* which carry bile in the opposite direction from the liver to the duodenum.

Blood from the portal vein and hepatic artery passes through the sinusoids where it is in intimate contact with the hepatocytes for the exchange of nutrients and metabolic products. The blood then flows into branches of the hepatic vein and thence into the inferior vena cava.

Fig. 15.1 **Liver (a) Diagram of liver lobule (b) Pig, H & E × 20 (c) Human, H & E × 20 (d) Diagram of simple acinus (e) Diagram of acinar agglomerate** (*illustrations opposite*)

Traditionally the structural unit of the liver was considered to be the conceptually simple *hepatic lobule*. More recently, it has been realised that the blood flow and function of the liver are more accurately represented by the unit structure known as the *hepatic acinus*.

The hepatic lobule (a) is roughly hexagonal in shape and is centred on a *terminal hepatic venule* (*centrilobular venule*) **V**. The portal tracts **T** are positioned at the angles of the hexagon. The blood from the portal vein and hepatic artery branches in the portal tracts flows to the central vein. Clearly this concept is flawed as blood from the portal tracts really flows away in all directions. In some species, such as the pig (b), the lobule is outlined by bands of fibrous tissue giving a well-defined structural unit. In humans (c) and most other species, no such clear structural definition exists, although lobules can be roughly outlined by the hexagonal array of portal tracts **T** arranged around a terminal hepatic venule **V**.

The *hepatic acinus* (d) is a more accurate representation of liver function although it is much more difficult to define histologically. The acinus is a roughly berry-shaped unit of liver parenchyma centred on a portal tract. The acinus lies between two or more terminal hepatic venules and blood flows from the portal tracts through the sinusoids to the venules. The acinus is divided into *zones 1, 2 and 3* and the hepatocytes in these zones have different metabolic functions. Zone 1 is closest to the portal tract and receives the most oxygenated blood, while zone 3 is furthest away and receives least oxygen. Zone 3 is thus most susceptible to ischaemic injury.

Simple acini are grouped into *complex acini* which are in turn grouped into *acinar agglomerates*; these are supplied by one branch each of the portal artery and hepatic vein. Although the entire structure looks on paper like a bunch of grapes, it must be remembered that this is a functional grouping and in reality the hepatic parenchyma is smooth and continuous.

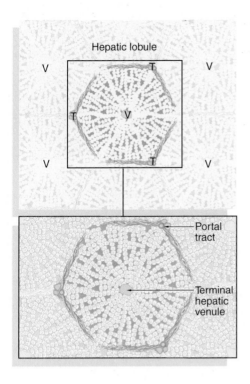

Hepatic lobule

Portal tract

Terminal hepatic venule

(a)

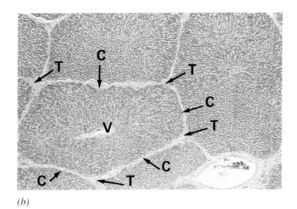

(b)

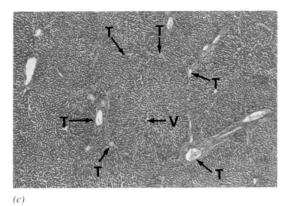

(c)

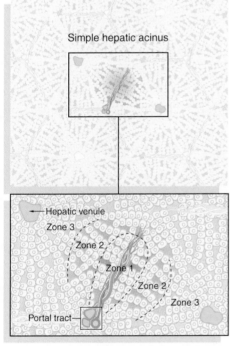

Simple hepatic acinus

Hepatic venule
Zone 3
Zone 2
Zone 1
Zone 2
Zone 3
Portal tract

(d)

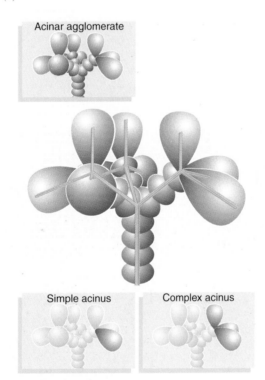

Acinar agglomerate

Simple acinus

Complex acinus

(e)

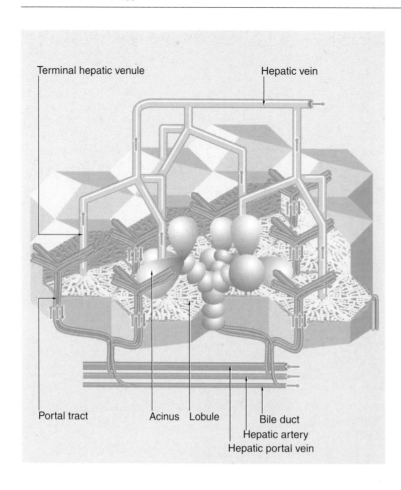

Terminal hepatic venule

Hepatic vein

Portal tract   Acinus   Lobule   Bile duct
Hepatic artery
Hepatic portal vein

Fig. 15.2 Hepatic vasculature and biliary system

This schematic diagram shows the arrangement of the hepatic vascular and bile collecting systems.

The hepatic portal vein and hepatic artery branch repeatedly within the liver. Their terminal branches run within the portal tracts and empty into the sinusoids. Blood from both systems then percolates between the branching plates of hepatocytes in the sinusoids, which converge to drain into a *terminal hepatic (centrilobular) venule*. These drain to *intercalated veins* and thence to the hepatic vein which drains into the inferior vena cava.

Bile is secreted into a network of minute *bile canaliculi* situated between the plasma membranes of adjacent hepatocytes; the canaliculi are too small to be represented in this diagram. The canalicular network then drains into a system of bile collecting ducts located in the portal tracts. Bile flows through the extrahepatic biliary tree and ultimately to the duodenum. The flow of bile in the biliary tree is thus in the opposite direction to the blood in the vessels of the portal tracts.

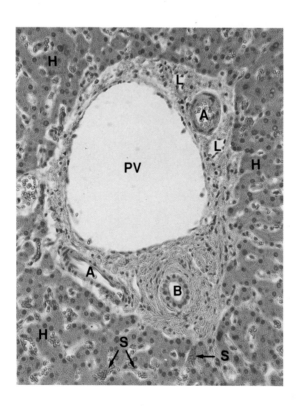

Fig. 15.3 Portal tract H & E × 150

This micrograph focuses on a typical portal tract containing three main structures in a fibrous stroma. The largest is a terminal branch of the hepatic portal vein **PV** (*terminal portal venule*) which has a very thin wall lined by flattened endothelial cells. Smaller diameter thick-walled vessels with the typical structure of arterioles are terminal branches of the hepatic artery **A**.

A network of bile canaliculi is located within each plate of hepatocytes but these are far too small to be seen at this magnification. These drain into bile collecting ducts lined by simple cuboidal or columnar epithelium, known as the *canals of Hering*, which in turn drain into the *bile ductules* **B**. The bile ductules are usually located at the periphery of the tract and are approximately the same size as the arterioles. The bile ductules merge to form larger, more centrally located *trabecular ducts* which drain via *intrahepatic ducts* into the *right and left hepatic ducts*, the *common hepatic duct* and thence to the duodenum via the *common bile duct*. Because these three structures are always found in the portal tracts, the tracts are often referred to as *portal triads*. Lymphatics **L** are also present in the portal tracts, but since their walls are delicate and often collapsed they are less easily identified.

Surrounding the portal tract are anastomosing plates of hepatocytes **H**, between which are the hepatic sinusoids **S** receiving blood from both the hepatic portal and hepatic arterial systems. The layer of hepatocytes immediately bordering the portal tract is known as the *limiting plate*.

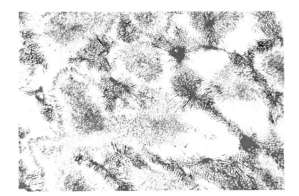

Fig. 15.4 **Liver** Perfusion method × 20

This preparation shows one of the techniques used by early histologists in mapping hepatic blood flow. The hepatic portal vein (supplying the liver) has been perfused with a red dye and the hepatic vein (draining the liver) has been back-perfused with a blue dye. Thus it can be seen how a hepatic lobule is defined by a number of portal tracts peripherally (stained red) with blood draining to a single terminal hepatic venule (stained blue) at the centre. Alternatively, an hepatic acinus is centred around a portal tract with blood radiating outwards to drain into a number of terminal hepatic venules.

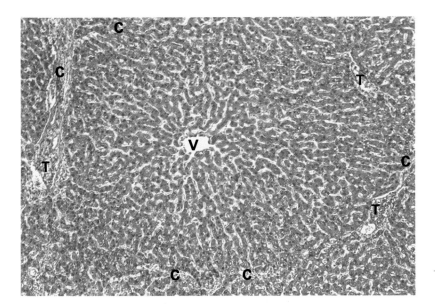

Fig. 15.5 **Liver lobule** H & E × 75

This micrograph illustrates a single human liver lobule and includes parts of a number of hepatic acini, each centred on a portal tract. The irregular hexagonal boundary of the lobule is defined by portal tracts **T** and sparse collagenous tissue **C**. Sinusoids originate at the lobule margin and course between plates of hepatocytes to converge upon the terminal hepatic venule **V**. The plates of hepatocytes are usually only one cell thick and each hepatocyte is thus exposed to blood on at least two sides. The plates of hepatocytes branch and anastomose to form a three-dimensional structure like a sponge.

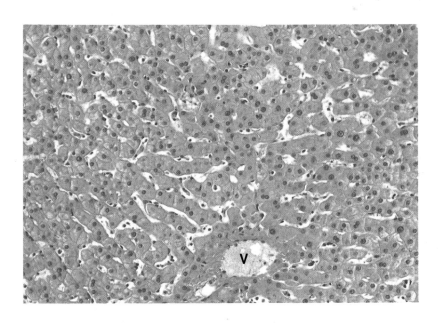

Fig. 15.6 **Liver parenchyma** H & E × 150

The arrangement of hepatocytes within the liver parenchyma can be readily seen at this magnification. The hepatocytes form flat, anastomosing plates usually only one cell thick. The sinusoids carry blood sluggishly towards the terminal hepatic venule **V**. The sinusoids are lined by a discontinuous, fenestrated endothelium, which has no basement membrane and which is separated from the hepatocytes by a narrow space (*space of Disse*), which drains into the lymphatics of the portal tracts.

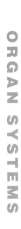

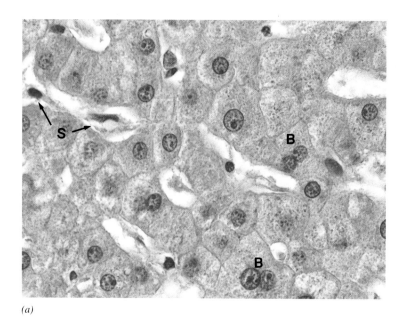

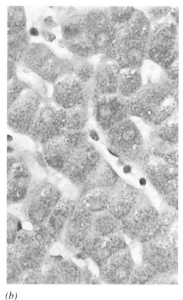

(a)   *(b)*

Fig. 15.7   **Hepatocytes** (a) H & E × 600 (b) PAS/haematoxylin × 400

Hepatocytes are large polyhedral cells with round nuclei with peripherally dispersed chromatin and prominent nucleoli. The nuclei vary greatly in size, reflecting an unusual cellular feature; more than half the hepatocytes contain twice the normal (diploid) complement of chromosomes within a single nucleus (i.e. they are tetraploid) and some contain four or even eight times this amount (polyploid). Binucleate cells **B** are also common in normal liver.

The extensive cytoplasm has a variable appearance depending on the nutritional status of the individual. When well-nourished, hepatocytes store significant quantities of glycogen and process large quantities of lipid. Both of these metabolites are partially removed during routine histological preparation, leaving irregular unstained areas within the cytoplasm. The cytoplasm is otherwise strongly eosinophilic due to numerous mitochondria with a fine basophilic granularity due to extensive free ribosomes and rough ER. Fine brown granules of the 'wear and tear' pigment lipofuscin (see Fig. 1.14) are present in variable amounts, increasing with age. All these features are seen in micrograph (a).

Sinusoid lining cells **S** are readily distinguishable from hepatocytes by their flattened condensed nuclei and attenuated poorly stained cytoplasm.

Micrograph (b) demonstrates the presence within the hepatocytes of glycogen granules which, being polysaccharide, are PAS-positive, i.e. stain magenta; the nuclei are counterstained blue.

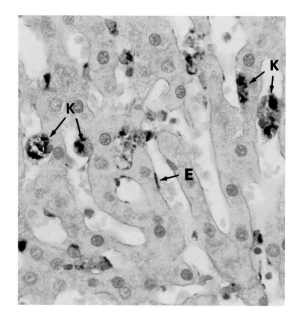

Fig. 15.8   **Sinusoid lining cells**
Perl's Prussian blue × 48

The sinusoid lining cells include at least three cell types. The majority are endothelial cells **E** with flat darkly stained nuclei and thin fenestrated cytoplasm. Scattered among the endothelial cells are large plump phagocytic cells with ovoid nuclei. Known as *Kupffer cells* **K**, these form part of the monocyte–macrophage defence system (see Chs 3 and 4) and, with the spleen, participate in the removal of spent erythrocytes and other particulate debris from the circulation. The phagocytic capability of the Kupffer cells can be demonstrated when they are 'fed', either artificially or under pathological conditions, with appropriate particulate matter. The animal used for this preparation was injected intravenously with a particulate iron-sugar compound, which with this staining method is demonstrated as a dark deposit within the sinusoid lining cells.

The third cell type, known variously as *stellate cells, Ito cells* or *hepatic lipocytes*, cannot be easily distinguished by light microscopy. These recently discovered cells have lipid droplets containing vitamin A in their cytoplasm. These cells have the dual functions of vitamin A storage and production of extracellular matrix and collagen. During liver injury, these cells are thought to produce greatly increased amounts of collagen causing the fibrosis so characteristic of hepatic cirrhosis.

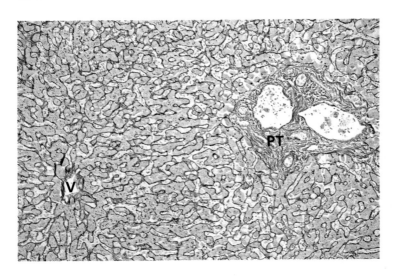

Fig. 15.9 Liver
Reticulin method × 75

Hepatocytes and sinusoid lining cells are supported by a fine meshwork of reticulin fibres (collagen type III, stained black in this preparation), which merge with the sparse collagenous supporting tissue of the portal tracts **PT** and terminal hepatic venules **V**. At the periphery of the liver, the reticulin becomes continuous with a thin but tough collagenous capsule, *Glisson's capsule*, which invests the external surface of the liver.

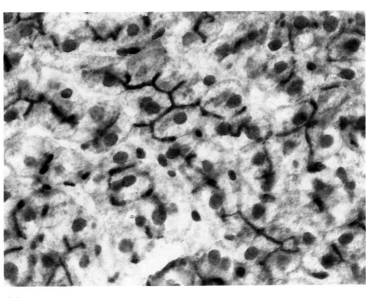

(a)

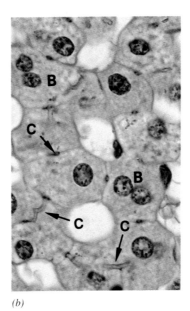

(b)

Fig. 15.10 Bile canaliculi (a) Enzyme histochemical method for ATPase × 480 (b) Iron haematoxylin × 480

Bile is synthesised by all hepatocytes and secreted into a system of minute canaliculi which form an anastomosing network within the plates of hepatocytes. The canaliculi have no discrete structure of their own but consist merely of fine channels formed by the plasma membranes of adjacent hepatocytes; the ultrastructural features are shown in Figure 15.12. Bile canaliculi of adjacent hepatocyte plates merge to form *canals of Hering* before draining into the bile ductules of the portal tracts.

The hepatocyte plasma membranes forming the walls of the canaliculi contain the enzyme ATPase, which

suggests that bile secretion is an energy-dependent process. A histochemical method for ATPase has been used in micrograph (a) to demonstrate bile canaliculi (stained brown), which are difficult to demonstrate with routine light microscopy methods. Within each hepatocyte plate, the canaliculi form a regular hexagonal network reminiscent of chicken wire, each hexagon enclosing a single hepatocyte. In micrograph (b), iron has been deposited in the walls of the canaliculi **C**. Note two binucleate hepatocytes **B**.

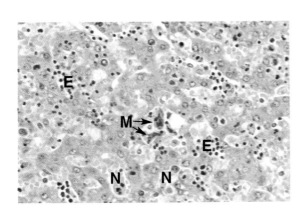

Fig. 15.11 Fetal liver H & E × 100

In fetal life, the liver and spleen are important sites of haemopoeisis (see Ch. 3). When haemopoeisis in bone marrow begins, some time after the fourth month of gestation, the importance of the liver and spleen for this function gradually declines.

In this micrograph of fetal liver, the hepatocyte plates are two cells thick, a normal finding up to the age of about 7 years. The sinusoids are packed with blood precursors, including megakaryocytes **M** and erythroid **E** and myeloid precursors **N**.

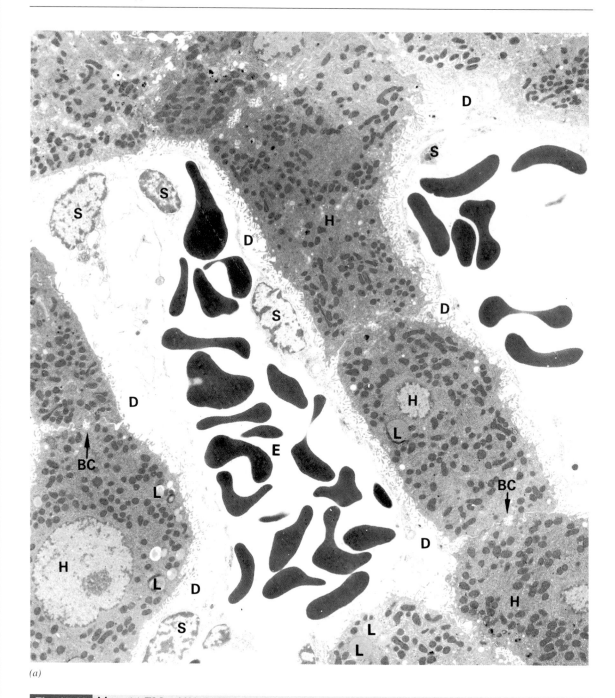

(a)

Fig. 15.12 Liver (a) EM × 4400 (b) EM × 15 200 (*opposite*)

These micrographs demonstrate the main ultrastructural features of the liver. Hepatocytes **H** are exposed on each side to the sinusoids lined by a discontinuous layer of sinusoid lining cells **S**. These are supported by the fine reticulin framework of the liver (see Fig. 15.9) with the *space of Disse* **D** between the lining cells and the hepatocyte surface. Via the gaps in the sinusoid lining, the space of Disse is continuous with the sinusoid lumen, thus bathing the hepatocyte surface with plasma. Numerous irregular microvilli **Mv** extend from the hepatocyte surface into the space of Disse, greatly increasing the surface area for metabolic exchange. Between the bases of the microvilli are coated pits involved in endocytosis. Erythrocytes **E** can be seen within the sinusoids.

Reflecting their extraordinary range of biosynthetic and degradative activities, the hepatocyte cytoplasm (b) is crowded with organelles, particularly rough endoplasmic reticulum **rER**, smooth endoplasmic reticulum **sER**, Golgi stacks, free ribosomes, mitochondria **M**, lysosomes **Ly** and peroxisomes. Lipid droplets **L** and glycogen rosettes are present in variable numbers depending on nutritional status.

Bile canaliculi **BC** are seen to be formed from the plasma membranes of adjacent hepatocytes, the plasma membranes being tightly bound by junctional complexes **J**; small microvilli project into the canaliculi. The subjacent cytoplasm contains a network of actin filaments, contraction of which reduces canalicular diameter, thus reducing flow rate.

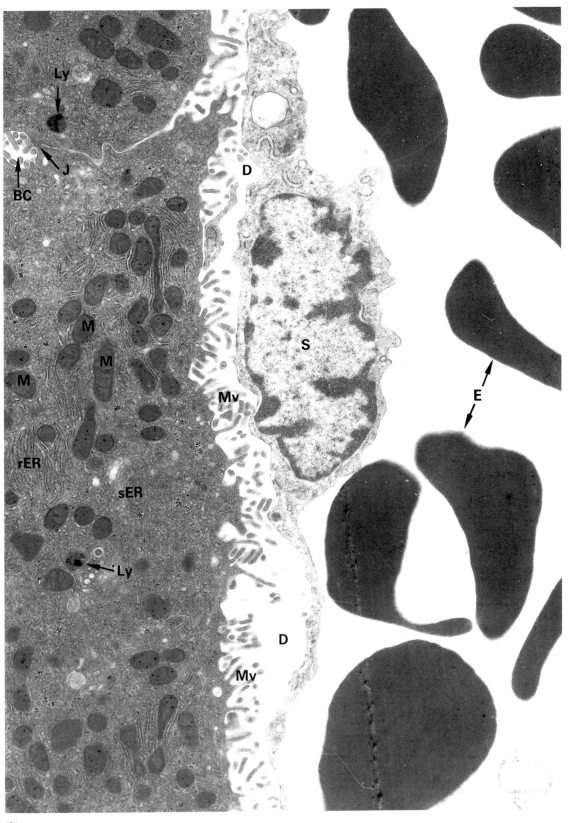

(b)

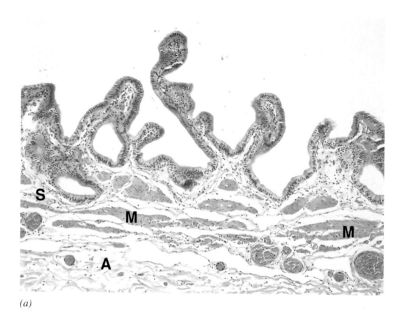

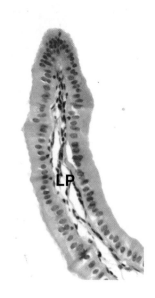

(a)   *(b)*

Fig. 15.13 Gall bladder (a) H & E × 30
(b) H & E × 100 (c) H & E × 10

The intrahepatic bile collecting system merges to form
right and *left hepatic ducts*, which join creating a single
large duct, the *common hepatic duct*. On leaving the
liver, this is joined by the *cystic duct* which drains the
gall bladder. The *common bile duct* so formed joins
the *pancreatic duct* to form the short *ampulla of Vater*
before entering the duodenum. Bile draining down the
common hepatic duct is shunted into the gall bladder
where it is stored and concentrated. The major bile ducts
outwith the liver are collectively called the *extrahepatic
biliary tree*.

The gall bladder is a muscular sac lined by a simple
columnar epithelium; it has a capacity of about 100 ml
in humans. The presence of lipid in the duodenum
promotes the secretion of the hormone cholecystokinin-
pancreozymin (CCK) by endocrine cells of the duodenal
mucosa, stimulating contraction of the gall bladder and
forcing bile into the duodenum. Bile is an emulsifying
agent facilitating the hydrolysis of dietary lipids by
pancreatic lipases.

Micrograph (a) shows the wall of a gall bladder in the
non-distended state in which the mucosa is thrown up into
many folds. The relatively loose submucosa **S** is rich in
elastic fibres, blood vessels and lymphatics, which drain
water reabsorbed from bile during the concentration
process. The fibres of the muscular layer **M** are arranged
in longitudinal, transverse and oblique orientations but do
not form distinct layers. Externally, there is a thick
collagenous adventitial (serosal) coat **A** conveying the
larger blood and lymphatic vessels. In the neck of the gall
bladder and in the extrahepatic biliary tree, mucous
glands are found in the submucosa; mucus may provide a
protective surface film for the biliary tract.

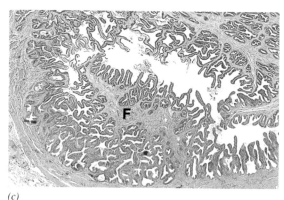

(c)

At high magnification in micrograph (b), the simple
epithelial lining of the gall bladder is seen to consist of very
tall columnar cells with basally located nuclei; numerous
short irregular microvilli account for the unevenness of
the luminal surface. The lining cells concentrate bile
five- to 10-fold by an active process, the resulting water
passing into lymphatics in the lamina propria **LP**.

Micrograph (c) illustrates the wall of the cystic duct
which is formed into a twisted mucosa-covered fold **F**
known as the *spiral valve of Heister*.

The flow of bile and pancreatic juice into the
duodenum is controlled by the complex arrangement of
smooth muscle known as the *sphincter of Oddi*. The
components of this structure include the *choledochal
spincter* at the distal end of the common bile duct, the
pancreatic sphincter at the end of the pancreatic duct and
a meshwork of muscle fibres around the ampulla. This
arrangement controls the flow of bile and pancreatic juice
into the duodenum and at the same time prevents reflux of
bile and pancreatic juice into the wrong parts of the duct
system. When the choledochal sphincter is closed, bile is
directed into the gall bladder where it is concentrated.

Pancreas

The pancreas is a large gland which, like the liver, develops embryologically as an outgrowth of the primitive foregut. The pancreas has both exocrine and endocrine components; the endocrine pancreas is described in detail in Chapter 17. The exocrine pancreas, which forms the bulk of the gland, secretes an enzyme-rich alkaline fluid into the duodenum via the *pancreatic duct*. The high pH of pancreatic secretions is due to a high content of bicarbonate ions and serves to neutralise the acidic chyme as it enters the small intestine from the stomach. The pancreatic enzymes degrade proteins, carbohydrates, lipids and nucleic acids by the process of luminal digestion (see Fig. 14.16). Like pepsin in the stomach, the pancreatic proteolytic enzymes *trypsin* and *chymo-trypsin* are secreted in an inactive form. *Enterokinase*, an enzyme secreted by the duodenal mucosa, activates protrypsin to form trypsin; trypsin then activates prochymotrypsin to form chymotrypsin. This mechanism prevents autodigestion of the pancreas. The other pancreatic enzymes are secreted in the active form.

Pancreatic secretion occurs continuously, the rate being modulated by hormonal and nervous influences. *Secretin*, a hormone released by neuroendocrine cells scattered in the duodenum, promotes the secretion of copious watery fluid rich in bicarbonate. Cholecystokinin-pancreozymin (CCK), also derived from duodenal neuroendocrine cells, stimulates the secretion of enzyme-rich pancreatic fluid. Gastrin, secreted by endocrine cells of the pyloric mucosa, has a similar action on the pancreas to that of CCK. The pancreas is richly inner-vated by the autonomic nervous system, but the effect of this on pancreatic secretion is not well understood.

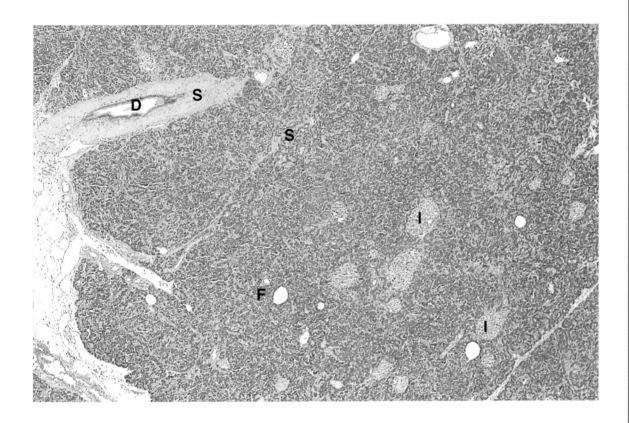

Fig. 15.14   Pancreas **H & E** × 45

The pancreas is a lobulated gland invested by a thin collagenous capsule which extends as delicate septa **S** between the lobules. The exocrine component of the pancreas consists of closely packed secretory acini which drain into a highly branched duct system. Most of the secretion drains into the main pancreatic duct, which joins the common bile duct to drain into the duodenum via the ampulla of Vater; in most people, a small *accessory pancreatic duct* drains into the duodenum more proximally. *Interlobular ducts* **D** can be seen in this micrograph; their surrounding supporting tissue reinforces the septal framework.

The endocrine tissue of the pancreas forms *islets of Langerhans* **I** of various sizes scattered throughout the exocrine tissue. Occasional fat cells **F** are scattered throughout the parenchyma. These are scanty in young adults but are seen in increasing numbers in older people, reflecting the natural atrophy of the gland with age.

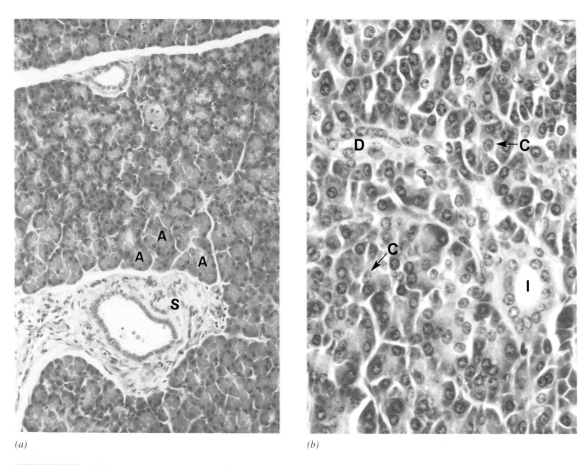

(a) *(b)*

Fig. 15.15 **Exocrine pancreas (a) H & E × 200 (b) H & E × 450 (c) EM × 8500 (*opposite*)**

Details of the pancreatic acini and duct system can be seen in these micrographs. Each acinus is made up of an irregular cluster of pyramid-shaped secretory cells, the apices of which surround a minute central lumen which represents the terminal end of the duct system. The smallest of the tributaries are known as *intercalated ducts*. Adjacent acini are separated by inconspicuous supporting tissue containing numerous capillaries. In histological section, the interacinar spaces tend to appear wider than they do in vivo, due to a fixation artefact. The intercalated ducts drain into small *intralobular ducts*, which in turn drain into the *interlobular ducts* in the septa of the gland. The intercalated ducts are lined by simple low cuboidal epithelium, which becomes stratified cuboidal in the larger ducts. With increasing size, the ducts are invested by a progressively thicker layer of dense collagenous supporting tissue; the wall of the main pancreatic duct contains smooth muscle.

Micrograph (a) shows the general arrangement of the glandular acini **A**. An intralobular duct is seen in upper midfield and a larger interlobular duct in lower midfield, the latter having a much broader sheath of supporting tissue **S**.

At higher magnification in micrograph (b), the cells of each pancreatic acinus have a roughly triangular shape in section, their apices projecting towards a central lumen of a minute duct. The acinar cells are typical protein-secreting (zymogenic) cells. The nuclei are basally located and surrounded by basophilic cytoplasm

crammed with rough endoplasmic reticulum; the apices of the cells are packed with eosinophilic zymogen secretory granules. The centres of the acini frequently contain one or more nuclei of *centroacinar cells* **C** with pale nuclei and sparse pale-stained cytoplasm; these represent the terminal lining cells of intercalated ducts. Cells of similar appearance can be seen between the acini and are those of intercalated ducts **D** passing to join the larger intralobular ducts **I**. The cells lining the intercalated ducts secrete water and bicarbonate ions into the pancreatic juice.

The electron micrograph (c) opposite illustrates part of a pancreatic acinus with its central lumen **L**. The pyramid-shaped secretory cells have round basally located nuclei with dispersed chromatin and prominent nucleoli **Nu**, both characteristic features of highly active cells. The basal cytoplasm is packed with lamellar profiles of rough endoplasmic reticulum **rER**, among which elongated mitochondria **M** are scattered. A large Golgi apparatus **G** is located in a supranuclear position and is responsible for packaging enzymes synthesised on the rough endoplasmic reticulum to form zymogen granules. Newly packed zymogen granules Z_1 are large and much less electron-dense than the smaller mature granules Z_2 which aggregate in the apical cytoplasm. Zymogen granules are released into the acinar lumen by exocytosis; small irregular microvilli associated with this process are seen projecting into the lumen. Note small capillaries **C**, a fibroblast **F** and collagen **Coll** in the fine supporting tissue which surrounds the acinus.

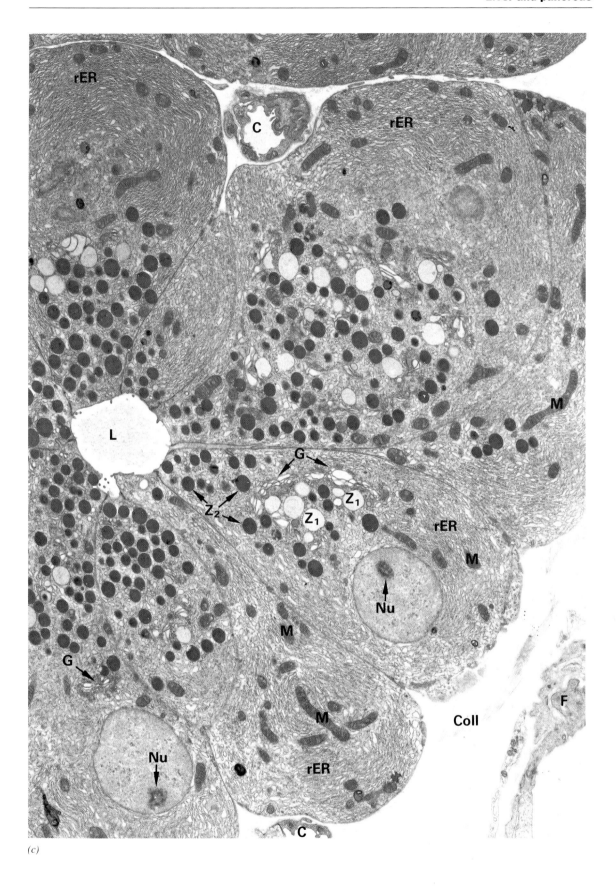

(c)

16. Urinary system

Introduction

The principal function of the urinary system is the maintenance of water and electrolyte homeostasis, which requires that any input into the system is balanced by an equivalent output. The urinary system provides the mechanism by which excess water and electrolytes are eliminated from the body. A second major function of the urinary system is the excretion of many toxic metabolic waste products, particularly the nitrogenous compounds urea and creatinine; this function is intimately related to water and electrolyte elimination which provides an appropriate fluid vehicle. The end product of these processes is *urine*. Since all body fluids are maintained in dynamic equilibrium with one another by the circulatory system, any adjustment in the composition of the blood results in similar changes in the other fluid compartments of the body. Thus regulation of the osmotic concentration of blood plasma by the kidneys (*osmoregulation*) ensures the osmotic regulation of all other body fluids.

The functional and structural unit of the kidney, the *nephron*, consists of a *renal corpuscle* plus a long folded *renal tubule*. The human kidney contains approximately one million nephrons. Nephrons perform the functions of osmoregulation and excretion by the following processes:

- Filtration of most small molecules from blood plasma to form an ultrafiltrate of plasma.
- Selective reabsorption of most of the water and some other molecules from the ultrafiltrate, leaving behind excess and waste materials to be excreted.
- Secretion of some excretory products directly from blood into the urine.
- Maintenance of the acid–base balance by selective secretion of H^+ ions into the urine.

The kidney also participates in other homeostatic mechanisms either by production or by modification of various hormones:

- *Renin*, synthesised in the kidney, is a component of the *renin–angiotensin–aldosterone* mechanism which controls blood pressure.
- *Erythropoietin*, synthesised in the kidney, stimulates the production of erythrocytes in the bone marrow and thus regulates the oxygen-carrying capacity of the blood.
- *Vitamin D*, which regulates calcium balance, is converted to an active form in the kidney.

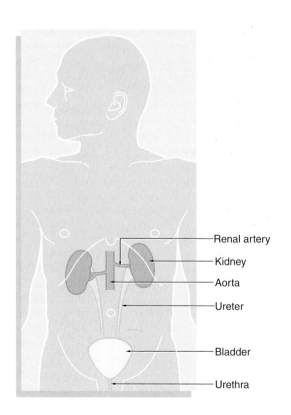

Renal artery
Kidney
Aorta
Ureter
Bladder
Urethra

Fig. 16.1 The urinary system

The urinary system comprises two *kidneys*, two *ureters*, a *bladder* and a *urethra*. Urine is produced in the kidneys and flows down the ureters to the bladder where it is stored until voided via the urethra. The kidneys and ureters are found in the retroperitoneum while the urinary bladder is in the anterior part of the pelvis.

Blood is supplied to each kidney by the *renal arteries*, which arise from the aorta. One or more *renal veins* drains each kidney to the inferior vena cava. The total blood volume of the body is circulated through the kidneys about 300 times each day.

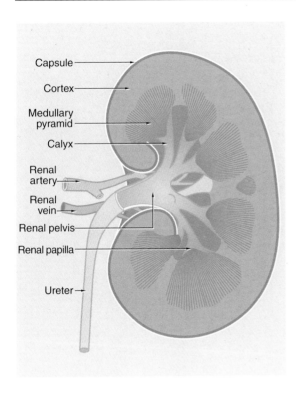

Capsule
Cortex
Medullary pyramid
Calyx
Renal artery
Renal vein
Renal pelvis
Renal papilla
Ureter

Fig. 16.2 Kidney

The kidney is a bean-shaped organ lying in the upper retroperitoneal area and oriented with the *hilum* directed medially. In adults the kidney measures 10–12 cm. The hilum is the site of entry and exit of the renal blood vessels and the ureter.

The archetypal kidney of lower mammals consists of a single lobe made up of a *medullary pyramid* (which is really cone-shaped), the base of which is enveloped by the cortex containing the renal corpuscles and the proximal and distal parts of the tubules. Nephrons arise in the cortex and then loop down into the medulla for a variable distance, returning again to the cortex. From here they drain into *collecting ducts* which descend again into the medulla to discharge urine from the apex of the medullary pyramid. The apical part of the pyramid is enveloped by a funnel-shaped *renal pelvis* which represents the dilated proximal part of the ureter; that part of the medullary pyramid surrounded by the pelvis is known as the *renal papilla*.

The human kidney is made up of 10–18 lobes. In the adult the cortical components of the lobes are fused so that the cortex forms a continuous smooth outer zone which extends down between the pyramids. The *renal medulla* is made up of multiple medullary pyramids separated by medullary extensions of the cortex. Each renal papilla is surrounded by a branch of the renal pelvis called a *calyx*, the whole urinary collecting system within the kidney being described as the *pelvicalyceal system*.

The kidney is invested by a tough fibrous capsule, which is surrounded by a thick layer of perinephric fat which provides some protection from trauma.

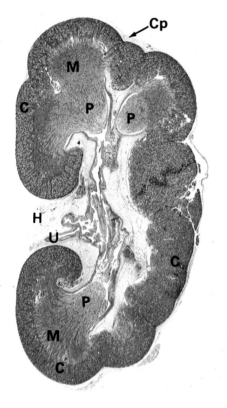

Cp
M
C
P
P
H
U
C
P
M
C

Fig. 16.3 Kidney H & E × 3

This micrograph of a kidney from a stillborn child illustrates at low power the features of the kidney described in Figure 16.2. The kidney of a baby has been chosen as it is small enough to section and photograph as a whole. Furthermore its convex surface is irregular, reflecting the development of the many lobes making up the organ. In histological section, only a single plane through the pelvicalyceal system can be visualised. This plane of section includes the axes of three lobes, the papilla **P** of each one projecting into the central pelvicalyceal space; this drains into the ureter **U** which leaves the kidney via the hilum **H**.

The darker stained cortex **C** can be clearly differentiated from the paler stained medulla **M**. The cortex contains large numbers of tiny spheroidal structures, the developing renal corpuscles (see Fig. 16.4). The medullary pyramids are characterised by the numerous tubules converging towards the tips of the renal papillae. Note the continuity of the cortex throughout the outer zone of the kidney and the cortical extension between the two medullary pyramids at the top of the field. The fibrous capsule **Cp** of the kidney is continuous at the hilum with supporting tissue, which packs the spaces between the hilar structures. In adults, the hilum contains significant quantities of adipose tissue. The renal artery and vein also pass through the hilum but are not seen in this plane of section.

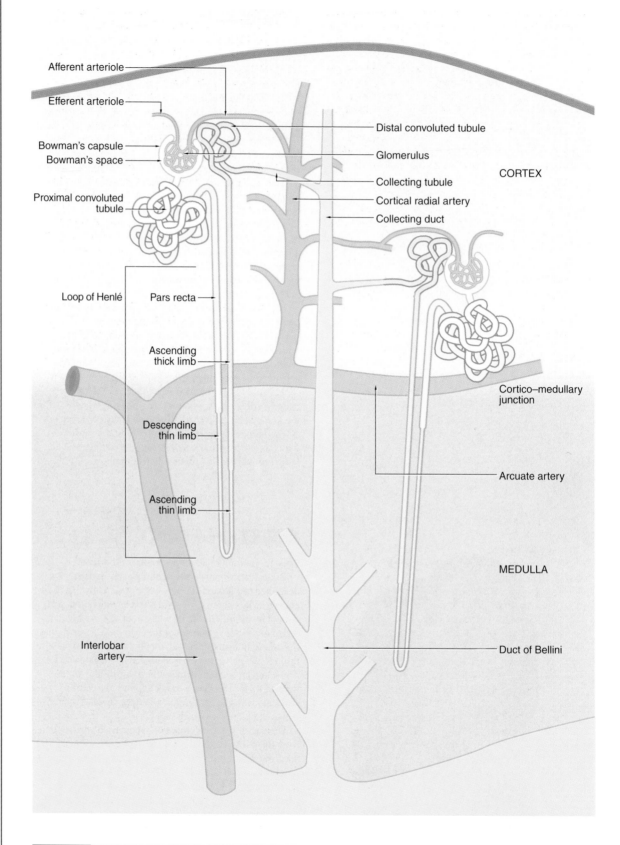

Afferent arteriole

Efferent arteriole

Bowman's capsule

Bowman's space

Proximal convoluted tubule

Loop of Henlé

Pars recta

Ascending thick limb

Descending thin limb

Ascending thin limb

Interlobar artery

Distal convoluted tubule

Glomerulus

CORTEX

Collecting tubule

Cortical radial artery

Collecting duct

Cortico–medullary junction

Arcuate artery

MEDULLA

Duct of Bellini

Fig. 16.4 Basic organisation of the nephron, collecting system and renal vasculature

The nephron and collecting system

The nephron, the functional unit of the kidney, consists of two major components, the *renal corpuscle* and the *renal tubule*.

Renal corpuscle. The renal corpuscle is responsible for the filtration of plasma and is a combination of two structures, *Bowman's capsule* and the *glomerulus*.

Bowman's capsule consists of a single layer of flattened cells resting on a basement membrane; it is derived from the distended, blind end of the renal tubule.

The glomerulus is a globular network of anastomosing capillaries which invaginates Bowman's capsule (see Fig. 16.8). Within the capsule, the glomerulus is invested by a layer of epithelial cells called *podocytes*, which constitute the *visceral layer of Bowman's capsule*; the visceral layer is reflected around the vascular stalk of the glomerulus to become continuous with the *parietal layer* which constitutes Bowman's capsule proper. The space between the visceral and parietal layers is known as *Bowman's space* and is continuous with the lumen of the renal tubule; the parietal epithelium of Bowman's capsule is continuous with the epithelium lining the renal tubule.

In the renal corpuscle, water and low molecular weight constituents of plasma are filtered from the glomerular capillaries into Bowman's space to form the *glomerular ultrafiltrate*, which then passes into the renal tubule. Thus the filtration barrier between the capillary lumen and Bowman's space consists of the capillary endothelium, the podocyte layer and their common basement membrane known as the *glomerular basement membrane* (see Fig. 16.14).

The *afferent arteriole*, which supplies the glomerulus, and the *efferent arteriole*, which drains it, enter and leave the corpuscle at the *vascular pole* which is usually situated opposite the entrance to the renal tubule, the *urinary pole* (see Fig. 16.7).

Renal tubule. The renal tubule extends from Bowman's capsule to its junction with a *collecting duct*. The renal tubule is up to 55 mm long in humans and is lined by a single layer of epithelial cells. The primary function of the renal tubule is the selective reabsorption of water, inorganic ions and other molecules from the glomerular filtrate. In addition, some inorganic ions are secreted directly from blood into the lumen of the tubule. In humans, glomerular filtrate is produced at a steady rate of approximately 120 ml/min; of this, all but about 1 ml is reabsorbed by the renal tubules. The renal tubule has a convoluted shape and has four distinct histophysiological zones, each of which has a different role in tubular function.

1. *The proximal convoluted tubule* (*PCT*) is the longest, most convoluted section of the tubule and is responsible for the reabsorption of approximately 65% of the ions and water of the glomerular filtrate. PCTs are confined to the renal cortex and make up the greater part of its bulk.
2. *The loop of Henle* includes the distal straight part of the proximal tubule, the *pars recta*, the *thin descending and ascending limbs*, and the *thick ascending limb*. The difference between these parts is due to differences in the epithelial lining. The thin segments of the loop of Henle dip down into the medulla where they form a hairpin bend. The length of the loop of Henle varies from short to long depending on the location of the renal corpuscle of the particular nephron. The corpuscles of short-looped nephrons tend to be located in the superficial and midcortical regions, the loops extending very little beyond the corticomedullary junction. Long-looped nephrons are mainly associated with juxtamedullary corpuscles; a small proportion of long loops almost reach the tips of the renal papillae but successively greater numbers turn back at higher levels as necessitated by the tapering shape of the medullary pyramids. The limbs of the loop of Henle are closely associated with parallel wide capillary loops, the *vasa recta* (not shown in this diagram), which arise from the efferent arterioles of glomeruli located near the corticomedullary junction. The vasa recta descend into the medulla then loop

back on themselves to drain into veins at the junction of the medulla and cortex. The main function of the loops of Henle is to generate a high osmotic pressure in the extracellular fluid of the renal medulla; the mechanism by which this is achieved is known as the *counter-current multiplier system* (see Fig. 16.21). In some animals the loop of Henle plays a major role in reabsorption of water from the glomerular filtrate back into the circulation via the vasa recta; however, this function is of lesser importance in the human kidney.
3. *The distal convoluted tubule* (*DCT*) is a continuation of the thick limb of the loop of Henle after its return from the medulla. Shorter and less convoluted than the PCT, the DCT is responsible for reabsorption of sodium ions by an active process which is controlled by the adrenocortical hormone *aldosterone*. Sodium reabsorption is coupled with the secretion of hydrogen or potassium ions into the DCT, the secretion of hydrogen ions resulting in a net loss of acid from the body.
4. *The collecting tubule* is the straight terminal portion of the nephron, several collecting tubules converging to form a *collecting duct*. The collecting ducts descend through the cortex in parallel bundles called *medullary rays* (see Fig. 16.5), progressively merging in the medulla to form the large *ducts of Bellini* which open at the tips of the renal papillae to discharge urine into the pelvicalyceal system. The collecting tubules and ducts are not normally permeable to water. However, in the presence of *antidiuretic hormone* (*ADH*) secreted by the posterior pituitary, the collecting tubules and ducts become permeable to water, which is then drawn out by the high osmotic pressure generated by the counter-current multiplier system into the interstitial tissues of the medulla. From here water is returned to the general circulation via the vasa recta. The loops of Henle and ADH thus provide a mechanism for the production of urine which is hypertonic with respect to plasma.

The nephron arises embryologically from the *nephrogenic blastema* and the collecting ducts from the *ureteric bud*. There is some question as to which the collecting tubules are derived from.

Renal vasculature
Each kidney is supplied by a single renal artery which divides in the hilum into two main branches. Each of these gives rise to several *interlobar arteries*, which ascend between the pyramids to the corticomedullary junction. Here they branch to form the *arcuate arteries*, which run in an arc-like course parallel to the capsule of the kidney. The arcuate arteries give rise to numerous *cortical radial* (*interlobular*) *arteries*, which radiate towards the capsule, branching to form the afferent arterioles of the glomeruli.

As previously described, the vasa recta form a continuation of the efferent arterioles of juxtamedullary glomeruli and form the microcirculation of the renal medulla. The efferent arterioles of the rest of the cortex divide to form the plexus of capillaries that surround the tubules of the renal cortex. The cortical and medullary capillaries drain via *cortical radial* (*interlobular*) *veins* to *arcuate veins* at the cortico-medullary junction and thence to the *renal vein*.

ORGAN SYSTEMS

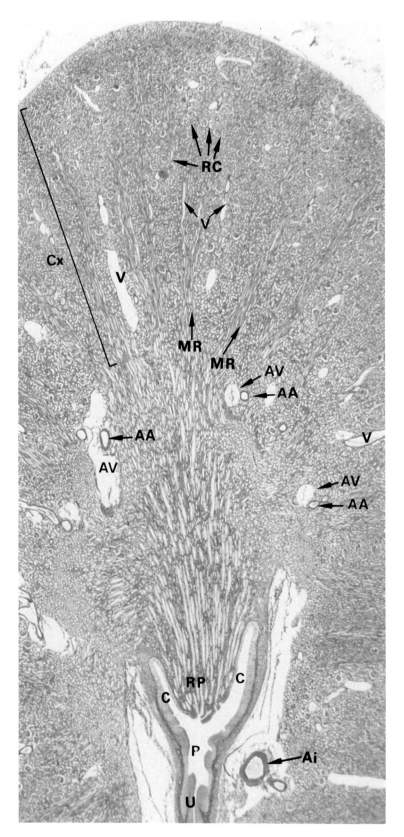

Fig. 16.5 Kidney (monkey)
Jones' methenamine silver
H & E × 12

The basic geography of the kidney can be seen in this unilobular kidney which has been sectioned through the axis of the medullary pyramid. Note the cup-shaped calyx **C** surrounding the renal papilla **RP** and converging via the pelvis **P** onto the ureter **U**.

In the cortex **Cx**, numerous renal corpuscles **RC** (200 μm in diameter) are just visible at this magnification. The corpuscles tend to be arranged in parallel rows at right angles to the capsule, separated by cortical radial arteries from which they derive their blood supply. Cortical radial arteries are too narrow to be identified at this magnification but a number of their accompanying thin-walled cortical radial veins **V** are easily seen.

Most of the cortical parenchyma surrounding the renal corpuscles consists of proximal and distal convoluted tubules. From the cortex, pale stained *medullary rays* **MR** radiate towards the medulla; they consist of collecting tubules and ducts draining nephrons located high in the cortex. The collecting ducts merge in the medulla to form the larger ducts of Bellini which converge towards the tip of the renal papilla. Although not visible at this magnification, long loops of Henle dip into the medulla between, and parallel with, the collecting ducts. The long, straight vasa recta also dip down into the medulla alongside the loops of Henle; these vessels, too small to be seen at this magnification, absorb water from the loops of Henle and collecting ducts.

The corticomedullary junction is marked by several arcuate arteries **AA** and their associated thin-walled arcuate veins **AV**. Note a large interlobar branch of the renal artery **Ai** in the hilar supporting tissue.

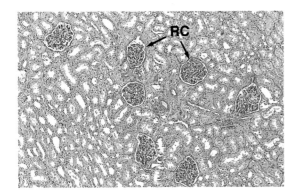

Fig. 16.6 **Renal cortex** H & E × 40

Higher magnification reveals more details of the cortical parenchyma. Renal corpuscles **RC** appear as dense rounded structures, the *glomeruli*, surrounded by narrow Bowman's spaces. Even at this magnification, it is evident that the tubules making up the bulk of the parenchyma between the renal corpuscles differ from one another in diameter, shape and staining intensity. The cortical tubules mainly consist of proximal convoluted tubules with smaller numbers of distal convoluted tubules and collecting tubules.

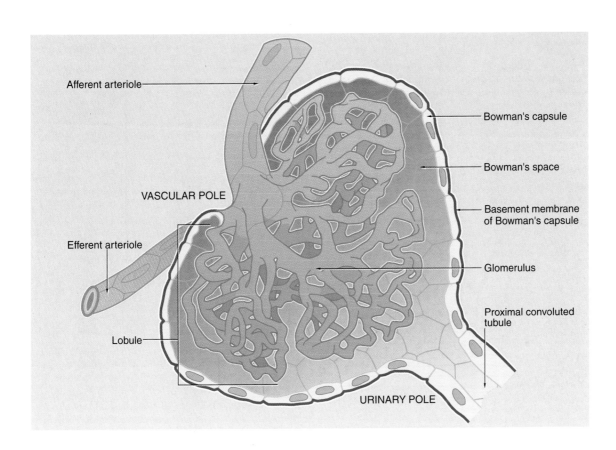

Fig. 16.7 **Renal corpuscle**

The main structural features of the renal corpuscle are demonstrated in this idealised diagram.

The relatively wide diameter afferent arteriole enters Bowman's capsule at the vascular pole of the renal corpuscle and then branches to form an anastomosing network of glomerular capillaries, each major branch giving rise to a *lobule*. The glomerulus is thus suspended in Bowman's space from the vascular pole. Although not shown in this diagram, the spaces between the capillary loops in each glomerular lobule are filled by basement membrane-like material called *mesangium*, which contains mesangial cells.

The efferent vessel draining the glomerulus is unusual in that it has the structure of an arteriole and is thus called the efferent arteriole (rather than the efferent venule). The efferent arteriole is of smaller diameter than the afferent arteriole and a pressure gradient is thus maintained which drives the filtration of plasma into Bowman's space.

The layer of podocytes investing the glomerular capillaries (visceral layer of Bowman's capsule) is not shown in this diagram. At the vascular pole, the podocyte layer is reflected to become continuous with the epithelium of Bowman's capsule proper, which in turn becomes continuous with the first part of the renal tubule, the proximal convoluted tubule.

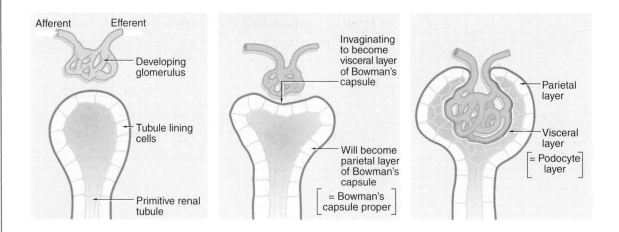

Fig. 16.8 Development of the renal corpuscle

This diagram illustrates in a highly schematic manner the mode of development of the renal corpuscle. The tubules develop from the embryological *metanephros* as blind-ended tubes consisting of a single layer of cuboidal epithelium. The ends of the tubules dilate and become invaginated by a tiny mass of mesodermal tissue which differentiates to form the glomerulus. The layer of invaginated epithelium flattens and differentiates into podocytes which become closely applied to the surface of the knot of glomerular capillaries. Most of the intervening tissue disappears so that the basement membrane of

glomerular endothelial cells and podocytes effectively fuse, forming the glomerular basement membrane. A small amount of tissue remains to support the capillary loops and differentiates to form the mesangium. Where the mesangium stretches between the capillary loops, its urinary surface is invested by podocyte cytoplasm with underlying basement membrane. When examining ultrathin light microscope specimens (e.g. Fig. 16.11) and electron micrographs (e.g. Fig. 16.14), the podocytes, endothelial cells and mesangium are identified most easily by tracing out the glomerular basement membrane.

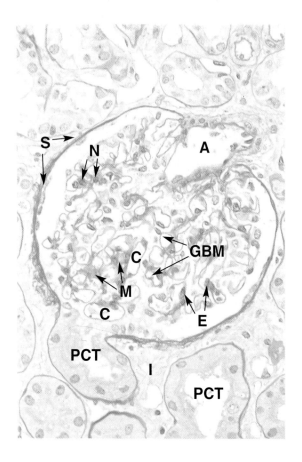

Fig. 16.9 Renal corpuscle PAS × 300

This renal corpuscle has been sectioned through the vascular pole and shows the afferent arteriole **A** entering the glomerulus. The efferent arteriole is not seen in this plane of section. At the opposite pole (the urinary pole) the start of the proximal convoluted tubule **PCT** can be identified. Other proximal convoluted tubules can be seen cut in various planes of section embedded in the renal interstitium **I**. Glomerular capillaries **C** are cut in transverse, longitudinal and oblique sections. The numerous nuclei in the glomerulus are those of capillary endothelial cells, mesangial cells and podocytes.

The PAS stain picks out the glomerular basement membrane **GBM** and the mesangium **M** which consists of basement membrane-like material. Mesangial cells are found embedded within the mesangium but only their nuclei **N** can be discerned by this staining method. The capillary lumina are lined by endothelial cells **E**.

Note the flattened nuclei of the squamous cells **S** lining Bowman's capsule. The squamous epithelium becomes continuous with the epithelium of the proximal convoluted tubule.

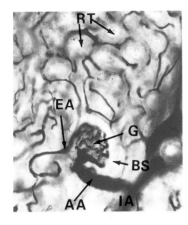

Fig. 16.10 **Blood supply of the glomerulus**
Carmine-gelatine perfused × 128

This section is from a kidney which has been perfused with a red dye in order to demonstrate the renal blood supply; the nephrons remain unstained.

An interlobular artery **IA** can be seen branching to form the afferent arteriole **AA** of a glomerulus **G**. The efferent arteriole **EA** leaving the glomerulus is of much smaller diameter than the afferent arteriole, an arrangement which maintains pressure within glomerular capillaries necessary for blood plasma to be filtered into Bowman's space **BS**. Blood pressure within the glomerulus is controlled by variation of the diameter of the afferent and efferent arterioles.

In the superficial and midcortex as shown here, efferent arterioles give rise to a network of capillaries which surround the renal tubules **RT**; towards the medulla, efferent arterioles give rise to the vasa recta. Molecules reabsorbed from glomerular filtrate are returned to the general circulation via this capillary network which drains into the renal venous system.

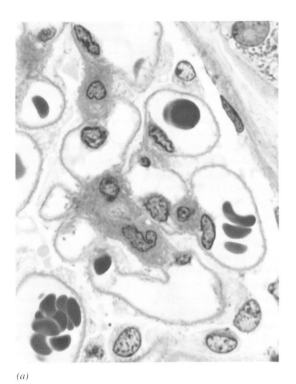

(a)

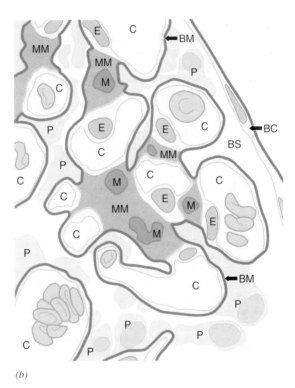

(b)

Fig. 16.11 **Glomerulus** (a) Thin section, toluidine blue × 1200 (b) Explanatory diagram

Using resin-embedding techniques it is possible to cut thin sections (approximately 0.5–1.0 μm thick) which permit much greater resolution at high magnification.

In this preparation, the glomerular capillaries **C**, some of which contain erythrocytes, are defined by the prominent glomerular basement membranes **BM**. Occasional capillary endothelial cell nuclei **E** are seen bulging into the capillary lumina. Mesangium **MM** consists of material similar to basement membrane and contains mesangial cells **M**. Mesangial cells, which are probably modified pericytes, have a number of functions, including phagocytosis, contractility by virtue of their cytoplasmic actin and myosin filaments, and secretion of various vasoactive substances. The last two functions can alter the diameter of capillaries and therefore control glomerular blood flow. The mesangium is separated from the capillary lumen only by a thin layer of fenestrated endothelial cell cytoplasm, the basement membrane of which merges with the mesangial stroma. The podocytes and their basement membrane invest the outer surface of the mesangium. Thus particulate matter from blood may pass into the mesangium where it can be phagocytosed and degraded by mesangial cells.

Podocytes **P** also invest the capillary loops exposed to Bowman's space **BS**. The podocytes have extensive branching pale stained cytoplasm and large round pale stained nuclei. Note the nuclei of two squamous cells of Bowman's capsule **BC**.

Fig. 16.12 The glomerular filter

During filtration of plasma from glomerular capillaries into the renal tubule, the filtrate passes through three layers: capillary endothelium, glomerular basement membrane and the podocyte layer. All contribute to the filtration process.

- The capillary endothelium contains numerous large round fenestrations (70–100 nm in diameter) which occupy about 20% of the endothelial surface area. In adults the fenestrations do not exhibit diaphragms as in fenestrated capillaries elsewhere in the body (see Fig. 8.14). Another unusual feature is that the luminal surface of the endothelium is negatively charged due to a surface layer of a glycoprotein called *podocalyxin*.
- The glomerular basement membrane (240–340 nm) is much thicker than other basement membranes and appears to be elaborated by both capillary endothelial cells and podocytes. As with basement membranes elsewhere (see Ch. 4), it consists of a feltwork of type IV collagen, structural glycoproteins (fibronectin and laminin) and proteoglycans rich in heparan sulphate, the interstices of this highly cross-linked structure being occupied by water molecules. By electron microscopy, the glomerular basement membrane consists of three layers, a dense central layer, the *lamina densa*, with a thinner electron-lucent layer on either side of it, the *lamina rara interna* under the endothelium and the *lamina rara externa* supporting the podocytes. Both laminae rarae are negatively charged.
- The podocytes have long cytoplasmic extensions called *primary processes* which embrace the capillaries, giving rise to short *secondary foot processes (pedicels)* which interdigitate with those of other primary processes. The secondary foot processes are directly applied to the lamina rara externa and bound to it by fine filaments. The gaps between adjacent secondary foot processes, known as *filtration slits*, are of uniform width (25 nm) and are bridged by a delicate electron-dense diaphragm 4 nm thick. A layer of negatively charged *podocalyxin* covers the urinary surface of the podocytes including the filtration slits. Podocyte cytoplasm contains actin filaments as well as lysosomes and microtubules and thus, as well as elaborating glomerular basement membrane, the podocytes also seem to have contractile and phagocytic functions.

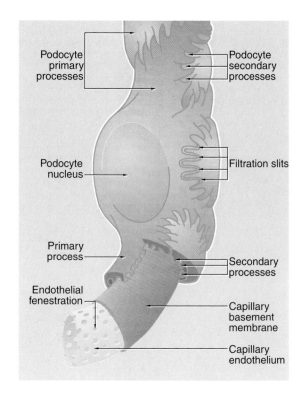

As mentioned at the outset, all layers contribute to the selective filtration process. Clinical evidence demonstrates that free haemoglobin (MW 65 000) and smaller molecules pass freely through the glomerular filter, whereas albumin (MW 68 000) and larger molecules are retained. For macromolecules, three factors determine permeability, namely electrical charge, size and configuration. Negatively charged (cationic) molecules are blocked by the negatively charged endothelial cell coat and laminae rarae of the basement membrane, whilst the meshwork of the lamina densa of the basement membrane discriminates on the basis of molecular size and configuration. The filtration slit diaphragm restricts the passage of any large molecules but its main role is in controlling water flow which is also held back by the colloidal osmotic pressure of retained albumin and other large molecules. The phagocytic function of the podocytes is to remove any large molecules which become trapped in the outer layers of the filter. Molecules trapped on the endothelial side are phagocytosed by mesangial cells.

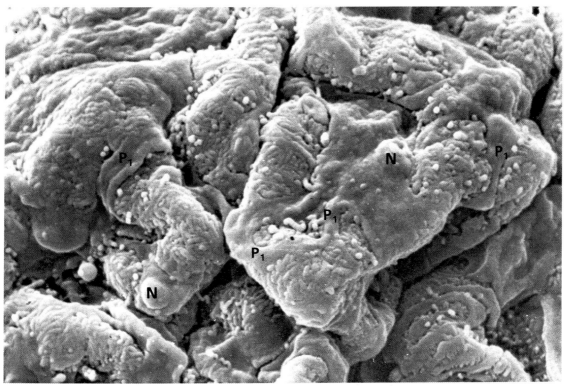

(a)

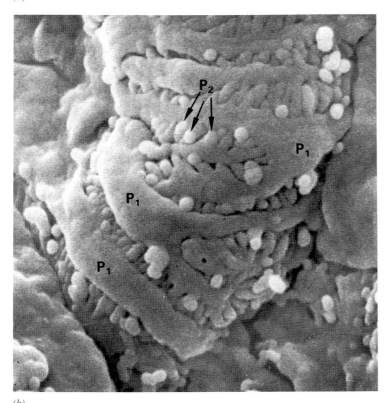

(b)

Fig. 16.13 **Glomerulus**
SEM, (a) × 1500 (b) × 6000

Scanning electron microscopy readily demonstrates the three-dimensional relationships of podocytes and their processes which extend like octopus tentacles over the whole surface of the glomerulus.

Micrograph (a) shows part of a glomerular capillary tuft. The capillaries are enveloped by podocytes which have large flattened cell bodies and bulging nuclei **N**. Each podocyte has several long primary processes P_1 which embrace one or more capillaries. Each primary process has numerous secondary foot processes (pedicels) which rest on the lamina rara externa of the glomerular basement membrane.

At higher magnification in micrograph (b), the secondary foot processes P_2 can be seen as extensions of the large primary processes P_1. The secondary foot processes interdigitate with those of other primary processes separated by filtration slits of uniform width.

ORGAN SYSTEMS

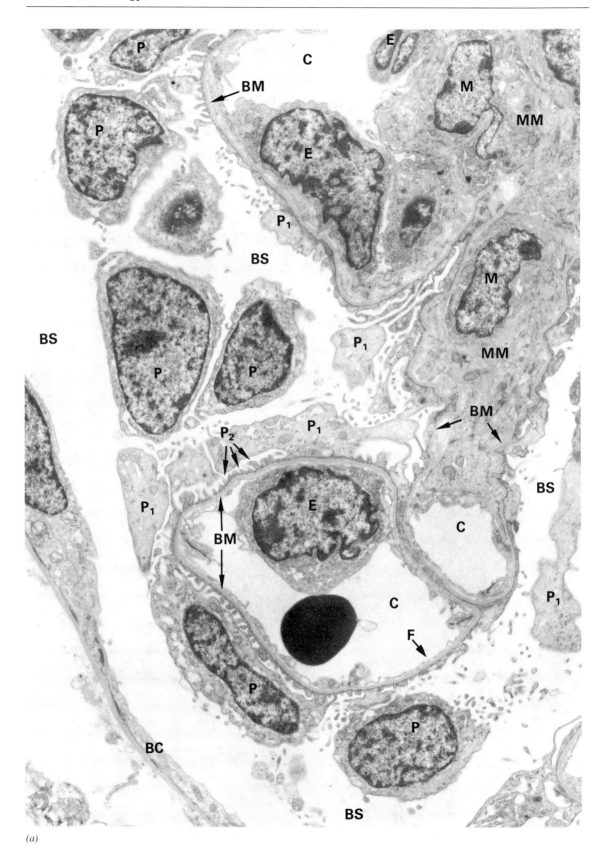

(a)

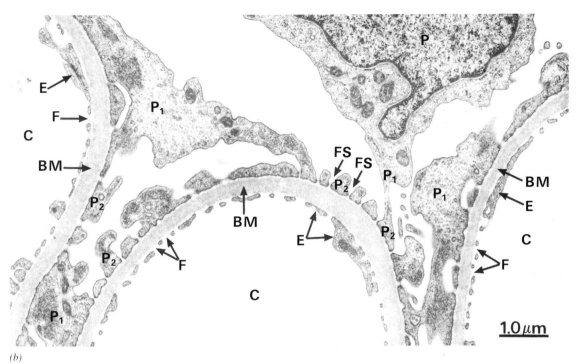

(b)

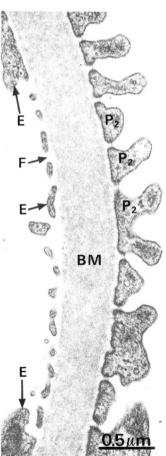

(c)

Fig. 16.14 **Glomerulus**
(a) EM × 4800 *(opposite)* **(b) EM × 14 000 (c) EM × 30 000**

Micrograph (a) shows several capillary loops **C** recognisable by their content of erythrocytes. The capillaries are lined by a thin layer of fenestrated endothelial cytoplasm, and endothelial cell nuclei **E** can be seen bulging into the capillary lumina; capillary endothelial fenestrations **F** are better seen at higher magnification in micrographs (b) and (c). The nuclei of several podocytes **P** can be seen, their primary processes **P₁** giving rise to numerous secondary foot processes **P₂** which rest on the glomerular basement membrane **BM**. At right midfield a branched mesangial stalk comprising mesangial cells **M** and dense mesangial matrix **MM** provides support for the capillary loops. The mesangium is separated from the capillary lumen only by the cytoplasm of the endothelial cells, while the podocytes and their basement membrane continue around the mesangial stalk separating it from Bowman's space. Part of Bowman's capsule **BC** is seen at the periphery, consisting of a squamous epithelial cell and underlying basement membrane. Each parietal epithelial cell has a single central cilium (not seen in this plane of section).
Note the labyrinth of Bowman's space **BS** ramifying throughout the glomerulus.

Micrograph (b), shows three glomerular capillaries **C** lined by attenuated endothelial cytoplasm **E** with wide fenestrations **F**. A podocyte **P** extends several primary foot processes **P₁** onto the capillaries, these in turn giving rise to multiple secondary foot processes **P₂** separated by filtration slits **FS**. A common basement membrane **BM** separates the podocytes and capillary endothelium. The thickness of the basement membrane appears variable but this is due to the slightly oblique plane of section; the basement membranes are in fact of uniform width.

With further magnification in micrograph (c), the three components of the glomerular filter are seen. The fenestrated capillary endothelium **E** is closely applied to the luminal surface of the glomerular basement membrane **BM**; on the opposite side are podocyte secondary foot processes **P₂**, separated by filtration slits of uniform width and bridged by fine electron-dense diaphragms. The wide central lamina densa of the glomerular basement membrane can be seen bordered on each side by a narrow lamina rara.

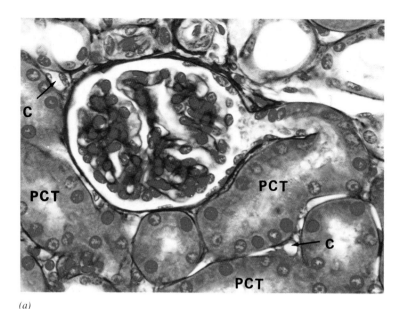
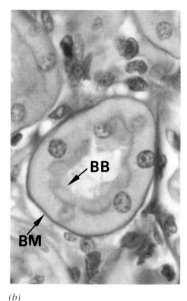

(a) *(b)*

Fig. 16.15 **Proximal convoluted tubule**
(a) Azan × 480 (b) PAS/haematoxylin × 800 (c) EM × 600 *(opposite above)*, (d) EM × 8500 *(opposite below)*

The proximal convoluted tubule (PCT) is a coiled tube measuring approximately 14 mm in length and sections of PCT thus dominate the parenchyma of the renal cortex. Approximately 65% of the glomerular filtrate is reabsorbed from the PCT, a function which is reflected in the structure of the epithelial lining.

Micrograph (a) shows a proximal convoluted tubule **PCT** arising from a renal corpuscle; convolutions of the PCT are also seen in longitudinal, oblique and transverse sections. The simple cuboidal epithelium has a prominent blue stained brush border of tall microvilli. This increases the surface area of plasma membrane some 20-fold. The cytoplasm of PCT epithelial cells stains intensely due to a high content of organelles, principally mitochondria. The basement membrane of the tubules stains blue with this staining method as do the glomerular basement membranes and that of Bowman's capsule.

The PAS staining method has been used in micrograph (b) to demonstrate the prominent brush border **BB** projecting into the lumen of the PCT. The brush border is PAS-positive since the surfaces of the microvilli are coated with a particularly dense glycocalyx (see Fig. 1.2) which is thought to afford physical and chemical protection to the microvilli. Like those elsewhere, the basement membrane **BM** supporting the tubular epithelium is strongly PAS-positive. In both micrographs, note that the epithelial cells of the PCT have round nuclei with prominent nucleoli.

A rich network of capillaries **C** arising from the efferent arteriole of the glomerulus (see Fig. 16.10) surrounds the proximal tubules and returns molecules reabsorbed from the glomerular filtrate back into the general circulation.

In micrograph (c), electron microscopy of the proximal tubule reveals profuse tall microvilli **Mv** constituting the brush border seen with light microscopy. The cytoplasm immediately beneath the brush border contains many pinocytotic vesicles **V** and lysosomes **L** which are involved in reabsorption and degradation of small amounts of protein that have leaked through the glomerular filter. Reabsorbed solutes are transported into surrounding capillaries **Cap** with attenuated endothelium **E** resting on a very thin basement membrane **BM**$_E$; note the narrow intervening supporting tissue layer **S**.

The epithelial cells of the PCT form multiple lateral processes **P** (micrograph (d)) which interdigitate with each other to form a complex *lateral intercellular space*, which has a plasma membrane area equivalent to the luminal plasma membrane. The lateral intercellular space is separated from the lumen of the PCT by a ring of junctional complexes **J** near the luminal surface. These lateral interdigitations were previously thought to be basal infoldings of the basal plasma membrane. The mitochondria **M** in these processes are elongated and arranged at right angles to the basement membrane **BM**. These mitochondria supply ATP for the active transport of Na$^+$ by the Na$^+$-K$^+$ ATPase (sodium pump) located in the basolateral plasma membrane. Thus active transport of Na$^+$ occurs across the plasma membrane into the lateral intercellular space. This active transport of Na$^+$ out of the cell is accompanied by facilitated transport into the cells of Na$^+$, glucose and amino acids by means of transport proteins found in the membrane of the brush border. Almost 100% of the filtered glucose and amino acids is reabsorbed by the PCT.

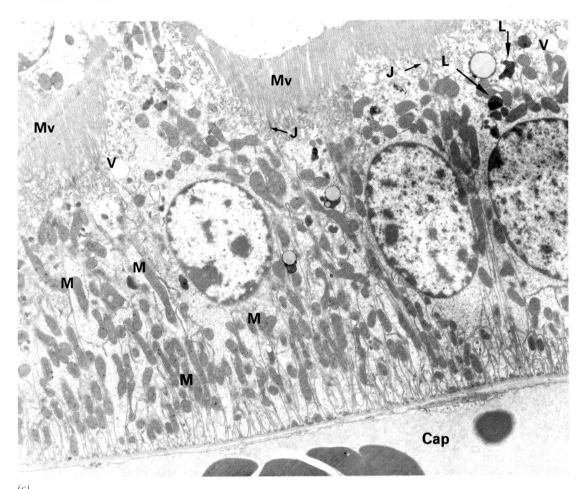

(c)

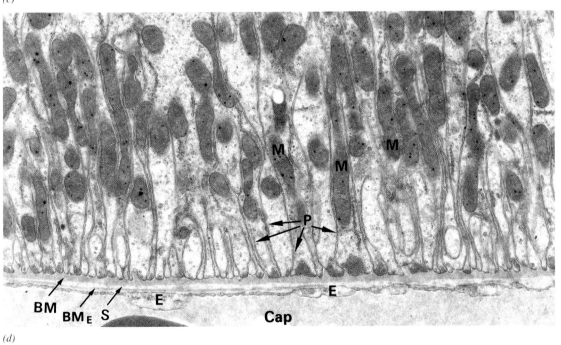

(d)

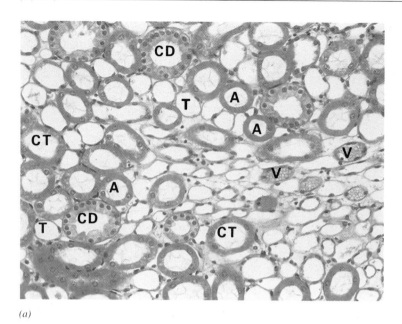

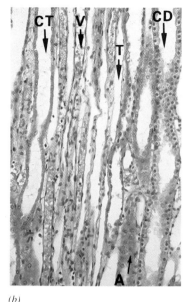

(a)   *(b)*

Fig. 16.16   **Loop of Henle** (a) H & E, TS × 198 (b) H & E, LS × 100

The loop of Henle is made up of four parts:

- the *pars recta* of the proximal tubule
- the *thin descending limb*
- the *thin ascending limb*
- the *thick ascending limb*.

The pars recta is the second, straight part of the proximal tubule which extends down into the outer medulla. There is an abrupt transition to the thin descending limb, which loops down into the medulla for a variable distance. The thin limbs of juxtamedullary nephrons extend down to the inner medulla before turning back on themselves, while those in the outer cortex only extend a short way into the medulla. After the hairpin bend, the tubule becomes the thin ascending limb for a short distance before abruptly changing into the thick ascending limb. Thus the thin descending limb is longer than the thin ascending limb. The loops of Henle are best seen in sections of renal medulla. In addition to loops of Henle, the medulla also contains the vasa recta, collecting tubules and collecting ducts. All these structures are seen in these micrographs and may be distinguished by the following features.

The thin limbs **T** have a simple squamous epithelium but may be differentiated from the vasa recta **V** by the absence of erythrocytes and their regular rounded shape in transverse section. The thick ascending limbs **A** are lined by low cuboidal epithelium and are also round in cross-section. Neither thick nor thin limbs of the loop of Henle have a brush border. Collecting tubules **CT** have a similar epithelial lining to the ascending limbs but are wider and less regular in shape. The collecting ducts **CD** are easily recognised by their large diameter and pale stained columnar epithelial lining.

The function of the loop of Henle is to produce an increasing osmotic gradient from the cortex to the tip of the renal papilla by the *counter-current multiplier mechanism* (see Fig. 16.21). In brief, the parts of the loop of Henle with a thick (cuboidal) epithelium participate in active transport of various ions and molecules out of the lumen and into the interstitium. On the other hand, the thin limbs are lined by a flattened squamous epithelium which has no capacity for active transport. The thin descending limb allows free diffusion of H_2O but is fairly impermeable to NaCl, while the thin ascending limb is permeable to NaCl but not to H_2O. The vasa recta take up water from the medullary interstitium and return it to the general circulation.

As the urine flows into the thick ascending limb, active transport of NaCl again occurs and this correlates with the appearances of the epithelium. Here the cuboidal epithelium exhibits basolateral processes which interdigitate with each other forming an extensive intercelluar space in a similar manner to the PCT. The active transport process is fuelled by ATP produced by the many mitochondria found in these processes. The thick ascending limb is also impermeable to water which may be related to its thick glycocalyx composed of the glycoprotein, Tamm–Horsfall protein.

The interstitium of the inner medulla in some species, including humans, contains unusual cells called *lipid laden interstitial cells* arranged at right angles to the tubules and vasa recta and bound tightly to one another. The function of these cells is not yet clear but they may be involved in the production of prostaglandins and/or hormones which regulate blood pressure.

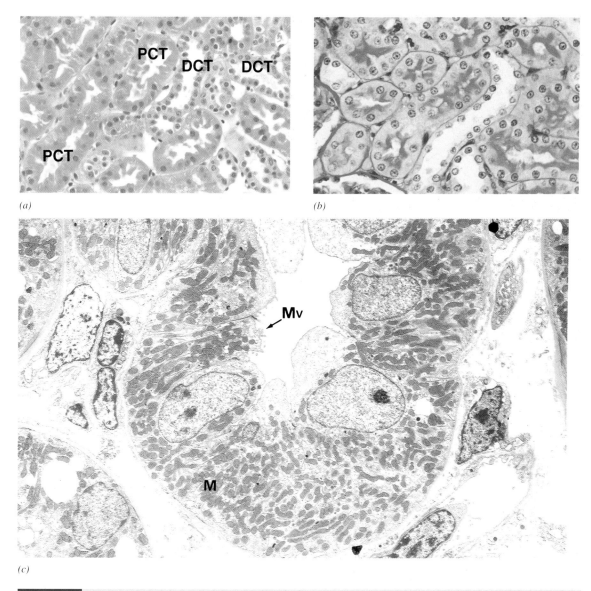

(a)

(b)

(c)

Fig. 16.17 **Distal convoluted tubule** (a) H & E × 200 (b) PAS/haematoxylin × 480 (c) EM × 3000

The distal tubule is a continuation of the thick ascending limb of the loop of Henle after its return to the cortex and forms the third segment of the renal tubule. Distal tubules are thus found within the cortex among the proximal convoluted tubules. The first part of the distal tubule forms the macula densa (see Fig 16.18) while the remainder makes up the distal convoluted tubule (DCT).

The DCT is mainly involved in reabsorption of sodium ions from the tubular fluid. The process is directly coupled to the secretion of hydrogen and potassium ions into the tubular fluid, one hydrogen ion or one potassium ion being secreted for every sodium ion reabsorbed; in this way the DCT plays an important role in acid–base balance. This process is controlled by the hormone *aldosterone* secreted by the adrenal cortex. A certain amount of potassium is also reabsorbed in the DCT.

As seen in micrograph (a), distal convoluted tubules **DCT** may be differentiated from proximal convoluted tubules **PCT** by the absence of a brush border, a larger more clearly defined lumen, more nuclei per cross-section (since DCT cells are smaller than PCT cells) and paler cytoplasm (due to fewer organelles). In addition, sections

of DCT are much less numerous than sections of PCT since the DCT is a much shorter segment of the renal tubule than the PCT.

Micrograph (b) differentiates between proximal and distal convoluted tubules on the basis of the presence or absence of a brush border. The PCT has a profuse PAS-positive brush border (see Fig. 16.15) which is absent from the DCT.

The distal convoluted tubule has many ultrastructural features in common with the proximal convoluted tubule (c), in particular the lateral cell interdigitations, and large numbers of mitochondria **M**. The basolateral plasma membrane contains the Na^+-K^+ ATPase which drives active transport of Na^+ ions. The most striking difference is that the DCT lacks a brush border, having only a few irregular microvilli **Mv** at the luminal surface. The DCT cells have less cytoplasm than those of the PCT although the nucleus is of about the same size and consequently occupies much more of the cell. The nuclei of the DCT cells lie close to the luminal surface and tend to bulge into the lumen; the overlying cytoplasm is devoid of mitochondria but contains large numbers of tiny vesicles.

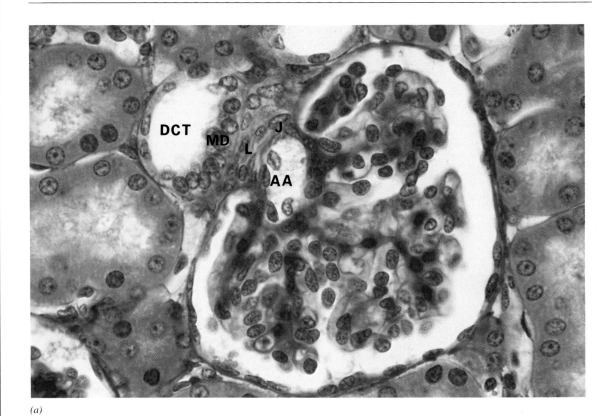

(a)

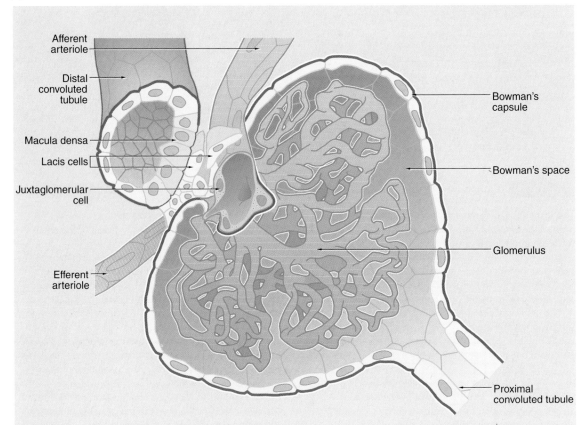

(b)

Fig. 16.18 Juxtaglomerular apparatus (a) Azan × 640 *(opposite above)*
(b) Explanatory diagram *(opposite below)* (c) Blood pressure control system *(below left)*

The *juxtaglomerular apparatus (JGA)* is a specialisation of the glomerular afferent arteriole **AA** and the distal convoluted tubule **DCT** of the same nephron and is involved in the regulation of systemic blood pressure via the *renin–angiotensin–aldosterone mechanism*.

The juxtaglomerular apparatus is made up of three components: the *macula densa* of the DCT, renin-secreting *juxtaglomerular cells* of the afferent arteriole and *extraglomerular mesangial cells*.

Macula densa. On returning to the cortex from the renal medulla, the ascending thick limb of the loop of Henle becomes the first part of the distal tubule and comes to lie in the angle between the afferent and efferent arterioles at the vascular pole of the glomerulus. The macula densa **MD** is an area of closely packed, specialised cells lining the DCT where it abuts the glomerular vascular pole. Compared with other DCT lining cells, the cells of the macula densa are taller and have larger more prominent nuclei which are situated towards the luminal surface. Mitochondria are scattered throughout the cytoplasm and Na⁺ pump activity is absent. The basement membrane between the macula and underlying cells is extremely thin.

The cells of the macula densa are thought to be sensitive to the concentration of sodium ions in the fluid within the DCT; a decrease in systemic blood pressure results in decreased production of glomerular filtrate and hence decreased concentration of sodium ions in the distal tubular fluid.

Juxtaglomerular cells. Juxtaglomerular cells **J** are specialised smooth muscle cells of the wall of the afferent arteriole forming a cluster around it just before it enters the glomerulus. Juxtaglomerular cell cytoplasm contains immature and mature membrane-bound granules of the enzyme *renin*.

Extraglomerular mesangial cells. Also called *Goormaghtigh cells* or *lacis cells* **L**, these cells form a conical mass, the apex of which is continuous with the mesangium of the glomerulus; laterally it is bounded by the afferent and efferent arterioles and its base abuts the macula densa. The lacis cells are flat and elongated with extensive fine cytoplasmic processes extending from their ends and surrounded by a network ('lacis') of mesangial material. Despite their central location in the JGA, the function of the extraglomerular mesangial cells is not yet clear. The current theory is that these cells participate in the *tubuloglomerular feedback mechanism* by which changes in Na⁺ concentration at the macula densa give rise to signals which directly control glomerular blood flow. The extraglomerular mesangial cells are thought to be responsible for transmission of a signal arising in the macula densa to the intraglomerular mesangial cells which then contract or relax to make the capillary loops narrower or wider.

Role of the JGA in the control of blood pressure

The juxtaglomerular apparatus is believed to act as both a baroreceptor and a chemoreceptor; controlling systemic blood pressure by the secretion of renin by the juxtaglomerular cells.

The juxtaglomerular cells are suitably placed to monitor systemic blood pressure, with a fall in blood pressure resulting in renin secretion. Reduction in blood pressure results in reduced glomerular filtration and consequently a lower concentration of sodium ions in the DCT. Acting as chemoreceptors, the cells of the macula densa in some way then promote renin secretion.

Renin diffuses into the bloodstream catalysing the conversion of *angiotensinogen*, an alpha₂-globulin synthesised by the liver, into the decapeptide *angiotensin I*. In the lungs, *angiotensin converting enzyme* cleaves two amino acids from angiotensin I to form *angiotensin II* which is a potent vasoconstrictor.

Angiotensin II raises blood pressure in three ways: constriction of peripheral blood vessels, release of aldosterone from the adrenal cortex and via a direct effect on the renal tubules where it promotes the reabsorption of sodium ions (and therefore water) from the DCT, thus expanding the plasma volume and increasing blood pressure.

As mentioned above, the tubuloglomerular feedback mechanism is also thought to operate at a local level to control glomerular blood flow and therefore indirectly systemic blood pressure.

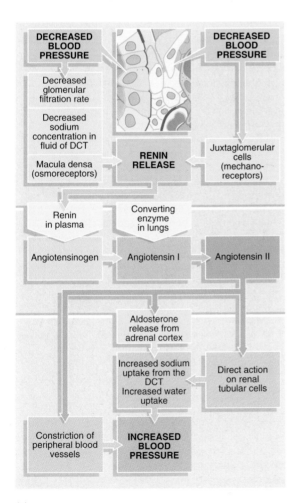

(c)

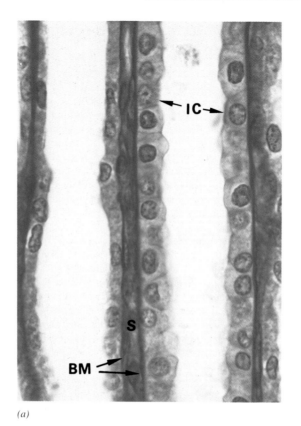

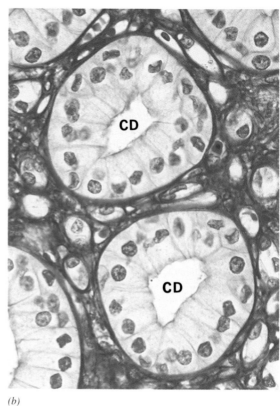

(a)   *(b)*

Fig. 16.19   Collecting tubules and ducts   (a) Azan × 750 (b) Azan × 480

The *collecting tubule*, or *connecting segment*, joins the distal convoluted tubule to the collecting duct. Several collecting tubules merge to form each collecting duct. The collecting tubules and ducts descend in the medullary rays (see Fig. 16.5) towards the renal medulla where they progressively merge to form the large ducts of Bellini which drain urine from the tip of the renal papilla into the pelvicalyceal system.

The collecting tubules and ducts concentrate urine by passive reabsorption of water into the medullary interstitium following the osmotic gradient created by the counter-current multiplier system of the loops of Henle (see Fig. 16.21). The vasa recta return this water to the general circulation. The amount of water reabsorbed is controlled by *antidiuretic hormone* (*ADH*, *vasopressin*) secreted by the posterior pituitary in response to dehydration. ADH acts by increasing the permeability to water of the collecting tubule and ducts, resulting in retention of water by the body and the production of hypertonic urine. Conversely, ADH secretion is inhibited by water overload and an increased volume of hypotonic urine is thus produced. The collecting tubules and ducts are also the site of H^+ secretion and therefore important in the maintenance of acid–base balance.

The simple columnar epithelium of the collecting ducts consists of two cell types, *principal cells* and *intercalated cells*. Principal cells have pale cytoplasm with scanty organelles with luminal short microvilli and a single cilium. There are prominent basal infoldings of the basolateral plasma membrane but no lateral

interdigitations. Principal cells actively reabsorb Na^+ and secrete K^+ as well as reabsorbing water. Intercalated cells have darker cytoplasm due to the content of multiple mitochondria, polyribosomes and membrane-bound vesicles. These cells function to secrete H^+ and reabsorb bicarbonate and are thus important in acid–base homeostasis. The number of intercalated cells varies between different parts of the collecting duct and they are virtually absent in the inner medullary segment.

The collecting tubules are lined by a mixture of DCT cells, collecting tubule cells, principal cells and intercalated cells. Overall the epithelium is cuboidal and becomes increasingly tall distally until it merges with the columnar epithelium of the collecting duct.

Micrograph (a) illustrates two collecting tubules in the renal cortex, the tubule on the left being more proximal and the tubule on the right more distal as shown by the flatter cuboidal lining of the former. The majority of the lining cells are relatively poorly stained. The different cell types cannot be differentiated by light microscopy, except for a small number of dark intercalated cells **IC** (with microvillous surface). Note the blue stained tubular basement membranes **BM** and narrow intervening supporting tissue **S** mainly occupied by capillaries.

Micrograph (b) is from the renal medulla and illustrates two collecting ducts **CD** surrounded by loops of Henle and vasa recta which cannot be readily distinguished from one another. In the medullary portion of the collecting ducts, principal cells are predominant and no intercalated cells can be seen in this section.

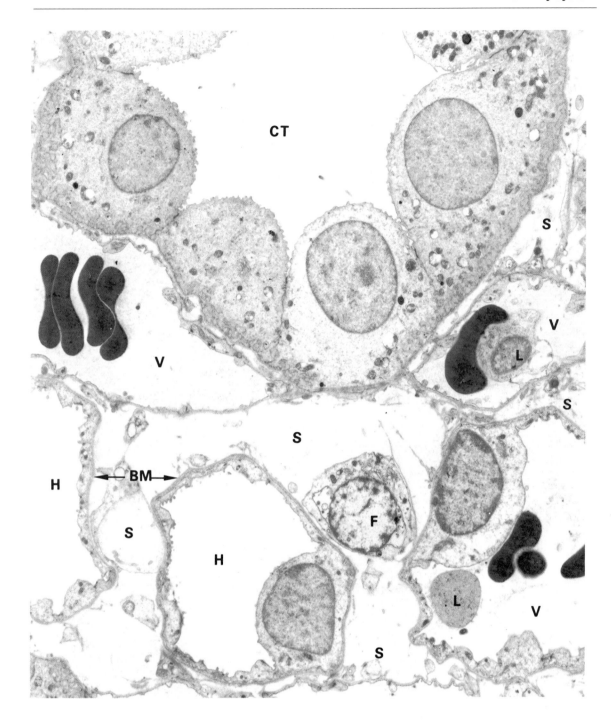

Fig. 16.20 Renal medulla (rat) EM × 4000

This micrograph from the outer medulla illustrates the ultrastructural features of a collecting tubule **CT**, thin loops of Henle **H** and vasa recta **V**.

The collecting tubule in this section is lined mainly by principal cells whose basal mitochondria associated with infoldings of the plasma membrane can just be identified at this power. The cells of the thin limbs of loops of Henle are similar to capillary endothelial cells in structure, most of the wall consisting of a thin irregular layer of cytoplasm with a few very short luminal microvilli and

the nucleus bulging into the lumen. The epithelium is supported by a thin basement membrane **BM**. The vasa recta can only be readily distinguished from the thin limbs by their content of erythrocytes, occasional leucocytes **L** and precipitated plasma proteins.

Lying between the vasa recta and nephrons is delicate interstitial supporting tissue **S** containing a little collagen, scattered fibroblasts **F** and their slender cytoplasmic processes.

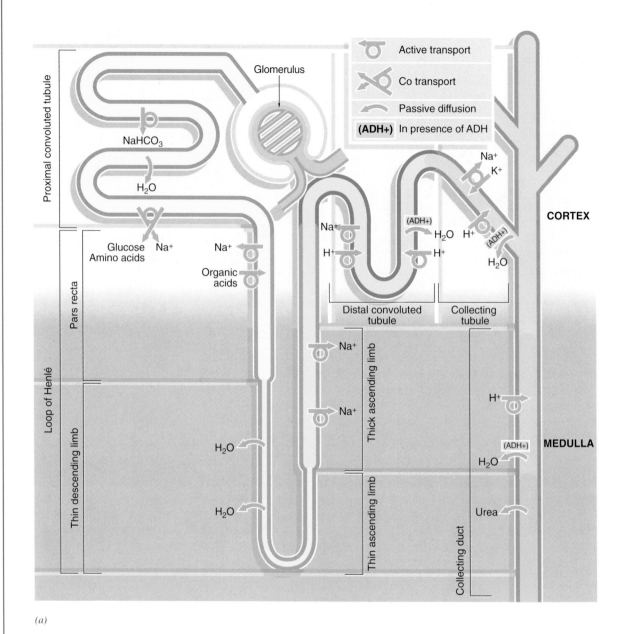

(a)

Fig. 16.21 (a) Summary diagram of activities of different parts of the tubule
(b) Comparison of epithelial structure in different parts of the renal tubule *(opposite)*

The function of the renal tubule is to transform an ultrafiltrate of plasma into a concentrated solution of waste products such as urea, creatinine, excess H^+ and K^+ and many other substances. At the same time the tubule conserves essential water, Na^+, bicarbonate, amino acids, glucose and low molecular weight proteins. This complex procedure is carried out by a variety of mechanisms in different segments of the tubule including active transport, co-transport, passive diffusion, facilitated diffusion (see Ch. 1) and differential permeability of different parts of the tubule.

The ability of the tubule to produce a highly concentrated urine is dependent on the high osmolarity of the renal medulla which is created by the unique structure of the loops of Henle and vasa recta dipping down into the medulla, known as the counter-current multiplier mechanism. In the presence of ADH, which renders the collecting tubule and duct permeable to water, the high osmolarity of the renal medulla draws water passively out of the tubule and into the medulla where it is carried away

by the vasa recta. The counter-current multiplier mechanism is set up by the ability of the thick ascending limb of the loop of Henle to pump large amounts of NaCl into the interstitium against a concentration gradient whilst remaining impermeable to water. The thin descending limb is permeable to water but not NaCl and water is reabsorbed into the medulla resulting in hyperosmolar urine reaching the hairpin bend of the loop. This water, however, is removed by the vasa recta. The hyperosmolarity of the medulla is also partly due to the high concentrations of urea resulting from passive diffusion of urea from the medullary collecting duct into the interstitium along its concentration gradient.

Diagram (a) outlines the major movements of solutes and water into and out of the different parts of the renal tubule. For further detail of these processes the reader is referred to current physiology texts. Diagram (b) gives the major morphological features of the epithelium of the different segments of the tubule and correlates them with function.

Part of tubule	Type of epithelium	Special features	Functional significance
Proximal convoluted tubule	Simple cuboidal	Microvilli (brush border) Extensive basolateral interdigitations Plentiful mitochondria	Facilitated diffusion glucose, amino acids Na^+ pump Energy for active transport
Pars recta of proximal tubule	Simple cuboidal	Microvilli (brush border) No basolateral interdigitations	Secretion of organic acids
Thin descending/ascending limbs	Simple squamous	No basolateral interdigitations or microvilli Mitochondria scanty	No active transport Low energy requirement
Thick ascending limb	Simple cuboidal	Microvilli absent Extensive basolateral interdigitations	No facilitated diffusion Active transport of Na^+
Distal convoluted tubule (DCT)	Simple cuboidal	Extensive basolateral interdigitations Mitochondria plentiful	Active transport of Na^+ Energy for active transport
Collecting tubule	Simple cuboidal	Principal cells Intercalated cells DCT cells Collecting tubule cells	Na^+ reabsorption, ADH-dependent water reabsorption, K^+ secretion Acid–base balance, K^+ reabsorption Active transport of Na^+
Cortical collecting duct	Simple columnar	Principal cells Intercalated cells	Na^+ reabsorption, ADH-dependent water reabsorption, K^+ secretion Acid–base balance, K^+ reabsorption
Medullary collecting duct	Simple columnar	Mainly principal cells	ADH-dependent water reabsorption

(b)

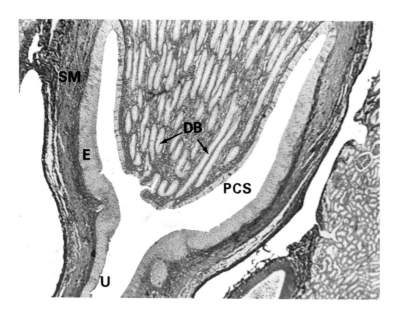

Fig. 16.22 Renal papilla (monkey) Azan × 30

The renal papilla forms the apex of the medullary pyramid where it projects into the pelvicalyceal space **PCS**. Ducts of Bellini **DB**, the largest of the collecting ducts, converge to drain urine through a number of holes (*cribriform area*) at the tip of the papilla. Between the ducts are the longest loops of Henle and vasa recta, not visible at this magnification. This papilla is a simple papilla, but at the poles of the kidney the papillae are often fused to form complex papillae.

The pelvicalyceal system represents the proximal end of the ureter **U** and as such is lined by typical urinary (transitional) epithelium **E**. The wall of the pelvis contains smooth muscle **SM** which is continuous with that of the ureter.

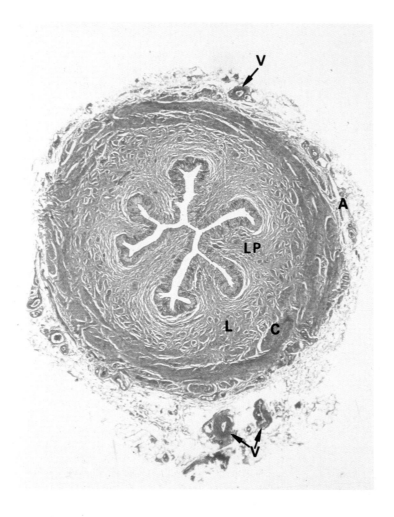

Fig. 16.23 Ureter Masson's trichrome × 18

The ureters are muscular tubes, which carry urine from the kidneys to the bladder. Urine is conducted from the pelvicalyceal system as a bolus, which is propelled by peristaltic action of the ureteric wall. The wall of the ureter contains two layers of smooth muscle arranged as an inner elongated spiral but traditionally known as the longitudinal layer **L** and an outer tight spiral traditionally described as the circular layer **C**. Another outer longitudinal layer is present in the lower third of the ureter. However, in reality the three layers are often difficult to distinguish from each other.

The lumen of the ureter is lined by *transitional epithelium* (*urothelium*), which is thrown up into folds in the relaxed state allowing the ureter to dilate during the passage of a bolus of urine. Beneath the epithelium is a broad collagenous lamina propria **LP**, the collagen fibres of which are stained greenish-blue in this preparation. Surrounding the muscular wall is a loose collagenous adventitia **A** containing blood vessels **V**, lymphatics and nerves.

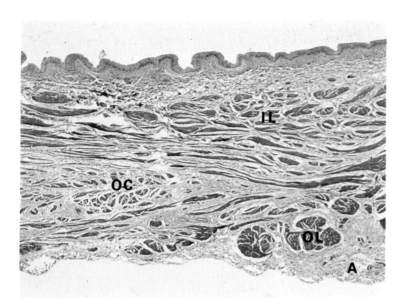

Fig. 16.24 Bladder
Masson's trichrome × 12

The general structure of the bladder wall resembles that of the lower third of the ureters. The wall of the bladder consists of three loosely arranged layers of smooth muscle and elastic fibres which contract during micturition. Note the inner longitudinal **IL**, outer circular **OC** and outermost longitudinal **OL** layers of smooth muscle. As in the ureter, the layers are often difficult to distinguish. The transitional epithelium lining the bladder is thrown into many folds in the relaxed state. The outer adventitial coat **A** contains arteries, veins and lymphatics.

The urethra, the final conducting portion of the urinary tract, is discussed as part of the male reproductive tract in Chapter 18.

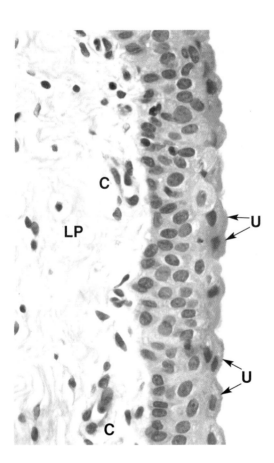

Fig. 16.25 Urinary epithelium H & E × 450

Transitional epithelium, also called urothelium, is found only within the conducting passages of the urinary system for which it is especially adapted. The epithelium is stratified, comprising three to six layers of cells, the number of layers being greatest when the epithelium is least distended at the time of fixation. The specimen shown here is typical and is taken from a non-distended bladder.

The cells of the basal layer are compact and cuboidal or columnar in form, while those of the intermediate layers are more polygonal. The surface cells are often called *umbrella cells* **U** and have unique features which allow them to maintain the impermeability of the epithelium to urine even when at full stretch. This permeability barrier also prevents water from being drawn through the epithelium into hypertonic urine. The umbrella cells are large and ovoid with round nuclei and plentiful eosinophilic cytoplasm; some surface cells are binucleate. The surface outline has a characteristic scalloped appearance and the superficial cytoplasm is fuzzy, indistinct and more intensely stained than the rest of the cytoplasm.

Ultrastructural studies have revealed that much of the surface plasma membrane consists of thickened inflexible *plaques*, often called *asymmetrical unit membrane*, interspersed with narrow zones of normal membrane. These normal areas act as 'hinges', allowing sections of the membrane to fold inwards somewhat like a concertina, forming deep clefts and stacks of flattened *fusiform vesicles*. This structure allows the umbrella cells to expand greatly when the bladder is distended and the epithelium is at full stretch. The concertina folds unfold and the fusiform vesicles become incorporated into the membrane so as to allow greatly increased surface area without loss of integrity of the surface layer. Plentiful junctional complexes between the cells maintain the cohesion of adjacent cells.

Urinary epithelium rests on a basement membrane which is often too thin to be resolved by light microscopy. The loose lamina propria **LP** containing capillaries **C** is seen underlying the epithelium.

17. The endocrine glands

Introduction

Endocrine glands are responsible for the synthesis and secretion of chemical messengers known as *hormones*. Hormones may be disseminated throughout the body by the bloodstream where they may act on specific *target organs* or affect a wide range of organs and tissues. Other hormones act locally, often arriving at their site of action by way of a specialised microcirculation. In conjunction with the nervous system, hormones coordinate and integrate the functions of all the physiological systems.

As a general rule, endocrine glands are composed of islands of secretory cells of epithelial origin with intervening supporting tissue, which is rich in blood and lymphatic capillaries. The secretory cells discharge their hormone product into the interstitial spaces from which they are rapidly absorbed into the circulatory system. Unlike exocrine glands (see Ch. 5), endocrine glands have no duct system and are therefore sometimes called the *ductless glands*.

Reflecting their active synthetic function, endocrine secretory cells are usually characterised by prominent nuclei and abundant cytoplasmic organelles, especially mitochondria, endoplasmic reticulum, Golgi bodies and secretory vesicles.

Some endocrine glands exist in the form of discrete organs, e.g. pituitary, thyroid, parathyroid and adrenal glands. Other endocrine tissues are found in association with exocrine glands, e.g. pancreas, or within complex organs, e.g. kidney, testis, ovary, placenta, brain and the gastrointestinal tract. This chapter deals with the pituitary, thyroid, parathyroids, adrenals, endocrine pancreas, pineal and the gastrointestinal and respiratory endocrine systems; other endocrine tissues are discussed with the organs with which they are associated.

Pituitary gland

The *pituitary gland*, also known as the *hypophysis*, is found at the base of the brain. It secretes a variety of hormones, which mediate non-neural mechanisms by which the central nervous system integrates and controls many body functions. The pituitary hormones fall into two functional groups:

- Hormones which act directly on non-endocrine tissues: growth hormone (GH), prolactin, antidiuretic hormone (ADH), oxytocin and melanocyte stimulating hormone (MSH).
- Hormones which modulate the secretory activity of other endocrine glands (*trophic hormones*): thyroid stimulating hormone (TSH), adrenocorticotrophic hormone (ACTH) and the gonadotrophic hormones, follicle stimulating hormone (FSH) and luteinising hormone (LH).

Thus the thyroid gland, adrenal cortex and gonads may be described as *pituitary-dependent endocrine glands*.

The secretion of all pituitary hormones is directly controlled by the hypothalamus which is under the influence of nervous stimuli from higher centres in the CNS and controlled by feedback from the levels of circulating hormones produced by the pituitary-dependent glands. Thus the pituitary gland plays a central role in integrating the nervous and endocrine systems.

The pituitary gland is a small, slightly elongated organ, approximately 1 cm in diameter, lying immediately beneath the third ventricle in a bony cavity, the *sella turcica*, in the base of the skull. The gland is divided into anterior and posterior parts, which have entirely different embryological origins, functions and control mechanisms.

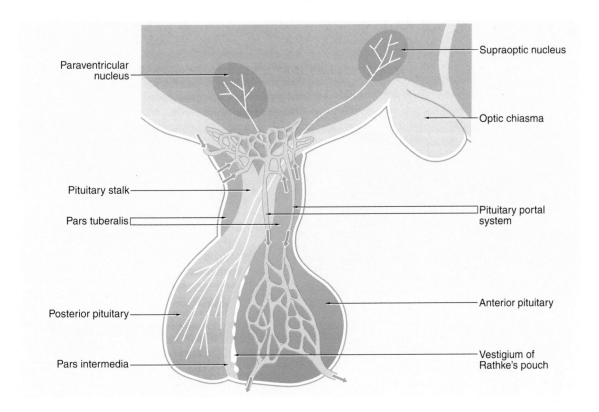

Paraventricular nucleus

Supraoptic nucleus

Optic chiasma

Pituitary stalk

Pars tuberalis

Pituitary portal system

Anterior pituitary

Posterior pituitary

Vestigium of Rathke's pouch

Pars intermedia

Fig. 17.1 **Pituitary gland**

The anterior and posterior parts of the pituitary originate from different embryological sources and this is reflected in their structure and function.

- The **posterior pituitary**, also called the *neurohypophysis* or *pars nervosa* is derived from a downgrowth of nervous tissue from the hypothalamus to which it remains joined by the *pituitary stalk*.
- The **anterior pituitary** arises as an epithelial upgrowth from the roof of the primitive oral cavity, known as *Rathke's pouch*. This specialised glandular epithelium is wrapped around the anterior aspect of the posterior pituitary and is often called the *adenohypophysis*. The adenohypophysis may contain a cleft or group of cyst-like spaces which represent the vestigial lumen of Rathke's pouch. This vestigial cleft divides the major part of the anterior pituitary from a thin zone of tissue lying against the posterior pituitary, known as the *pars intermedia*. An extension of the adenohypophysis surrounds the neural stalk and is known as the *pars tuberalis*.

The type and mode of secretion of the posterior pituitary differ greatly from that of the anterior pituitary. The posterior pituitary secretes two hormones, *antidiuretic hormone* (ADH), also called *vasopressin*, and the hormone *oxytocin*, both of which act directly on non-endocrine tissues. ADH is synthesised in the neurone cell bodies of the *supraoptic nucleus*, and oxytocin is synthesised in those of the *paraventricular nucleus* of the hypothalamus. Bound to glycoproteins, the hormones pass down the axons of the hypothalamopituitary tract through the pituitary stalk to the posterior pituitary where

they are stored in the distended terminal parts of the axons. Release of posterior pituitary hormones is controlled directly by nervous impulses passing down the axons from the hypothalamus; a process known as *neurosecretion*.

The anterior pituitary has the typical structure of epithelial-derived endocrine glands elsewhere in the body. It secretes both trophic and direct action hormones:

- *Trophic hormones*: thyroid stimulating hormone (TSH), adrenocorticotrophic hormone (ACTH), and the gonadotrophic hormones, follicle stimulating hormone (FSH) and luteinising hormone (LH).
- *Direct action hormones*: growth hormone (GH) and prolactin. (Recent evidence suggests that prolactin has a trophic action on the endocrine tissues of the ovary in some animals.)

Hypothalamic control of anterior pituitary secretion is mediated by specific hypothalamic releasing hormones, e.g. *thyroid stimulating hormone releasing hormone* (TSHRH); exceptions to this rule are prolactin secretion, which is under the inhibitory control of *dopamine*, and secretion of growth hormone which is controlled by both releasing and inhibitory hormones. These releasing and inhibitory hormones are conducted from the *median hypothalamic eminence* to the anterior pituitary by a unique system of *portal veins* (the *pituitary portal system*).

The pars intermedia synthesises and secretes melanocyte stimulating hormone (MSH); in humans, the pars intermedia is rudimentary and the physiological importance of MSH and the control of its secretion are poorly understood.

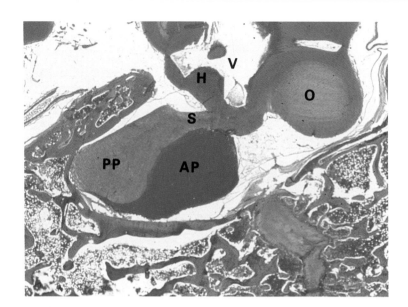

Fig. 17.2 **Pituitary gland (monkey)** H & E × 12

This micrograph from a midline section through the brain and cranial floor illustrates the pituitary gland in situ. The pituitary sits in a bony depression in the sphenoid bone, called the *sella turcica*. The two major components of the gland, the anterior pituitary **AP** and the posterior pituitary **PP**, are easily seen at this magnification. The posterior pituitary is connected to the hypothalamus **H** by the pituitary stalk **S** and, like the hypothalamus, is composed of nervous tissue. Note the close proximity of the third ventricle **V** above the hypothalamus and the optic chiasma **O** anteriorly.

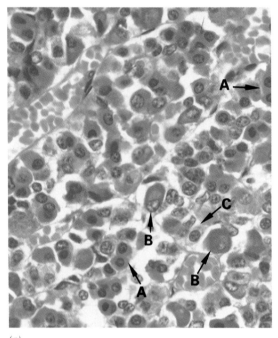

(a)

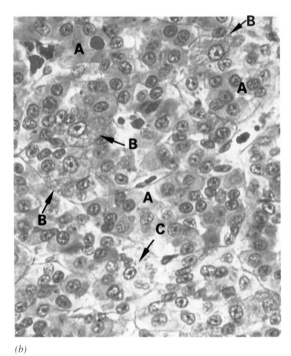

(b)

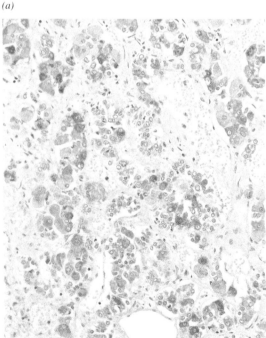

(c)

Fig. 17.3 **Anterior pituitary**
(a) H & E × 480 (b) Modified Azan × 480
(c) Immunoperoxidase for LH × 150
(d) EM × 4270 *(illustration opposite)*

The secretory cells of the anterior pituitary have been traditionally classified into two groups, *chromophils* and *chromophobes*, according to their affinities for histological stains. The chromophils are subdivided into *acidophils* and *basophils* according to their staining properties. For example, in micrograph (b), acidophils **A** are stained orange and basophils **B** are stained blue. In H & E preparations (micrograph a), the distinction between them is much less obvious. The chromophobes **C** are the smallest cell type in the anterior pituitary and contain few cytoplasmic granules; they have little affinity for either acidic or basic dyes and probably represent resting or degranulated chromophil cells.

The secretory cells of the anterior pituitary form branching cords which are surrounded by a rich network of sinusoidal capillaries supported by a delicate stroma containing reticulin and fine collagen fibres. Reflecting their epithelial nature, the clumps of secretory

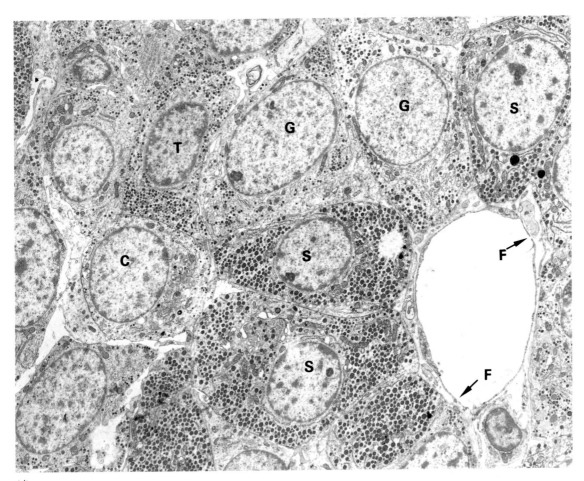

(d)

cells are surrounded by basement membranes which stain blue in preparation (b).

Traditional histological methods of studying the pituitary have been superseded by specific immunohistochemical techniques by which five types of cells are defined according to their secretory product. Micrograph (c) shows a section of anterior pituitary stained by the immunoperoxidase technique for luteinising hormone. The brown stained LH-containing cells can be seen scattered at random among the other cells types. The different cell types are now named as follows:

- **Somatotrophs**, the cells responsible for growth hormone secretion, are the most numerous, making up almost half of the bulk of the anterior pituitary.
- **Mammotrophs (lactotrophs)**, the prolactin secreting cells, comprise up to 20% of the anterior pituitary, increasing in number during pregnancy; prolactin controls milk production during lactation.
- **Corticotrophs** secrete ACTH (*corticotrophin*) and constitute about 20% of the anterior pituitary mass. ACTH is a polypeptide which becomes split from a much larger peptide molecule known as *pro-opiomelanocortin*. *Lipotropins* (involved in regulation of lipid metabolism), *endorphins* (endogenous opioids) and various species of MSH can be derived from the same molecule; the last explains the hyperpigmentation associated with excessive ACTH secretion.
- **Thyrotrophs**, which secrete TSH (*thyrotrophin*), are much less numerous, making up only about 5% of the gland.
- **Gonadotrophs**, the cells responsible for the secretion of FSH and LH, make up the remaining 5% of the anterior pituitary.

The somatotrophs and mammotrophs represent the acidophils of traditional light microscopy, the basophils being the thyrotrophs, gonadotrophs and the corticotrophs. In general one cell produces a single hormone, although LH- and FSH-containing secretory granules have been demonstrated within a single cell. The different cell types are not evenly distributed throughout the gland, but rather particular cell types tend to congregate in particular zones of the gland.

The secretory granules of each cell type have a characteristic size, shape and electron density by which the different cell types can be recognised with electron microscopy as in micrograph (d). Somatotrophs **S** are packed with secretory granules of moderate size. Thyrotrophs **T** have smaller granules which tend to be more peripherally located. Gonadotrophs **G** are large cells with secretory granules of variable size. Corticotrophs **C** have sparse secretory granules located at the extreme periphery of the cell.

The endothelial lining of capillaries in endocrine tissue is characteristically fenestrated (see Fig. 8.14) facilitating the passage of hormones into the sinusoids. Note the fenestrations **F** in the sinusoid seen in micrograph (d).

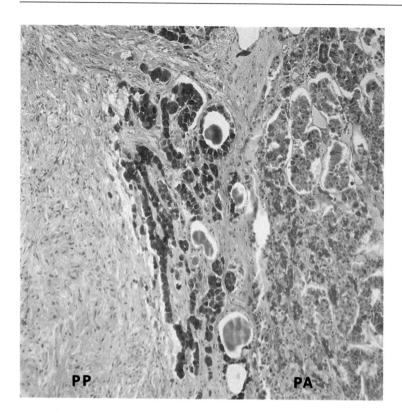

Fig. 17.4 Pituitary: pars intermedia Isamine blue/eosin × 100

The pars intermedia, like the anterior pituitary, is derived embryologically from Rathke's pouch. The cells, which are similar to corticotrophs, are basophilic (stained blue) and form irregular clumps lying between the pars anterior **PA** and pars posterior **PP** but tending to spill out into the neural tissue of the pars posterior. Small cystic spaces filled with eosinophilic material may be seen representing the residuum of Rathke's pouch. The pars intermedia is poorly developed in humans (as in this specimen) but relatively well developed in other mammals and some lower species.

Ultrastructurally, the cells of the pars intermedia contain secretory granules similar to corticotrophs, and pro-opiomelanocortin is synthesised and split into a number of fragments including ACTH, two types of MSH, endorphins and lipotrophins. MSH promotes melanin synthesis by skin melanocytes, thereby increasing skin pigmentation.

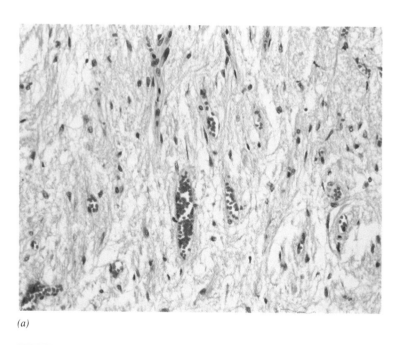

(a)

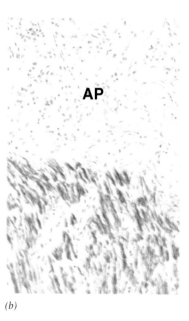

(b)

Fig. 17.5 Posterior pituitary (a) H & E × 200 (b) Immunoperoxidase × 100

The posterior pituitary contains the non-myelinated axons of neurosecretory cells, the cell bodies of which are located in the hypothalamus. The neurosecretory axons are supported by cells called *pituicytes*, which are similar in structure and function to the neuroglial cells of the central nervous system (see Figs 7.2 to 7.24). Most of the nuclei seen in micrograph (a) are those of pituicytes. The axons of the neural cells are indistinguishable from the cytoplasm of the pituicytes in H & E preparations but can be demonstrated using the immunoperoxidase technique (micrograph b). Here an antibody to neurofilament protein (NFP), an intermediate filament characteristic of nerve cells, highlights the axons, which are seen stained brown in the lower half of the micrograph. There is an abrupt transition to anterior pituitary **AP**, which is composed of epithelial cells containing no NFP. A rich network of small fenestrated capillaries pervades the posterior pituitary.

Thyroid gland

The thyroid gland is a butterfly-shaped endocrine gland lying in the neck in front of the upper part of the trachea. The thyroid gland produces hormones of two types:

- Iodine-containing hormones *tri-iodothyronine* (T_3) and *thyroxine* (*tetra-iodothyronine*, T_4); T_4 is converted to T_3 in the general circulation by removal of one iodothyronine unit although a small amount of T_3 is secreted directly. T_3 is much more potent than T_4 and appears to be the metabolically active form of the hormone. Thyroid hormone regulates the basal metabolic rate and has an important influence on growth and maturation particularly of nerve tissue. The secretion of these hormones is regulated by TSH secreted by the anterior pituitary.
- The polypeptide hormone *calcitonin*; this hormone regulates blood calcium levels in conjunction with parathyroid hormone. Calcitonin lowers blood calcium levels by inhibiting the rate of decalcification of bone by osteoclastic resorption and by stimulating osteoblastic activity. Control of calcitonin secretion is dependent only on blood calcium levels and is independent of pituitary and parathyroid hormone levels.

The thyroid gland is unique among the human endocrine glands in that it stores large amounts of hormone in an inactive form within extracellular compartments in the centre of follicles; in contrast, other endocrine glands store only small quantities of hormones in intracellular sites.

The main bulk of the gland develops from an epithelial downgrowth from the fetal tongue whereas the calcitonin-secreting cells are derived from the ultimobranchial element of the fourth branchial pouch.

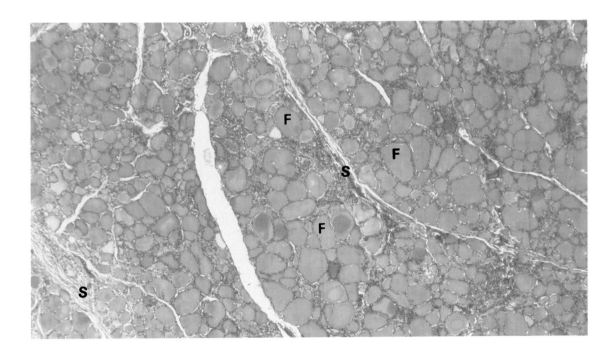

Fig. 17.6 Thyroid gland H & E × 12

The functional units of the thyroid gland are the *thyroid follicles*, spheroidal structures composed of a single layer of cuboidal epithelial cells bounded by a basement membrane (see also Fig. 5.30). As seen in this micrograph of a normal active thyroid, the follicles F are variable in size and contain a homogeneous colloid material which is stained pink in this preparation.

The thyroid gland is enveloped by a fibrous capsule from which fine collagenous septa S extend into the gland, dividing it into lobules. The septa convey a rich blood supply together with lymphatics and nerves; during histological preparation, the lobules tend to shrink, as seen here, leaving artefactual spaces in the septal planes.

ORGAN SYSTEMS

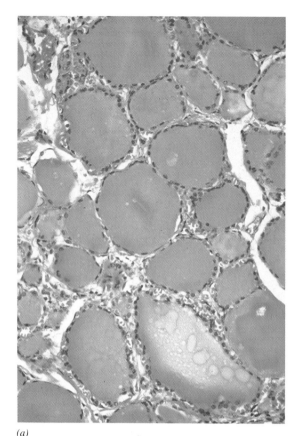

(a)

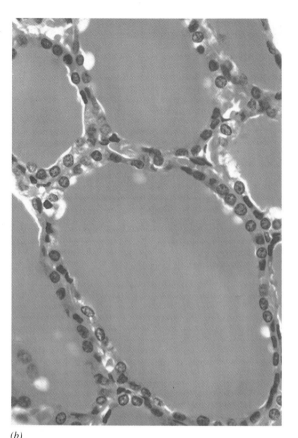

(b)

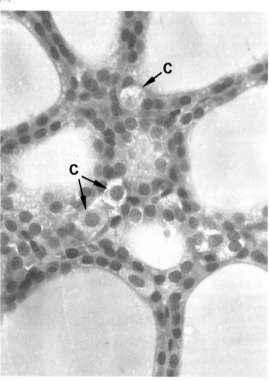

(c)

Fig. 17.7 Thyroid gland
(a) Human, H & E × 240 (b) Human, H & E × 480
(c) Dog, H & E × 480

Thyroid follicles are lined by a simple cuboidal epithelium, which is responsible for the synthesis and secretion of the iodine-containing hormones T_3, and T_4. Thyroid follicles are filled with a glycoprotein complex called *thyroglobulin* (*thyroid colloid*) which stores the thyroid hormones prior to secretion. The size of the follicles and their lining cells tends to vary according to the state of activity of the gland. Actively secreting thyroid tissue is composed of smaller follicles lined by tall cuboidal/columnar cells, while less active tissue is characterised by larger follicles lined by flattened epithelial cells and containing large amounts of stored colloid.

The second secretory cell type is found in the thyroid gland as single cells scattered among the follicular cells within the basement membrane of the follicles. These cells were first described in the dog in which they have an extensive unstained cytoplasm and are therefore called *C cells* (*clear cells*), also occasionally *parafollicular cells* C. This characteristic feature is seen in micrograph (c). In other mammals, including humans, C cells are usually much less distinctive, with pale granular cytoplasm, and are often difficult to distinguish in H & E sections. C cells synthesise and secrete the hormone calcitonin in direct response to raised blood calcium levels and have the structural and functional characteristics of neuroendocrine cells.

C cells have a different embryological origin from the follicular cells and in some species constitute a discrete endocrine organ called the ultimobranchial body. C cells are only found in the middle third of the lateral lobes of the thyroid.

ORGAN SYSTEMS

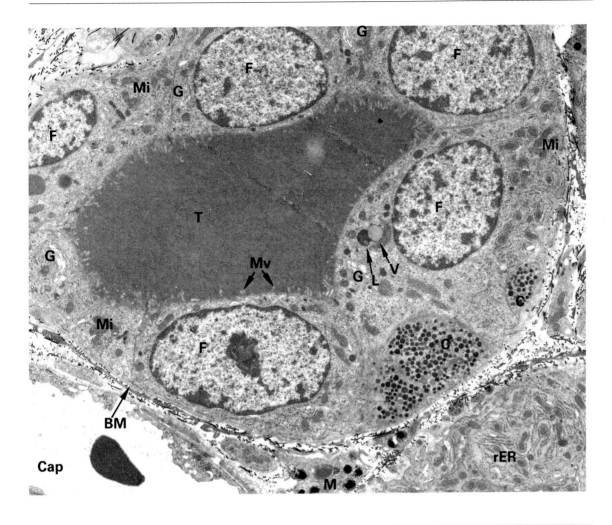

Fig. 17.8 **Thyroid follicle (rat)** EM × 6800

This micrograph demonstrates a thyroid follicle composed of cuboidal follicular cells **F** surrounding a lumen containing the homogeneous colloid, thyroglobulin **T**. A basement membrane **BM** delineates the follicle. Two portions of the cytoplasm of a C cell **C** are seen within the follicular epithelium typically located on the basement membrane and not exposed to the follicular lumen. The cytoplasm contains numerous electron-dense secretory granules of the hormone calcitonin. A fenestrated capillary **Cap** containing an erythrocyte is closely applied to the follicular basement membrane. Part of a mast cell **M** is seen in the interfollicular supporting tissue.

Follicular cells concentrate iodide from the blood by means of an iodide pump in the basal plasma membrane. Within the cell, iodide is oxidised to iodine and transported to the follicular plasma membrane where it is released into the follicular lumen. The glycoprotein thyroglobulin is synthesised in the rough endoplasmic reticulum, glycosylated and packaged by the Golgi apparatus, then released into the follicular lumen by exocytosis. Within the follicular lumen (not within the follicular cells), iodine combines with tyrosine residues of the thyroglobulin to form the hormones tri-iodothyronine

(T_3) and tetra-iodothyronine (thyroxine, T_4) which remain bound to the glycoprotein in an inactive form.

Secretion of these hormones involves pinocytosis of the thyroglobulin–hormone complex to form cytoplasmic vacuoles; the vacuoles then fuse with lysosomes of the follicular cell cytoplasm and hydrolytic enzymes cleave the hormone from the thyroglobulin. The hormones are released in the basal cytoplasm from which they diffuse into the bloodstream. The synthetic and secretory activity of the thyroid gland is dependent on thyroid stimulating hormone (TSH) secreted by the anterior pituitary.

In this micrograph, rough endoplasmic reticulum **rER** is best demonstrated in the basal aspect of a secretory cell of an adjacent follicle. Mitochondria **Mi** are closely associated with the endoplasmic reticulum and are also scattered throughout the cytoplasm. Golgi complexes **G** are a prominent feature. Small microvilli **Mv** associated with the exocytosis of thyroglobulin and the endocytosis of the thyroglobulin–hormone complex protrude into the follicular lumen. In one cell a vacuole **V** of thyroglobulin–hormone is seen about to fuse with a large lysosome **L**. Electron-dense lysosomes are also seen scattered throughout the cytoplasm.

ORGAN SYSTEMS

Parathyroid gland

The parathyroid glands are small oval endocrine glands closely associated with the thyroid gland. In mammals, there are usually two pairs of glands, one pair situated on the posterior surface of the thyroid gland on each side, although occasional individuals possess five or even six parathyroids. The embryological origins of the parathyroid glands are the third and fourth branchial (pharyngeal) pouches. The parathyroid glands regulate serum calcium and phosphate levels via *parathyroid hormone (parathormone, PTH)*.

Parathyroid hormone raises serum calcium levels in three ways:

- Direct action on bone, increasing the rate of osteoclastic resorption and promoting breakdown of the bone matrix.
- Direct action on the kidney, increasing the renal tubular reabsorption of calcium ions and inhibiting the reabsorption of phosphate ions from the glomerular filtrate.
- Promotion of the absorption of calcium from the small intestine; this effect involves vitamin D.

Secretion of parathyroid hormone is stimulated by a decrease in blood calcium levels. In conjunction with calcitonin secreted by the C cells of the thyroid gland, blood calcium levels are maintained within narrow limits. Parathyroid hormone is the most important regulator of blood calcium levels and is essential to life, whereas calcitonin appears to provide a complementary mechanism for fine adjustment and is not essential to life.

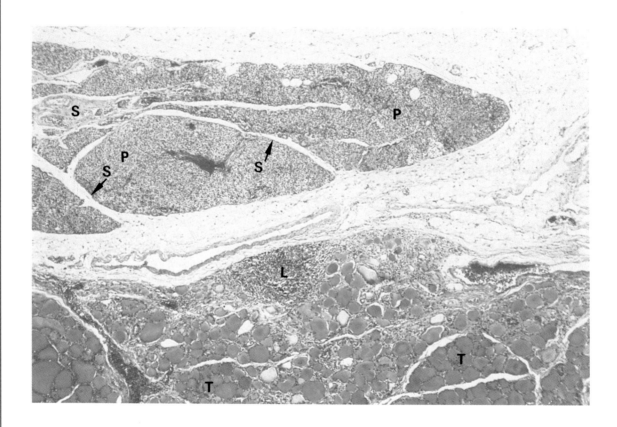

Fig. 17.9   **Parathyroid gland** H & E × 45

This micrograph shows a parathyroid gland **P**, characteristically embedded in the capsule of a thyroid gland **T**. Some parathyroids are actually found embedded in the thyroid. The thin fibrous capsule of the parathyroid gland gives rise to delicate septa **S** which divide the parenchyma into nodules of secretory cells; as seen here they are very prone to shrinkage artefact during histological preparation. The septa carry blood vessels, lymphatics and nerves.

Note that in this specimen from a 55-year-old woman, there is some infiltration of the thyroid by lymphocytes **L**; this is a common feature of the ageing thyroid gland, and is often of little clinical significance.

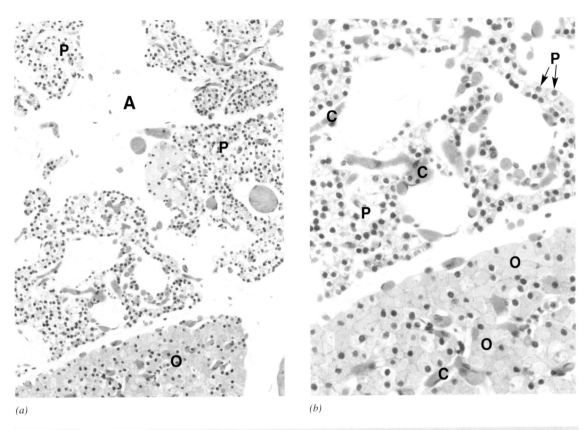

(a)   *(b)*

Fig. 17.10   **Parathyroid gland** (a) H & E × 150 (b) H & E × 300

Micrograph (a) is a medium power view of normal adult parathyroid showing the glandular elements intermixed with adipose tissue **A**, which begins to accumulate after puberty and makes up 25–40% of the total tissue in normal adults. The glandular cells are of two types: *chief* or *principal cells* **P** and *oxyphil cells* **O**. The glandular cells are arranged as clusters, ribbons or glands.

At higher power, in micrograph (b), the chief cells **P**, are small with round central nuclei and pale eosinophilic or clear cytoplasm. These are the cells which synthesise and secrete PTH. The staining intensity of the cytoplasm depends on whether the cells are actively secreting PTH, in which case the cytoplasm contains plentiful rough endoplasmic reticulum and stains strongly. On the other hand, resting cells have pale cytoplasm and make up about 80% of the total in normal adults.

Oxyphil cells **O**, which tend to occur in nodules, have copious eosinophilic cytoplasm which ultrastructurally is seen to be packed with mitochondria. These cell do not secrete PTH and increase in number with age.

Note the many delicate capillaries **C** between the nests of endocrine cells.

Adrenal gland

The adrenal (suprarenal) glands are small flattened endocrine glands which are closely applied to the upper pole of each kidney. In mammals, the adrenal gland contains two functionally different types of endocrine tissue which have distinctly different embryological origins; in some lower animals, these two components exist as separate endocrine glands. The two components of the adrenal gland are the *adrenal cortex* and *adrenal medulla*.

- **Adrenal cortex.** The adrenal cortex has a similar embryological origin to the gonads and, like them, secretes a variety of *steroid hormones* all structurally related to their common precursor, *cholesterol*. The adrenal steroids may be divided into three functional classes, *mineralocorticoids*, *glucocorticoids* and *sex hormones*. The mineralocorticoids are concerned with electrolyte and fluid homeostasis. The glucocorticoids have a wide range of effects on carbohydrate, protein and lipid metabolism. Small quantities of sex hormones are secreted by the adrenal cortex and supplement gonadal sex hormone secretion.
- **Adrenal medulla.** Embryologically, the adrenal medulla has a similar origin to that of the sympathetic nervous system and may be considered as a highly specialised adjunct of this system. The adrenal medulla secretes the catecholamine hormones, *adrenaline* (*epinephrine*) and *noradrenaline* (*norepinephrine*).

The control of hormone secretion differs markedly between the cortex and medulla. Glucocorticoid secretion is mainly regulated by the pituitary trophic hormone ACTH, while mineralocorticoid secretion is under the control of the renin–angiotensin system (see Ch. 16). In contrast, the secretion of adrenal medullary

ORGAN SYSTEMS

catecholamines is directly controlled by the sympathetic nervous system. The function of the adrenal medulla is to reinforce the action of the sympathetic nervous system under conditions of stress, the direct nervous control of adrenal medullary secretion permitting a rapid response.

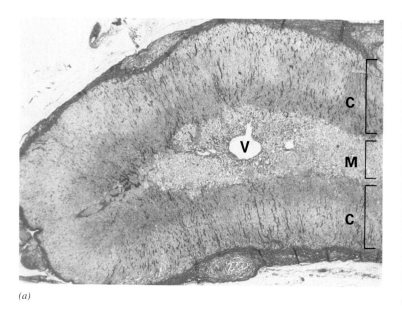

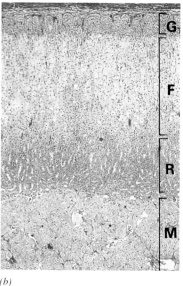

(a) *(b)*

Fig. 17.11 **Adrenal gland** (a) Azan × 12 (b) Azan × 20

At low magnification, the adrenal gland is seen to be divided into an outer cortex **C** and a pale stained inner medulla **M**. A dense fibrous tissue capsule, stained blue in this preparation, invests the gland and provides external support for a delicate collagenous framework supporting the secretory cells. A prominent vein **V** is characteristically located in the centre of the medulla.

At higher magnification in micrograph (b), the adrenal cortex can be seen to consist of three histological zones which are named according to the arrangement of the secretory cells: *zona glomerulosa*, *zona fasciculata* and *zona reticularis*.

The zona glomerulosa **G** lying beneath the capsule contains secretory cells arranged in rounded clusters. The intermediate zona fasciculata **F** consists of parallel cords of secretory cells disposed at right angles to the capsule. The zona reticularis **R**, which lies adjacent to the medulla **M**, consists of small closely packed cells arranged in irregular cords. Often the borders of the zones are less regular and less easily recognised than in this specimen.

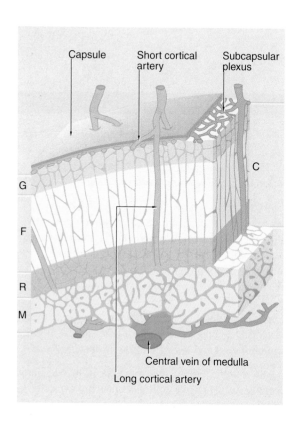

Fig. 17.12 **Blood supply of the adrenal**

The adrenal gland is supplied by the *superior*, *middle* and *inferior suprarenal* arteries, which form a plexus just under the capsule of the gland.

The vascular system of the cortex **C** consists of an anastomosing network of capillary sinusoids supplied by branches of the subcapsular plexus, known as *short cortical arteries*. The sinusoids descend between the cords of secretory cells in the zona fasciculata **F** into a deep plexus in the zona reticularis **R** before draining into small venules which converge upon the central vein of the medulla **M**. The central medullary veins contain longitudinal bundles of smooth muscle between which the cortical venules enter; contraction of this smooth muscle is thought to dam back cortical blood and thus regulate flow.

The medulla is supplied by *long cortical arteries* which descend from the subcapsular plexus through the cortex into the medulla where they ramify into a rich network of dilated capillaries surrounding the medullary secretory cells. The medullary capillaries also drain into the central vein of the medulla. Thus the secretory cells of the medulla are exposed to fresh arterial blood as well as blood rich in adrenocorticosteroids, which are believed to have an important influence on the synthesis of adrenaline by the medulla.

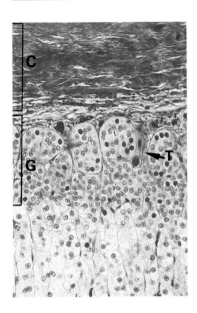

Fig. 17.13 **Adrenal cortex: zona glomerulosa** Azan × 128

The zona glomerulosa **G**, which often forms an incomplete layer, is composed of secretory cells arranged in irregular ovoid clusters separated by delicate trabeculae containing wide diameter capillaries; the collagen of the capsule **C** and trabeculae **T** stains blue with Azan. The secretory cells have round strongly stained nuclei and less cytoplasm than the adjacent zona fasciculata. The cytoplasm is acidophilic giving the darker stained appearance of this zone when seen at lower magnification (see Fig. 17.11). The cytoplasm of the secretory cells contains plentiful smooth endoplasmic reticulum and numerous mitochondria. Lipid droplets, which are the basic substrate for steroid synthesis, are much less common than in the zona fasciculata.

The zona glomerulosa secretes the mineralocorticoid hormones, principally *aldosterone*. As described in Chapter 16, aldosterone secretion is controlled by the renin–angiotensin system which is in turn regulated by the macula densa of the distal renal tubule. Aldosterone acts directly on the renal tubules to increase sodium and therefore water retention, thus increasing extracellular fluid volume and therefore arterial blood pressure. Aldosterone secretion is independent of ACTH.

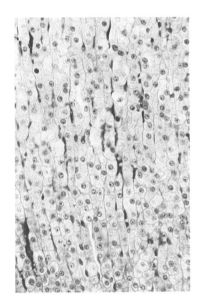

Fig. 17.14 **Adrenal cortex: zona fasciculata** Azan × 128

The zona fasciculata is the middle and broadest of the three zones of the adrenal cortex. It consists of narrow radially arranged cords of secretory cells, often only one cell thick, separated by fine strands of supporting tissue containing wide diameter capillaries. The secretory cells have abundant poorly stained cytoplasm. The cytoplasm is rich in smooth endoplasmic reticulum, mitochondria and lipid droplets. The lipid droplets give the cytoplasm a pale foamy appearance.

The zona fasciculata secretes glucocorticoid hormones, principally *cortisol*, which has wide-ranging metabolic effects. Reflecting the name glucocorticoid, an important metabolic effect is to raise blood glucose levels and increase cellular synthesis of glycogen. These effects on carbohydrate metabolism are complemented by increased breakdown of proteins and liberation of lipid from tissue stores.

Cortisol secretion is controlled by the hypothalamus via the anterior pituitary hormone ACTH. By this means, many stimuli, including stress, promote secretion of glucocorticoids which adjust body metabolism appropriately.

The zona fasciculata is also the site of secretion of small amounts of androgenic sex hormones.

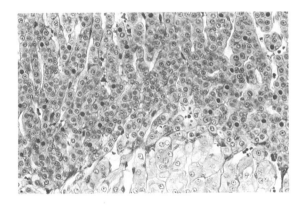

Fig. 17.15 **Adrenal cortex: zona reticularis** Azan × 128

The zona reticularis is the thin innermost zone of the adrenal cortex. It consists of an irregular network of branching cords and clusters of glandular cells separated by numerous wide diameter capillaries. The glandular cells are much smaller than those of the adjacent zona fasciculata, and the cytoplasm, which contains few lipid droplets, stains more strongly. The brown wear and tear pigment lipofuscin (see Fig. 1.14) is a characteristic feature of H & E stained specimens.

The zona reticularis secretes small quantities of androgens and glucocorticoids. The width of the zona reticularis varies under different physiological conditions.

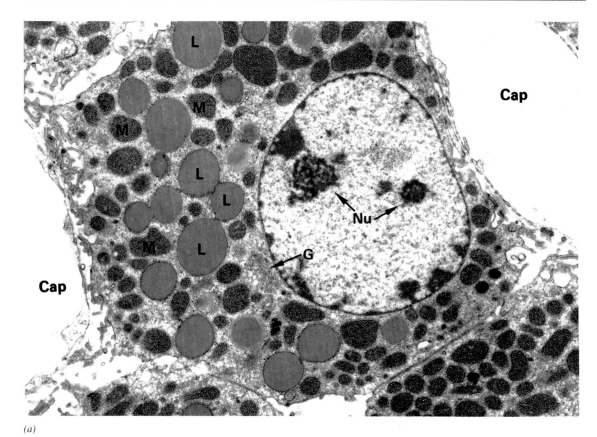

(a)

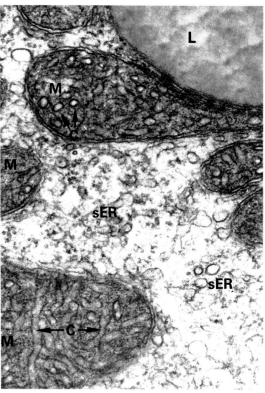

(b)

Fig. 17.16 Steroid-secreting cell
(a) EM × 8500 (b) EM × 110 500

These micrographs illustrate the typical ultrastructural features of steroid-secreting cells which are seen not only in the cells of the adrenal cortex but also in the steroid-secreting cells of the ovaries and testes (see Chs 18 and 19). At low magnification in micrograph (a), a secretory cell is seen intimately associated with fenestrated capillaries **Cap**. Note the short microvillous projections of the secretory cell plasma membrane subjacent to the capillary endothelium. The rounded secretory cell nucleus is characterised by one or more prominent nucleoli **Nu**.

The abundant cytoplasm contains many large lipid droplets **L** containing stored cholesterol esters. A small Golgi apparatus **G** is seen close to the nucleus. Numerous variably shaped mitochondria **M** crowd the cytoplasm. As seen in micrograph (b) at high magnification, the mitochondria **M** have unusual, tubular cristae **C**. The cytoplasm contains a prolific system of smooth endoplasmic reticulum **sER**.

Synthesis of steroid hormones begins with the liberation of cholesterol esters from lipid droplets. The cholesterol molecule is modified to form a wide range of steroid hormones by enzyme systems found in the smooth endoplasmic reticulum and in the mitochondria.

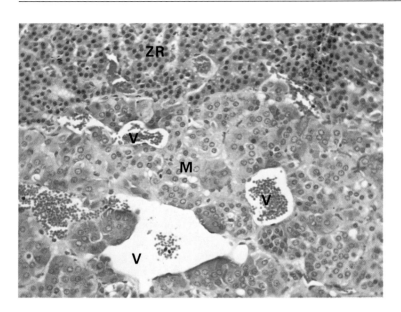

Fig. 17.17 Adrenal medulla H & E × 198

The adrenal medulla **M** is composed of closely packed clusters of secretory cells supported by a fine collagenous network containing numerous wide diameter capillaries. Many venous channels **V** draining blood from the sinusoids of the cortex pass through the medulla towards the central medullary vein (see Fig. 17.11).

The secretory cells of the adrenal medulla have large nuclei and extensive strongly basophilic, faintly granular cytoplasm which contains scanty endoplasmic reticulum and no stored lipid. Note the contrasting eosinophilic cytoplasm of the cells of the adjacent zona reticularis **ZR** of the cortex.

The adrenal medulla secretes the catecholamine hormones *noradrenaline* and *adrenaline* under the direct control of the sympathetic nervous system. Adrenal medullary hormones are not secreted continuously but are stored in membrane-bound dense core cytoplasmic granules and released only in response to nervous stimulation in a manner similar to the release of neurotransmitter substances from nerve endings. The dense core secretory granules give rise to the cytoplasmic granularity just detectable by light microscopy.

Recent investigations show that the adrenal medulla is also responsible for the secretion of *enkephalins*, opioid peptides involved in control of pain.

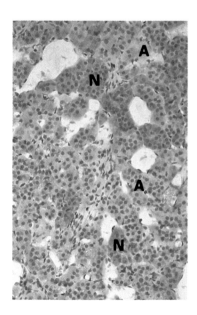

Fig. 17.18 Adrenal medulla Chrome salt fixation H & E × 800

When fixed in chrome salts, the stored catecholamine granules of adrenal medullary cells are oxidised to a brown colour; consequently the name *chromaffin cells* was often applied to the secretory cells of the adrenal medulla.

Some adrenal medullary cells synthesise noradrenaline; however, the majority synthesise adrenaline by the addition of a further N-methyl group to noradrenaline. The enzyme responsible for this conversion is induced by cortisol percolating down from the cortex. Those cells containing noradrenaline **N** exhibit a much more strongly positive chromaffin reaction than adrenaline-secreting cells **A**.

Secretion of catecholamines by the adrenal medulla is controlled by preganglionic neurones of the sympathetic nervous system; thus the secretory cells of the adrenal medulla are functionally equivalent to the postganglionic neurones of the sympathetic nervous system. Acute physical and psychological stresses initiate release of adrenal medullary hormones. The released catecholamines act on adrenergic receptors throughout the body, particularly in the heart and blood vessels, bronchioles, visceral muscle and skeletal muscle, producing physiological effects very familiar to those who have ever taken a viva voce examination. Adrenaline also has potent metabolic effects such as the promotion of glycogenolysis in liver and skeletal muscle, thus releasing a readily available energy source during stress situations.

Endocrine pancreas

The pancreas is not only a major exocrine gland (see Ch. 15) but also has important endocrine functions.

The embryonic epithelium of the pancreatic ducts consists of both potential exocrine and endocrine cells. During development, the endocrine cells migrate from the duct system and aggregate around capillaries to form isolated clusters of cells, known as *islets of Langerhans*, scattered throughout the exocrine glandular tissue. The islets vary in size and are most numerous in the tail of the pancreas. The islets contain a variety of cell types each responsible for secretion of one type of polypeptide hormone.

The main secretory products of the endocrine pancreas are *insulin* and *glucagon*, polypeptide hormones which play an important role in carbohydrate metabolism. Insulin promotes the uptake of glucose by most cells, particularly those of the liver, skeletal muscle and adipose tissue, thus lowering plasma glucose concentration. In general, glucagon has metabolic effects that oppose the actions of insulin. Apart from their role in carbohydrate metabolism, these hormones have a wide variety of other effects on energy metabolism, growth and development.

At least four other types of endocrine cells are present in the islets or else scattered singly or in small groups between the exocrine acini and along the ducts. Their secretory products include *somatostatin* (which has a wide variety of effects on gastrointestinal function and may also inhibit insulin and glucagon secretion), *vasoactive intestinal peptide* (*VIP*) and *pancreatic polypeptide* (*PP*). Another cell type, the enterochromaffin (EC) cell, appears to secrete several different peptides including *motilin, serotonin* and *substance P*.

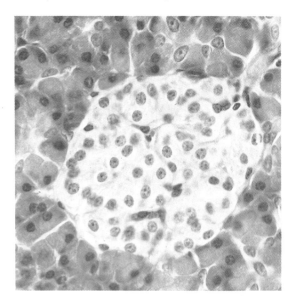

Fig. 17.19 | Islet of Langerhans H & E × 480

The islets of Langerhans are composed of groups of up to 3000 secretory cells supported by a fine collagenous network containing numerous fenestrated capillaries. A delicate capsule surrounds each islet. The endocrine cells are small with a pale stained granular cytoplasm; in contrast, the large cells of the surrounding pancreatic acini stain strongly. This difference in staining intensity reflects the relatively greater amount of rough endoplasmic reticulum in the exocrine cells, which secrete large quantities of protein (see Figs 15.15c).

The endocrine pancreas contains secretory cells of several types; however, in H & E stained preparations, the cell types are indistinguishable from one another and special staining methods are required to differentiate between them. Traditionally, the glucagon-, insulin- and somatostatin-secreting cells have been designated as *alpha, beta* and *delta cells*, respectively. However, with the advent of simple techniques (such as immunoperoxidase) for identification of secretory products, it is most appropriate to identify cells by their products.

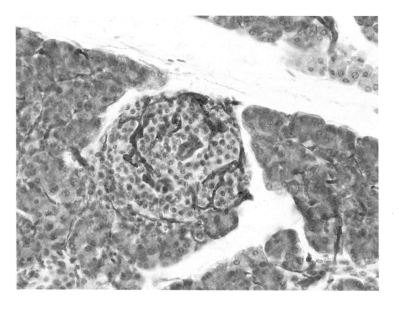

Fig. 17.20 | Blood supply of the endocrine pancreas Carmine perfused/ haematoxylin × 128

This specimen was perfused with a red dye before fixation to demonstrate the rich blood supply of the pancreatic islets. Each islet is supplied by as many as three arterioles, which ramify into a highly branched network of fenestrated capillaries, into which the hormones produced in the islet are secreted. The islet is drained by about six venules passing between the exocrine acini to the interlobular veins.

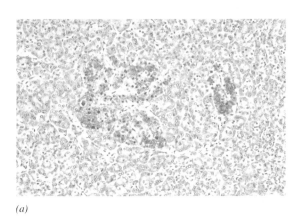

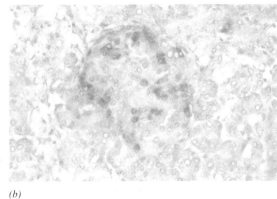

(a)   *(b)*

Fig. 17.21   **Islet of Langerhans**
(a) Immunoperoxidase for insulin × 100 (b) Immunoperoxidase for glucagon × 200

In the past, empirical staining methods were used to demonstrate the different cell types in the islets of Langerhans. These have now been superseded by the immunoperoxidase technique which is able to detect specific intercellular products, in this case insulin and glucagon. The insulin-producing *beta cells*, which constitute over 60% of the cells in the islet, are stained brown in micrograph (a). Beta cells are distributed throughout the islet while in contrast, glucagon-producing *alpha cells* (about 25% of the total) are arranged around the periphery (b). Other hormone-producing cells are unstained in these micrographs. The close proximity of these cells facilitates their interaction for control of blood glucose levels and other metabolic functions.

Insulin, a small protein, is synthesized in the rough endoplasmic reticulum as *preproinsulin* which is then cleaved to form *proinsulin*. Proinsulin is cleaved again, this time in the Golgi apparatus, to form insulin, which is then packaged with a small amount of uncleaved proinsulin into membrane-bound secretory granules which remain in the cytoplasm until insulin secretion is triggered.

Pineal gland

The pineal gland is a small organ, 6–8 mm long, which represents an evagination of the posterior part of the roof of the third ventricle in the midline. The pineal is connected to the brain via a short stalk containing nerve fibres, many of which communicate with the hypothalamus. In reptiles and other lower vertebrates, the pineal lies at or near the skin surface where it functions as a photoreceptor organ secreting the hormone *melatonin* which lightens skin colour by its action on melanophores, pigmented cells analogous to melanocytes in mammals.

Melatonin synthesis from the amino acid tryptophan is induced by darkness and inhibited by light. It functions as a *neuroendocrine transducer*, in that information received by the retina in the form of light is converted by the pineal into the chemical signal melatonin. Recent research has demonstrated a wide range of actions of this interesting hormone. It is now known that melatonin regulates the circadian rhythms of the body; hence its popularity with those lucky enough to be able to suffer the effects of 'jetlag'. Its secretion during the hours of darkness causes a hypnotic effect. It also probably has a variety of functions in the regulation of reproductive processes including the onset of puberty in humans and seasonal reproduction in animals. Other possible functions include effects on ageing and regulation of the immune system.

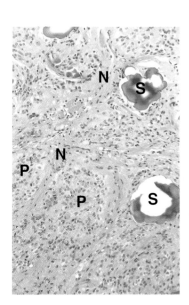

Fig. 17.22   **Pineal gland H & E × 100**

The pineal consists of two main cell types: *pinealocytes* (*pineal chief cells*) and *neuroglial cells*. Pinealocytes **P** are highly modified neurones arranged in clusters and cords surrounded by a rich network of fenestrated capillaries. Pinealocytes have round nuclei with prominent nucleoli and granular cytoplasm, and many highly branched processes, some of which terminate near or upon blood vessels. The cytoplasmic granules of pinealocytes contain melatonin and its precursor, serotonin.

The neuroglial cells **N**, which are similar to the astrocytes of the rest of the CNS, are dispersed between the clusters of pinealocytes and in association with capillaries.

A characteristic feature of the ageing pineal is the presence of basophilic extracellular bodies called *pineal sand* **S** consisting of concentric layers of calcium and magnesium phosphate in an organic matrix. The calcified pineal can be seen on X-rays of the skull and its position can be a useful guide to pathological conditions causing the midline to be displaced to one side.

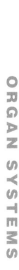

The gastrointestinal endocrine system

Neuroendocrine cells are found scattered in the mucosa of the gastrointestinal tract and in the pancreatic and biliary ducts. These cells secrete more than 20 different peptide and amine hormones including gastrin, secretin, CCK, serotonin, enteroglucagon, somatostatin, substance P, vasoactive intestinal peptide (VIP), bombesin, gastric inhibitory polypeptide (GIP), motilin and pancreatic polypeptide (PP). These hormones constitute a system of interacting mediators, which collectively regulate and coordinate most aspects of gastrointestinal activity in concert with the autonomic nervous system.

While some of these substances are true *endocrine hormones*, acting at a distance from their site of origin, others are locally acting mediators known as *paracrine hormones*. A third mechanism of action (*neurocrine*) is by neurotransmitter activity and indeed some of these substances also act as neurotransmitters within the central nervous system (gastrin, VIP, CCK and many others).

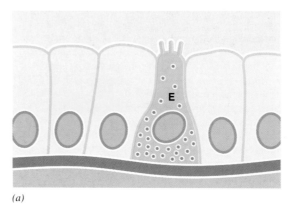
(a)

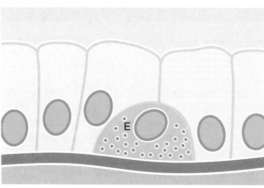
(b)

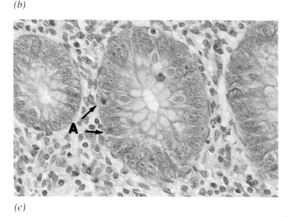
(c)

Fig. 17.23 Mucosal neuroendocrine cells
(a) Open type (b) Closed type
(c) Alkaline diazo method × 320

The endocrine cells **E** may be located at any level in the mucosa from the base of glands to the tips of villi. The cells exposed to the tract lumen may be receptive to gastrointestinal contents; these are termed the *open type* (a). Other endocrine cells are deep to the surface, the *closed type* (b), and may be receptive to changes in local tissue environment. The cells responsible for the secretion of a particular hormone tend to be located in a particular anatomical region in the tract but there is considerable overlap in distribution, e.g. gastrin-secreting cells are found in the body of the stomach, the duodenum and the pancreas.

Early methods for demonstrating these cells, which are difficult to detect with routine H & E staining, involved the use of silver or chromium salts. These cells were divided into two types, *argentaffin cells* (silver reducing) and *argyrophil cells* (silver absorbing). Like the catecholamine-secreting 'chromaffin' cells of the adrenal medulla (see Fig. 17.18), both these cell types could be stained specifically with chromium salts and thus the gastrointestinal endocrine cells became collectively known as *enterochromaffin cells*. These classifications were subsequently found to be of little functional significance and currently the term enterochromaffin cell is only applied to a specific cell type which secretes serotonin (5-hydroxytryptamine). Another empirical histochemical method has been used in (c) to demonstrate neuroendocrine cells in the colon (stained reddish brown **A**). Their deep position in the epithelium indicates that these cells are probably of the closed type.

Current practice is to name these cells according to their major secretory product (e.g. gastrin cells in the stomach). The cells and their products are now easily identified using the immunoperoxidase technique. Examples of these are shown in the relevant chapters (see Figs 12.10b and 14.13c).

The respiratory endocrine system

The lower respiratory tract contains scattered peptide- and amine-secreting endocrine cells analogous to those in the gastrointestinal tract, which are probably involved in local and autonomically mediated regulation of respiratory tract function particularly in early childhood. The endocrine cells are scattered individually in the epithelium or in clumps protruding into the airway and have a variety of secretory products including serotonin, calcitonin, bombesin and leu-enkephalin.

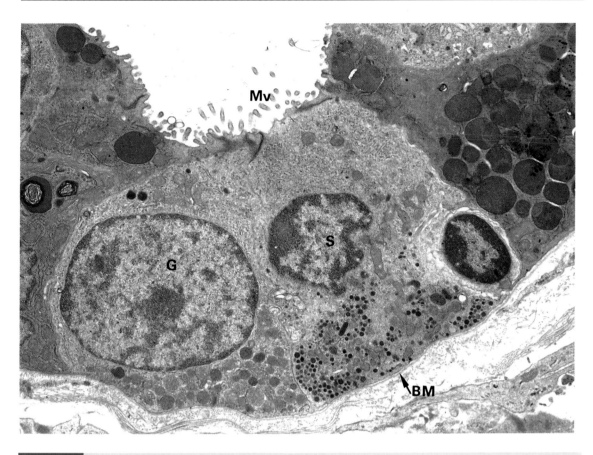

Fig. 17.24 **Gastrointestinal neuroendocrine cells** EM × 8300

This micrograph shows two cells from the human pylorus, both of which exhibit the typical characteristics of open-type gastrointestinal neuroendocrine cells. The cell marked **G** is a gastrin secreting cell recognised on the basis of its large moderately dense secretory granules. The adjacent endocrine cell marked **S** contains much smaller and more dense granules of somatostatin which has a broad range of actions including the inhibition of secretion of insulin, glucagon and many gastrointestinal hormones. Open-type neuroendocrine cells are usually pyramidal in shape, the apex extending to the tract lumen and the base resting on the basement membrane **BM**. The apical surface forms a few microvilli **Mv**, which may receive stimuli from the tract lumen. Secretory granules are aggregated in the basal cytoplasm from which they are released into the underlying extracellular space, diffusing into the capillaries of the lamina propria. Typically, the cytoplasm contains only a few short profiles of rough endoplasmic reticulum and numerous free ribosomes. Closed-type neuroendocrine cells are usually rounded and lack the polarity of the open type but otherwise have similar ultrastructural features.

The diffuse neuroendocrine concept

The concept of a diffuse neuroendocrine system has been refined and modified over many years. First recognised over 60 years ago, this group of cells was defined by their ability to take up amines and decarboxylate them and thus earned the inelegant name APUD cells (for amine uptake and decarboxylation). Tumours arising from these cells were accordingly named 'APUDomas'. However, it was subsequently shown that not all the cells in the group exhibited this function and the term APUD is thankfully falling into disuse. Similarly, at one time all the cells in the group were thought to be derived embryologically from the neural crest. Again rigorous testing of this theory has demonstrated that some of these cells are derived from endoderm (in particular those belonging to the gastrointestinal tract). The current consensus defines these cells according to functional and structural characteristics as follows:

- The cells produce amines or peptides with hormone-like activity and/or neurotransmitters.
- The cells possess synaptic vesicle-like structures or neurosecretory-type granules (*dense core vesicles,* see Fig. 7.21).
- The products of the cells are released by exocytosis in response to external stimuli.

The neuroendocrine group of cells includes cells forming part of recognised endocrine glands such as adrenal medullary cells, thyroid C cells, cells of the islets of Langerhans, ACTH- and MSH-producing cells of the pituitary as well as the diffusely scattered neuroendocrine cells of the gastrointestinal, respiratory and urogenital tracts. Also included in the group are the renin-secreting cells of the juxtaglomerular apparatus of the kidney and the chemoreceptor cells of the carotid body.

18. Male reproductive system

Introduction

The male reproductive system may be divided into four major functional components:

- The *testes* or male gonads, paired organs lying in the scrotal sac, are responsible for production of the male gametes, *spermatozoa*, and secretion of male sex hormones, principally *testosterone*.
- A paired system of ducts, each consisting of *ductuli efferentes*, *epididymis*, *ductus deferens* and *ejaculatory duct*, collect, store and conduct spermatozoa from each testis. The ejaculatory ducts converge on the *urethra* from which spermatozoa are expelled into the female reproductive tract during copulation.
- Two exocrine glands, the paired *seminal vesicles* and the single *prostate gland*, secrete a nutritive and lubricating fluid medium called *seminal fluid* in which spermatozoa are conveyed to the female reproductive tract. *Semen*, the fluid expelled during ejaculation, consists of seminal fluid and spermatozoa, plus some desquamated duct lining cells.
- The *penis* is the organ of copulation. A pair of small accessory glands, the *bulbourethral glands of Cowper*, secrete a fluid which lubricates the urethra for the passage of semen during ejaculation.

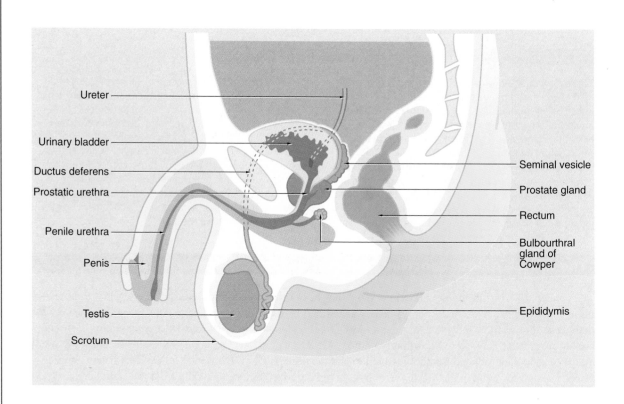

Fig. 18.1 Male reproductive system

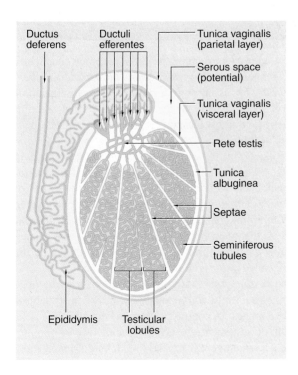

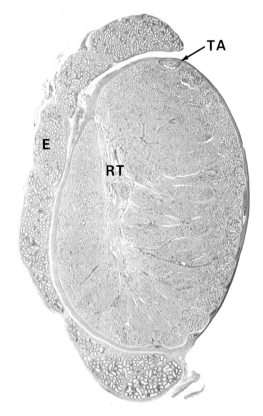

(a)

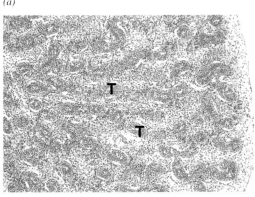

(b)

Fig. 18.2 Testis

During embryological development, each testis with the first part of its duct system, blood vessels, lymphatics and nerves, descends along a tortuous path from the posterior wall of the peritoneal cavity to the scrotum. During migration, the testis carries with it an investing layer of peritoneum so that in the scrotum the testis is almost completely surrounded by a double layer of mesothelium enclosing a potential space. This double lining is called the *tunica vaginalis* and, like the pleura, consists of *visceral* and *parietal layers* separated by a thin layer of serous fluid. The fluid is secreted by the mesothelial cells and acts as a lubricant, allowing the testis to move freely in the scrotal sac.

The visceral layer of the tunica vaginalis rests on the capsule of the testis, the *tunica albuginea*, which gives rise to numerous incomplete collagenous septa. These divide the testis into about 250 *testicular lobules*. Within each lobule there are one to four highly convoluted tubes, the *seminiferous tubules*, in which spermatozoa are produced. The seminiferous tubules converge upon a plexus of channels, the *rete testis*. From the rete testis, 15 to 20 small ducts, called the *ductuli efferentes*, conduct spermatozoa to the extremely tortuous first part of the *ductus deferens*, which is known as the *epididymis*.

Fig. 18.3 Testis
(a) Monkey, H & E × 3 (b) Human fetus, H & E × 10

Micrograph (a) illustrates the macroscopic features of a testis; cut in the sagittal plane, it shows the relationship of the epididymis **E** which lies on its posterior aspect. The testis is packed with coiled seminiferous tubules, which can just be seen in various planes of section at this magnification. Groups of up to four seminiferous tubules are segregated into testicular lobules; the interlobular septa are so delicate as to be barely seen at this magnification. The dense fibrous capsule which invests the testis, and which is continuous with many of the interlobular septa, is called the *tunica albuginea* **TA** since it appears white macroscopically. The tunica albuginea contains fibroblasts and myofibroblasts, particularly in the posterior aspect, which subject the seminiferous tissue to rhythmic contractions. The deepest layer of the tunica albuginea consists of loose connective tissue containing blood and lymphatic vessels, sometimes called the *tunica vasculosa*.

Spermatozoa pass from the seminiferous tubules into the rete testis **RT** which is connected to the epididymis via the ductuli efferentes at the upper posterior pole of the testis; the ductuli are not included in the plane of this section. The epididymis is a tightly coiled tube, which forms a compact mass extending down the whole length of the posterior surface of the testis. The epididymis is the major site of storage of newly formed spermatozoa. At the lower pole of the testis, the epididymal tube becomes continuous with the relatively straight ductus (vas) deferens, which is not seen in this section.

Micrograph (b) is of human fetal testis of 18 weeks' gestation. At this stage the tubular nature of the radially arranged seminiferous tubules **T** is much more obvious before significant coiling has occurred. The tubules contain spermatogonia and Sertoli cells. Production of gametes, however, does not begin until after puberty.

ORGAN SYSTEMS

Gametogenesis

In all somatic cells, cell division (mitosis) results in the formation of two daughter cells, each one genetically identical to the mother cell. Somatic cells contain a full complement of chromosomes (the ***diploid number***) which function as homologous pairs (see Ch. 2). The process of sexual reproduction involves the fusion of specialised male and female cells called ***gametes*** to form a ***zygote***, which has the diploid number of chromosomes. Each gamete contains only half the diploid number of chromosomes, one representative of each pair; this half complement of chromosomes is known as the ***haploid number***.

The production of haploid cells involves a unique form of cell division called ***meiosis***, which occurs only in the germ cells of the gonads during the formation of gametes; meiotic cell division is thus also called ***gametogenesis***. Meiosis involves two cell division cycles of which only the first is preceded by duplication of chromosomes (see Ch. 2). Thus, meiotic cell division of a single diploid germ cell gives rise to four haploid gametes. In the male, each of the four gametes undergoes morphological development into a mature ***spermatozoon***. In contrast, in the female, unequal distribution of the cytoplasm during meiosis results in one gamete gaining almost all the cytoplasm from the mother cell, whilst the other three acquire almost no cytoplasm; the large gamete matures to form an ***ovum*** and the other three, called ***polar bodies***, degenerate.

The primitive germ cells of the male, the ***spermatogonia***, are present only in small numbers in the male gonads before sexual maturity. After puberty, spermatogonia multiply continuously by mitosis to provide a supply of cells, which then undergo meiosis to form male gametes. In contrast, the germ cells of the female, called ***oogonia***, multiply by mitosis only during early fetal development, thereby producing a fixed complement of cells with the potential to undergo gametogenesis. Gametogenesis in the female is discussed more fully in Chapter 19. The production of male gametes is called ***spermatogenesis*** and the subsequent development of the male gamete into a motile spermatozoon is called ***spermiogenesis***, the whole process taking approximately 70 days; both these processes occur within the testes although final maturation of spermatozoa occurs in the epididymis.

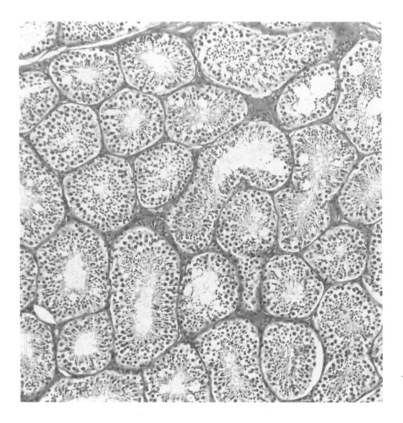

Fig. 18.4 **Seminiferous tubules** H & E × 100

This micrograph illustrates seminiferous tubules cut in various planes of section. The seminiferous tubules are highly convoluted and lined by a stratified epithelium which consists of two distinct populations of cells:

- Cells in various stages of spermatogenesis and spermiogenesis are collectively referred to as the ***spermatogenic series***.
- Non-spermatogenic cells called ***Sertoli cells*** support and nourish the developing spermatozoa. The Sertoli cells, by virtue of their intercellular adhesions, divide the seminiferous epithelium into two compartments, known as the ***basal*** and ***adluminal*** compartments.

In the interstitial spaces between the tubules, endocrine cells called ***Leydig cells*** are found either singly or in groups in the supporting tissue.

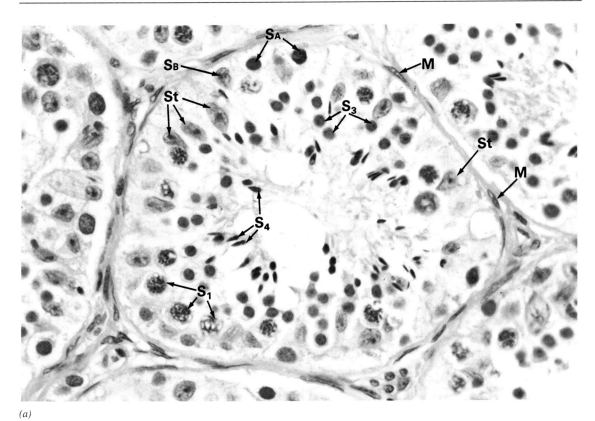

(a)

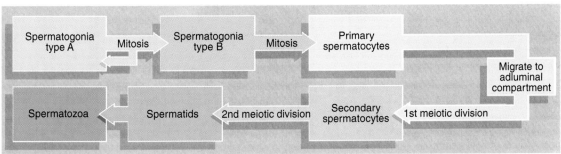

(b)

Fig. 18.5 **Seminiferous tubule** (a) H & E × 640 (b) Diagram

Micrograph (a) illustrates an adult seminiferous tubule cut in transverse section. The processes of spermatogenesis and spermiogenesis are synchronised, with waves of activity occurring sequentially along the length of each tubule. Thus in a single cross-section of a tubule, not all development phases will be represented (b).

The undifferentiated germ cells, found in the basal compartment of the seminiferous tubule, are called *type A spermatogonia*. These go through several cycles of mitosis to produce further type A spermatogonia, which maintain the germ cell pool, and *type B spermatogonia*, which are committed to production of spermatozoa. Spermatogonia type A S_A are characterised by a large round or oval nucleus with condensed chromatin; peripheral nucleoli and a nuclear vacuole may be prominent. Spermatogonia type B S_B have dispersed chromatin, central nucleoli, and no nuclear vacuole. Both types of spermatogonia have sparse poorly stained cytoplasm.

Type B spermatogonia undergo further mitotic divisions to produce *primary spermatocytes*. These migrate to the adluminal compartment of the seminiferous tubule before commencing the first meiotic division. Primary spermatocytes S_1 are readily recognised by their copious cytoplasm and large nuclei containing coarse

clumps or thin threads of chromatin; dividing cells may be seen. In humans, the first meiotic division cycle takes approximately 3 weeks to complete, after which time the daughter cells become known as *secondary spermatocytes*. The smaller secondary spermatocytes rapidly undergo the second meiotic division and are therefore seldom seen.

The gametes thus produced, called *spermatids* S_3, then proceed through the long maturation process known as spermiogenesis to become recognisable as spermatozoa. During this process, the nuclei of the spermatids assume the small pointed form of spermatozoa S_4 (see Fig. 18.7). Examination of different sections of the tubules of a normal testis shows about half the spermatogenic cells to be in the late spermatid stage.

During the developmental process, the cells of the spermatogenic series are supported by Sertoli cells **St**, whose nuclei are usually found towards the basement membrane of the seminiferous tubule. The Sertoli cell nucleus is typically triangular or ovoid in shape with a prominent nucleolus and dispersed chromatin.

The basal layer of germinal cells is supported by a basement membrane, which is surrounded by a lamina propria containing several layers of spindle-shaped myofibroblasts **M** and fibroblasts.

ORGAN SYSTEMS

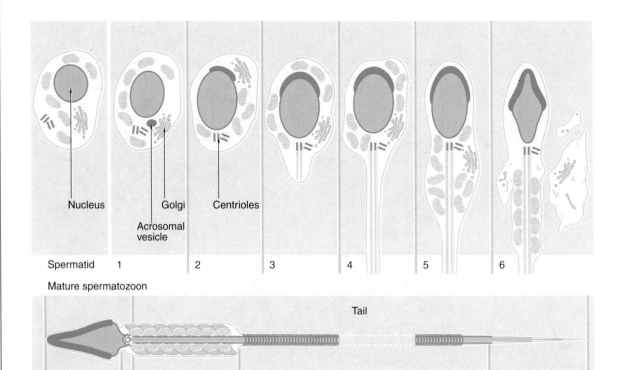

| Spermatid | 1 | 2 | 3 | 4 | 5 | 6 |

Labels: Nucleus, Golgi, Centrioles, Acrosomal vesicle

Mature spermatozoon

Tail

Head | Neck | Middle piece | Principal piece | End piece

Fig. 18.6 **Spermiogenesis**

Spermiogenesis is the process by which spermatids, the gametes produced by meiotic division, are transformed into motile mature spermatozoa. This involves the following major stages:

1. The Golgi apparatus elaborates a large vesicle, the *acrosomal vesicle*, which accumulates carbohydrates and hydrolytic enzymes.
2. The acrosomal vesicle becomes applied to one pole of the progressively elongating nucleus to form a structure known as the *acrosomal head cap*.
3. Meanwhile, both centrioles migrate to the end of the cell opposite to the acrosomal head cap; the centriole aligned parallel to the long axis of the nucleus elongates to form a flagellum which has a basic structure similar to that of the cilium (see Fig. 5.15).
4. As the flagellum elongates, nine *coarse fibrils*, which may contain contractile proteins, become arranged longitudinally around the core of the flagellum. Further rib-like fibrils then become disposed circumferentially around the whole flagellum.
5. The cytoplasm migrates to surround the first part of the flagellum. The remainder of the flagellum appears to project from the cell but in fact remains surrounded by plasma membrane. This migration of cytoplasm thus concentrates mitochondria in the flagellar region.
6. As the flagellum elongates, excess cytoplasm is phagocytosed by the enveloping Sertoli cell prior to release of the spermatid into the lumen.

The mitochondria become arranged in a helical manner around the fibrils, which surround the first part of the flagellum.

The structure of fully formed spermatozoa varies in detail from species to species, but conforms to the basic structure seen in this diagram of a human spermatozoon.

Throughout the entire developmental process from spermatogonia to spermatozoa, hundreds of spermatids remain connected to one another by narrow cytoplasmic bridges which only break down upon release of spermatozoa into the lumen of the seminiferous tubule. This explains the synchronous development of spermatozoa at any one part of the tubule.

Sertoli cells are important in the regulation of spermatogenesis and spermiogenesis. Sertoli cells form tight junctions with each other as well as with the developing germ cells. It is well established that high concentrations of androgen hormones secreted by Leydig cells of the testicular interstitium (see Fig. 18.9) are essential for production and maturation of spermatogenic cells. Sertoli cells secrete an androgen-binding protein, which transports testosterone and dihydrotestosterone to the lumen of the seminiferous tubule. These hormones are also necessary for function of the epithelium of the rete testis and epididymis; production of this binding protein is believed to be dependent on the pituitary gonadotrophin, follicle stimulating hormone (FSH).

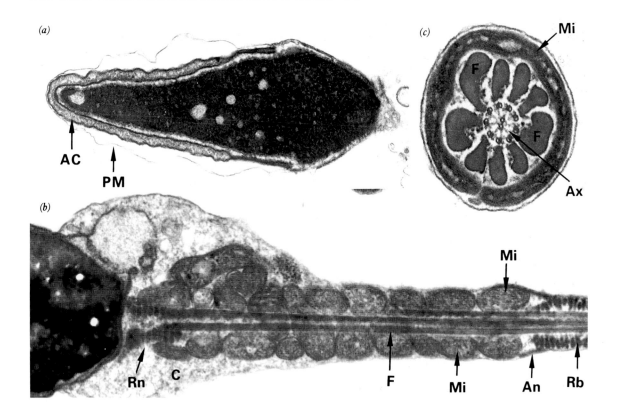

Fig. 18.7 Spermatozoa (a) Head: EM, LS × 14 000
(b) Neck (middle piece and principal piece): EM, LS × 17 000 (c) (middle piece): EM, TS × 48 000

The ultrastructural features of human spermatozoa are shown in these micrographs. The spermatozoon is an extremely elongated cell (about 65 μm long) consisting of three main components, the *head*, *neck* and *tail*. The tail is subdivided into three segments, the *middle piece*, *principal piece* and *end piece* (see Fig. 18.6).

The head is the most variable structure between different mammalian species. In humans, the head is about 7 μm long and has a flattened pear shape. As seen in micrograph (a), the nucleus, which occupies most of the head, is composed of very condensed chromatin; in humans, this contains a variable number of areas of dispersed chromatin called *nuclear vacuoles*. Surrounding the anterior two-thirds of the nucleus is the acrosomal cap **AC**, a flattened membrane-bound vesicle containing a range of glycoproteins and a variety of hydrolytic enzymes, principally *hyaluronidase*; the enzymes disaggregate the cells of the corona radiata and dissolve the zona pellucida during fertilisation (see Ch. 19). Note the plasma membrane **PM**, which has become partially separated during preparation.

The neck is a very short segment connecting the head with the tail. It contains vestiges of the centrioles, one of which gives rise to the axoneme **Ax** of the flagellum which is seen in micrograph (c). The axoneme has the standard 'nine plus two' arrangement of microtubule doublets seen in cilia (see Fig. 5.15). The axoneme of the neck is surrounded by several condensed fibrous rings **Rn** seen in micrograph (b). In human spermatozoa, a significant amount of cytoplasm **C** often remains in the neck region.

The middle piece, the first part of the tail, is about the same length as the head and consists of the flagellar axoneme surrounded by nine *coarse (outer dense) fibres* **F** arranged longitudinally. External to this core, elongated mitochondria **Mi** are arranged in a tightly packed helix providing the energy required for flagellar movement. A fibrous thickening beneath the plasma membrane, called the annulus **An**, prevents the mitochondria from slipping into the principal piece. The principal piece, which constitutes most of the tail length, consists of a central core, comprising the axoneme and the nine coarse fibres continuing from the middle piece. Surrounding this core are numerous fibrous ribs **Rb** arranged in a circular manner and seen in micrograph (b). Two of the longitudinal fibrils of the core are fused with the surrounding ribs so as to form *dorsal* and *ventral columns* extending throughout the length of the principal piece (not illustrated). This arrangement divides the principal piece longitudinally into two functional compartments, one containing three coarse fibrils and the other containing four. Little is known of the mechanism of flagellar motion but this asymmetry may account for the more powerful stroke of the tail in one direction, the so-called 'power stroke'; this can easily be observed in fresh, live preparations of spermatozoa viewed with the light microscope. The end piece, not shown in these micrographs, is merely a short tapering portion of the tail containing the axoneme only.

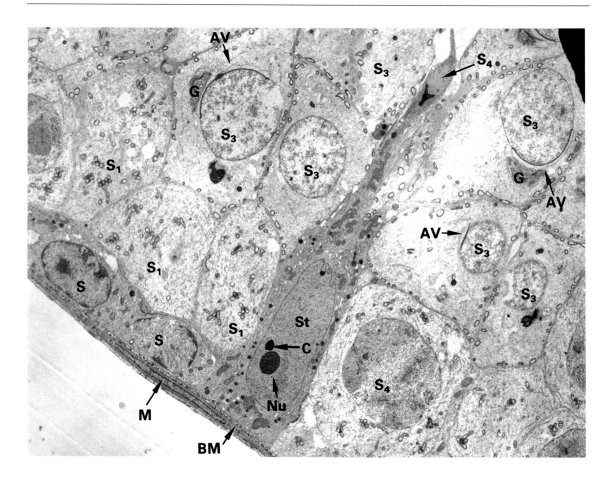

Fig. 18.8 Sertoli cell EM × 3400

The intimate relationship of a Sertoli cell **St** to cells of the spermatogenic series is demonstrated in this electron micrograph.

The Sertoli cell rests on the basement membrane **BM** of the seminiferous tubule and its cytoplasm extends to the lumen of the tubule. Sertoli cells have an extensive cytoplasm, which ramifies throughout the whole germinal epithelium enclosing all the cells of the spermatogenic series. The cytoplasmic outline of the Sertoli cell is thus highly irregular and constantly changing to permit the progressive movement of developing spermatozoa towards the luminal surface. The oval nucleus of the Sertoli cell is characteristically orientated at right angles to the basement membrane and often exhibits a deep indentation. A prominent nucleolus **Nu** is a constant feature and dense chromatin bodies **C** are often associated with the nucleolus. the cytoplasm contains a moderate number of mitochondria, lipid droplets and a small amount of rough endoplasmic reticulum. Plentiful smooth endoplasmic reticulum is also present as well as lamellar protein arrays known as Charcot–Bottcher crystals (not seen at this power).

Sertoli cells are bound to one another by junctional complexes containing extensive tight junctions (see Ch. 5). The junctional complex is located towards the basal layer of the spermatogenic epithelium so as to divide the tubule into *basal* and *adluminal compartments*. The latter contains the spermatids which are thus isolated by a *blood–testis barrier*. The Sertoli cells mediate all metabolic exchange with the systemic compartment. The function of this barrier is to prevent exposure of gametes, which are antigenically different from somatic cells, to the immune system, thus preventing an autoimmune response. Sertoli cells have multiple functions including:

- Secretion of factors which regulate spermatogenesis and spermiogenesis.
- Secretion of factors which regulate the function of Leydig cells and peritubular cells.
- Secretion of *inhibin* which regulates hormone production.
- Secretion of tubular fluid.
- Phagocytosis of discarded spermatid cytoplasm.

A variety of cells of the spermatogenic series are seen in this micrograph. Spermatogonia **S** rest upon the basement membrane beneath which is a myofibroblast **M**. Above the germ cell layer, primary spermatocytes S_1 are seen; secondary spermatocytes are short-lived and therefore rarely seen. Spermatids S_3 in different phases of spermiogenesis are seen in upper layers; these cells have developing acrosomal vesicles **AV** elaborated by a large Golgi apparatus **G** (see Fig. 18.6). At the luminal surface, the Sertoli cell envelops an almost fully formed spermatozoon S_4.

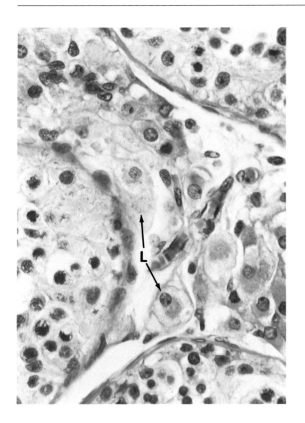

Fig. 18.9 Interstitial (Leydig) cells of the testis
H & E × 480

Leydig cells **L**, the principal cell type found in the interstitial supporting tissue between the seminiferous tubules, synthesise and secrete the male sex hormones and other non-steroid substances. They occur singly or in clumps and are embedded in the rich plexus of blood and lymph capillaries which surrounds the seminiferous tubules. The nucleus is round with dispersed chromatin and one or two nucleoli at the periphery. The extensive eosinophilic cytoplasm contains variable numbers of lipid vacuoles and seen by electron microscopy closely resembles the steroid-secreting cells of the adrenal cortex (see Fig. 17.16). In humans (and wild bush rats), but no other species, Leydig cells also contain elongated cytoplasmic *crystals of Reinke* which are large enough to be seen with light microscopy when suitably stained; these crystals are found only in adults but their function is unknown.

Testosterone is the main hormone secreted by Leydig cells. Testosterone is not only responsible for the development of male secondary sexual characteristics at puberty but is also essential for the continued function of the seminiferous epithelium. The secretory activity of Leydig cells is controlled by the pituitary gonadotrophic hormone, luteinising hormone, sometimes called *interstitial cell stimulating hormone* (ICSH) in the male.

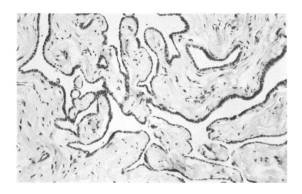

Fig. 18.10 Rete testis H & E × 128

The seminiferous tubules converge upon the *mediastinum testis*, which consists of a plexiform arrangement of channels, the *rete testis*, surrounded by highly vascular collagenous supporting tissue containing myoid cells. The rete testis is lined by a single layer of cuboidal epithelial cells with surface microvilli and a single cilium.

Myoid cell contraction helps to mix the spermatozoa and move them towards the epididymis. The lining epithelium reabsorbs protein and potassium from the seminal fluid. Ciliary activity is presumed to aid the progress of spermatozoa, which do not become motile until after maturation is completed in the epididymis.

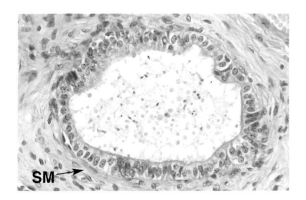

Fig. 18.11 Ductulus efferens H & E × 200

The rete testis drains into the head of the epididymis via some 15–20 convoluted ducts, the *ductuli efferentes*. The ductuli are lined by a single layer of epithelial cells, some of which are tall columnar and ciliated and others which are short and non-ciliated; both cell types often contain a brown pigment of unknown composition. Ciliary action in the ductuli propels the still non-motile spermatozoa towards the epididymis. The non-ciliated cells reabsorb some of the fluid produced by the testis. Basal cells, which do not reach the lumen, are also present and probably act as reserve cells. A thin band of circularly arranged smooth muscle **SM** surrounds each ductulus and aids propulsion of the spermatozoa towards the epididymis.

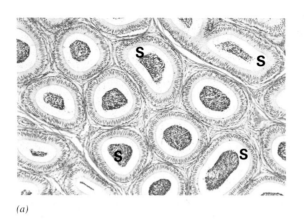

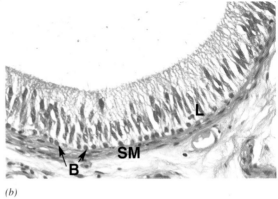

(a)   *(b)*

Fig. 18.12   Epididymis   (a) H & E × 50 (b) H & E × 200

The *epididymis* is a long extremely convoluted duct extending down the posterior aspect of the testis to the lower pole where it becomes the ductus deferens. The epididymis consists of a *head* at the upper pole of the testis, a *body* lying along the posterior margin and a *tail* at the lower pole of the testis. The major function of the epididymis is the accumulation, storage and maturation of spermatozoa **S**; in the epididymis, the spermatozoa develop motility.

The epididymis is a tube of smooth muscle lined by a pseudostratified epithelium. From the proximal to the distal end of the epididymis, the muscular wall increases from a single circular layer **SM**, as in these micrographs, to three layers organised in the same manner as in the ductus deferens (see Fig. 18.13). Proximally, the smooth muscle exhibits slow rhythmic contractility which gently moves spermatozoa towards the ductus deferens.

Distally, the smooth muscle is richly innervated by the sympathetic nervous system which produces intense contractions of the lower part of the epididymis during ejaculation.

The epithelial lining of the epididymis exhibits a gradual transition from a tall pseudostratified columnar form in the head, as seen in micrograph (b), to a shorter pseudostratified form at the tail. The principal cells of the epididymal epithelium bear tufts of very long microvilli, inappropriately called *stereocilia* (see Fig. 5.17), which are thought to be involved in absorption of an excess of fluid accompanying the spermatozoa from the testis. The ultrastructure of the cells strongly suggests an additional secretory function, but the nature of epididymal secretory products, if any, remains unknown. Basal cells **B** as well as occasional lymphocytes **L** may be seen within the epithelium.

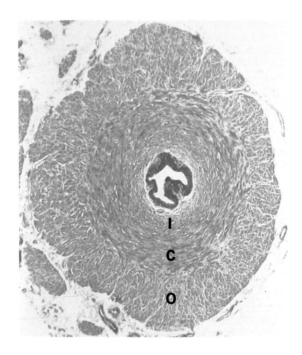

Fig. 18.13   Ductus deferens   H & E × 30

The *ductus* (or *vas*) *deferens*, which conducts spermatozoa from the epididymis to the urethra, is a thick-walled muscular tube consisting of inner **I** and outer **O** longitudinal layers and a thick intermediate circular layer **C**. Like the distal part of the epididymis, the ductus deferens is innervated by the sympathetic nervous system, producing strong peristaltic contractions to expel its contents into the urethra during ejaculation.

The ductus deferens is lined by a pseudostratified columnar epithelium similar to that of the epididymis (see Fig. 18.12); the epithelial lining and its supporting lamina propria are thrown into longitudinal folds, permitting expansion of the duct during ejaculation. The dilated distal portion of each ductus deferens, known as the *ampulla*, receives a short duct draining the seminal vesicle, thus forming the short *ejaculatory duct*; the ejaculatory ducts from each side converge to join the urethra as it passes through the prostate gland.

This specimen was obtained at operation for male sterilisation (*vasectomy*).

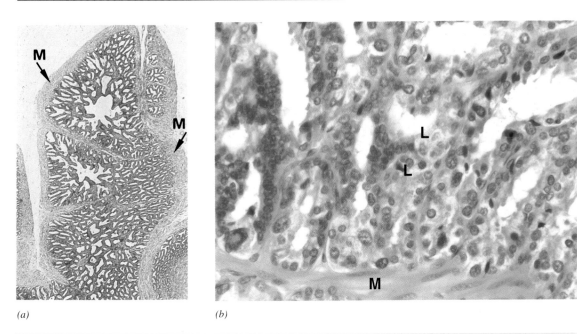

(a)   *(b)*

Fig. 18.14 | **Seminal vesicle** (a) H & E × 10 (b) H & E × 300

Each seminal vesicle is a complex glandular diverticulum of the associated ductus deferens. Between them the seminal vesicles secrete up to 85% of the total volume of seminal fluid, most of the rest being secreted by the prostate gland. The lumen of each seminal vesicle is highly irregular and recessed, giving a honeycombed appearance at low magnification.

The epithelial lining is usually of a pseudostratified tall columnar type and consists of secretory cells with lipid droplets in the cytoplasm giving it a foamy appearance. The seminal vesicles produce a yellowish viscid alkaline fluid containing a wide range of substances, including

fructose, fibrinogen, vitamin C and prostaglandins. The epithelial cells often contain brown lipofuscin granules **L** and characteristically have rather variable nuclear shape and size. Both of these features are seen in micrograph (b). Although not thought to store spermatozoa, seminal vesicles are often seen to contain spermatozoa which have probably entered by reflux from the ampulla. The prominent muscular wall **M** is arranged into inner circular and outer longitudinal layers and is supplied by the sympathetic nervous system; during ejaculation, muscle contraction forces secretions from the seminal vesicles into the urethra via the ampullae.

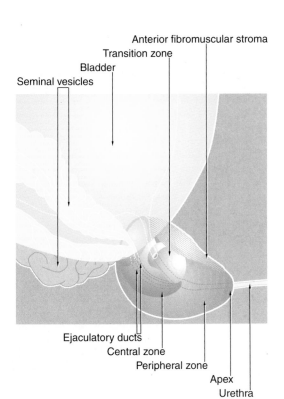

Anterior fibromuscular stroma
Transition zone
Bladder
Seminal vesicles

Ejaculatory ducts
Central zone
Peripheral zone
Apex
Urethra

Fig. 18.15 | **Prostate gland**

The prostate gland, which in young adults is about the size of a walnut, surrounds the bladder neck and the first part of the urethra, known as the *prostatic urethra*. The urethra courses through the prostate to become the *membranous urethra* at the apex of the prostate. In the substance of the gland, the urethra merges with the ejaculatory ducts and at this point angles forwards.

The prostate consists of branched tubulo-acinar glands embedded in a fibromuscular stroma. There is a partial capsule enclosing the posterior and lateral aspects of the prostate but the anterior and apical surfaces are bounded by the *anterior fibromuscular stroma*, a part of the gland consisting, as the name implies, only of collagenous stroma and muscle fibres.

In the past the prostate was described as consisting of a number of ill-defined lobes. However, this terminology has been replaced by the concept of prostate zones and the gland is now described as consisting of four zones of unequal size:

- The *transition zone* surrounds the proximal prostatic urethra and comprises about 5% of the glandular tissue.
- The *central zone* (20%) surrounds the ejaculatory ducts.
- The *peripheral zone* makes up the bulk of the gland (approximately 70%).
- The *anterior fibromuscular stroma* contains no glandular tissue and lies anteriorly.

ORGAN SYSTEMS

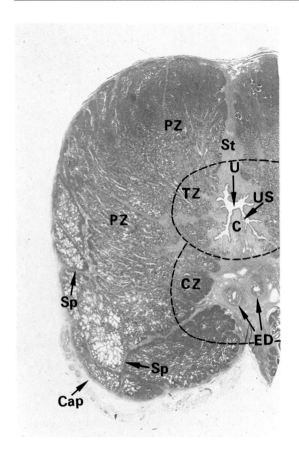

Fig. 18.16 Prostate gland (dog) H & E × 5

This low power view of the prostate of a dog shows the general architectural features of the gland. The urethra **U** lies centrally surrounded by a fibrous stroma **St**. The ejaculatory ducts **ED** also lie in this central stroma as they course towards their junction with the prostatic urethra. The zones of the prostate are not clearly demarcated from each other anatomically. Partial fibrous septa **Sp** separate the gland into lobules. The transition zone **TZ** surrounds the first part of the prostatic urethra. The central zone **CZ** lies posterior to the transition zone and encircles the ejaculatory ducts. The peripheral zone **PZ** makes up the main bulk of the gland. The ducts of the peripheral zone glands empty into the posterolateral recesses of the urethra on either side of the *verumontanum (urethral crest)* **C**.

The different zones of the prostate are important because they tend to be the sites of different disease processes. Most cases of carcinoma of the prostate arise in the peripheral zone while the transition zone harbours almost all cases of benign nodular hyperplasia.

At this power the anterior fibromuscular stroma appears continuous with the capsule and its content of muscle fibres cannot be discerned.

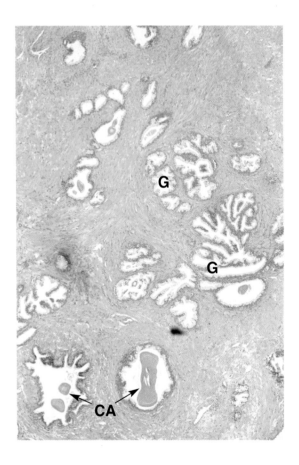

Fig. 18.17 Human prostate H & E × 30

At intermediate power, the branching nature of the prostatic glands **G** is more apparent. The glands are irregularly shaped with the epithelium forming folds, which allow for expansion of the glands by secretions. This gives the epithelium a papillary appearance.

The secretory product of the prostate, which makes up about half of the seminal fluid volume, is thin and milky; it is rich in citric acid and hydrolytic enzymes, notably fibrinolysin, which liquefies coagulated semen after it has been deposited within the female genital tract. Lamellated glycoprotein masses called *corpora amylacea* **CA** are a feature of increasing age, becoming progressively calcified to form *prostatic concretions*.

The stroma of the prostate consists of dense collagen, fibroblasts and haphazardly arranged smooth muscle fibres which, like those of the seminal vesicles and the rest of the tract, are innervated by the sympathetic nervous system which stimulates powerful contractions during ejaculation. Towards the apex of the gland the anterior fibromuscular stroma also contains skeletal muscle fibres.

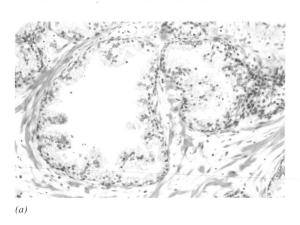
(a)

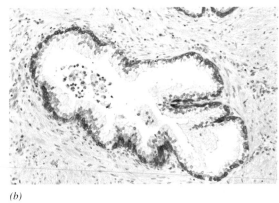
(b)

Fig. 18.18 Human prostate (a) H & E × 50 (b) Immunoperoxidase × 50

The epithelium of the prostate glands consists of a double layer of cells. The luminal layer is made up of tall columnar secretory cells with basal nuclei (a). Between the secretory cells and the basement membrane lies a layer of flattened basal cells, which probably act as reserve cells replacing dead secretory cells. The basal cell layer is often incomplete and may be hard to detect on routine H & E stained sections. However, these cells produce a type of high molecular weight keratin not found in the secretory cells. Micrograph (b) is an immunoperoxidase preparation using an antibody to this particular keratin which highlights the basal cells (stained brown).

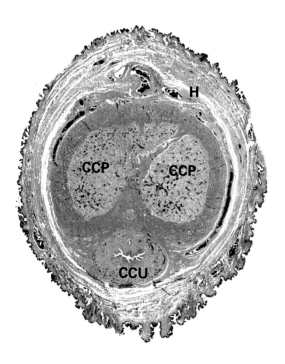

Fig. 18.19 Penis H & E × 3

This transverse section through the penis of an adult human male demonstrates the general arrangement of the penile tissues. The penis consists of three cylindrical masses of erectile tissue including the paired *corpora cavernosa penis* **CCP** in the dorsal aspect and the midline *corpus spongiosum* (sometimes called the *corpus cavernosum urethrae* **CCU**) which surrounds and supports the penile urethra and distally forms the *glans penis*. Condensed fibroelastic tissue, the *tunica albuginea* invests the cavernous bodies. It is thickest around the corpora cavernosa penis which are incompletely separated by a midline septum. This dense collagenous tissue is continuous with the very loose hypodermis **H** which allows the thin penile skin to move freely over the underlying structures. Note the prominent blood vessels of the hypodermis.

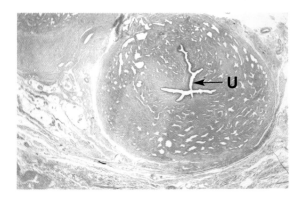

Fig. 18.20 Corpus cavernosum urethra H & E × 5

The erectile tissue of the penis consists of broad vascular lacunae or cavernous sinuses supported by trabeculae of fibroelastic tissue containing smooth muscle fibres. The lacunae are lined by non-fenestrated vascular endothelium. The penile urethra **U** has an irregular outline due to the presence of deep outpocketings which are continuous with the ducts of simple acinar glands, the *para-urethral glands* (not seen at this power).

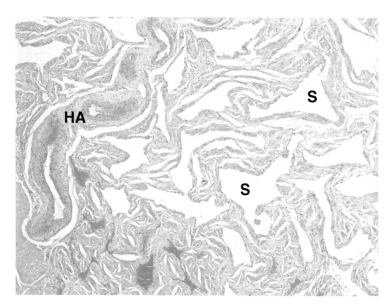

Fig. 18.21 **Penile erectile tissue** H & E × 30

The vascular sinuses **S** of the cavernous bodies of the penis are supplied by numerous anastomosing thick-walled arteries and arterioles called *helicine arteries* **HA** since they follow a spiral course in the flaccid state. Blood drains from the sinuses via veins which lie immediately beneath the dense fibroelastic tissue investing the cavernous bodies. During erection, dilatation of the helicine arteries, mediated by the parasympathetic nervous system, results in engorgement of the vascular sinuses, which enlarge, compressing and restricting venous outflow. The process is enhanced by relaxation of smooth muscle cells in the trabeculae of the cavernous bodies.

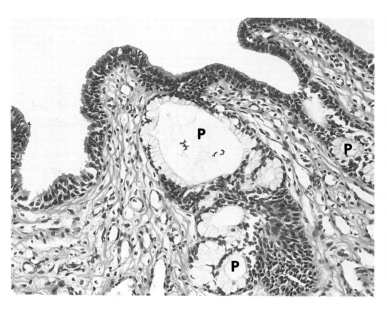

Fig. 18.22 **Penile urethra** H & E × 200

Apart from the prostatic urethra, which is lined by transitional epithelium, the male urethra is lined by stratified or pseudostratified columnar epithelium, although small areas of stratified squamous epithelium may also be found in human adult males. The external opening (*urethral meatus*) is lined by stratified squamous epithelium, which becomes continuous with the epithelium of the glans.

The urethra is lubricated by mucoid secretions from the para-urethral glands **P** and the *bulbo-urethral glands of Cowper* (see Fig. 18.1) which have a similar, but more discrete, organisation.

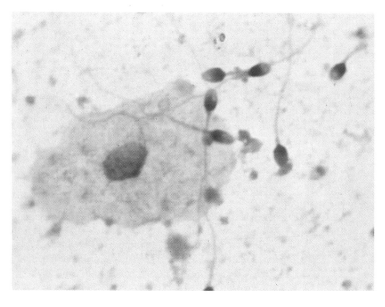

Fig. 18.23 **Semen** H & E × 1200

Semen, the product of ejaculation, consists of spermatozoa and seminal fluid which is derived principally from the seminal vesicles and prostate gland. The volume of each human ejaculate is about 3.5 ml containing from 50 to 150 million spermatozoa per ml. In normal fertile human males, up to 25% of the ejaculated spermatozoa are abnormal or degenerate forms. By the time of ejaculation, spermatozoa have matured and acquired the property of motility; nevertheless, they remain incapable of fertilising an ovum until after undergoing a process called *capacitation* within the female genital tract. Metabolites for motility are provided in the form of fructose and citrate in the seminal fluid. Note that desquamated cells, prostatic concretions and other urinary tract debris are normal constituents of semen.

19. Female reproductive system

Introduction

The female reproductive system has six major functions:

- production of female gametes, the *ova*, by the process of *oogenesis*
- reception of male gametes, the spermatozoa
- provision of a suitable environment for the fertilisation of ova by spermatozoa
- provision of an environment for the development of the fetus
- a means for the expulsion of the developed fetus to the external environment
- nutrition of the newborn.

These functions are all integrated by an elegant system of hormonal and nervous mechanisms. The female reproductive system may be divided into three structural units on the basis of function:

- **The ovaries**, which are the site of oogenesis, are paired organs lying on either side of the uterus adjacent to the lateral wall of the pelvis. In sexually mature mammals, ova are released, by the process of *ovulation*, in a cyclical manner either seasonally or at regular intervals throughout the year. This cycle is suspended during pregnancy. The ovaries are also endocrine organs producing the hormones *oestrogen* and *progesterone*. Both ovulation and ovarian hormone production are controlled by the cyclical release from the anterior pituitary of the gonadotrophic hormones, *luteinising hormone* (LH) and *follicle stimulating hormone* (FSH). Oestrogen and progesterone in turn regulate LH and FSH production by feedback mechanisms. Thus ovulation is coordinated with preparation of the uterus to receive the fertilised ovum.
- **The genital tract** extends from near the ovaries to an opening at the external surface and provides an environment for reception of male gametes, fertilisation of ova, development of the fetus and expulsion of the fetus at birth. The genital tract begins with a pair of *Fallopian tubes*, also called *oviducts* or *uterine tubes*, which conduct ova from the ovaries to the uterus where fetal development occurs. Fertilisation of ova by spermatozoa occurs within the Fallopian tubes. The uterus is a muscular organ, the mucosal lining of which undergoes cyclical proliferation under the influence of ovarian hormones. This provides a suitable environment for implantation of the fertilised ovum and subsequent development of the placenta via which the developing fetus is nourished throughout gestation. At birth (*parturition*), strong contractions of the muscular uterine wall expel the fetus through the *cervix* into the birth canal or *vagina*. The vagina is an expansile muscular tube specialised for the passage of the fetus to the external environment and the reception of the penis during coitus. At the external opening of the vagina are thick folds of skin, the *labia*, which along with the *clitoris* constitute the vulva.
- **The breasts** are highly modified apocrine sweat glands which, in the female, develop at puberty and regress at menopause. During pregnancy, the secretory components expand greatly in size and number in preparation for milk production (*lactation*).

In the non-pregnant state, the female reproductive system undergoes continuous cyclical changes from puberty to menopause. When ovulation is not followed by the implantation of a fertilised ovum, the thickened mucosal lining, the *endometrium*, regresses and a new ovulation cycle commences. In humans, the thickened endometrium is shed in a period of bleeding known as *menstruation*; the first day of bleeding marks the beginning of a new cycle of endometrial proliferation which is known as the *menstrual cycle*. In humans, the standard menstrual cycle is of 28 days duration but there is considerable variation among normal individuals. Ovulation usually occurs at the midpoint of the cycle.

In other mammals, the proliferated uterine mucosa is absorbed rather than shed and the female is receptive to the male only during the period of ovulation which is known as *oestrus* (or heat). The remaining part of the cycle is called the *dioestrus* and the whole cycle is known as the *oestrus cycle*.

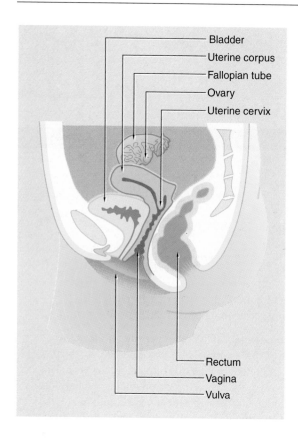

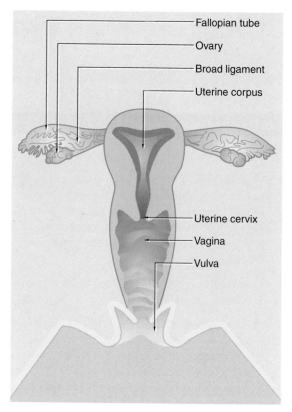

Fig. 19.1 Female reproductive system *(sagittal section)*

Fig. 19.2 Female reproductive system *(coronal view)*

Fig. 19.3 Ovary *(illustrations opposite)* (a) Monkey, Azan × 18 (b) Human, H & E × 8

The ovaries of all mammals have a similar basic structure. Their overall appearance, however, varies considerably in accordance with species differences in the ovarian cycle and the stage in the cycle at which the ovary is examined. These micrographs compare the ovarian appearance of the monkey with that of the human.

The ovaries, which are some 3–5 cm long in humans, have a flattened ovoid shape. The body of the ovary consists of spindle-shaped cells, fine collagen fibres and ground substance which together constitute the *ovarian stroma*. The stromal cells resemble fibroblasts but some contain lipid droplets. Bundles of smooth muscle cells are also scattered throughout the stroma. In the peripheral zone of the stroma, known as the *cortex*, are numerous *follicles* which contain female gametes in various stages of development. In addition, there may also be post-ovulatory follicles of various kinds, namely *corpora lutea* (responsible for oestrogen and progesterone production, see Fig. 19.8), degenerate and former corpora lutea (*corpora albicantes*, see Fig. 19.11) and degenerate (atretic) follicles (see Fig. 19.10).

The superficial cortex is more fibrotic than the deep cortex and is often called the *tunica albuginea*. However, unlike the testis, this is not an anatomically distinct capsule. On the surface of the ovary is an epithelial covering, misleadingly called *germinal epithelium*, which is a continuation of the peritoneum.

In the monkey ovary, numerous follicles **F** are seen in various sizes and states of development. In contrast,

developing follicles are difficult to see in the human ovary (b) at this magnification; this human ovary is dominated by an active corpus luteum **CL** and several degenerating corpora lutea **D** and corpora albicantes **A**.

The central zone of the ovarian stroma, the *medulla* **M**, is highly vascular and contains *hilus cells* which are morphologically very similar to Leydig cells of the testis. The ovarian artery (a branch of the aorta) and ovarian branches of the uterine artery form anastomoses in the *mesovarium* and the *broad ligament* **L**. From this arterial plexus approximately 10 coiled arteries, the *helicine arteries* **H** enter the hilum of the ovary, shown in micrograph (a). Smaller branches form a plexus at the corticomedullary junction, giving rise to straight cortical arterioles which radiate into the cortex. Here they branch and anastomose to form vascular arcades which give rise to a rich network of capillaries around the follicles. Venous drainage follows the course of the arterial system, the medullary veins being particularly large and tortuous. Lymphatics arise in the perifollicular stroma, draining to larger vessels which coil around the medullary veins. Innervation of the ovary is by sympathetic fibres which not only supply blood vessels but also terminate on smooth muscle cells in the stroma around the follicles, possibly playing some part in follicular maturation and ovulation. In micrograph (b), the nearby Fallopian tube **Ft** is included in the plane of section.

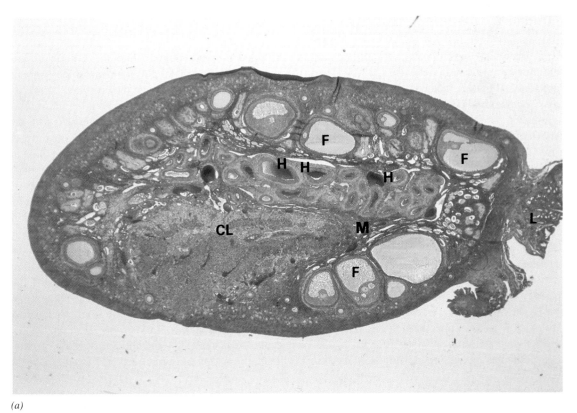

(a)

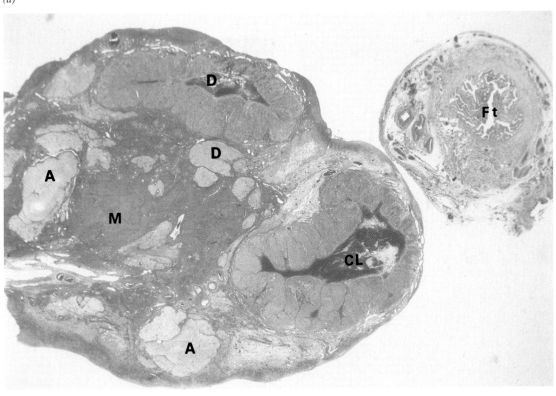

(b)

Follicular development

During early fetal development, primordial germ cells called *oogonia* migrate into the ovarian cortex where they multiply by mitosis. By the fourth and fifth months of human fetal development, some oogonia enlarge and assume the potential for development into mature gametes. At this stage they become known as *primary oocytes* and commence the first stage of meiotic division (see Ch. 2). By the seventh month of fetal development, the primary oocytes become encapsulated by a single layer of flattened *follicular cells* to form *primordial follicles*, of which there are some 400 000 in the human ovary at birth. This encapsulation arrests the first meiotic division and no further development of primordial follicles then occurs until after the female reaches sexual maturity. The process of meiotic division is only completed during follicular maturation leading up to ovulation and fertilisation. Thus all the female germ cells are present at birth but the process of meiotic division is only completed some 15–50 years later! In contrast, in males, meiotic division of germ cells commences only after sexual maturity, and formation and maturation of spermatozoa are accomplished within about 70 days (see Ch. 18). Female germ cells may undergo degeneration (*atresia*) at any stage of follicular maturation.

During each ovarian cycle, a cohort of up to 20 primordial follicles is activated to begin the maturation process; nevertheless, usually only one follicle reaches full maturity and undergoes ovulation whilst the remainder regress before this point. The reason for this apparent wastage is unclear; during maturation, however, the follicles have an endocrine function which may be far beyond the capacity of a single follicle and the primary purpose of the other follicles may be to act as an endocrine gland.

Follicular maturation involves changes in the oocyte, the follicular cells and the surrounding stromal tissue. Follicular maturation is stimulated by FSH (follicle stimulating hormone) secreted by the anterior pituitary gland.

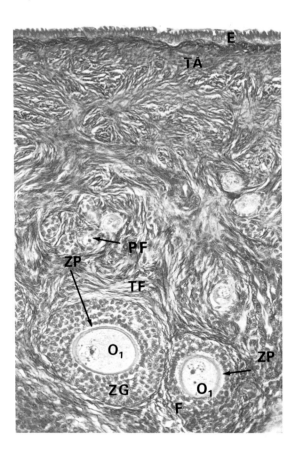

Fig. 19.4   Ovarian cortex Azan × 120

This micrograph, taken from a monkey, shows the typical appearance of follicles in the ovarian cortex and illustrates several stages in early follicular development.

In the mature ovary, undeveloped follicles exist as *primordial follicles* **PF** which are composed of a *primary oocyte* surrounded by a single layer of flattened follicular cells. The primary oocyte has a large nucleus with dispersed finely granular chromatin, a prominent nucleolus and little cytoplasm.

At the lower right of the field, a primordial follicle has been stimulated, increasing in size to form a *primary follicle*; its oocyte O_1 has greatly enlarged and the follicular cells **F** have multiplied by mitosis and become cuboidal in shape; they are now known as *granulosa cells*. A thick homogeneous layer of glycoprotein and acid proteoglycans, the *zona pellucida* **ZP**, develops between the oocyte and the follicular cells; both cell types probably contribute to its formation.

With further follicular development as seen in the large follicle at lower left, the surrounding stromal cells begin to form an organised layer around the follicle called the *theca folliculi* **TF** separated from the granulosa cells by a basement membrane. Theca cells are derived from the fibroblast-like cells of the ovarian stroma. The primary follicle continues to enlarge and the granulosa cells continue to proliferate, forming a layer several cells thick called the *zona granulosa* **ZG**.

Note also in this micrograph, the fibrous tunica albuginea **TA** and the single layer of cuboidal or columnar epithelial cells **E** on the surface of the ovary. This epithelial layer is continuous with the mesothelial lining of the peritoneal cavity and was formerly known as the *germinal epithelium* from the mistaken belief that these cells were the origin of the female germ cells.

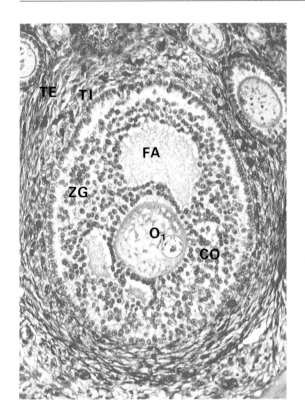

Fig. 19.5 Secondary follicle Azan × 120

Primary follicles continue to develop to form *secondary follicles* and acquire the features seen in this micrograph; by now they are usually situated deeper in the ovarian cortex.

The zona granulosa **ZG** continues to proliferate and within it appear small fluid-filled spaces that fuse to form the *follicular antrum* **FA**, in which follicular fluid accumulates. At this stage, the oocyte O_1 has almost reached its full size and becomes situated eccentrically in a thickened area of the granulosa called the *cumulus oophorus* **CO**.

At the periphery of the follicle, the theca folliculi has developed two layers, the *theca interna* **TI**, comprising several layers of rounded cells, and the less well-defined *theca externa* **TE** consisting of spindle-shaped cells which merge with the surrounding stroma.

The cells of the theca interna have the features of typical steroid-secreting cells (see Fig. 17.16) and secrete oestrogen precursors (e.g. androstenedione), oestrogen and, in the preovulatory stage, progesterone. In the ovary these steroid-secreting cells are often described as *luteinised*. Follicular hormones promote proliferation of the endometrium in readiness for the implantation of a fertilised ovum. The theca externa is composed of flattened stromal cells and has no endocrine function. The granulosa cells also produce hormones from the stage of antral formation onwards; oestrogen is produced from precursors secreted by the theca interna as well as small amounts of intrafollicular FSH and (at ovulation) the FSH inhibitor, *inhibin F*.

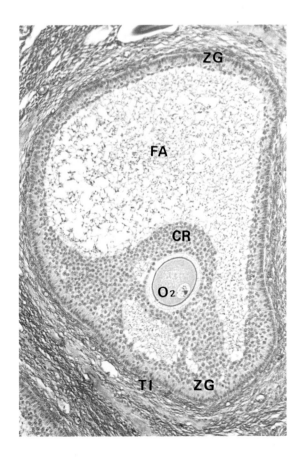

Fig. 19.6 Graafian follicle Azan × 75

Approaching maturity, further growth of the oocyte ceases and the first meiotic division is completed just before ovulation. At this stage, the oocyte becomes known as the *secondary oocyte* and commences the second meiotic division. The first polar body (see Ch. 2), containing very little cytoplasm, remains inconspicuously within the zona pellucida. The follicular antrum **FA** enlarges markedly and the zona granulosa **ZG** now forms a layer of even thickness around the periphery of the follicle. The cumulus oophorus diminishes leaving the oocyte O_2 surrounded by a layer several cells thick, the *corona radiata* **CR**, which remains attached to the zona granulosa by thin bridges of cells. Before ovulation, these bridges break down and the oocyte, surrounded by the corona radiata, floats free inside the follicle. Note the surrounding theca interna **TI** consisting of plump luteinised cells. By this stage the follicle has reached between 1.5 and 2.5 cm in diameter and bulges under the ovarian surface. The overlying surface epithelial cells are flattened and atrophic and the thin intervening stroma becomes degenerate and avascular.

At ovulation, the mature follicle ruptures and the ovum, comprising the secondary oocyte, zona pellucida and corona radiata, is expelled into the peritoneal cavity near the entrance to the Fallopian tube. The second meiotic division of the oocyte is not completed until after penetration of the ovum by a spermatozoon.

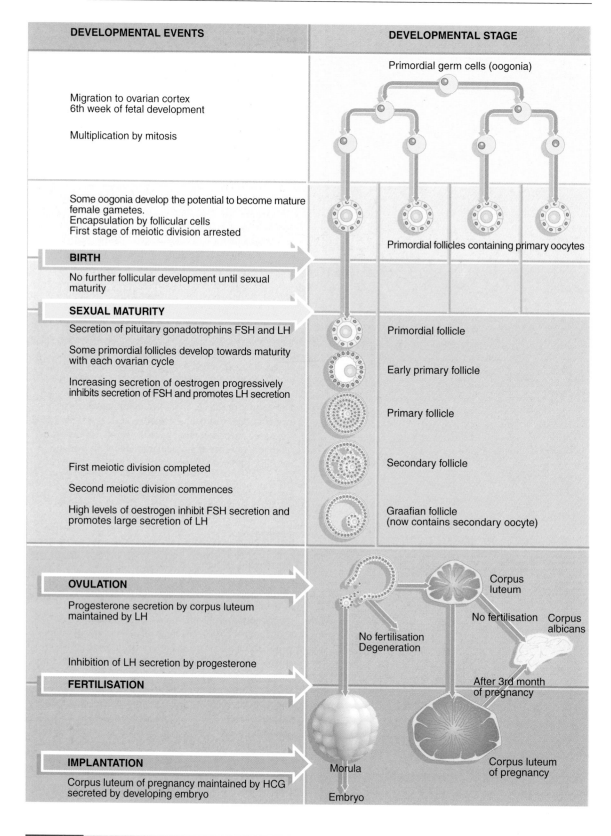

DEVELOPMENTAL EVENTS	DEVELOPMENTAL STAGE
	Primordial germ cells (oogonia)
Migration to ovarian cortex 6th week of fetal development Multiplication by mitosis	
Some oogonia develop the potential to become mature female gametes. Encapsulation by follicular cells First stage of meiotic division arrested	Primordial follicles containing primary oocytes
BIRTH	
No further follicular development until sexual maturity	
SEXUAL MATURITY	
Secretion of pituitary gonadotrophins FSH and LH	Primordial follicle
Some primordial follicles develop towards maturity with each ovarian cycle	Early primary follicle
Increasing secretion of oestrogen progressively inhibits secretion of FSH and promotes LH secretion	Primary follicle
First meiotic division completed	Secondary follicle
Second meiotic division commences	
High levels of oestrogen inhibit FSH secretion and promotes large secretion of LH	Graafian follicle (now contains secondary oocyte)
OVULATION	Corpus luteum
Progesterone secretion by corpus luteum maintained by LH	No fertilisation Corpus albicans No fertilisation Degeneration
Inhibition of LH secretion by progesterone	After 3rd month of pregnancy
FERTILISATION	
IMPLANTATION	Morula Corpus luteum of pregnancy
Corpus luteum of pregnancy maintained by HCG secreted by developing embryo	Embryo

Fig. 19.7   **Follicular development**

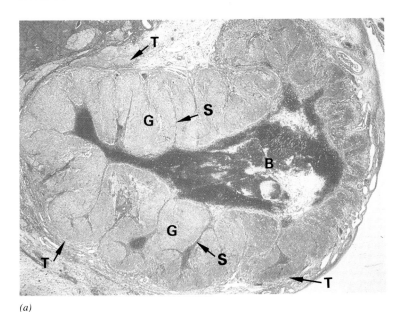
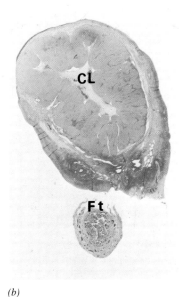

(a) *(b)*

Fig. 19.8 | **Corpus luteum** (a) H & E × 42 (b) H & E × 3

Following ovulation, the ruptured follicle collapses and fills with a blood clot to form the ***corpus luteum of menstruation*** which has a brief career as an endocrine organ. The corpus luteum of menstruation is about the same size as the antecedent ovulatory follicle, i.e. 1.5–2.5 cm. Under the influence of luteinising hormone (LH) secreted by the anterior pituitary, granulosa cells increase greatly in size and begin secretion of progesterone. The granulosa cells acquire the characteristics of steroid-secreting cells. Their copious cytoplasm contains plentiful smooth endoplasmic reticulum, abundant mitochondria, lipid droplets and some lipofuscin, giving the corpus luteum a yellow colour macroscopically. The granulosa cells are now called ***granulosa lutein cells***. Progesterone promotes secretion by glands in the uterine endometrium which have by now greatly proliferated under the influence of the oestrogens secreted by the follicle before ovulation (see Figs 19.15–19.16). This provides a suitable environment for the implantation of a fertilised ovum.

The cells of the theca interna also increase somewhat in size and acquire similar cytoplasmic features to the luteinised granulosa cells. Although interrupted by ovulation, these cells (as well as the granulosa cells) continue to secrete oestrogens, which are necessary to maintain the thickened uterine mucosa. These cells become known as ***theca lutein cells***.

The basement membrane between the zona granulosa and theca interna breaks down and these layers are invaded by capillaries and larger vessels from the theca externa to form a rich vascular network characteristic of endocrine glands.

Progesterone production by the corpus luteum is dependent on LH from the anterior pituitary, but rising progesterone levels inhibit LH production. Without the continuing stimulus of LH, the corpus luteum cannot be maintained and 12–14 days after ovulation it regresses, ultimately forming a functionless ***corpus albicans*** (see Fig. 19.11). Once the corpus luteum regresses, secretion of both oestrogen and progesterone ceases. Without these hormones the endometrial lining of the uterus collapses, resulting in the onset of menstruation.

Implantation of a fertilised ovum in the uterine wall interrupts the integrated ovarian and menstrual cycles. After implantation, a hormone called ***human chorionic gonadotrophin (HCG)*** is secreted into the maternal circulation by the developing placenta. HCG has an analogous function to LH and maintains the function of the corpus luteum in secreting oestrogen and progesterone until about the 12th week of pregnancy. After this time, the ***corpus luteum of pregnancy*** slowly regresses to form a functionless corpus albicans and the placenta takes over the major role of oestrogen and progesterone secretion until parturition.

Micrograph (a) shows a corpus luteum of menstruation. In the centre, the remnant of the post-ovulatory blood clot **B** is seen surrounded by a broad zone of granulosa lutein cells **G** penetrated by septa **S** containing the larger blood vessels. Peripherally, a thin zone of theca lutein cells **T** can be seen. Externally, the corpus luteum is bounded by a zone of condensed stromal tissue representing the theca externa of the antecedent Graafian follicle.

Micrograph (b) shows a human ovary during the first trimester of pregnancy. The corpus luteum **CL** is greatly enlarged compared with that of the second half of the menstrual cycle and by now occupies most of the ovary. The organisation of the corpus luteum of pregnancy is similar to that of menstruation. Note the adjacent Fallopian tube **Ft**.

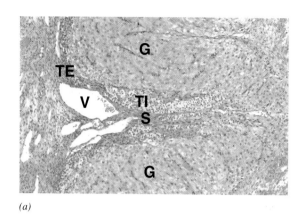

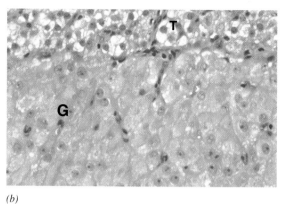

(a)   *(b)*

Fig. 19.9   Corpus luteum (a) H & E × 50 (b) H & E × 100

Micrograph (a) shows the margin of a corpus luteum at intermediate magnification. Most of the field is occupied by granulosa lutein cells **G**, the large polygonal cells containing abundant pale eosinophilic (pink stained) cytoplasm and small round nuclei. At the periphery are theca cells which also extend in a finger-like extension forming a sheath **S** around blood vessels **V**. The theca externa cells **TE** have darker stained cytoplasm while the luteinised theca interna cells **TI** have pale cytoplasm due to their content of lipid droplets.

At high magnification in micrograph (b), granulosa lutein cells **G** may be compared with theca lutein cells **T**. The eosinophilic cytoplasm of the granulosa lutein cells contains numerous small lipid droplets which give rise to the vacuolated appearance seen in this preparation; their large spherical nuclei contain one or two prominent nucleoli. Theca lutein cells are smaller, with a more densely staining cytoplasm but with larger lipid vacuoles; their ovoid nucleus has a single large nucleolus. The ultrastructure of the endocrine cells of the corpus luteum is characteristic of all steroid secretory cells (see Fig. 17.16).

As previously described, the granulosa lutein cells secrete progesterone (and a small amount of oestrogen) and the theca lutein cells secrete oestrogen precursors which are converted to oestrogen by the granulosa cells.

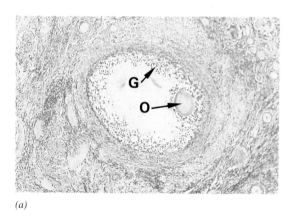

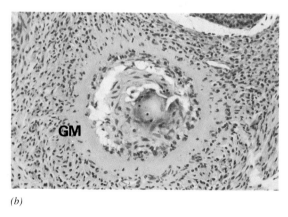

(a)   *(b)*

Fig. 19.10   Atretic follicles (a) H & E × 128 (b) H & E × 128

The process of follicular atresia (degeneration) may occur at any stage in the development of the ovum. By the sixth month of development, the fetal ovary contains several million primordial follicles, yet by the time of birth less than half a million remain. Atresia continues until puberty and thereafter through the reproductive years.

In addition, with each ovarian cycle approximately 20 follicles begin to mature, usually all but one becoming atretic at some stage before complete maturity.

The histological appearance of **atretic follicles** varies enormously, depending on the stage of development reached and the progress of atresia. The atretic follicle seen in micrograph (a) is a secondary follicle in early atresia; the oocyte **O** has degenerated and the granulosa cells **G** have begun to disaggregate. Advanced atresia, as seen in micrograph (b), is characterised by gross thickening of the basement membrane between the granulosa cells and the theca interna, forming the so-called **glassy membrane GM**. Atretic follicles are ultimately replaced completely by collagenous tissue known as the **corpus fibrosum**. Most corpora fibrosa eventually disappear completely. In the postmenopausal woman, primordial follicles are absent and the cortex consists of stroma and corpora albicantes only, with no developing follicles. The postmenopausal ovary is smaller than that in premenopausal women and is usually described as atrophic.

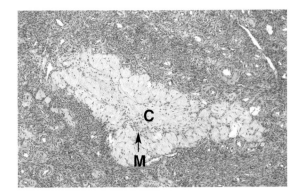

Fig. 19.11 Corpus albicans H & E × 50

The corpus albicans **C** is the inactive fibrous tissue mass which forms following the involution of a corpus luteum. The secretory cells of the degenerate corpus luteum undergo autolysis and are phagocytosed by macrophages **M**, a few of which, containing cytoplasmic haemosiderin pigment, can be seen here. The vascular supporting tissue regresses to form a relatively acellular collagenous scar containing a few fibroblasts.

In the human ovary, corpora albicantes are a dominant feature, increasing in number with age and often appearing to occupy almost the whole ovarian stroma. However, most regress completely leaving no trace; otherwise the postmenopausal ovary would contain approximately 500 corpora albicantes.

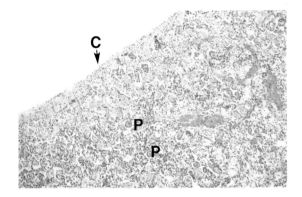

Fig. 19.12 Fetal ovary H & E × 50

In this micrograph of ovary from a term fetus, the ovarian cortex is seen to be packed with primordial follicles **P**. The surrounding stoma is much more delicate than in an adult woman and the ovarian capsule **C** is thin. These ova are arrested in the first meiotic division and remain so until the onset of puberty signals the waves of maturation of follicles which occur with each cycle in the reproductive years.

The genital tract

The genital tract consists of the Fallopian tubes, uterus and vagina, all of which have the same basic structure: a wall of smooth muscle, an inner mucosal lining and an outer layer of loose supporting tissue. The mucosal and muscular components vary greatly according to their location and functional requirements; the whole tract undergoes cyclical changes under the influence of ovarian hormones released during the ovarian cycle.

The cyclical changes in the genital tract facilitate the entry of ova into the Fallopian tube, the passage of spermatozoa through the uterine cervix and into the Fallopian tube, the passage of the fertilised ovum into the uterus and the implantation and development of the fertilised ovum in the mucosal lining (endometrium) of the uterus. Implantation of a fertilised ovum results in the secretion of hormones which inhibit the ovarian cycle and produce the changes in the genital tract necessary for fetal development and parturition.

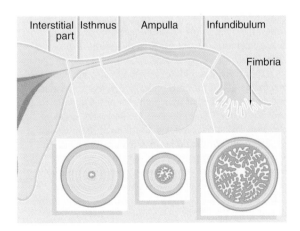

Fig. 19.13 Fallopian tubes

The *Fallopian tubes* (also called *uterine tubes* or *oviducts*) conduct ova from the surface of the ovaries to the uterine cavity and are also the site of fertilisation by spermatozoa. The Fallopian tube is shaped like an elongated funnel and is divided anatomically into four parts as shown in the diagram.

The *infundibulum* moves so as to overlie the site of rupture of the Graafian follicle at ovulation; finger-like projections called *fimbriae* extending from the end of the tube envelop the ovulation site and direct the ovum into the tube. Movement of the ovum down the tube is mediated by gentle peristaltic action of the longitudinal and circular smooth muscle layers of the oviduct wall; this is aided by a current of fluid propelled by the action of the ciliated epithelium lining the tube. Fertilisation usually occurs in the *ampulla*.

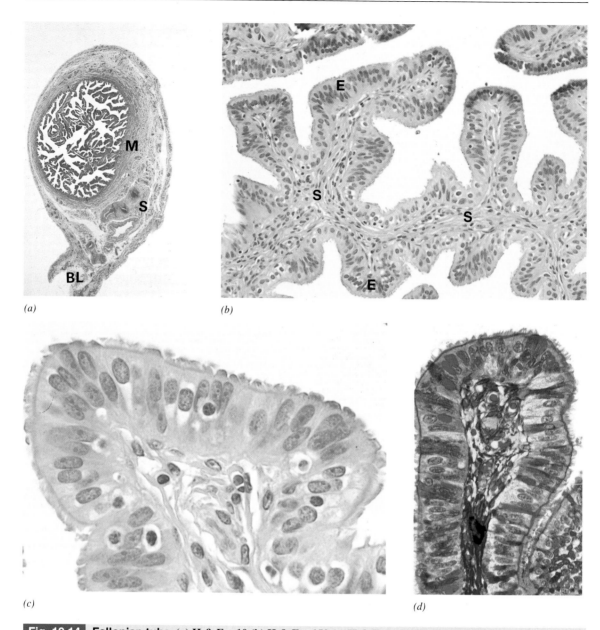

Fig. 19.14 **Fallopian tube** (a) H & E × 10 (b) H & E × 150 (c) H & E × 600 (d) Azan × 320

The mucosal lining of the Fallopian tube is thrown into a labyrinth of branching, longitudinal folds which provide a suitable environment for fertilisation. This feature is most prominent in the ampullary part of the tube as shown in micrograph (a) which is from a specimen obtained during female sterilisation. Note also in this micrograph, the muscular wall **M** and the vascular supporting tissue of the serosa **S** which is continuous with the broad ligament **BL**. The serosal layer and broad ligament have a surface lining of mesothelium. The muscular wall has two layers, an inner circular and an outer longitudinal, not discernible at this power.

Micrograph (b) focuses on one of the mucosal folds of the ampulla. These have a branching core of vascular supporting tissue **S** and are invested by a single layer of tall columnar epithelial cells **E**.

Micrograph (c) shows the tip of a mucosal fold at high magnification. The columnar cells of the epithelium are of three types, *ciliated*, *non-ciliated secretory* and *intercalated cells*. The non-ciliated cells produce a secretion which is propelled towards the uterus by the wave-like beating of the cilia of the ciliated cells, carrying with it the ovum. This secretion probably also has a role in the nutrition and protection of the ovum. The intercalated cells may be a morphologic variant of the secretory cells. The ratio of ciliated to non-ciliated cells and the height of the cells undergo cyclical variations under the influence of ovarian hormones. The ciliated cells are generally shorter than the secretory cells, making the epithelial surface somewhat irregular in outline. Scattered intraepithelial lymphocytes are also present. Micrograph (d) employs a method which stains the secretory cells blue. Note that the collagen of the core of lamina propria is also stained blue.

The human menstrual cycle

The uterus is a flattened pear-shaped organ approximately 7 cm long in the non-pregnant state. Its mucosal lining, the *endometrium*, provides the environment for fetal development; the thick smooth muscle wall, the *myometrium*, expands greatly during pregnancy and provides protection for the fetus and a mechanism for the expulsion of the fetus at parturition.

The endometrial lining of the uterine cavity consists of a pseudostratified columnar ciliated epithelium supported by a cellular stroma containing numerous simple tubular glands. Under the influence of oestrogen and progesterone secreted by follicles during the ovarian cycle, the endometrium undergoes regular cyclical changes so as to offer a suitable environment for implantation of a fertilised ovum. For successful implantation, the fertilised ovum requires an easily penetrable, highly vascular tissue and an abundant supply of glycogen for nutrition until vascular connections are established with the maternal vasculature.

The cycle of changes in the endometrium proceeds through two distinct phases, proliferation and secretion; these changes involve both the epithelium and supporting stroma.

- **The proliferative phase**: the endometrial stroma proliferates becoming thicker and richly vascularised. The simple tubular glands proliferate to form numerous glands which begin secretion coincident with ovulation. The proliferative phase is initiated and sustained until ovulation by the increasing production of oestrogens from developing ovarian follicles.
- **The secretory phase**: release of progesterone from the corpus luteum after ovulation promotes production of a copious thick glycogen-rich secretion by the endometrial glands.

Unless implantation of a fertilised ovum occurs, the continuing production of progesterone is inhibited by negative feedback upon the anterior pituitary, thus suppressing LH release and leading to involution of the corpus luteum. In the absence of progesterone, the endometrium cannot be maintained and most of it is shed during the period of bleeding known as *menstruation*. Reactivation of FSH secretion initiates a new cycle of follicular development and oestrogen secretion; this in turn, initiates a new cycle of proliferation of the endometrium from the endometrial remnants of the previous cycle. Although the process of menstruation represents the end-point of the cycle of endometrial changes, the first day of menstruation also marks the beginning of a new proliferative phase. Furthermore, as the most easily recognisable point it is usually taken to mark the first day of the 28-day menstrual cycle. Menstruation lasts on average 5 days; the proliferative phase continues until about the 14th day when ovulation occurs and the secretory phase begins. The secretory phase culminates at the onset of menstruation on about the 28th day.

The endometrium is divided into three histologically and functionally distinct layers. The deepest or basal layer, the *stratum basalis*, adjacent to the myometrium, undergoes little change during the menstrual cycle and is not shed during menstruation. The broad intermediate layer is characterised by a stroma with a spongy appearance and is called the *stratum spongiosum*. The thinner superficial layer which has a compact stromal appearance is known as the *stratum compactum*. The compact and spongy layers exhibit dramatic changes throughout the cycle and both are shed during menstruation; hence they are jointly referred to as the *stratum functionalis*.

The arrangement of the arterial supply of the endometrium has important influences on the menstrual cycle. Branches of the uterine arteries pass through the myometrium and immediately divide into two different types of arteries, *straight arteries* and *spiral arteries*. Straight arteries are short and pass a small distance into the endometrium, then bifurcating to form a plexus supplying the stratum basalis. Spiral arteries are long, coiled and thick-walled and pass to the surface of the endometrium giving off numerous branches which give rise to a capillary plexus around the glands and in the stratum compactum. Unlike the straight arteries, the spiral arteries are responsive to the hormonal changes of the menstrual cycle. The withdrawal of progesterone secretion at the end of the cycle causes the spiral arteries to constrict and this precipitates an *ischaemic phase* which immediately precedes menstruation.

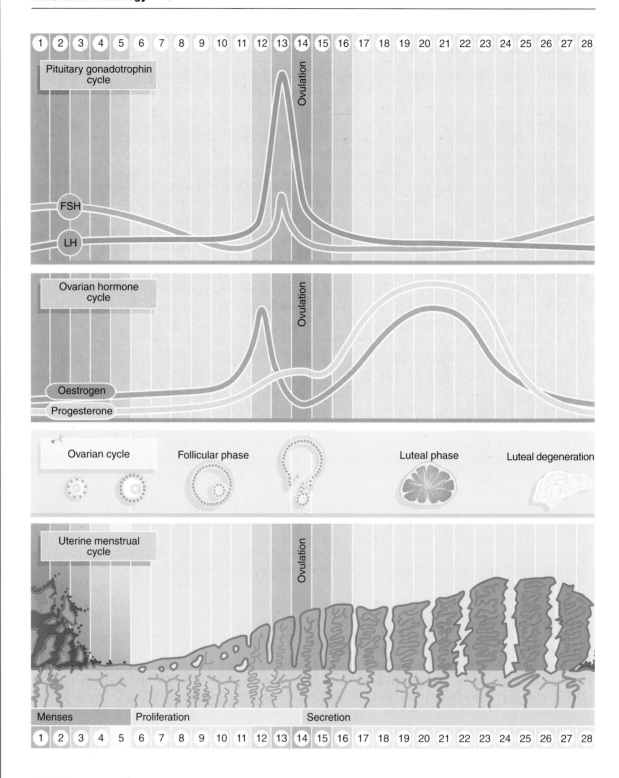

Fig. 19.15   The hormonal integration of the ovarian and menstrual cycles

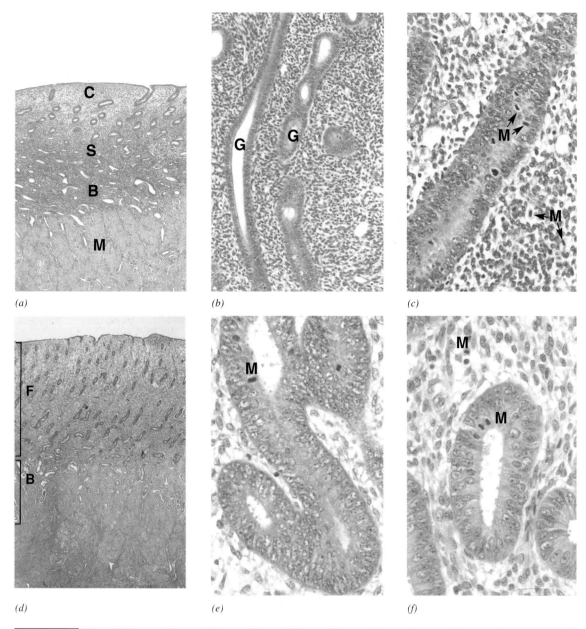

(a) (b) (c) (d) (e) (f)

Fig. 19.16 **Proliferative endometrium** Early phase: (a) H & E × 20 (b) H & E × 100 (c) H & E × 200; Late phase: (d) H & E × 10 (e) H & E × 100 (f) H & E × 200

Micrograph (a) illustrates early proliferative endometrium at low magnification. At the bottom of the field is the muscular wall, the myometrium **M**. The relatively thin endometrium consists of the stratum basalis **B**, stratum spongiosum **S** and stratum compactum **C**. The glands at this stage are fairly sparse and straight. As the glands, stroma and vessels proliferate, the endometrium gradually becomes thicker. By day 5–6 of the cycle the surface epithelium has regenerated. During the proliferative phase the epithelial cells acquire microvilli and cilia as well as the cytoplasmic organelles required for the secretory phase.

At higher magnification in micrograph (b), the straight tubular form of the endometrial glands **G** can be seen. At very high magnification in micrograph (c), the proliferating glandular epithelium is seen to consist of columnar cells with basally located nuclei exhibiting prominent nucleoli. Mitotic figures **M** can be seen both

in the epithelium and in the stroma. Note the highly cellular stroma, almost devoid of collagen fibres.

By the late proliferative stage, shown at low magnification in micrograph (d), the endometrium has doubled in thickness. Note that in contrast to the stratum functionalis **F**, the appearance of the stratum basalis **B** is little changed when compared with the early proliferative phase. With further magnification, micrograph (e) shows that the tubular glands are now becoming coiled and more closely packed. At very high magnification in micrograph (f), mitotic figures **M** are more prevalent in both the glandular epithelium and the supporting stroma. The stroma is also somewhat oedematous at this stage. During the proliferative phase there is a continuum of change which makes the precise dating of the cycle inaccurate in histological specimens. Lymphocytes and occasional lymphoid aggregates are a normal feature of late proliferative phase endometrium.

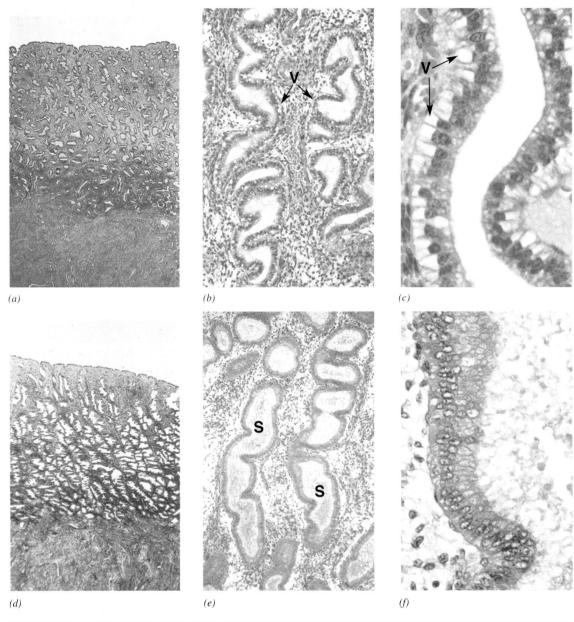

Fig. 19.17 **Secretory endometrium** Early phase: (a) H & E × 8 (b) H & E × 50
(c) H & E × 200; Late phase: (d) H & E × 8 (e) H & E × 50 (f) H & E × 300

Ovulation marks the onset of the secretory phase although endometrial proliferation continues for several days. At low magnification in micrograph (a), the coiled appearance of the glands is now more pronounced and the endometrium approaches its maximum thickness.

Under the influence of progesterone, the glandular epithelium is stimulated to synthesise glycogen. Initially the glycogen accumulates to form vacuoles **V** in the basal aspect of the cells, thus displacing the nuclei towards the centre of the now tall columnar cells. This *basal vacuolation* of the cells appears on day 16 and is the characteristic feature of early secretory endometrium as seen at intermediate and high magnification in micrographs (b) and (c), respectively. Glycogen is an important source of nutrition for the fertilised ovum.

As seen at low magnification in micrograph (d), the late secretory phase is characterised by a saw-tooth appearance of the glands which contain copious thick glycogen and glycoprotein-rich secretions **S**. This rather ragged, tortuous coiling is shown at higher magnification in micrograph (e).

At very high magnification in micrograph (f), the cells have cytoplasmic vacuoles above the nucleus. These vacuoles contain glycogen and glycoproteins which are secreted into the glandular lumen by apocrine-type secretion. Mitotic figures are absent. The stroma is by now at its most vascular and interstitial fluid begins to accumulate between the stromal cells. *Endometrial stromal granulocytes*, which are probably large granular lymphocytes, are found in the stroma at this stage.

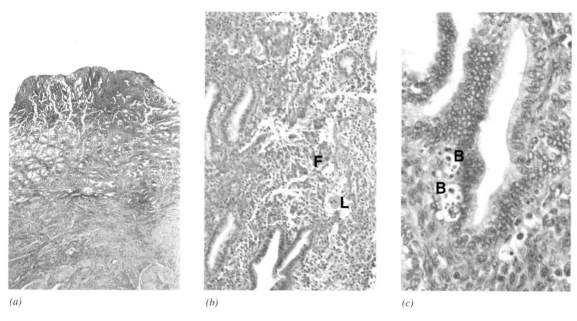

(a)　　　　　　　　　　　*(b)*　　　　　　　　　　*(c)*

Fig. 19.18 Endometrium: onset of menstruation (a) H & E × 8 (b) H & E × 100 (c) H & E × 300

In the absence of implantation of a fertilised ovum, degeneration of the corpus luteum results in cessation of oestrogen and progesterone secretion which initiates phases of spasmodic constriction in the spiral arterioles of the endometrial stratum functionalis **F**. The resulting ischaemia is initially manifest by degeneration of the superficial layers of the endometrium and leakage of blood **L** into the stroma; this is seen in micrographs (a) and (b). Stromal cells disaggregate and the endometrial glands collapse. These features are indicative of early necrosis of glands and stroma. At high magnification in micrograph (c), nuclear debris of endometrial cells **B** can be seen at the onset of menstruation. These cells have died by apoptosis (see Ch. 2).

Further ischaemia leads to degeneration of the whole stratum functionalis which is progressively shed as *menses*. Menses is thus composed of blood, necrotic epithelium and stroma. Normally, menstrual blood does not clot due to the local release of inhibitory (anticoagulant) factors and its expulsion is enhanced by endometrial contractions. By day 3–4 of menstruation most of the stratum functionalis has been shed and proliferation of the basal layer of the endometrium has commenced.

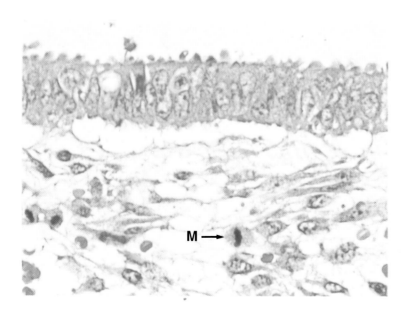

Fig. 19.19 Endometrial surface H & E × 600

This micrograph illustrates the surface epithelium of the endometrium which is tall columnar in form. Some of the cells bear cilia, the remainder having surface microvilli. Stromal cells have plump spindle-shaped nuclei and scanty cytoplasm. In this micrograph they are separated by oedema fluid, a normal feature of late proliferative endometrium. The specimen was obtained during the proliferative phase and mitotic figures **M** are frequent in the stroma.

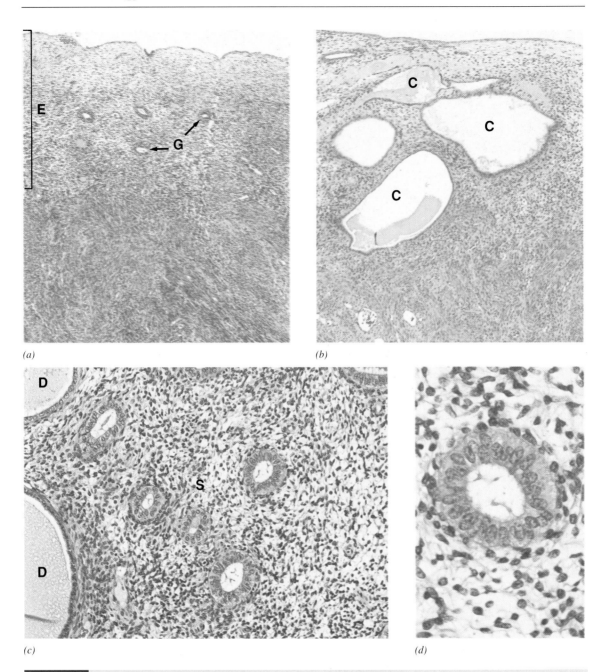

(a) *(b)*

(c) *(d)*

Fig. 19.20 **Post menopausal endometrium** (a) H & E × 60 (b) H & E × 60 (c) H & E × 150 (d) H & E × 400

After the menopause, the cyclical production of oestrogen and progesterone from the ovaries ceases and the whole genital tract undergoes atrophic changes. As seen in micrograph (a), the endometrium **E** is thin, consisting only of the stratum basalis, and the glands **G** are sparse and inactive. As shown in micrograph (b), in some women the glands become dilated to form cystic spaces **C**; the reason for this is unknown but this appearance is so common as to be considered a normal variant.

As shown at higher magnifications in micrographs (c) and (d), the glandular epithelial cells are cuboidal or low columnar with no features of proliferation (i.e. no mitotic figures) or secretory activity. The epithelium which lines cystically dilated glands **D**, as shown in micrograph (c), is often flattened. The stroma **S** is much less cellular and contains more collagen fibres than during the reproductive years and no mitotic activity is seen.

The myometrium also becomes atrophic after the menopause and the uterus shrinks to half its former size.

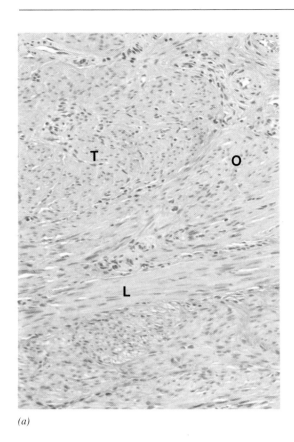

(a)

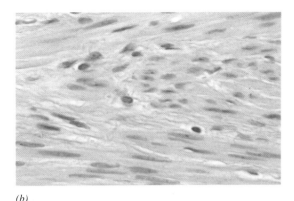

(b)

Fig. 19.21 Myometrium
(a) H & E × 150 (b) H & E × 400

The main bulk of the uterus consists of smooth muscle, the myometrium, which is composed of interlacing bundles of long slender fibres arranged in ill-defined layers; this is readily seen in micrograph (a) which contains bundles of fibres in transverse **T**, longitudinal **L**, and oblique sections **O**. Within the muscle is a rich network of arteries and veins supported by dense collagenous tissue. Micrograph (b) shows detail of the smooth muscle cells at high magnification, highlighting the closeness with which the muscle fibres are packed.

During pregnancy, in response to increased levels of oestrogens, the myometrium increases greatly in size, mainly by increasing cell size (*hypertrophy*), although some increase in cell numbers (*hyperplasia*) due to cell division may also occur.

At parturition, strong contractions of the myometrium are reinforced by the action of the hormone oxytocin secreted by the posterior pituitary. These contractions expel the fetus from the uterus and also constrict the blood supply to the placenta, thus precipitating its detachment from the uterine wall.

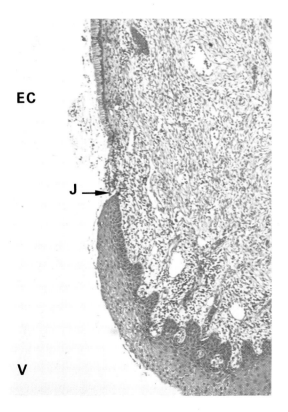

Fig. 19.22 Uterine cervix H & E × 200

The uterine cervix protrudes into the upper vagina and contains the *endocervical canal* linking the uterine cavity with the vagina. The function of the cervix is to admit spermatozoa to the genital tract at the time when fertilisation is possible, i.e. around the time of ovulation, but at other times, including pregnancy, its function is to protect the uterus and upper tract from bacterial invasion. In addition, the cervix must be capable of great dilatation to permit the passage of the fetus during parturition.

As seen in this micrograph, the endocervical canal **EC** is lined by a single layer of tall columnar mucus-secreting cells. Where the cervix is exposed to the more hostile environment of the vagina **V**, the *ectocervix*, it is lined by thick stratified squamous epithelium as in the rest of the vagina. The cells of the ectocervix often have clear cytoplasm due to their high glycogen content (not apparent in this specimen). The junction **J** between the vaginal and endocervical epithelium is quite abrupt and is normally located at the external os, the point at which the endocervical canal opens into the vagina.

The main bulk of the cervix is composed of tough, collagenous tissue containing relatively little smooth muscle. Beneath the squamocolumnar junction, the cervical stroma is often infiltrated with leucocytes forming part of the defence against ingress of microorganisms.

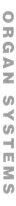

ORGAN SYSTEMS

Fig. 19.23 Cervical cytology Papanicolaou method × 400

The cervical stroma is influenced by the ovarian hormones, particularly oestrogens, which soften the tissues by reducing collagenous cross-linkages and increasing uptake of water by the ground substance. At its most extreme, this provides the means by which the cervix stretches, thins and dilates in late pregnancy and during parturition. To a much lesser extent, similar changes occur during the normal menstrual cycle. One effect of this is that the volume of the cervical stroma varies during each cycle causing eversion of the columnar epithelium near the squamocolumnar junction and exposing it to the vaginal environment; this *ectropion* is known colloquially as 'cervical erosions'. This induces the growth of stratified squamous epithelium (*squamous metaplasia*) over the exposed area, considered a normal variant in women of reproductive age. The importance of this *transformation zone* is that it may undergo malignant change, causing cancer of the cervix.

This area can be studied by scraping cells from the surface using various types of spatula or brush, smearing them on a glass slide and staining them by the Papanicolaou method (*cervical smear* or *Pap test*); this technique is known as *exfoliative cytology* and is demonstrated here from a normal healthy cervix. The surface cells of the stratified squamous epithelium have contracted nuclei and are stained pink due to the cytoplasmic keratin; the deeper cells have plump nuclei of normal appearance and the cytoplasm is stained blue/green. An adequate Pap smear should also contain some endocervical cells (demonstrating that the transformation zone has been adequately sampled) as well as cervical mucin and inflammatory cells.

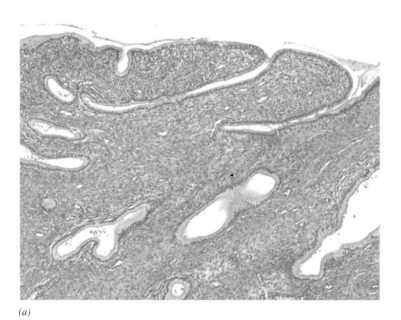

(a)

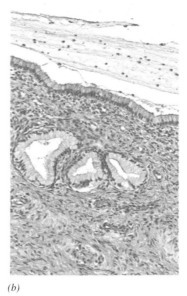

(b)

Fig. 19.24 Endocervix (a) H & E × 60 (b) H & E × 100

As seen in micrograph (a), the mucus-secreting epithelial lining of the endocervical canal is thrown into deep furrows and tunnels giving the appearance in two dimensions of branched tubular glands – hence the rather inaccurate term *endocervical glands*. The columnar mucus-secreting cells lining the 'glands' are shown at higher magnification in micrograph (b). Note the leucocytic infiltrate in the superficial stroma and the presence of leucocytes in the endocervical mucus on the surface.

During the menstrual cycle, the endocervical glands undergo cyclical changes in secretory activity. In the proliferative phase, rising levels of oestrogen promote secretion of thin watery mucus which permits the passage of spermatozoa into the uterus around the period of ovulation. Following ovulation, the cervical mucus becomes highly viscid forming a plug which inhibits the entry of microorganisms (and spermatozoa) from the vagina; this is particularly important should pregnancy occur.

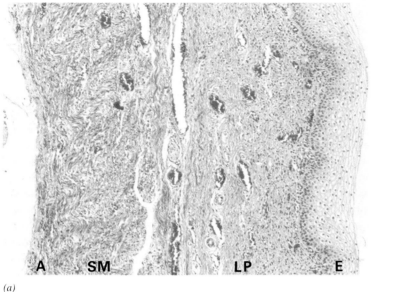
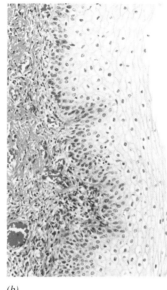

(a) *(b)*

Fig. 19.25 **Vagina** (a) Masson's trichrome × 75 (b) Masson's trichrome × 128

The vagina is a fibromuscular canal and, as seen in micrograph (à), the wall consists of a mucosal layer lined by stratified squamous epithelium **E**, a layer of smooth muscle **SM** and an outer adventitial layer **A**. In the relaxed state, the vaginal wall collapses to obliterate the lumen and the vaginal epithelium is thrown up into folds. The dense lamina propria **LP** contains many elastic fibres, has a rich plexus of small veins and is devoid of glands. The vagina is lubricated by cervical mucus, a fluid transudate from the rich vascular network of the lamina propria and mucus secreted by glands of the labia minora. The smooth muscle bundles of the muscular layer are arranged in ill-defined inner circular and outer longitudinal layers. The adventitial layer of the vagina is not lined by mesothelium but merges with the adventitial layers of the bladder anteriorly and rectum posteriorly.

The combination of a muscular layer and a highly elastic lamina propria permits the gross distension which occurs during parturition. Conversely, after coitus, involuntary contraction of the smooth muscle layer ensures that a pool of semen remains in the cervical region. Thick elastic fibres in the outer adventitial layer also facilitate these functions.

Micrograph (b) illustrates the stratified squamous epithelium which lines the vagina. During the menstrual cycle, this epithelium undergoes cyclical changes in glycogen levels. Throughout the cycle, the superficial cells produce glycogen which is anaerobically metabolised by vaginal commensal bacteria to form lactic acid which inhibits the growth of pathogenic microorganisms.

The placenta

The placenta is formed from elements of the membranes which surround the developing fetus as well as the uterine endometrium and provides the means for physiological exchange between the fetal and maternal circulations. The structure of the placenta varies greatly from one species to another and the following discussion is thus necessarily confined to the human placenta. At various stages during fetal development, the placenta performs a remarkable range of functions until the fetal organs become functional. These include gaseous exchange, excretion, maintenance of homeostasis, hormone secretion, haemopoiesis and hepatic metabolic functions.

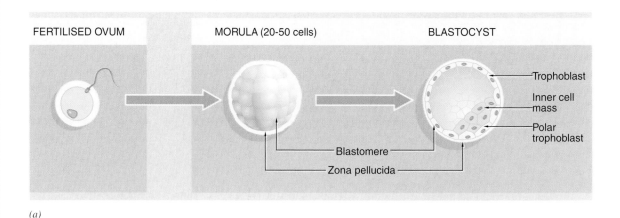

FERTILISED OVUM   MORULA (20-50 cells)   BLASTOCYST

Trophoblast
Inner cell mass
Polar trophoblast
Blastomere
Zona pellucida

(a)

Fig. 19.26 **Fertilisation and implantation** **(a) Diagram above (b) Diagram opposite**

Within about 12 hours after ovulation, fertilisation of an ovum by a spermatozoon occurs in the ampulla of the Fallopian tube with the formation of a *zygote*; the zona pellucida remains intact (see Fig. 19.4). Within 24 hours, the zygote undergoes its first mitotic cell division, the process continuing over the next 4–5 days until there are some 20–50 cells called *blastomeres*, each with a small portion of the original cytoplasm. The mass, now called a *morula* (for its resemblance to a mulberry), remains enclosed by the now thinning zona pellucida through which it is nourished by diffusion of oxygen and low molecular weight metabolites from Fallopian tube secretions.

By now the morula has reached the uterus and begins to absorb uterine fluid forming a central cavity. The *blastocyst*, as it is now known, consists of a peripheral layer of blastomeres forming the *trophoblast*, with a mass of cells at one aspect, the *polar trophoblast*, bulging into the central lumen and known as the *inner cell mass*. The trophoblast (along with a maternal contribution) eventually gives rise to the placenta whilst the inner cell mass develops into the future embryo. By this time, the blastocyst has grown to about twice the size of the original ovum and the zona pellucida has become quite thin. When the blastocyst has been within the uterine cavity for 2–3 days, implantation occurs. The polar trophoblast invades the endometrium so that by the 10th day after ovulation the blastocyst is completely buried. Dissolution of the zona pellucida brings the endometrium into direct contact with the trophoblast which undergoes rapid growth and differentiation.

The trophoblast gives rise to two layers, an inner *cytotrophoblast layer* of mononuclear cells and an outer *syncytiotrophoblast* layer derived by fusion of cytotrophoblast cells to form a continuous multinucleate syncytium in which there is no internal cytoplasmic demarcation by plasma membranes. The cytotrophoblast remains as a single layer of stem cells whereas the syncytiotrophoblast becomes increasingly broad and develops finger-like projections into the endometrium. A third type of trophoblast known as *intermediate trophoblast* has histological features intermediate between cytotrophoblast and syncytiotrophoblast and has a major role in invading the endometrium. Within a short time, a sponge-like network of spaces called lacunae develops within the syncytiotrophoblast, initially filled with tissue fluid and uterine secretions. Soon afterwards,

invasion by the intermediate trophoblast causes disintegration of endometrial capillaries with leakage of maternal blood into the lacunae. Progressively the trophoblast envelops maternal capillaries, expanding the lacunar network and establishing an arterial supply and venous drainage system.

By now, the syncytiotrophoblast also secretes a variety of hormones including *human chorionic gonadotrophin* (*HCG*), *human chorionic somatotrophin* (previously human placental lactogen, HPL), *oestrogen* and *progesterone* which are necessary to sustain the endometrial tissues. In the meantime, the blastocyst cavity becomes filled with *extraembryonic mesoderm* (mesenchyme) which completely surrounds the early embryo developing from the inner cell mass. The embryo by now comprises plates of *embryonic endoderm* and *ectoderm* on either side of which lie the *yolk sac* and *amniotic cavities* enclosed by *extraembryonic endoderm* and *extraembrionic ectoderm*, respectively. Subsequently, a cavity forms within the extraembryonic mesoderm, this *extraembryonic coelom* eventually surrounds the developing embryo which remains attached to the trophoblast by a *connecting stalk* of extraembryonic mesoderm. The trophoblast, along with the mesodermal layer remaining beneath it, now constitutes the *chorion*.

Meanwhile the *trabeculae* of syncytiotrophoblast and intermediate trophoblast between the lacunae are invaded by columns of cytotrophoblastic cells called *primary chorionic villi* which grow out to the periphery and spread out over the interface between the trophoblast and endometrium forming the *cytotrophoblast shell*. Extraembryonic mesoderm now invades the primary villi which thus develop a mesenchymal core, becoming known as *secondary chorionic villi*.

By about 2 weeks after implantation (i.e. about 20 days after fertilisation), primitive blood vessels begin to develop in the chorionic mesoderm simultaneously with development of the primitive embryonic circulatory system, the embryo now being too large to rely on mere diffusion for its growth and metabolic requirements. When the mesenchymal cores of the villi become vascularised they become known as *tertiary villi* (not illustrated).

The form of the placenta is essentially established by the end of the fourth month after which the placenta grows in diameter, complementing growth in the size of the uterus.

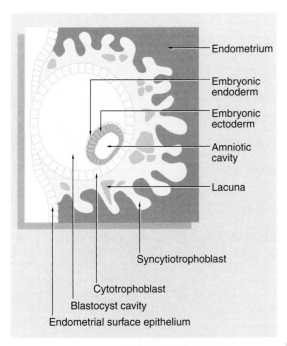

Endometrium

Embryonic endoderm

Embryonic ectoderm

Amniotic cavity

Lacuna

Syncytiotrophoblast

Cytotrophoblast

Blastocyst cavity

Endometrial surface epithelium

IMPLANTATION OF BLASTOCYST

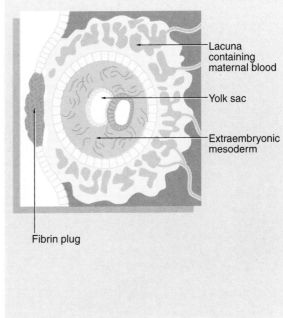

Lacuna containing maternal blood

Yolk sac

Extraembryonic mesoderm

Fibrin plug

EXTRAEMBRYONIC MESODERM REPLACES THE BLASTOCYST CAVITY

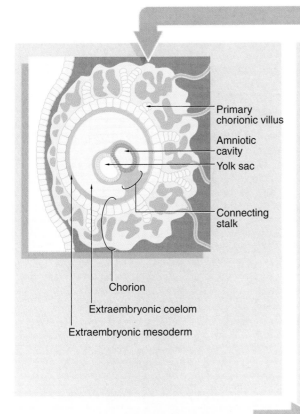

Primary chorionic villus

Amniotic cavity

Yolk sac

Connecting stalk

Chorion

Extraembryonic coelom

Extraembryonic mesoderm

CHORIONIC VESICLE FORMATION

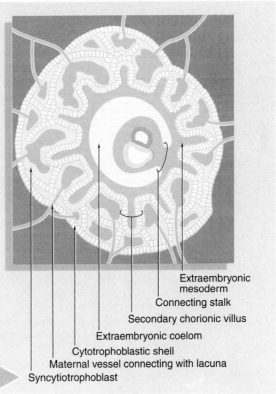

Extraembryonic mesoderm

Connecting stalk

Secondary chorionic villus

Extraembryonic coelom

Cytotrophoblastic shell

Maternal vessel connecting with lacuna

Syncytiotrophoblast

(b)

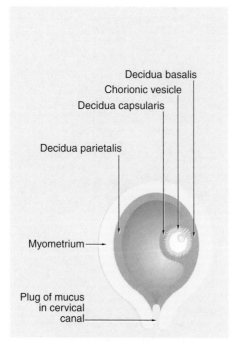

Decidua basalis
Chorionic vesicle
Decidua capsularis

Decidua parietalis

Myometrium

Plug of mucus
in cervical
canal

EARLY PLACENTATION

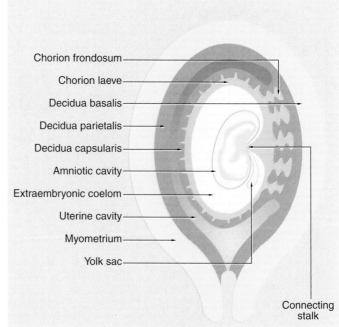

Chorion frondosum
Chorion laeve
Decidua basalis
Decidua parietalis
Decidua capsularis
Amniotic cavity
Extraembryonic coelom
Uterine cavity
Myometrium
Yolk sac

Connecting
stalk

LATER PLACENTATION

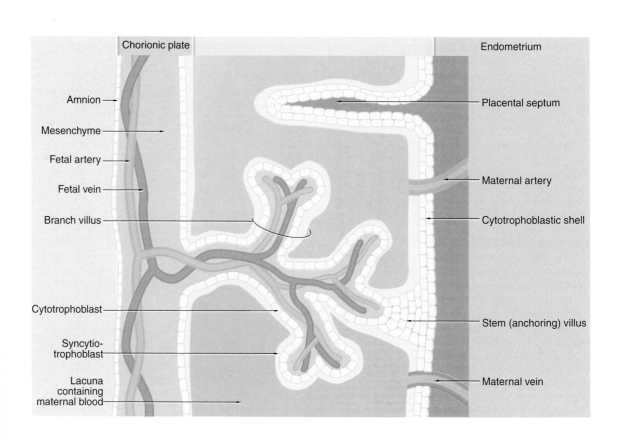

Chorionic plate

Amnion
Mesenchyme
Fetal artery
Fetal vein
Branch villus

Cytotrophoblast

Syncytio-
trophoblast

Lacuna
containing
maternal blood

Endometrium

Placental septum

Maternal artery

Cytotrophoblastic shell

Stem (anchoring) villus

Maternal vein

Fig. 19.27 **Decidua formation and early placental development** *(illustrations opposite, above)*

During the process of implantation, secretion by the syncytiotrophoblast of HCG (which is functionally analogous to luteinising hormone) interrupts the ovarian cycle. This results in growth and proliferation of stromal cells of the endometrial stratum functionalis at the implantation site into large polyhedral *decidual cells*, a change which has already begun in the late secretory phase. The *decidua* beneath the developing embryo is known as the *decidua basalis* and with the trophoblast will form the future placenta; that overlying the embryo is known as the *decidua capsularis* and the decidual lining of the rest of the uterus is called the *decidua parietalis*. Ultimately, expansion of the embryo and its enveloping fluid-filled membrane system results in fusion of the opposed capsular and parietal layers of the decidua with complete obliteration of the uterine cavity.

During the first 2 months of embryological development the chorion grows fairly uniformly around the whole periphery of the vesicle. From the third month, the chorion in contact with the decidua basalis develops extensive frond-like villous outgrowths into the decidua becoming known as the *chorion frondosum*, whilst the superficial chorion in contact with the decidua capsularis atrophies to become the smooth *chorion laeve*. Progressively, the chorion frondosum and decidua basalis develop into the flattened placenta and the vessels connecting the chorion to the embryonic circulation become the umbilical cord.

Fig. 19.28 **Structure of placental villi** *(illustration opposite, below)*

From the time maternal blood appears within the trophoblastic lacunae, the trabeculae between the lacunae become increasingly robust with *stem villi* forming anchorage points with the cytotrophoblastic shell. Side branches grow out into the lacunae, progressively forming a complex villous structure. Each villus contains a mesenchymal core containing capillaries served by afferent and efferent fetal blood vessels. Between the villous capillaries and the maternal blood is a continuous layer of syncytiotrophoblast supported by a layer of proliferating cytotrophoblast cells. From the fourth month onwards, the cytotrophoblast layer becomes atrophic.

As more and more branches are added to the villous tree, the villi become smaller and smaller and the tissue barrier between fetal capillaries and maternal blood is greatly diminished.

As the placenta develops, the decidua basalis regresses so that all that remains are a number of anastomosing septa of maternal supporting tissue projecting into the cytotrophoblastic shell. When the placenta is shed immediately after childbirth, its maternal surface is seen to be divided into about 20 irregular segments called *cotyledons* which are demarcated from each other by the positions of the former maternal (placental) septa.

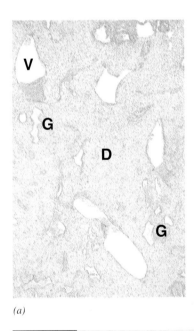
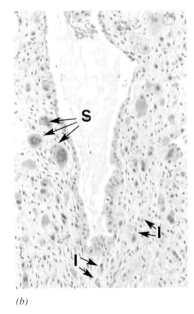
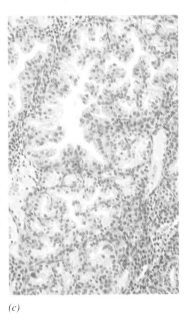

(a)   *(b)*   *(c)*

Fig. 19.29 **Decidua (a) H & E × 20 (b) H & E × 100 (c) H & E × 200**

Micrograph (a) illustrates decidual change **D** in the endometrial stroma. The decidual cells proliferate and enlarge greatly, their cytoplasm staining pink (eosinophilia) due to the presence of numerous mitochondria and intermediate filaments. Dilated blood vessels **V** and endometrial glands **G** are apparent.

At higher power in micrograph (b), multinucleated syncytiotrophoblast cells **S** can be seen infiltrating the decidua. Intermediate trophoblast cells **I** are actually present in greater numbers than syncytiotrophoblast but are less easily identified. In the centre of the field is a dilated gland.

Micrograph (c) shows the deeper part of the endometrium in pregnancy. Here the decidual reaction is inconspicuous but the secretory nature of the glands is greatly exaggerated; it is thus often called *hypersecretory endometrium*. Note the prominent infolding of the glandular epithelium and the vacuolation of the epithelial cell cytoplasm.

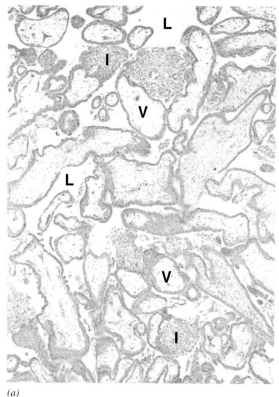

(a)

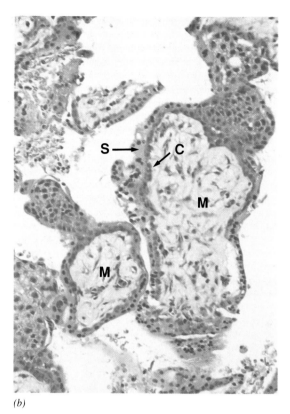

(b)

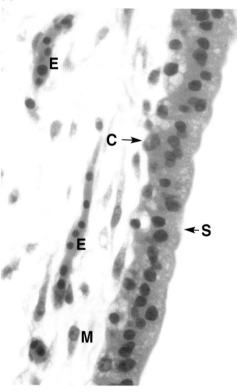

(c)

Fig. 19.30 Early placenta
(a) H & E × 50 (b) H & E × 150 (c) H & E × 300

This series of micrographs at increasing magnification shows a placenta at about 6 weeks gestational age. Nucleated fetal erythrocytes **E**, which in humans persist until 9 weeks gestational age, can be seen in the capillary in micrograph (c).

At low magnification in micrograph (a), the main feature is the large numbers of villi **V** projecting into the lacuna system **L** which in vivo would be filled with maternal blood; some villi show evidence of branching. Solid cores of cytotrophoblast and intermediate trophoblast **I** can be seen extending away from the villi to form new branches.

With further magnification in micrograph (b), the villi are seen to have a cellular core of mesenchyme **M**. The villi are invested by trophoblast comprising an inner layer of cytotrophoblast cells **C** and a broader, outer syncytiotrophoblast layer **S**. In some areas, solid buds of trophoblast can be seen forming branches. The specimen is a little broken up as it is derived from a curettage specimen following incomplete spontaneous abortion.

Micrograph (c) focuses on the margin of a villus at high magnification, the cellular preservation being again less than ideal due to its origin from a spontaneous abortion. The syncytiotrophoblast layer **S** can be distinguished from the single layer of cytotrophoblast cells **C** which are smaller. The mesenchymal cells **M** are large, with extensive branching cytoplasmic processes, and the intercellular matrix is mucoid due to its high glycosaminoglycan content.

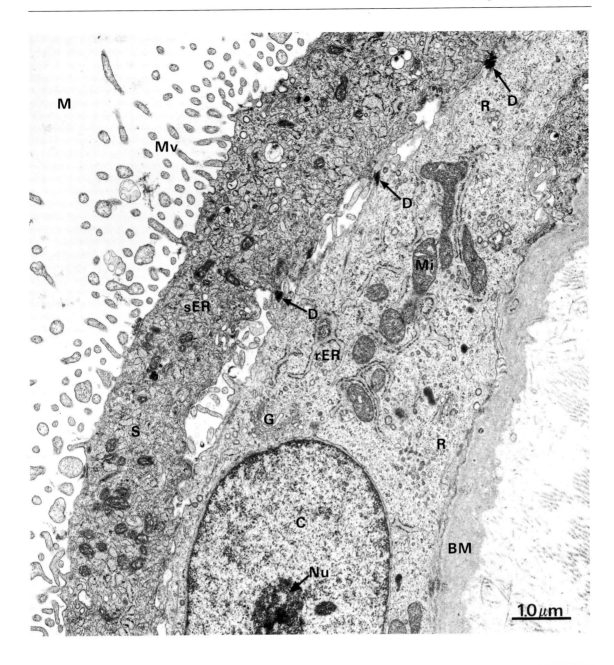

Fig. 19.31 Trophoblast EM × 16 000

This micrograph shows the general ultrastructural features of the trophoblastic components; these show considerable variation from one region to another and from early to late stages of placental function.

The syncytiotrophoblast **S** typically presents large numbers of irregular microvilli **Mv** to the maternal blood spaces **M** greatly enhancing the surface area for physiological exchange. The plasma membranes of the microvilli incorporate a wide variety of enzymes and receptors involved in membrane transfer processes as well as receptors for many hormones and growth factors. Microfilaments extend into the microvilli from a cytoskeletal network concentrated immediately below the free surface. Some areas of the syncytiotrophoblast contain rough endoplasmic reticulum whilst in others,

such as shown here, smooth endoplasmic reticulum **sER** predominates, presumably involved in steroid hormone synthesis.

The cytotrophoblast layer **C** has ultrastructural features of relatively undifferentiated stem cells exhibiting profiles of rough endoplasmic reticulum **rER**, a well-defined Golgi appatatus **G**, relatively few mitochondria **Mi** and numerous polyribosomes **R**. The nucleus is typically large with dispersed chromatin and nucleoli **Nu**. The cytotrophoblast is typically tightly bound to the overlying syncytiotrophoblast by desmosomes **D** but in some areas, as in this specimen, spaces can be seen between the cell layers; the reason for this is unclear. Separating the cytotrophoblast from the underlying collagenous stroma is a relatively thick basement membrane **BM**.

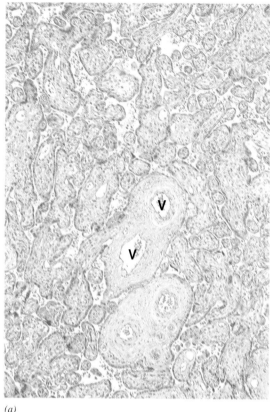

(a)

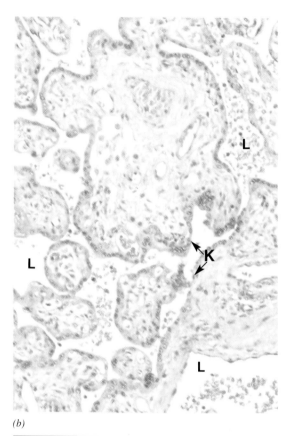

(b)

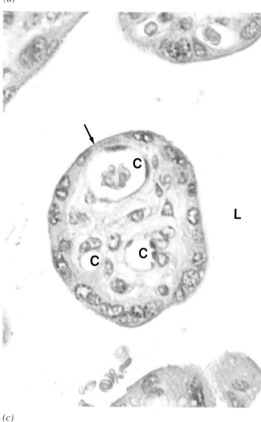

(c)

Fig. 19.32 Term placenta
(a) H & E × 60 (b) H & E × 150 (c) H & E × 600

These micrographs illustrate placenta from a full-term fetus.

At low magnification in micrograph (a), huge numbers of villi can be seen cut in various planes of section and varying in diameter from large main stem villi to very small terminal branch villi. Compared with early placenta shown in Figure 19.30(a), the villous pattern is much more highly developed and the average villous diameter is much smaller, reflecting the extensive branching growth of the villi as the placenta enlarges. Note the large vessels **V** in the biggest villi.

Micrograph (b) demonstrates the branching nature of the villi at higher magnification. Compare the marked vascularity of the villous cores with that of the much earlier placenta in Figure 19.30(b) and the greatly increased villous surface area exposed to the lacunae **L** filled with maternal blood. A feature of the term placenta is the syncytial knot **K**, where syncytiotrophoblast nuclei are aggregated together in clusters leaving zones of thin cytoplasm devoid of nuclei between.

Micrograph (c) focuses on a small branch villus and highlights the proximity of blood in fetal capillaries **C** to maternal blood in the surrounding lacuna **L**. The trophoblast is reduced to a thin layer of syncytiotrophoblast only and the capillaries tend to be located in the periphery of the core. The diffusion barrier between maternal and fetal circulations comprises five layers, namely: trophoblast, trophoblast basement membrane, core supporting tissue, capillary endothelial basement membrane and endothelium. In many cases (as marked by the arrow), fetal capillaries are so close to the trophoblast that their basement membranes fuse, reducing the diffusion barrier to only three layers.

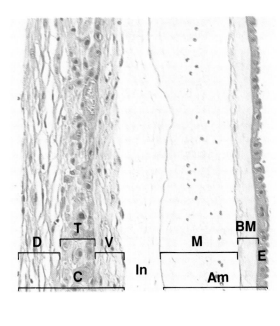

Fig. 19.33   Fetal membranes H & E × 150

During early development, the embryo is surrounded by the extraembryonic coelom (see Fig. 19.27) but later this becomes obliterated as the amniotic cavity expands to surround the fetus. The outer mesenchymal layer of the amnion then comes to lie in contact with (and often fuses with) the inner mesenchymal layer of the chorion forming the *chorio-amnion* or fetal membranes. The two layers are often difficult to separate from one another at birth.

The amniotic membrane **Am** comprises a single layer of epithelial cells **E** derived from extraembryonic ectoderm resting on a thick basement membrane **BM**; beneath this is a delicate avascular mesenchymal layer **M** which is a remnant of the extraembryonic mesoderm. The chorionic membrane **C** consists of three layers. A vascular collagenous inner layer **V** is also derived from extraembryonic mesoderm; the *intermediate zone* **In** seen here separating it from the amnion represents the remnant of the extraembryonic coelom and varies greatly in thickness. The trophoblast **T** of the chorion laeve is represented by the middle layer of eosinophilic epithelial cells, and the outermost vascular collagenous layer **D** is of maternal origin representing the decidua capsularis (see Fig. 19.27).

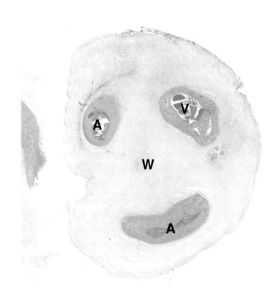

(a)

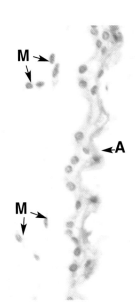

(b)

Fig. 19.34   Umbilical cord (a) H & E × 7.5 (b) H & E × 300

The development of the umbilical cord begins with the formation of the extraembryonic coelom which almost surrounds the early embryo and which remains attached to the chorion by the connecting stalk of mesenchyme (see Fig. 19.26). With further embryonic development, the site of attachment of the connecting stalk becomes located ventrally, just caudal to the point where the *vitello-intestinal* duct connects the *yolk sac* to the mid-gut. As the embryo grows, the amniotic sac expands greatly, filling the extraembryonic coelom and compressing the vitello-intestinal duct and yolk sac remnant (surrounded by a sleeve of extraembryonic coelom) up against the connecting stalk. These structures ultimately fuse to form

the umbilical cord which now is surrounded by the amnion and amniotic cavity.

By the middle of the fifth month, the remnants of the vitello-intestinal duct, yolk sac and sheath of extraembryonic coelom atrophy and disappear. As seen in micrograph (a), all that remains are two umbilical arteries **A** and a single umbilical vein **V** embedded in mesenchyme consisting mainly of ground substance and known as *Wharton's jelly* **W**. Mesenchymal cells **M** and surface amnion **A** are shown at high magnification in micrograph (b). The umbilical arteries convey deoxygenated fetal blood to the placenta whilst the umbilical vein conveys oxygenated blood back to the fetus.

The breasts

The breasts (mammary glands) are highly modified apocrine sweat glands (see Fig. 9.16) which develop embryologically along two lines, the *milk lines*, extending from the axillae to the groins. In humans, only one gland develops on each side of the thorax, although accessory breast tissue may be found anywhere along the milk lines.

The breasts of both sexes follow a similar course of development until puberty, after which the female breasts develop under the influence of pituitary, ovarian and other hormones. Until the menopause, the breasts undergo cyclical changes in activity which are controlled by the hormones of the ovarian cycle. After menopause, the breasts, like the other female reproductive tissues, undergo progressive atrophy and involution.

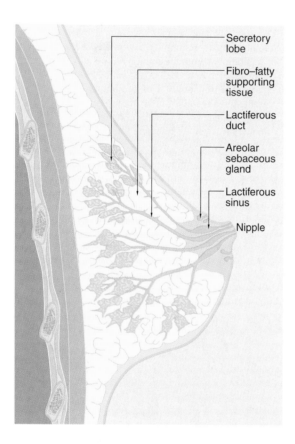

Secretory lobe

Fibro–fatty supporting tissue

Lactiferous duct

Areolar sebaceous gland

Lactiferous sinus

Nipple

Fig. 19.35   Structure of the breast

This highly schematic diagram illustrates the general organisation of the breast. Each breast consists of 15–25 independent glandular units called *breast lobes*, each consisting of a compound tubulo-acinar gland (see Fig. 5.28). The lobes are embedded in a mass of adipose tissue which is subdivided by collagenous septa. More robust fibrous septa separate the territory of each lobe.

The lobes are arranged radially at different depths around the nipple, a single large duct, the *lactiferous duct*, draining each lobe via a separate opening on the surface of the nipple. Immediately before opening onto the surface, the duct forms a dilatation called the *lactiferous sinus*. The nipple contains bands of smooth muscle orientated in parallel to the lactiferous ducts and circularly near the base; contraction of this muscle causes erection of the nipple.

Within each lobe of the breast, the main duct branches repeatedly to form a number of *terminal ducts*, each of which leads to a *lobule* consisting of multiple *acini*. Each terminal duct and its associated lobule is called a *terminal duct–lobular unit*. The lobules are separated by moderately dense collagenous *interlobular* tissue, whereas the *intralobular* supporting tissue surrounding the ducts within each lobule is less collagenous and more vascular. The skin surrounding the nipple, the *areola*, is pigmented and contains sebaceous glands which are not associated with hair follicles. The secretions of these glands probably help to protect the nipple and areola during suckling.

Fig. 19.36   Breast *(illustrations opposite)*
(a) H & E × 30 (b) H & E × 60 (c) H & E × 150 (d) H & E × 400 (e) H & E × 400 (f) Immunoperoxidase × 100

These micrographs show breast tissue from a non-pregnant woman of reproductive age. Micrograph (a) shows two terminal duct–lobular units (TDLU) at low magnification. The extensive branching duct system is surrounded by relatively dense fibrous interlobular tissue **F**, at the periphery of which is adipose tissue **A**. The interlacing (reticular) arrangement of the coarse collagen of the interlobular tissue is seen at higher magnification in micrograph (b) as is the arborising duct system of the lobule.

Micrograph (c) focuses on a peripheral branching part of the lobule at higher magnification showing well the loose vascular intralobular supporting tissue between the ducts. The ducts and acini are lined by two layers of cells, a luminal layer of epithelial cells and a basal layer of flattened myoepithelial cells. In the larger ducts, as shown in micrograph (d), the luminal epithelial cells **E** are tall columnar type whereas in the smaller ducts and acini shown in micrograph (e) the epithelial cells are cuboidal. A discontinuous layer of stellate myoepithelial cells **M** with pale cytoplasm surrounds the ductal lining cells. In micrograph (f), which uses the imunoperoxidase technique to stain the myoepithelial cells for actin, the extent and number of the myoepithelial cells (stained brown) are apparent. During the reproductive years, the duct epithelium undergoes mild cyclical changes under the influence of ovarian hormones. Early in the cycle, the duct lumina are not clearly evident but later in the cycle they become more prominent and may contain an eosinophilic secretion.

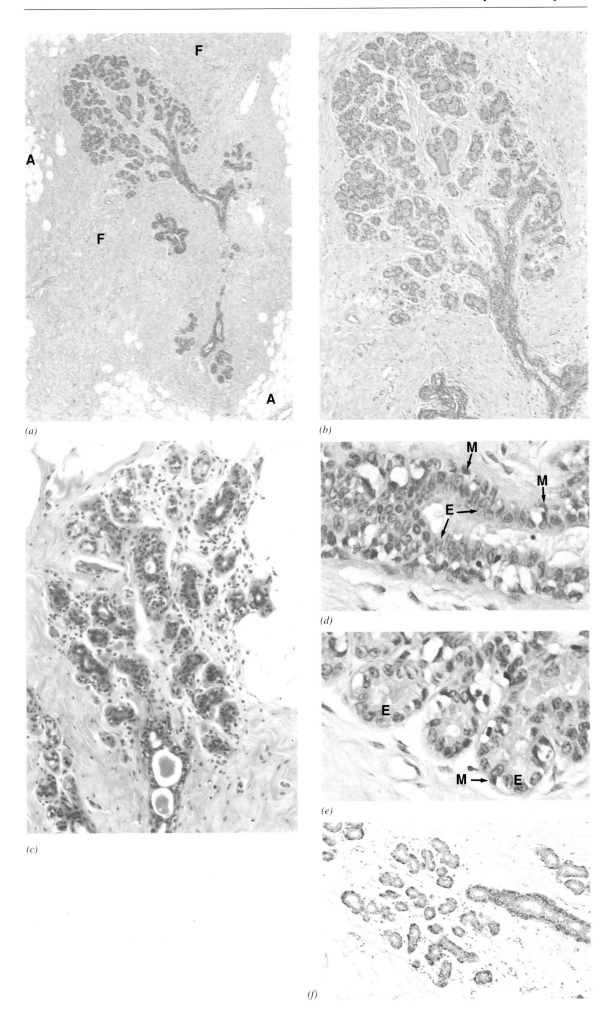

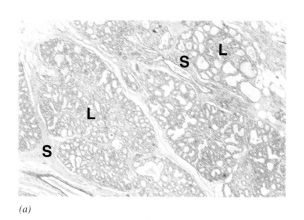
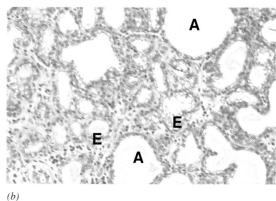

(a) *(b)*

Fig. 19.37 **Breast during pregnancy** (a) H & E × 20 (b) H & E × 100

Under the influence of oestrogens and progesterone produced by the corpus luteum and later by the placenta, the terminal duct epithelium proliferates to form greatly increased numbers of secretory acini. Breast proliferation is also dependent on prolactin, human chorionic somatomammotropin (a prolactin-like hormone produced by the placenta), thyroid hormone and corticosteroids.

At low magnification in micrograph (a), the breast lobules **L** are seen to have enlarged greatly at the expense of the intralobular tissue and interlobar adipose tissue although septa **S** of interlobular tissue still remain. At higher magnification in (b) the acini **A** are dilated. The lining epithelial cells **E** vary from cuboidal to low columnar and contain cytoplasmic vacuoles. The intralobular stroma is much less prominent and contains an infiltrate of lymphocytes, eosinophils and plasma cells

As pregnancy progresses, the acini begin to secrete a protein-rich fluid called ***colostrum***, the accumulation of which dilates the acinar and duct lumina as seen in micrograph (b). Colostrum is the form of breast secretion available during the first few days after birth; it contains a laxative substance and maternal antibodies. Unlike milk, colostrum contains little lipid. Breast secretion is controlled by the hormone prolactin. During pregnancy, prolactin secretion progressively increases but its activity is suppressed by high levels of circulating oestrogens and progesterone.

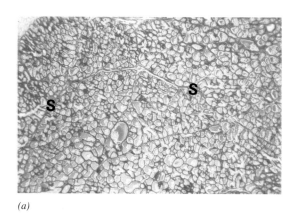
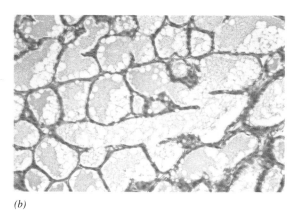

(a) *(b)*

Fig. 19.38 **Lactating breast** (a) H & E × 20 (b) H & E × 128

After parturition, the levels of circulating progesterone and oestrogens, which inhibit milk secretion, fall precipitously. Prolactin stimulates milk production in conjunction with several other hormones.

As seen in micrograph (a), the lactating breast is composed almost entirely of acini distended with milk, the interlobular tissue now being reduced to thin septa **S** between the lobules. At higher magnification in (b), the acini are seen to be filled with an eosinophilic material containing clear vacuoles caused by lipid droplets dissolved out during tissue preparation.

In micrograph (b) the epithelial cells are flattened and the acini distended by secretions. However, in different areas the epithelium may be thicker and the acinar lumina smaller.

Milk production proceeds for as long as suckling continues and can continue for some years after childbirth. The process is mediated by a neurohormonal reflex in which nipple stimulation by suckling causes release of prolactin from the anterior pituitary. A different neurohormonal reflex, also initiated by suckling, causes the release of the hormone oxytocin from the posterior pituitary. Oxytocin causes contraction of the myoepithelial cells which embrace the secretory acini and ducts, thus propelling milk into the lactiferous sinuses (milk 'let-down'). Withdrawal of the suckling stimulus, and hence the release of pituitary hormones at weaning, results in regression of the lactating breast and resumption of the ovarian cycle.

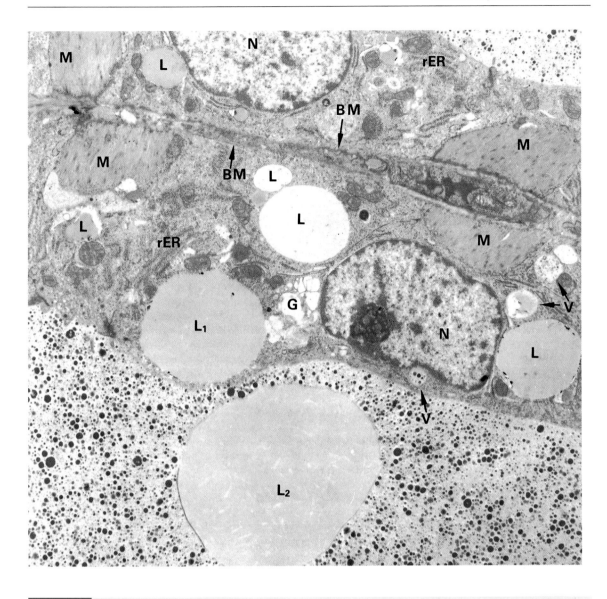

Fig. 19.39 **Lactating breast** EM × 9000

This micrograph shows two secretory cells of adjacent acini in a lactating breast. Their nuclei **N** are large with prominent nucleoli. Each acinus is bounded by a basement membrane **BM**, the basement membranes in this example being separated by only a shred of intralobular tissue. Between each basement membrane and the secretory cells are the cytoplasmic processes of myoepithelial cells **M**, contraction of which expels milk from the gland.

The composition of milk varies somewhat during lactation and even during each suckling episode but its main constituents are as follows: water (88%), ions (particularly sodium, potassium, chloride, calcium and phosphate), protein (1.5%, mainly lactalbumin and casein), carbohydrate (7%, mainly lactose), lipids (3.5%, mainly triglycerides), vitamins and antibodies (of the IgA class).

Secretion of different components of the milk occurs by different mechanisms. Water and some ions diffuse freely through the apical cell membrane. Proteins are synthesised on the rough endoplasmic reticulum **rER**, packaged in the Golgi apparatus **G** and secreted in

vacuoles **V** by exocytosis; protein in the milk is represented by small electron-dense granules. The Golgi apparatus is extensive and the protein-containing secretory vacuoles also contain a considerable amount of other less electron-dense material including lactose and calcium.

The cytoplasm of the secretory cells contains lipid droplets **L** of various sizes not bounded by membrane; these contain triglyceride, although whether this is derived directly from blood or synthesised in the secretory cells is uncertain. The lipid is discharged by apocrine secretion which involves the lipid droplet, surrounding cytoplasm and plasma membrane being cast off into the lumen. A large lipid droplet L_1 with thin overlying rim of cytoplasm can be seen in the lower acinus just prior to secretion; an even larger droplet L_2 surrounded by a remnant of cytoplasm and plasma membrane is seen in the lumen close by.

IgA, taken up by receptor-mediated endocytosis at the base of the cell from the bloodstream, is transported across the cell in small membranous vesicles and released by exocytosis into the milk.

20. Central nervous system

Introduction

The central nervous system (CNS) consists of the brain and spinal cord, which are composed of **neurones**, the supporting cells of the CNS (**glial cells**) and blood vessels. The histology of nervous tissue and the meninges which invest the CNS are described in Chapter 7.

Macroscopically, all parts of the CNS are made up of grey matter and white matter, the grey matter containing most of the neurone cell bodies and the white matter the axons; lipid in the myelin sheaths of the axons accounts for the white appearance of the white matter. The distribution of grey matter and white matter differs greatly from one part of the brain to another as does the morphology and arrangement of the neurones.

The histological methods used in the study of the CNS can be divided into four groups:

- **Techniques which demonstrate nuclei, cell bodies and their cytoplasmic contituents**. Such methods include routine stains such as H & E and more specific methods for demonstrating particular cytoplasmic constituents such as the Nissl method for RNA. These methods show minimal detail of axons and dendrites and the structure of white matter but are useful to highlight the arrangement of neurones, glial cells and blood vessels.
- **Myelin methods**, e.g. Weigart–Pal or Luxol fast blue, are routinely used in studying the arrangement of grey matter (nuclei) and white matter in the brain stem and spinal cord, as well as abnormalities of myelination. With myelin methods, the white matter stains strongly, the grey matter remaining unstained.
- **Immunohistochemical techniques** using antibodies against proteins specific to neurones, astrocytes, oligodendroglia or microglia are routinely used to delineate individual cell types, especially in examination of diseases of the nervous system.
- **Heavy metal impregnation methods**, applied to thick tissue sections, demonstrate overall cell morphology, especially the pattern of branching of axons and dendrites, permitting study of neuronal interconnections. These methods are rarely used today.

Within the CNS, specific terms are used to describe arrangements of cells and their connections:

- the arrangement of neurones over the surface of the brain is termed the **cortex**
- an arrangement of neuronal cells as a discrete unit is termed a **nucleus**.
- an arrangement of neuronal cells running along the spinal cord is termed a **column**
- a defined bundle of axons running in white matter is termed a **tract** or a **fascicle**.

The CNS develops through growth and complex folding, resulting in distinct convolutions visible on external surface and in sections. In the cerebral cortex, the crests of folds are termed **gyri** while the clefts between folds are termed **sulci**. In the cerebellum these folds are termed **folia**.

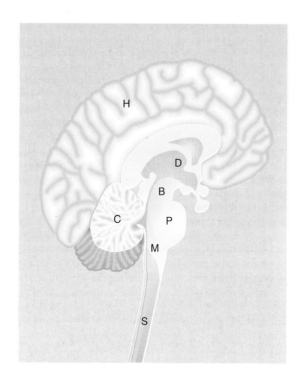

Fig. 20.1 Main anatomic divisions in the central nervous system

This diagram shows the brain and spinal cord viewed in a sagittal section. The main part of the brain consists of the paired cerebral hemispheres **H** which are invested by the cerebral cortex. Deep within the brain are large grey matter structures which form the diencephalon **D**. Included in this region are the basal ganglia and thalamus. The cerebral hemispheres are connected to structures below by the midbrain **B**. In this region there are important nuclei including the substantia nigra. The pons **P** connects to the medulla **M** as well as to the cerebellum **C**. The spinal cord **S** extends from the lower end of the medulla.

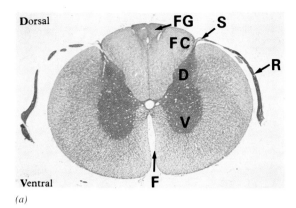

(a)

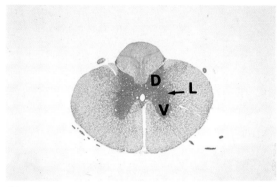

(b)

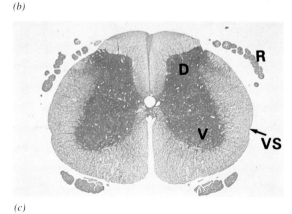

(c)

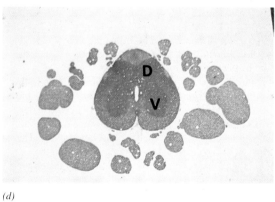

(d)

Fig. 20.2 Spinal cord (cat: Weigart–Pal × 10)
(a) Cervical (b) Thoracic (c) Lumbar (d) Sacral

The structure of the spinal cord is basically similar throughout its whole length, with the four main regions demonstrated in this series of micrographs.

In transverse section, the central mass of grey matter has the shape of a butterfly, the *ventral horns* **V** being most prominent and containing the cell bodies of the large lower motor neurones. The *dorsal horns* **D** are much less prominent and contain the cell bodies of small second order sensory neurones; these relay sensory information to the brain from primary afferent neurones for the modalities of temperature and pain whose cell bodies lie in the dorsal root ganglia. Small *lateral horns* **L**, which contain the cell bodies of preganglionic, sympathetic efferent neurones, are found in the thoracic and upper lumbar regions corresponding to the level of the sympathetic outflow from the cord. The volume of grey matter is much more extensive in the cervical and lumbar regions corresponding to the sensory and motor innervation of the limbs and this is reflected in the much greater diameter of the spinal cord in these areas. The *central canal* lies in the *central commissure* of grey matter; it is lined by ependymal cells and contains CSF.

The white matter of the spinal cord consists of ascending tracts of sensory fibres and descending motor tracts; passing up the spinal cord towards the brain, more and more fibres enter and leave the cord so that the volume of white matter increases progressively from the sacral to cervical regions.

Externally, the spinal cord has a deep *ventral median fissure* **F** but dorsally there is only a shallow dorsal *midline sulcus*. On each side, a *dorsolateral sulcus* **S** marks the line of entry of the dorsal nerve roots **R**, part of which can be seen in micrographs (a) and (c). The roughly triangular area of white matter between the dorsal horns represents the ascending *dorsal columns* which convey fibres for the senses of vibration, proprioception and discriminatory touch to the medulla where they synapse with second order sensory neurones in the *gracile* and *cuneate nuclei*. In the cervical region, each dorsal column is subdivided into two fascicles, the medial *fasciculus gracilis* **FG** conveying fibres from the lower limbs, and the lateral *fasciculus cuneatus* **FC** conveying fibres from the upper limbs.

Ventrolateral sulci **VS** may be discernible on each side as in micrograph (c), marking the sites of exit of the ventral nerve roots.

The ventrolateral white matter on each side is made up of various ascending and descending tracts, most notably the *lateral spinothalamic* tract (pain and temperature), *ventral spinothalamic tract* (light touch), *spinocerebellar tracts* and *corticospinal tract* (motor).

Like the brain, the spinal cord is invested by meninges, the outer surface of the dura mater being loosely connected to the periosteum of the vertebral canal by the denticulate ligaments, and the intervening epidural space being filled with loose adipose tissue and an extensive venous plexus. During development, the vertebral column lengthens to a greater degree than the enclosed spinal cord and the segmental levels of the lower part of the cord therefore lie above the corresponding intervertebral foramina. Consequently, below the cervical region, the nerve roots pursue an increasingly oblique course in the subarachnoid space before passing through the intervertebral foramina; thus they can be seen adjacent to the cord, particularly in the lumbar and sacral regions.

ORGAN SYSTEMS

Fig. 20.3 Medulla oblongata
(a) Upper to mid-level,
Weigart–Pal × 4
(b) Lower level, Weigart–Pal × 4

The medulla oblongata, the most distal part of the brain stem, can be roughly divided into upper and lower parts. At the upper medullary level shown in micrograph (a), the fourth ventricle **V** closes to become a narrow central canal which continues down into the spinal cord. Thus the medulla is often divided into an upper, open part and a lower, closed part. The myelin staining method employed in these preparations leaves grey matter relatively unstained.

The most obvious feature of the upper half of the medulla is the *inferior olivary nucleus* **O** with its peculiar convoluted appearance in transverse section; adjacent are the smaller *dorsal* **D** and *medial accessory olivary nuclei* **M** which complete the *inferior olivary complex*. The neurones of the inferior olivary complex relay central and spinal afferent stimuli to the cerebellar cortex.

All of the ascending (sensory) and descending (motor) pathways found in the spinal cord pass through the medulla, although their arrangement in the medulla differs considerably from that in the spinal cord. The most easily recognisable features of these pathways in the medulla are the gracile and cuneate nuclei and fasciculi, and the pyramids.

The dorsal white matter columns of the spinal cord convey ascending proprioceptive, vibration and discriminatory touch fibres from the lower limbs and upper limbs in the *fasciculus gracilis* **FG** and *fasciculus cuneatus* **FC** respectively. In the similarly situated *nucleus gracilis* and *nucleus cuneatus* in the dorsum of the medulla, these fibres synapse with cell bodies of second order neurones which then pass upwards to the thalamus via the *medial lemniscus* **ML** which lies medial to the olivary complex.

Axons originating in the motor cortex descend through the *internal capsule*, break up into small bundles

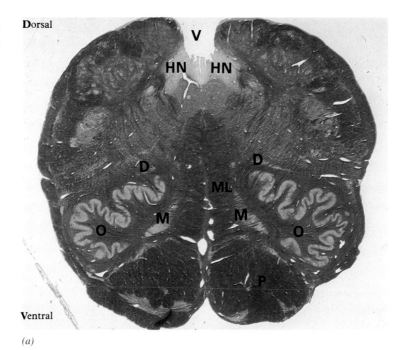

Dorsal

Ventral

(a)

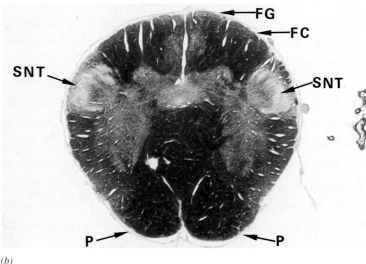

(b)

in the *pons*, then converge again in the medulla to form a prominent ventral pyramid **P** on each side of the medulla; in the pyramids, about 85% of fibres cross to the other side in the *decussation of the pyramids*.

The medulla also contains the various tracts and nuclei of the eighth to the twelfth cranial nerves as well as the *spinal nucleus* and *tract* of the *trigeminal nerve* which extends from the pons down into the upper cervical cord. The spinal nucleus of the trigeminal tract **SNT** is easily recognisable dorsolaterally throughout the medulla with its tract of white matter lying superficially. The *hypoglossal nucleus* **HN** can also be identified in micrograph (a). In the centre of the lower medulla, grey matter can be seen, still roughly resembling the characteristic butterfly shape seen in sections of the spinal cord; the ventral grey matter horns contain cell bodies of lower motor neurones running in the spinal accessory and first cervical nerves.

Dorsal

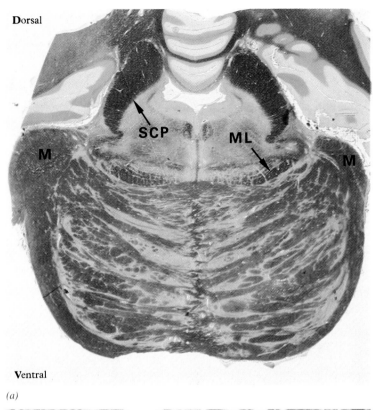

Ventral

(a)

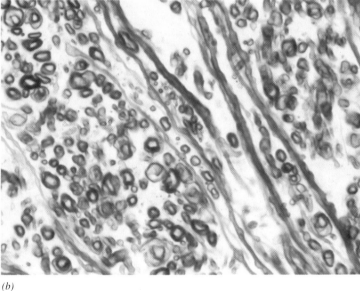

(b)

Fig. 20.4 **Pons**
(a) Mid-level, Weigart–Pal × 3
(b) Basal pons, Weigart–Pal × 480

The pons is the middle portion of the brain stem, lying between midbrain proximally and medulla distally. In transverse section, it comprises two parts, a bulky ventral region (the ***basal pons***) and a smaller dorsal (***tegmental***) region.

The basal pons consists of criss-crossed bundles of longitudinal and transverse fibres between which lie collections of neurone cell bodies known as ***pontine nuclei***. Micrograph (b) shows a small area of this region at high magnification, the myelin investing the axons being stained blue; neurone cell bodies are not stained and are therefore not identifiable. The longitudinal fibres of the basal pons consist of descending fibres of two main types. Firstly, there are axons from the motor cortex passing down to synapse with lower motor neurones of the ventral horns of the spinal cord; on leaving the pons, these axons converge to form the characteristic pyramids (pyramidal tracts) of the medulla. The second group of descending fibres originate in various areas of the cortex and synapse in the pontine nuclei from which fibres then pass in the transverse bundles, crossing the midline to enter the cerebellum via the ***middle peduncles*** **M**.

The dorsal tegmentum contains the ascending spinothalamic (sensory) tracts and the nuclei of the fifth, sixth and seventh cranial nerves. On each side, the ***medial lemniscus*** **ML** is readily identifiable; this represents the upward continuation of proprioceptive, vibration and fine touch pathways from the gracile and cuneate nuclei of the medulla. The cerebellar peduncles are a readily recognisable feature of the pons, the middle peduncle being still present in sections through the mid-pontine level as in micrograph (a); at this level the superior peduncles **SCP** are very prominent. The main bulk of the superior cerebellar peduncles is made up of fibres from the central nuclei of the cerebellum passing upwards to the thalamus and then projecting to the motor cortex.

ORGAN SYSTEMS

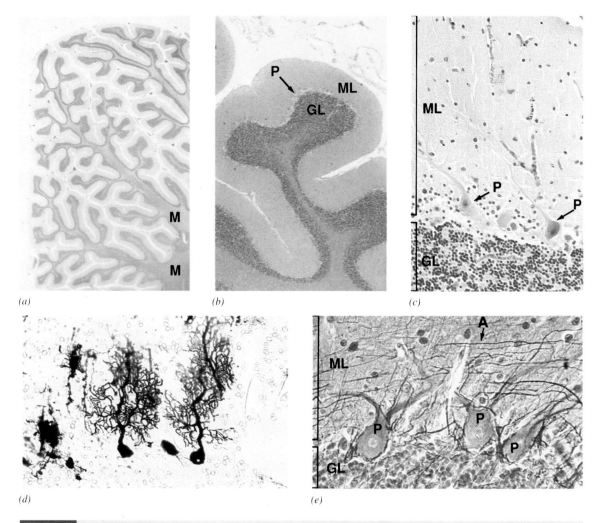

(a) (b) (c)

(d) (e)

Fig. 20.5 Cerebellum

(a) H & E × 4 (b) H & E × 20 (c) H & E × 320 (d) Golgi–Cox × 320 (e) Bielschowsky/neutral red × 600

The cerebellum, which coordinates muscular activity and maintains posture and equilibrium, consists of a cortex of grey matter with a central core of white matter containing four pairs of nuclei. Afferent and efferent fibres pass to and from the brain stem via inferior, middle and superior cerebellar peduncles linking medulla, pons and midbrain respectively.

As seen in micrograph (a), the cerebellar cortex forms a series of deeply convoluted folds or *folia* supported by a branching central medulla **M** of white matter. At higher magnification in micrograph (b), the cortex is seen to consist of three layers. The outer *molecular layer* **ML** contains relatively few neurones and large numbers of unmyelinated fibres. The inner *granular cell layer* **GL** is extremely cellular. Between the two is a single layer of huge neurones called *Purkinje cells* **P**.

Purkinje cells **P** are seen at higher magnification in micrograph (c); they have very large cell bodies, a relatively fine axon extending down through the granular cell layer **GL**, and an extensively branching dendritic system which arborises into the outer molecular layer **ML**. This extraordinary dendritic system is best demonstrated by heavy metal methods as in micrograph (d).

The deep granular cell layer of the cortex contains numerous small neurones, the non-myelinated axons of which pass outwards to the molecular layer where they bifurcate to run parallel to the surface to synapse with the dendrites of Purkinje cells. Micrograph (e) demonstrates the course of granular cell axons in the molecular layer. The axons **A** are stained black with silver and their cell bodies in the granular cell layer **GL** are counter-stained with neutral red. In addition to the Purkinje **P** and granular cells already described, there are three other types of small neurones in the cerebellar cortex, namely *stellate cells* and *basket cells* scattered in the molecular layer **ML** and *Golgi cells* scattered in the superficial part of the granular cell layer.

In simple terms, afferent fibres enter the cerebellum from the brain stem and then pass via the white matter core to make complex connections with granular cells, Purkinje dendrites and other neurones of the cerebellar cortex; these cortical cells also make numerous interconnections with each other within the molecular layer. The only efferent fibres from the cerebellar cortex are the Purkinje cell axons which pass down through the granular cell layer into the white matter where they synapse in the central nuclei of the cerebellum.

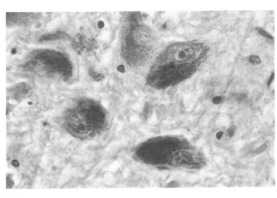

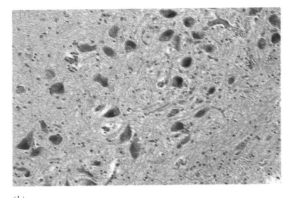

(a)   *(b)*

Fig. 20.6   **Substantia nigra**   (a) H & E × 100 (b) H & E × 400

The substantia nigra is a large mass of grey matter extending throughout the midbrain; on each side it divides the cerebral peduncles into dorsal and ventral parts and in sections of the midbrain, as in micrograph (a), it is easily recognised by the black pigment from which its name derives. The substantia nigra has extensive connections with the cortex, spinal cord, corpus striatum and reticular formation and appears to play an important part in the fine control of motor function.

The neurones of the substantia nigra are multipolar in form and in adults the cytoplasm contains numerous granules of neuromelanin pigment as seen in micrograph (b). The pigmented neurones of the substantia nigra contain ***dopamine*** which appears to act as a neurotransmitter causing inhibitory effects particularly on neurones in the corpus striatum.

DOPA (dihydroxyphenylalanine) is a precursor of dopamine and also of melanin, and the melanin of substantia nigra neurones may merely represent a residual product of normal metabolic activity; this is supported by the fact that very little melanin is present at birth, with the amount increasing considerably during childhood and thereafter rising at a slower rate into old age.

Parkinson's disease, a debilitating disorder characterised by tremor, muscular rigidity and impaired speed and precision of motor functions, is associated with degeneration of neurones in the substantia nigra and a marked reduction in dopamine synthesis. Symptoms can be alleviated by the drug L-dopa, a dopamine precursor which crosses the blood–brain barrier.

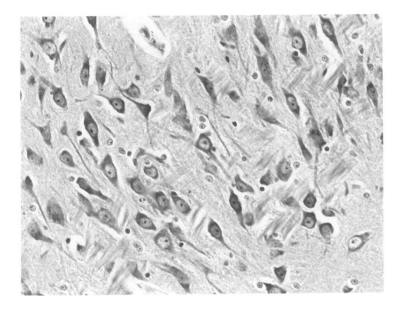

Fig. 20.7   **Thalamus**
H & E × 480

The thalami are large masses of grey matter lying on each side of the third ventricle and comprising the main bulk of the ***diencephalon***, the central core of the cerebrum. Functionally, the thalamus is subdivided into a large number of nuclei including reticular and motor nuclei as well as specific sensory nuclei containing the cell bodies of neurones with axons projecting to the cerebral cortex. The thalamus constitutes an extremely complex relay and integration centre for information from almost all parts of the CNS.

This micrograph shows the histological appearance of a typical thalamic nucleus consisting of a dense aggregation of neurone cell bodies criss-crossed by tracts of afferent and efferent nerve fibres.

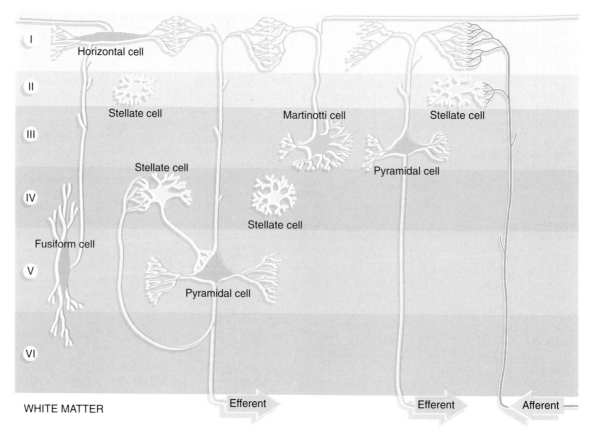

(a)

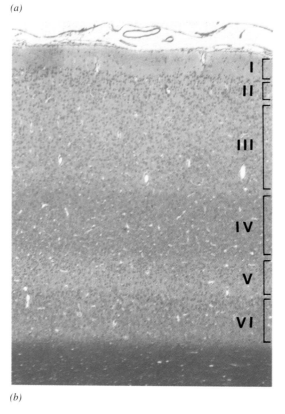

(b)

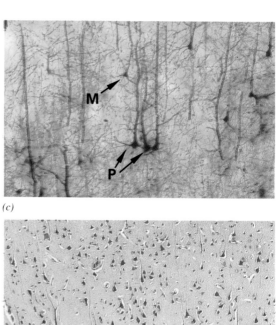

(c)

(d)

The cerebral hemispheres consist of a convoluted cortex of grey matter overlying the central medullary mass of white matter which conveys fibres between different parts of the cortex and to and from other parts of the CNS.

Histologically, the neurones of the cerebral cortex are divided into five different morphological types which are arranged in several layers. In submammalian species, the major function of the cortex concerns the sense of olfaction (smell) and the neurones are arranged into three layers. In mammals, there has evolved the so-called *neocortex* consisting of six layers of neurones. The neocortex includes the *sensory* and *motor areas* of the cortex as well as the *association cortex* and in humans constitutes about 90% of the cerebral cortex. The primitive three-layered pattern persists only in the olfactory cortex and cortical part of the limbic system in the temporal lobe.

Neurone types in the cerebral cortex

The five characteristic types of cortical neurone are shown diagrammatically in (a), the pyramidal and stellate cells being by far the most common type.

- *Pyramidal cells*, as their name implies, have pyramid-shaped cell bodies, the apex being directed towards the cortical surface. A slender axon arises from the base of the cell and passes into the underlying white matter, though in the case of small superficially located cells, the axon may synapse in the deep layers of the cortex. From the apex, a thick branching dendrite passes towards the surface where it has an array of fine dendritic branches. In addition, short dendrites arise from the edges of the base and ramify laterally. The size of the pyramidal cells varies from small to large, the smallest tending to lie more superficially. The huge upper motor neurones of the motor cortex, known as *Betz cells*, are the largest of the pyramidal cells in the cortex.
- *Stellate (granule) cells* are small neurones with a short vertical axon and several short branching dendrites, giving the cell body the shape of a star; basket and neurogliaform subtypes are also described. With routine histological methods, the cells look like small granules giving rise to their alternative name.
- *Cells of Martinotti* are small polygonal cells with a few short dendrites; the axon extends towards the surface and bifurcates to run horizontally, usually in the most superficial layer.
- *Fusiform cells* are spindle-shaped cells oriented at right angles to the surface of the cerebral cortex. The axon arises from the side of the cell body and passes superficially. Dendrites extend from each end of the cell body branching into deeper and more superficial layers.
- *Horizontal cells of Cajal* are small and spindle-shaped but oriented parallel to the surface. They are the least common cell type and are only found in the most superficial layer where their axons pass laterally to synapse with the dendrites of pyramidal cells.

In addition to neurones, the cortex contains supporting neuroglial cells, i.e. astrocytes, oligodendroglia and microglia.

Layers of the neocortex

As previously stated, the neurones in the neocortex are arranged into six layers, the layers differing in neurone morphology, size and population density. The layers merge with one another rather than being highly demarcated and vary somewhat from one region of the cortex to another depending on cortical thickness and function.

Micrograph (b) illustrates the typical layered appearance of the cerebral cortex, the more detailed characteristics of each layer being as follows:

I. *Plexiform (molecular) layer*. This most superficial layer mainly contains dendrites and axons of cortical neurones making synapses with one another; the sparse nuclei are those of neuroglia and occasional horizontal cells of Cajal.
II. *Outer granular layer*. A dense population of small pyramidal cells and stellate cells make up this thin layer which also contains various axons and dendritic connections from deeper layers.
III. *Pyramidal cell layer*. Pyramidal cells of moderate size predominate in this broad layer, the cells increasing in size deeper in the layer.
IV. *Inner granular layer*. This layer consists mainly of densely packed stellate cells.
V. *Ganglionic layer*. Large pyramidal cells and smaller numbers of stellate cells and cells of Martinotti make up this layer, the name of the layer originating from the huge pyramidal (ganglion) Betz cells of the motor cortex.
VI. *Multiform cell layer*. This is so named for the wide variety of differing morphological forms found in this layer. It contains numerous small pyramidal cells and cells of Martinotti, as well as stellate cells, especially superficially, and fusiform cells in the deeper part.

Micrograph (c) shows part of layer V; a thick section is employed, stained with a heavy metal impregnation technique which demonstrates considerable morphological detail. Several pyramidal cells **P** are easily identifiable, the principal dendrite of each (but not the axon) being included in the plane of section. A cell of Martinotti **M** can also be identified by its polygonal shape.

Micrograph (d) also shows layer V but in this case the section is thinner and stained by a routine histological method. In this example there is little morphological detail, nevertheless most of the cells are identifiable as pyramidal cells, increasing in size in the deeper part and including several very large cells.

The synaptic interconnections within the cortex are exceedingly complex, with any one neurone synapsing with several hundred others. However, there are several basic principles of cortical organisation and function:

- Functional units are disposed vertically, corresponding to the general orientation of axons and major dendrites.
- Afferent fibres (their cell bodies lying elsewhere in the CNS) generally synapse high in the cortex with dendrites of efferent neurones, the cell bodies of which lie in deeper layers of the cortex.
- Efferent pathways, typically the axons of pyramidal cells, tend to give off branches which pass back into more superficial layers to communicate with their own dendrites via interneuronal connections involving other cortical cell types.

21. Special sense organs

Introduction

The organs of special sense are highly sophisticated sensory receptors in which the specific neural receptors are incorporated in a non-neural structure which enhances and refines the reception of incoming stimuli. The eye and audiovestibular apparatus of the ear are the main special sense organs, but the gustatory (taste) and olfactory (smell) receptors are usually also included in this category.

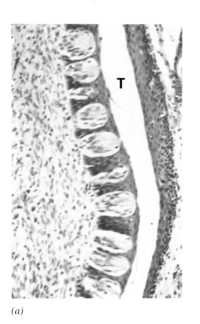

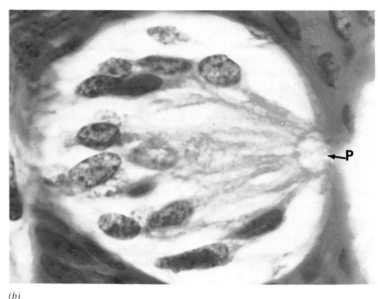

(a)   *(b)*

Fig. 21.1   **Taste buds** **(a) H & E × 128 (b) H & E × 1200**

Taste buds, the chemoreceptors for the sense of taste (*gustation*), are in humans mainly located in the epithelium of the circumvallate papillae of the tongue (see Fig. 13.12), although they are also found scattered in other parts of the tongue, palate, pharynx and epiglottis. In the circumvallate papillae, taste buds face into the deep troughs **T** surrounding the papillae as shown in micrograph (a). Serous glands, called the **glands of von Ebner**, secrete a serous fluid into the troughs to act as a solvent for taste provoking substances. The human tongue has approximately 3000 taste buds.

The taste bud is a barrel-shaped organ extending the full thickness of the epithelium and opening at the surface via the **taste pore** **P**. Each taste bud contains about 50 long spindle-shaped cells which extend from the basement membrane to the taste pore. Classically, two types of cell are described in the taste bud: light **gustatory cells** and dark **supporting** or **sustentacular cells**. A third cell type, the **basal cell**, is now generally recognised and may constitute the precursor of one or both of the other cell types. Both gustatory and sustentacular cells have

long microvilli extending into the taste pore which contains a glycoprotein substance thought to be secreted by the sustentacular cells.

Ultrastructural studies have shown that non-myelinated nerve fibres are associated with both cell types (see Fig. 13.12), but there appears to be a more intimate, synapse-like relationship between the nerve fibres and the gustatory cells. Although the gustatory cells are thought to be the taste receptors, the sustentacular cells may also serve some receptor function. Like the oral epithelium, all the cells of the taste bud, which represent highly specialised epithelial cells, are renewed continuously although the gustatory and sustentacular cells are replaced at different rates.

Four taste modalities are recognised: sweet, bitter, acid and salt. Each modality tends to be principally perceived in a specific region of the tongue; however, no structural differences have been demonstrated between taste buds from different areas. The sensations of taste and smell are closely associated and loss of olfactory sense is accompanied by diminished gustatory perception.

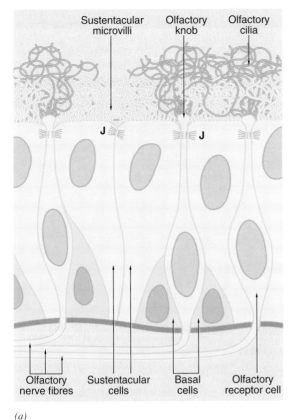

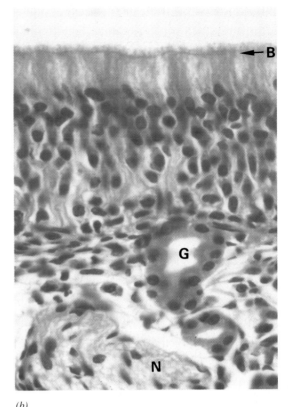

(a)   *(b)*

Fig. 21.2   **Olfactory receptors** (a) Schematic diagram (b) H & E × 720

The receptors for the sense of smell are located in a modified form of respiratory epithelium called *olfactory epithelium* in the nasal cavity; although extensive in some mammals such as the dog, the olfactory epithelium is restricted to a small area in the roof of the nasal cavity in humans. The olfactory epithelium is very tall, pseudostratified columnar in form and contains cells of three types: olfactory receptor cells, supporting epithelial (*sustentacular*) cells and basal epithelial cells.

The *olfactory receptor cells* are true bipolar neurones (see Fig. 7.2), the cell bodies of which are located in the middle stratum of the olfactory epithelium. A single dendritic process extends from the cell body to the free surface where it terminates as a small swelling, the *olfactory knob*, which gives rise to about a dozen extremely long modified cilia. These cilia, or olfactory hairs, contain the usual '9 plus 2' arrangement of microtubules in their proximal portion but become thinner distally where they contain variable numbers of single microtubules in different species. The cilia are non-motile and lie flattened against the epithelial surface in the surface mucous layer. The cilia are the sites of interaction between odiferous substances and the receptor cells. At the basal aspect, each receptor cell gives rise to a single fine non-myelinated axon which penetrates the basement membrane to join the axons of other receptor cells. The bundles of axons pass via about 20 small holes on each side of the *cribriform plate* of the ethmoid bone

to reach the *olfactory bulbs* of the forebrain where they synapse with second order sensory neurones.

The supporting or sustentacular cells are elongated with their tapered bases resting on the basement membrane. Many long microvilli extend from their luminal surfaces to form a tangled mat with the cilia of the receptor cells. At the luminal surface, the plasma membranes of the sustentacular and receptor cells are bound together by typical junctional complexes **J**. The functions of the sustentacular cells are poorly understood but they probably provide mechanical and physiological support for the receptor cells. The basal cells are small, conical cells which appear to be stem cells for both olfactory and sustentacular cells.

In histological section, it is difficult to distinguish individual cell types within the olfactory epithelium; however, the nuclei of sustentacular cells occupy the uppermost stratum, those of the receptor cells the middle stratum and those of the basal cells lie close to the basement membrane. Note the terminal bar **B** at the luminal surface representing junctional complexes; note also the tangled meshwork of microvilli and cilia on the surface.

The olfactory epithelium is supported by loose vascular tissue containing bundles of afferent nerve fibres **N** and numerous serous glands called *Bowman's glands* **G** which produce the watery surface secretions in which odiferous substances are dissolved.

The eye

The eye is a highly specialised organ of photoreception, a process which involves the conversion of different quanta of light energy into nerve action potentials.

The photoreceptors are modified dendrites of two types of nerve cells, **rod cells** and **cone cells**. The rods are integrated into a system which is receptive to light of differing intensity; this is perceived in a form analogous to a black and white photographic image. The cones are of three functional types receptive to the colours blue, green and red and constitute a system by which coloured images are seen. The rod and cone receptors and a system of integrating neurones are located in the inner layer of the eye, the **retina**. The remaining structures of the eye serve to support the retina or to focus images of the visual world upon the retina.

In addition, several accessory structures, namely the **eyelids, lacrimal gland** and **conjunctiva**, protect the eye from external damage.

Fig. 21.3 | The eye *(illustration opposite)*

The eye is made up of three basic layers: the outer **corneo-scleral layer**, the intermediate **uveal layer** (**uveal tract**) and the inner **retinal layer**.

Corneo-scleral layer. The corneo-scleral layer forms a tough, fibroelastic capsule which supports the eye. The posterior five-sixths, the **sclera**, is opaque and provides insertion for the extraocular muscles.

The anterior one-sixth, the **cornea**, is transparent and has a smaller radius of curvature than the sclera. The cornea is the principal refracting medium of the eye and roughly focuses an image onto the retina; the focusing power of the cornea depends mainly on the radius of curvature of its external surface. The corneo-scleral junction is known as the **limbus** and is marked internally and externally by a shallow depression.

Uveal layer. The middle layer, the uvea or uveal tract, is a highly vascular layer which is made up of three components: the **choroid, ciliary body** and the **iris**. The choroid lies between the sclera and retina in the posterior five-sixths of the eye. It provides nutritive support for the retina and is heavily pigmented, thus absorbing light which has passed through the retina. Anteriorly, the choroid merges with the ciliary body which is a circumferential thickening of the uvea lying beneath the limbus.

The ciliary body surrounds the coronal equator of the **lens** and is attached to it by the **suspensory ligament** or **zonule**. The lens is a biconvex transparent structure, the shape of which can be varied to provide fine focus of the corneal image upon the retina. The ciliary body contains smooth muscle, the tone of which controls the shape of the lens via the suspensory ligament. The lens, suspensory ligament and ciliary body partition the eye into a large posterior compartment and a smaller anterior compartment.

The iris, the third component of the uvea, forms a diaphragm extending in front of the lens from the ciliary body so as to incompletely divide the anterior compartment into two chambers; these are known by the terms **anterior** and **posterior chamber** (not to be confused with the anterior and posterior compartments mentioned above). The highly pigmented iris acts as an adjustable diaphragm which regulates the amount of light reaching the retina. The aperture of the iris is called the **pupil**.

The anterior and posterior chambers contain a watery fluid, the **aqueous humor**, which is secreted into the posterior chamber by the ciliary body and circulated through the pupil to drain into a canal at the angle of the anterior chamber, the **canal of Schlemm**. The aqueous humor is a source of nutrients for the non-vascular lens and cornea, and acts as an optical medium which is non-refractive with respect to the cornea. The pressure of aqueous humor maintains the shape of the cornea.

The large, posterior compartment of the eye contains a gelatinous mass known as the **vitreous body**, consisting of transparent **vitreous humor**. The vitreous body supports the lens and retina from within as well as providing an optical medium which is non-refractive with respect to the lens. In life, the vitreous body contains a canal which extends from the exit of the optic nerve to the posterior surface of the lens; this **hyaloid canal** represents the course of the hyaloid artery which supplies the vitreous body during embryological development. The vitreous body and hyaloid canal are rarely preserved in histological preparations.

Retinal layer. The photosensitive retina forms the inner lining of most of the posterior compartment of the eye and terminates along a scalloped line, the **ora serrata**, behind the ciliary body. Anterior to the ora serrata, the retinal layer continues as a non-photosensitive epithelial layer which lines the ciliary body and the posterior surface of the iris.

The visual axis of the eye passes through a depression in the retina called the **fovea** which is surrounded by a yellow pigmented zone, the **macula lutea**. The fovea is the area of greatest visual acuity.

Afferent nerve fibres from the retina converge to form the **optic nerve** which leaves the eye through a part of the sclera known as the **lamina cribrosa**. The retina overlying the lamina cribrosa, the **optic papilla** (**optic disc**), is devoid of photoreceptors and thus represents a blind spot.

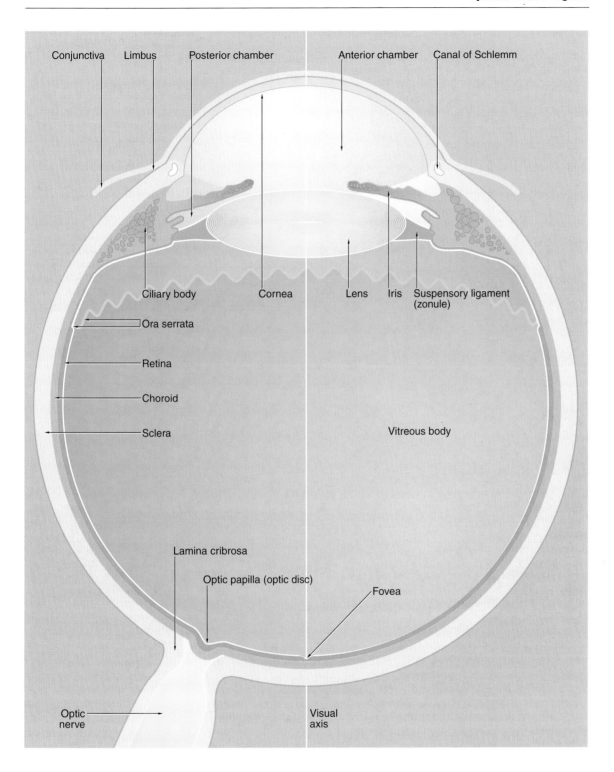

Conjunctiva Limbus Posterior chamber Anterior chamber Canal of Schlemm

Ciliary body Cornea Lens Iris Suspensory ligament (zonule)

Ora serrata

Retina

Choroid

Sclera Vitreous body

Lamina cribrosa

Optic papilla (optic disc) Fovea

Optic nerve Visual axis

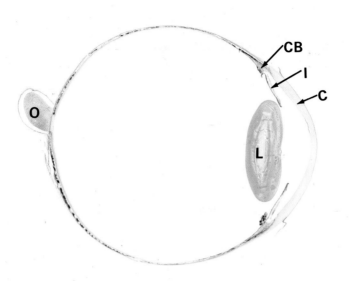

Fig. 21.4 **Eye (monkey)**
H & E × 5

This horizontal section shows the relative sizes of the components of the eye. At this magnification, the three layers making up the wall of the globe are not readily distinguishable although in the wall of the posterior compartment, the middle layer, the choroid, is recognisable by its high content of pigment.

The other uveal structures, the ciliary body **CB** and iris **I** are readily visible. The lens **L** has been artefactually distorted during preparation and the suspensory ligament by which it is attached to the ciliary body is not preserved. Note the relative thickness of the cornea **C**.

The optic nerve **O** is seen to penetrate the sclera medial to the visual axis; the fovea is not present in this plane of section.

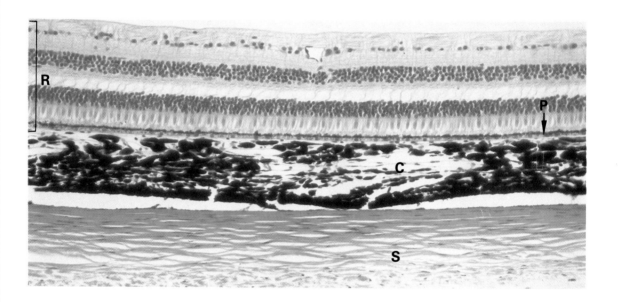

Fig. 21.5 **Wall of the eye** H & E × 300

The three layers of the wall of the eye are illustrated in this micrograph.

The inner photosensitive retina is a multilayered structure, the outermost limit of which is defined by a layer of pigmented epithelial cells **P**.

The choroid **C** is a layer of loose vascular supporting tissue lying between the sclera **S** externally and the retina **R** internally. The choroid and retina are separated by a membrane known as ***Bruch's membrane*** which is composed of the basement membranes of the pigmented epithelium of the retina and the endothelium of the choroid capillaries plus intervening layers of collagen and elastin fibres. The blood supply of the uveal layer of the eye is provided by branches of the ophthalmic artery which penetrates through the sclera. Larger vessels predominate in the superficial aspect of the choroid, with a rich capillary plexus in the deeper aspect providing nourishment for the outer layers of the retina by diffusion across Bruch's membrane. The choroid contains numerous large, heavily pigmented melanocytes which confer the dense pigmentation characteristic of the choroid. The pigment absorbs light rays passing through the retina and prevents interference due to light reflection.

The sclera consists of dense fibroelastic tissue, the fibres of which are arranged in bundles parallel to the surface. This layer contains little ground substance and few fibroblasts. The sclera varies in thickness, being thickest posteriorly and thinnest at the coronal equator of the globe.

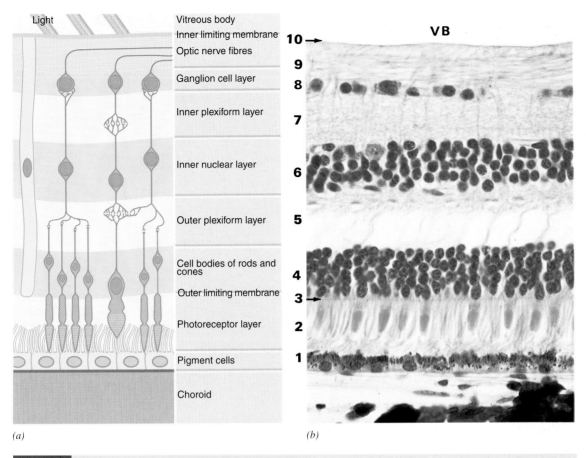

Light
Vitreous body
Inner limiting membrane
Optic nerve fibres
Ganglion cell layer
Inner plexiform layer
Inner nuclear layer
Outer plexiform layer
Cell bodies of rods and cones
Outer limiting membrane
Photoreceptor layer
Pigment cells
Choroid
VB

(a)   *(b)*

Fig. 21.6 **Retina** (a) Schematic diagram (b) H & E × 640

The retina is made up of three cell types: *neurones*, *pigmented epithelial cells* and *neurone support cells*. The neurones are divided into three functional groups, namely photoreceptor cells (rod cells and cone cells), the cells of afferent fibres passing in the optic nerve, and a group of neurones interposed between the first two types which integrate sensory input from the photoreceptors before transmission to the cerebral cortex. The integrating neurones are further subdivided into three types: *bipolar cells*, *horizontal cells* and *amacrine cells*.

Histologically, the retina is traditionally divided into 10 distinct histological layers, as shown in the micrograph; the distribution of the different cell types being illustrated in a highly schematic manner in the diagram.

The outermost layer (1) consists of the *pigmented epithelial cells* forming a single layer resting on Bruch's membrane which separates them from the choroid. The next layer is the *photoreceptor layer* made up of the rod and cone processes (2) with a thin eosinophilic structure known as the *outer limiting membrane* (3) separating them from a layer of densely packed nuclei described as the *outer nuclear layer* (4). The outer nuclear layer contains the cell bodies of the rod and cone photoreceptors. The almost featureless layer deep to this is known as the *outer plexiform layer* (5) and contains synaptic connections between the short axons of the photoreceptor cells and integrating neurones, the cell bodies of which lie in the *inner nuclear layer* (6). In the *inner plexiform layer* (7), the integrating neurones make synaptic connections with dendrites of neurones whose

axons form the optic tract. The cell bodies of the optic tract neurones (sometimes called *ganglion cells*) comprise the *ganglion cell layer* (8). Deep to this is the *layer of afferent fibres* (9) passing towards the optic disc to form the optic nerve. Finally, the *inner limiting membrane* (10) demarcates the innermost aspect of the retina from the *vitreous body* **VB**. Note in the diagram that only bipolar cells are represented in the integrating cell layer; this layer also contains the cell bodies of the horizontal and amacrine cells as illustrated in Figure 21.8. Note that light impinging on the retina passes through many layers before reaching the photoreceptor cells.

Towards the left of the diagram there is an extremely elongated support cell extending between inner and outer limiting membranes which has its nucleus in the same layer as the integrating neurones, the inner nuclear layer. These cells, known as *Muller cells*, are analogous to the neuroglia of the CNS and have long cytoplasmic processes which embrace and sometimes even encircle the retinal neurones filling all the intervening spaces. Muller cells provide structural support and may also mediate the transfer of essential metabolites such as glucose to the retinal neurones.

The outer limiting membrane is not a true membrane but merely represents the line of intercellular junctions between Muller cells and the photoreceptor cells (shown diagrammatically in Fig. 21.7). In contrast, the inner limiting membrane represents the basement membrane of the Muller cells resting on the vitreous body.

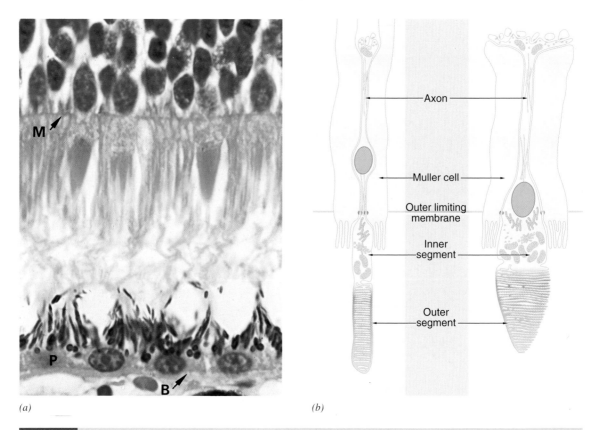

(a)   (b)

Fig. 21.7 | **Retinal photoreceptors** (a) H & E × 1200 (b) Schematic diagram

The rod and cone photoreceptor layer of the retina is shown at very high magnification in micrograph (a), the cell bodies of the rod and cone cells lying deep to the outer limiting membrane **M**. Peripherally, the rods and cones mingle with long microvilli extending from the pigmented epithelial cells **P**.

As shown in the diagram (b), the rod photoreceptors are long slender bipolar cells, the single dendrite of each cell extending beyond the outer limiting membrane as the rod proper. The rod proper consists of *inner* and *outer segments* connected by a thin eccentric strand of cytoplasm containing nine microtubule doublets similar to those of a cilium but without the inner pair of microtubules. The inner segment contains a prominent Golgi apparatus and many mitochondria. The outer segment has a regular cylindrical shape and contains a stack of flattened membranous discs which incorporate the pigment *rhodopsin* (visual purple). The membranous discs are continuously shed from the end of each rod and phagocytosed by the pigmented epithelial cells. The discs are continuously replaced from the inner part of the outer segment. In essence, the transduction process involves the interaction of light with rhodopsin molecules which promotes a conformational change in the rhodopsin molecule, thus initiating an action potential. The action potential then passes inwards along the dendrite and axon to the layer of integrating neurones.

Cones are similar in basic structure to the rods but they differ in several details. The outer segment of the cone is a long conical structure about two-thirds the length of a rod and containing a similar number of even more flattened membranous discs. Unlike the situation in the rods, however, the disc membrane is continuous with the

plasma membrane so that, on one side, the spaces between the discs are continuous with the extracellular environment (see diagram). The discs are not shed, although the tips of the cones are invested by processes of pigmented epithelial cells. The cones contain visual pigments similar to rhodopsin, receptive to blue, green and red light, and the mechanism of transduction is probably similar. The bodies of the cone cells are generally continuous with the inner segment of the cone proper without an intervening dendritic process and the nuclei of cone cells thus form a row immediately deep to the outer limiting membrane.

As seen in micrograph (a), the pigmented epithelial cells are cuboidal in shape with the nuclei located basally towards Bruch's membrane **B**. Apically, the cells are crammed with melanin granules, numerous mitochondria and lipofuscin, a residual product of phagocytosis (see Fig. 1.14). The pigmented cell microvilli, which are 5–7 μm long, extend between the photoreceptors and, with electron microscopy, are seen to contain membranous lamellae similar to those in the rod outer segments; these appear to disintegrate as they pass deeper into the pigmented cells. In addition to phagocytosis, the pigmented epithelial cells provide structural and metabolic support for the rods and cones and also absorb light, thus preventing back reflection.

During histological preparation, the retina frequently becomes detached from the wall of the eye and the plane of cleavage is usually between the rods and cones and the layer of pigmented epithelial cells corresponding to the cavity of the embryonic optic vesicle. This is also the plane along which the retina cleaves in the living eye in the pathological condition known as retinal detachment.

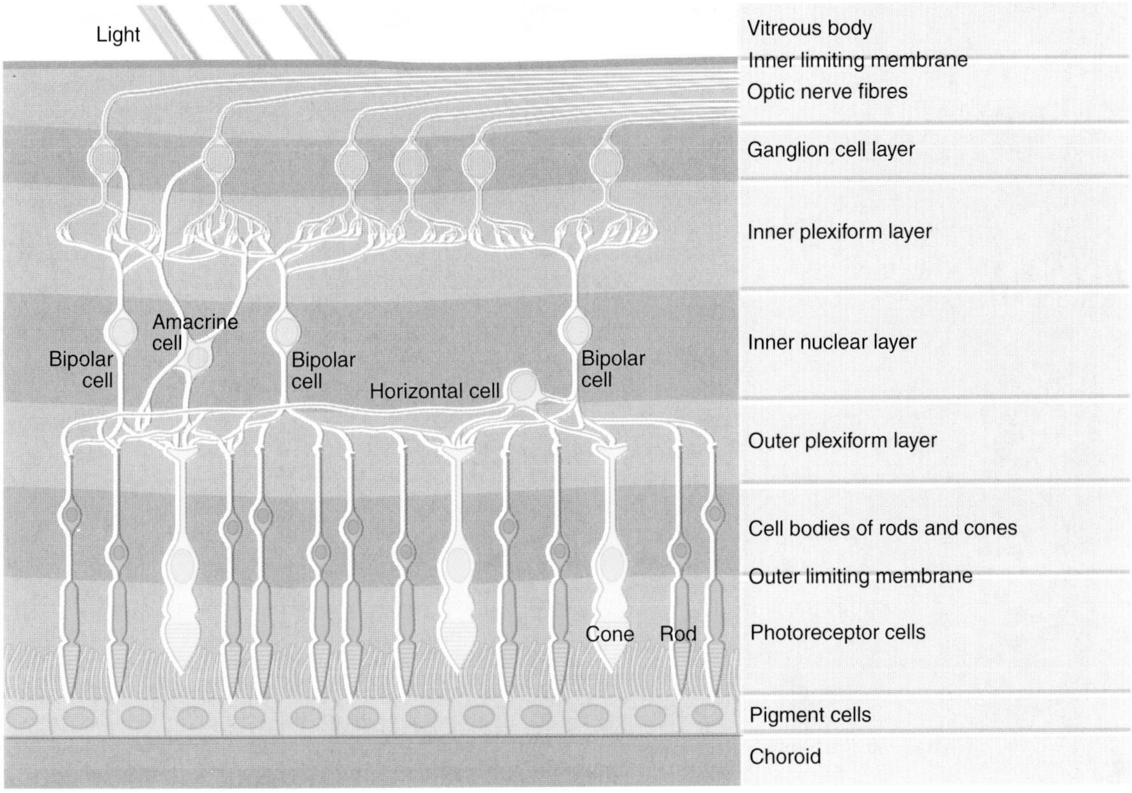

Light

Vitreous body
Inner limiting membrane
Optic nerve fibres

Ganglion cell layer

Inner plexiform layer

Inner nuclear layer

Outer plexiform layer

Cell bodies of rods and cones

Outer limiting membrane

Photoreceptor cells

Pigment cells

Choroid

Amacrine cell

Bipolar cell

Bipolar cell

Horizontal cell

Bipolar cell

Cone   Rod

Fig. 21.8 **Neuronal interconnections in the retina**

This diagram demonstrates the basic pattern of neuronal interconnections between the photoreceptor cells and the afferent neurones of the optic tract. The interneurones consist of three basic cell types, *bipolar cells*, *horizontal cells* and *amacrine cells*, their cell bodies all being located in the inner nuclear layer (along with those of the supporting Muller cells).

Bipolar cells, the most numerous of the integrating neurones, in general make direct connections between one or more photoreceptors and one or more optic tract neurones as well as with horizontal and amacrine cells. Horizontal cells have several short processes and one long process, the terminal branches of each making lateral connections between adjacent and more distant rods and cones in the outer plexiform layer. Horizontal cells also synapse with the dendrites of bipolar cells. The amacrine cells have numerous dendrites which make connections with bipolar and optic tract neurones in the inner plexiform layer, as well as making occasional feedback connections with photoreceptors in the outer plexiform layer.

As seen in Figure 21.7(b) opposite, the axons of the rod photoreceptors terminate in spherical processes into which are invaginated their small number of synaptic connections. In contrast, the cone photoreceptors have a flattened pedicle which accommodates hundreds of intercellular contacts.

In all, there are more than 100 million rods and 6 million cones. The cones are particularly dense in the macula and the immediately surrounding area and, in the fovea itself, the photoreceptors are almost exclusively cones. The density of both rods and cones diminishes towards the retinal periphery. The foveal cones have an almost one-to-one relationship with optic tract neurones giving maximal visual discrimination. There are only about 1 million optic tract neurones and the more peripheral the photoreceptors, the greater the number of photoreceptors synapsing with each optic tract neurone. This is consistent with the main function of the more peripheral receptors (predominantly rods) which is for determination of light and dark rather than fine two-point discrimination.

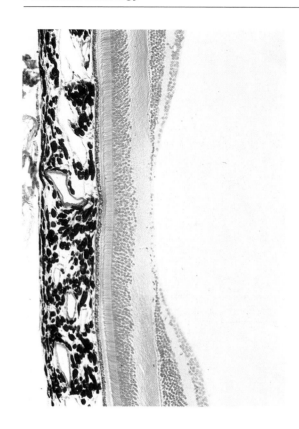

Fig. 21.9 Fovea Masson's trichrome × 320

The fovea is a conical depression in the retina corresponding to the point where the visual axis of the cornea and lens meets the retina and lying about 4 mm lateral and slightly inferior to the exit of the optic nerve fibres at the optic disc. Consequently, the fovea is the area subject to the least refractory distortion. To complement this, the foveal retina is modified to obtain the maximum photoreceptor sensitivity and is thus the area of the retina with the greatest visual discrimination; however, its function is poor in conditions of low light intensity. Surrounding the fovea is an ovoid yellow area about 1 mm wide called the *macula lutea*.

As seen in this micrograph, at the fovea the inner layers of the retina are flattened laterally so as to present the least barrier to light reaching the photoreceptors. Retinal blood vessels are absent at the fovea, as can be readily seen with the ophthalmoscope, and the brownish colour of the choroidal melanin shows through the much attenuated retina. At the fovea, the photoreceptors are almost exclusively cones which are elongated and closely packed (approximately 100 000 cones are contained in the fovea). Neuronal interconnections in the bipolar cell layer provide for a one-to-one ratio of these cones to optic nerve fibres which means that each foveal photoreceptor is individually represented at the visual cortex.

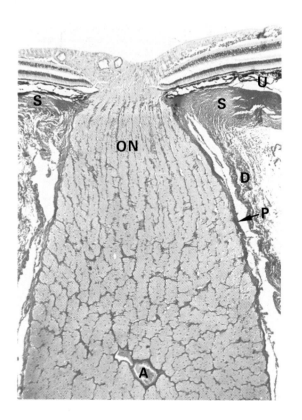

Fig. 21.10 Optic nerve
Haematoxylin/van Gieson × 30

The afferent fibres from the retina converge at a point medial to the fovea, the *optic papilla* or *optic disc*, fibres from the lateral quadrants sweeping above and below the macula to avoid the fovea. The fibres then penetrate the sclera **S** through the *lamina cribrosa* to form the optic nerve **ON**. Note the thickness of the optic tract layer overlying the disc and the absence of photoreceptor cells from the optic papilla which is thus a blind spot on the retina.

In their course across the retina, the afferent fibres are not myelinated as this would obstruct light passing to the photoreceptors. Myelination commences at the optic disc which imparts the white colour seen with the ophthalmoscope.

The optic nerve and retina develop embryologically as an outgrowth of the primitive forebrain, and thus the optic nerve is invested by meninges. The dura mater **D** becomes continuous with its developmental equivalent, the sclera, while the pia-arachnoid **P** continues into the eye as the uveal tract **U**.

The main blood supply of the retina is provided by the central artery of the retina **A**, a branch of the ophthalmic artery. This divides at the optic disc into four branches supplying the quadrants of the retina. These vessels course within the optic nerve fibre layer breaking up into a rich capillary network which drains back into a venous system closely following the course of the arterial supply. The vessels are confined to the optic nerve fibre layer, and more superficial layers are dependent on diffusion, the most peripheral retinal layers being supplied likewise from the choroid.

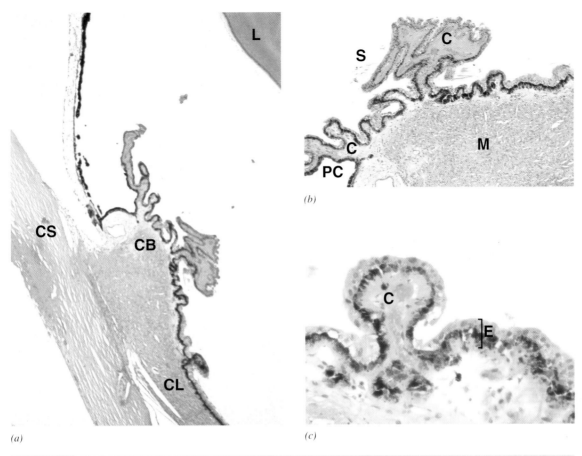

Fig. 21.11 **Ciliary body** (a) H & E × 30 (b) H & E × 50 (c) H & E × 200

The ciliary body is a circumferential structure which bulges into the eye between the ora serrata and the limbus (see Fig. 21.3). As seen in micrograph (a), the ciliary body **CB** represents the forward continuation of the choroid layer **CL** (uveal tract) of the posterior five-sixths of the wall of the eye and, like it, is highly vascular and contains a considerable amount of melanin pigment. Note the artefactual separation between the choroid and sclera in this specimen. Anteriorly, it is continuous with the third component of the uveal tract, the iris **I**, passing in front of the lens **L**.

As seen in micrograph (c), the ciliary body is lined with a double layer of cuboidal epithelium **E**. The deep layer is highly pigmented and represents a forward continuation of the pigmented epithelial layer of the retina, whilst the surface layer, which is not pigmented, is a non-photosensitive forward extension of the receptor layer of the retina.

The ciliary body is attached to the coronal equator of the lens by the suspensory ligament which consists of extremely fine collagenous strands which seldom remain intact after histological preparation; a few aggregated shreds of the suspensory ligament **S** are seen in micrograph (b). Tension in the suspensory ligament tends to flatten the lens which, in the relaxed state, assumes a more globular shape. The bulk of the ciliary body consists

of smooth muscle **M** arranged in such a manner that, when it contracts, tension upon the suspensory ligament is reduced, thus permitting the lens to assume a more convex shape. This mechanism permits fine focusing of images already roughly focused upon the retina by the cornea. The ciliary muscle is innervated by parasympathetic nerve fibres.

From that part of the ciliary body exposed to the angle of the posterior chamber **PC**, there project a number of branching epithelial folds called *ciliary processes* with a supporting tissue core rich in fenestrated capillaries **C**. The ciliary processes are responsible for the continuous production of aqueous humor which then circulates into the anterior chamber via the pupil. Aqueous humor is continuously reabsorbed into the *canal of Schlemm* **CS** seen at the angle of the anterior chamber in micrograph (a).

Aqueous humor is a clear, watery fluid somewhat similar in composition to CSF and hypotonic with respect to plasma. The production of aqueous humor is an active process mediated by the two epithelial layers lining the ciliary processes. Balanced rates of secretion and reabsorption of aqueous humor result in the maintenance of a constant intraocular pressure of about 15 mm of mercury which stabilises the lens and cornea. The flow of aqueous humor also provides for a continuous exchange of metabolites with the cells of the avascular cornea and lens.

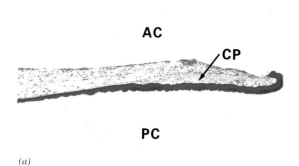

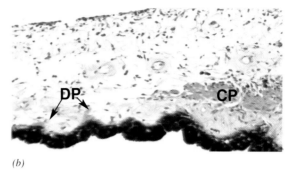

(a)   *(b)*

Fig. 21.12   Iris (a) H & E × 20 (b) H & E × 100

The iris is the most anterior part of the uveal layer of the eye. It arises from the ciliary body and forms a diaphragm in front of the lens, so dividing the anterior compartment of the eye into posterior **PC** and anterior chambers **AC** which communicate via the pupil. The pupillary edge of the iris rests on the anterior surface of the lens in life.

The main mass of the iris consists of loose, highly vascular tissue which is pigmented due to the presence of numerous melanocytes scattered in the stroma. The anterior surface of the iris is irregular and consists of a discontinuous layer of fibroblasts and melanocytes; in the fetus the surface is lined by endothelial cells but these disappear during early childhood. In contrast, the posterior surface is relatively smooth and is lined by epithelium which is derived embryologically as a continuation of the two layers which line the surface of the ciliary body. The surface layer, non-pigmented in the ciliary body, becomes heavily pigmented in the iris such

that the individual cells are completely obscured. The deep layer, pigmented in the ciliary body, is transformed in the iris into lightly pigmented myoepithelial cells which constitute the radially orientated *dilator pupillae muscle* **DP** of the iris. Even at high magnification (b), these myoepithelial cells are difficult to distinguish.

The *constrictor muscle of the pupil (constrictor pupillae)* **CP** consists of a band of circumferentially oriented smooth muscle fibres situated in the stroma near to the free edge of the iris. Like the smooth muscle of the ciliary body, the constrictor pupillae is innervated by the parasympathetic nervous system, whereas the myoepithelial cells of the dilator pupillae are innervated by the sympathetic nervous system.

The colour of the iris depends on the amount of pigment in the stroma, the amount of pigment in the posterior epithelial layer being relatively constant between individuals. Blue eyes contain little stromal pigment whereas brown eyes have much stromal pigment.

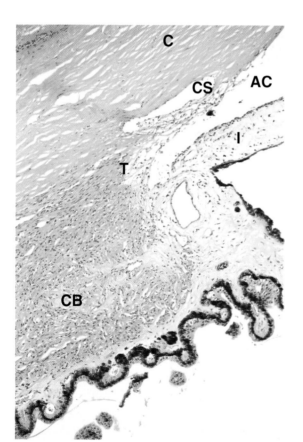

Fig. 21.13   Canal of Schlemm   H & E × 75

The canal of Schlemm **CS** is a circumferential canal lined by endothelium which is situated in the inner aspect of the corneal margin **C** immediately adjacent to the angle of the anterior chamber **AC**. At the angle of the anterior chamber there is a meshwork of fine collagenous trabeculae **T** lined by endothelium; aqueous humor percolates through the spaces between the trabeculae before reaching the canal of Schlemm. There is no direct communication between the trabecular spaces and the canal of Schlemm, and thus reabsorption of aqueous humor involves passage across two layers of endothelium and intervening supporting tissue. The mechanism of transport is not understood; disruption of this process leads to increased intraocular pressure as in the disease known as glaucoma. The canal of Schlemm drains via minute channels through the sclera into the episcleral venous system, a pressure gradient being maintained to prevent reflux of blood. Note the close relationship between the root of the iris **I** and the canal of Schlemm. The smooth muscle of the ciliary body **CB** is easily seen in this micrograph.

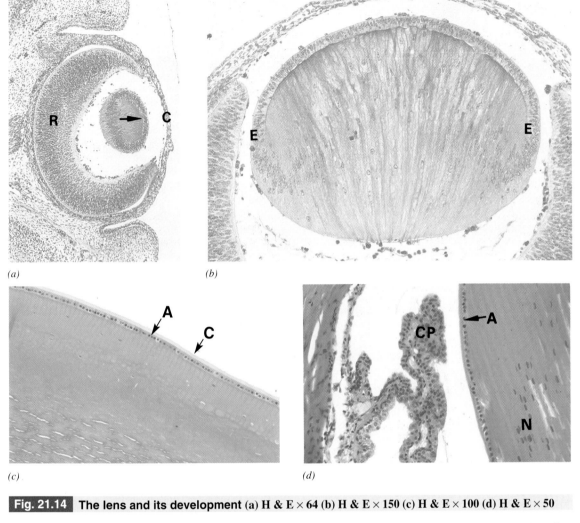

Fig. 21.14 The lens and its development (a) H & E × 64 (b) H & E × 150 (c) H & E × 100 (d) H & E × 50

The lens is an elastic biconvex structure which, although transparent and apparently amorphous, is almost entirely composed of living cells. The lens cells are highly modified epithelial cells derived embryologically from ectoderm which forms a depression, the *lens pit*, overlying the embryonic *optic vesicle*.

With further development, the lens pit becomes deeper, its margins fusing to form the *lens vesicle* which becomes detached from the surface and sinks deeper to become enveloped by the growing optic vesicle; at this stage the lens vesicle merely consists of a single layer of epithelial cells.

The posterior cells of the lens vesicle now become greatly elongated anteroposteriorly, filling the central cavity of the vesicle. This stage of development is shown in micrograph (a), the arrowhead marking the junction between posterior and anterior cells of the former lens vesicle. Note the developing cornea **C** and retina **R**. The lens cells in the central anteroposterior axis then undergo maturation, as seen in micrograph (b), losing their nuclei to become known as *lens fibres*. Proliferation of the cells at the lens equator **E** adds further fibres to the central mass, the growth process continuing at a slow rate even into old age.

When fully developed, the lens substance consists of 2000–3000 anucleate fibres, each stretching between anterior and posterior poles of the lens. The fibres have the shape of extremely elongated six-sided prisms, the more peripheral fibres curving to follow the anteroposterior surface contour of the lens. The lens fibres are packed with proteins called *crystallins* and the cell membranes of adjacent fibres are fused, leaving little intervening extracellular substance.

The whole lens is enveloped by a thick epithelial basement membrane forming the *lens capsule* which is connected via the suspensory ligament to the ciliary body. The anterior lens surface is covered by a single layer of cuboidal cells which retain their nuclei, this layer merging with the residual proliferative cells at the equatorial margin of the lens. This cell layer lies deep to the capsule and is absent posteriorly.

Micrograph (c) shows part of the mature lens including the anterior cuboidal epithelium **A** and lens capsule **C**. The lens substance is particularly prone to artefactual distortion during histological preparation. Micrograph (d) shows the equatorial region of the lens and nearby ciliary processes **CP**. Note the anterior epithelial layer **A** and nuclei **N** in the more recently formed peripheral fibres.

Fig. 21.15 Cornea H & E × 100

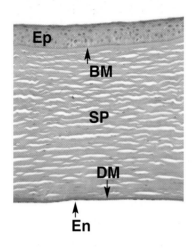

The cornea is the thick transparent portion of the corneo-scleral layer enclosing the anterior one-sixth of the eye. The fixed convexity of the external surface provides the principal mechanism for focusing images upon the retina.

The cornea is an avascular structure consisting of five layers. The outer surface is lined by stratified non-keratinised squamous epithelium **Ep** about five cells thick. This epithelium rests on a thin basal lamina supported by a specialised layer of corneal stroma known as *Bowman's membrane* **BM** which is particularly prominent in humans. The bulk of the cornea, the *substantia propria* or *stroma* **SP**, consists of a highly regular form of dense collagenous tissue forming thin lamellae. Fibroblasts and occasional lymphocytes are scattered in the ground substance between the lamellae. The inner surface of the cornea is lined by a layer of flattened endothelial cells **En** which are supported by a very thick elastic basement membrane known as *Descemet's membrane* **DM**. The *corneal* endothelium is highly active in pumping fluid from the substantia propria, preventing excessive hydration which would result in the cornea becoming opaque.

The cornea is sustained by diffusion of metabolites from the aqueous humor and the blood vessels of the limbus; some oxygen is derived directly from the external environment.

Fig. 21.16 Conjunctiva
Haematoxylin / van Gieson × 128

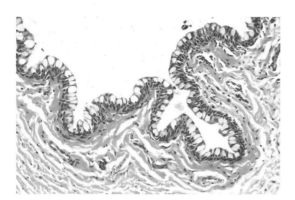

The conjunctiva is the epithelium which covers the exposed part of the sclera and inner surface of the eyelids. It is stratified columnar in form and for a stratified epithelium is unusual in that it contains goblet cells in the surface layers. Melanocytes are found in the basal layer. The conjunctival mucous secretions contribute to the protective layer on the exposed surface of the eye, and allow the eyelids to move freely over the eye.

Beneath the conjunctival epithelium is loose vascular supporting tissue.

Fig. 21.17 Lacrimal gland
H & E × 150

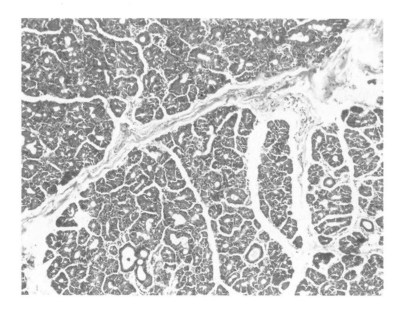

The lacrimal gland is responsible for the secretion of tears, a watery fluid containing the antibacterial enzyme *lysozyme* and electrolytes of similar concentration to plasma.

Histologically, the lacrimal glands are similar to the salivary glands in the lobular structure and compound tubulo-acinar form of the secretory units. The secretory cells have the typical appearance of serous (protein-secreting) cells with basally located nuclei and strongly stained granular cytoplasm.

Each gland drains via a dozen or more small ducts into the superior fornix. Tears drain to the inner aspect of the eye and then into the nasal cavity via the nasolacrimal duct.

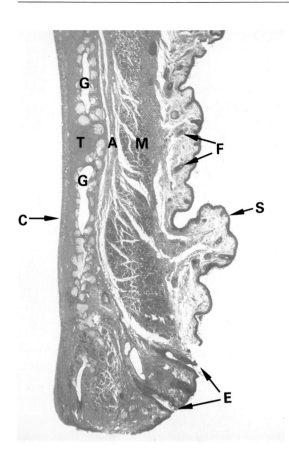

Each eyelid consists of a dense fibroelastic plate, the *tarsus* **T**, covered externally by thin, highly folded skin **S** and on the internal aspect by smooth conjunctiva **C**. The skin contains scattered fine hair follicles **F** and the underlying supporting tissue is extremely loose and devoid of fat.

Skeletal muscle **M** of *orbicularis oculi* (and *levator palpebrae* in the upper eyelid) lies immediately superficial to the tarsal plate and is separated from it by a layer of supporting tissue **A** which, in the upper lid, represents a forward continuation of the sub-aponeurotic layer of the scalp. The clinical importance of this is that blood or inflammatory exudates collecting above the scalp aponeurosis may track forward into the superficial planes of the eyelid; being extremely lax, this area may become markedly swollen. This supporting tissue layer also contains the sensory nerves of the eyelid.

Within the tarsal plate lie some 12–30 *tarsal (Meibomian) glands* **G** oriented vertically and opening at the free margin of the eyelid via minute foramina. These glands are modified sebaceous glands each consisting of a long central duct into which open numerous sebaceous acini. Associated with the eyelashes **E** are sebaceous glands known as the *glands of Zeis* and modified apocrine sweat glands known as the *glands of Moll*. Together, the glands of the eyelid produce an oily layer which is thought to cover the tear layer, thereby preventing evaporation of the tears.

The ear

The ear or vestibulo-cochlear apparatus has the dual sensory function of maintenance of equilibrium and hearing (stato-acoustic system).

Structurally the system may be divided into three parts, the *external ear*, the *middle ear* and the *internal ear*. The specific sensory receptors for both movement and sound are situated in a membranous structure located in the internal ear, while the external and middle ear are concerned with reception, transmission and amplification of incoming sound waves.

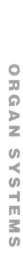

Fig. 21.19 **The ear** *(illustration opposite)*

The main structural elements of the vestibulo-cochlear apparatus are illustrated in this diagram.

External ear

The external ear is responsible for reception of sound waves which are funnelled onto the ear drum (***tympanic membrane***). It consists of the ***auricle (pinna)***, a modified horn-shaped structure composed of elastic cartilage covered by skin, which converges onto the ***external auditory meatus (canal)***. Elastic cartilage also forms the wall of the outer third of the canal whilst the inner two-thirds of the canal lie in the petrous part of the temporal bone. The canal is lined by hairy skin containing sebaceous glands and modified apocrine sweat glands which secrete a waxy material called ***cerumen***.

Middle ear

The middle ear is an air-filled cavity, the ***tympanic cavity***, located in the petrous temporal bone and is separated from the external auditory canal by the tympanic membrane. Sound waves impinging on the tympanic membrane are converted into mechanical vibrations which are then amplified by a system of levers made up of three small bones called ***ossicles*** (the ***malleus***, ***incus*** and ***stapes***) and transmitted to the fluid-filled inner ear cavity. The ossicles articulate with one another via synovial joints and the malleus and incus pivot on tiny ligaments which are attached to the wall of the middle ear cavity. Small slips of muscle, the ***tensor tympani*** and ***stapedius***, pass to the midpoint of the tympanic membrane and stapes bone, respectively, and damp down excessive vibrations which might otherwise damage the delicate auditory apparatus. The middle ear cavity communicates anteriorly with the nasopharynx via the ***auditory (Eustachian) tube*** which permits equalisation of pressure changes with the external environment. Posteriorly, the middle ear cavity communicates with numerous interconnected air spaces which lighten the mass of the mastoid part of the temporal bone. The whole of the middle ear and mastoid cavities are lined by simple squamous or cuboidal epithelium.

Internal ear

The internal ear consists of an interconnected fluid-filled ***membranous labyrinth*** lying within a labyrinth of spaces of complementary shape in the temporal bone (the ***osseous labyrinth***). The membranous labyrinth is bound down to the walls of the osseous labyrinth in various places but in the main is separated from the bony walls by a fluid-filled space. The fluid within the membranous labyrinth is known as ***endolymph*** and the fluid in the surrounding perimembranous space is known as ***perilymph***. The perimembranous space is directly connected with the subarachnoid space and, like the latter, is crossed by delicate fibrous strands and lined by squamous epithelium; the perilymphatic fluid is thus similar in composition to CSF. In contrast, the membranous labyrinth is a closed system with a sac, the ***endolymphatic sac***, lying in the subdural space of the underlying brain. The membranous labyrinth is lined by a simple epithelium except in the endolymphatic sac where the cells are columnar with morphological features, suggesting that this is the site of endolymph absorption.

The osseous labyrinth may be divided into three main areas:

- **The vestibule**. The central space of the osseous labyrinth is called the ***vestibule***; it gives rise to three semicircular canals posteriorly, and to the ***cochlea*** anteriorly. The vestibule contains two components of the membranous labyrinth, namely the ***utricle*** and the ***saccule***, which are connected by a short, Y-shaped duct from which arises the endolymphatic duct. The walls of the utricle and saccule each contain a specialised area of sensory receptor cells known as a ***macula*** (see Fig. 21.27) from which axons pass into the ***vestibular nerve*** as part of the sensory input for maintenance of equilibrium. Laterally, the vestibule is separated from the middle ear cavity by a thin bony plate containing two fenestrations, one oval and the other round in shape. The ***oval window*** is occluded by the base of the stirrup-shaped stapes bone and its surrounding ***annular ligament*** whereby vibrations are transmitted to the perilymph from the tympanic membrane via the ossicle chain. The ***round window*** is closed by a membrane similar to the tympanic membrane and it is thus sometimes described as the ***secondary tympanic membrane***. This membrane permits vibrations which have passed to sensory receptors for sound to be dissipated.

- **The semicircular canals**. Three semicircular canals arise from the posterior aspect of the vestibule, two being disposed in vertical planes at right angles to one another and the other in a near-horizontal plane. Within each semicircular canal is a semicircular membranous duct filled with endolymph and continuous at both ends with the utricle; near one end of each semicircular membranous duct is a dilated area called the ***ampulla***. In each ampulla, there is a ridge called the ***crista ampullaris*** (see Fig. 21.28) containing sensory receptors with axons converging on the vestibular nerve. Together with the receptors of the maculae of the utricle and saccule, these receptors form the sensory afferents for the maintenance of balance and equilibrium.

- **The cochlea**. The cochlea occupies a conical, spiral-shaped space in the temporal bone extending from the anterior aspect of the vestibule; the space is roughly similar in shape to that inside the shell of a cone-shaped snail. The membranous component of the cochlea arises from the saccule and spirals upwards with its blind end attached at the apex of the osseous space. The membranous canal is triangular in cross-section and attached to the bony walls of the cochlea in such a manner as to divide the osseous space into three spiral compartments (see Fig. 21.24). The middle compartment, the ***scala media***, contains endolymph, and the upper and lower compartments contain perilymph. At the base of the cochlea, the upper perilymph compartment is directly continuous with the perilymph of the vestibule and via this space, called the ***scala vestibuli***, vibrations pass through the perilymph towards the apex of the cochlea. At the apex, the scala vestibuli becomes continuous with the lower perilymphatic space of the cochlear spiral via a minute hole called the ***helicotrema***. This lower space terminates at the secondary tympanic membrane covering the round window and 'spent' vibrations are thus dissipated; the lower perilymphatic space is therefore known as the ***scala tympani***. The sensory receptors for sound are located in a spiral shaped structure known as the ***organ of Corti*** shown in detail in Figure 21.25.

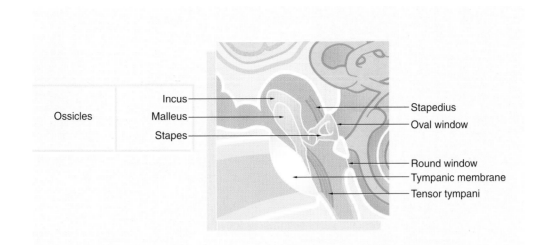

Ossicles
- Incus — Stapedius
- Malleus — Oval window
- Stapes

- Round window
- Tympanic membrane
- Tensor tympani

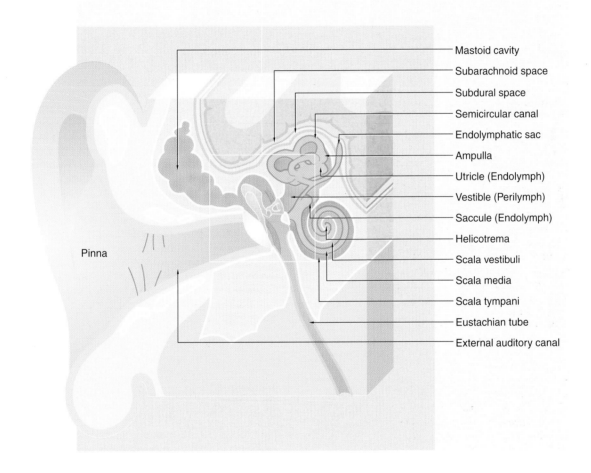

Pinna

- Mastoid cavity
- Subarachnoid space
- Subdural space
- Semicircular canal
- Endolymphatic sac
- Ampulla
- Utricle (Endolymph)
- Vestible (Perilymph)
- Saccule (Endolymph)
- Helicotrema
- Scala vestibuli
- Scala media
- Scala tympani
- Eustachian tube
- External auditory canal

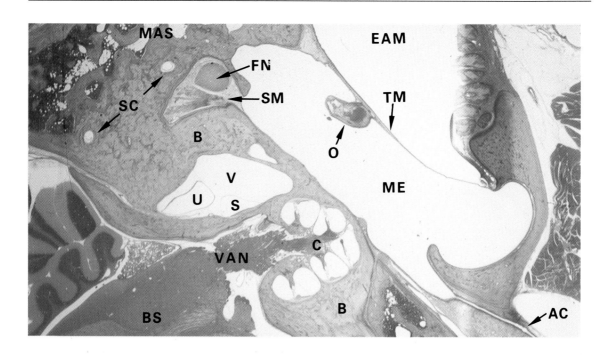

Fig. 21.20 | **The ear** H & E × 8

This micrograph shows a horizontal section through the vestibulo-cochlear apparatus which lies within the temporal bone **B**. The tympanic membrane **TM** can be seen stretched between the tympanic plate of the temporal bone anteriorly and the lateral part of the petrous temporal bone posteriorly, dividing the external auditory meatus **EAM** from the cavity of the middle ear **ME**. Part of one of the ossicles **O**, the handle of the malleus, can be seen attached to the inner aspect of the tympanic membrane. From the anterior aspect of the middle ear chamber, the auditory canal (Eustachian canal) **AC** passes forwards towards the nasopharynx; in the mastoid part of the temporal bone there are numerous irregular mastoid air spaces **MAS**.

Near the centre of the field is the vestibule of the inner ear **V** containing two delicate membranous structures, the utricle **U** and saccule **S** more anteriorly. Two of the semicircular canals **SC** can be identified deep in the posterior part of the petrous temporal bone. Immediately posterior to the middle ear cavity, the facial nerve **FN** is seen in transverse section as it passes inferiorly; just medial to it lies the stapedius muscle **SM**.

Anterior to the vestibule, the conical spiral of the cochlea **C** has been cut in longitudinal section through its central bony axis. From the base of the cochlea, the vestibulo-auditory nerve **VAN** passes towards the brain stem **BS**, behind which the cerebellum is easily recognisable.

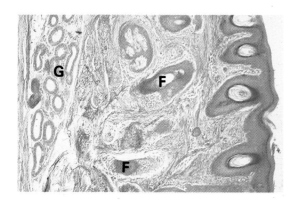

Fig. 21.21 **External auditory meatus** H & E × 100

The external auditory meatus is the canal leading from the auricle to the tympanic membrane. The wall of the outer third is formed by elastic cartilage whereas the inner two-thirds is formed by the temporal bone. The canal is lined by skin which is devoid of the usual dermal papillae and closely bound down to the underlying cartilage or bone by a dense collagenous dermis. The skin of the outer third (as shown here) has fine hairs and the dermis contains numerous coiled tubular *ceruminous glands* **G** which secrete wax (cerumen) and which represent specialised apocrine sweat glands. The ceruminous glands open directly onto the skin surface or into the sebaceous glands associated with hair follicles **F**. The meatal hairs provide protection from foreign bodies whilst the cerumen protects the skin of the external meatus from moisture and infection.

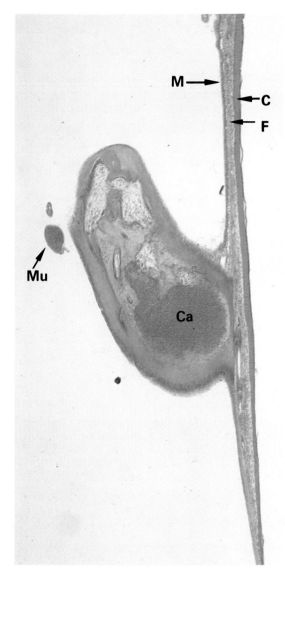

Fig. 21.22 Tympanic membrane and ossicle
H & E × 20

The tympanic membrane (ear drum) is a thin fibrous membrane separating the external auditory canal from the cavity of the middle ear. With the exception of a small triangular area superiorly, the ***pars flaccida***, the membrane is tense (***pars tensa***), being firmly attached to the surrounding bone by a fibrocartilaginous ring. The handle of the malleus is attached to the centre of the membrane, the chain of ossicles pulling the membrane slightly inwards.

The tympanic membrane is made up of three layers: an external ***cuticular layer***, an intermediate fibrous layer and an inner ***mucous layer***. The cuticular layer **C** consists of thin hairless skin, the epidermis being only about 10 cells thick and the basal layer being flat and devoid of the usual epidermal ridges. The thin dermis contains plump fibroblasts and a fine vascular network.

The intermediate fibrous layer **F** consists of an outer layer of fibres radiating from the centre of the membrane towards the circumference and an inner layer of fibres disposed circumferentially at the periphery. These fibres have long been assumed to be collagen associated with a fine meshwork of elastin; however, recent evidence suggests that the fibres are of a unique composition especially adapted for the function of the tympanic membrane.

The inner mucous layer **M** represents a continuation of the modified respiratory-type mucous membrane lining the middle ear cavity, but in this situation it is merely a single layer of cuboidal cells devoid of cilia and goblet cells. The underlying lamina propria is thin with a blood supply separate from that of the dermis of the cuticular layer. A similar modified respiratory-type mucosa invests the ossicles, small muscles and nerves exposed to the middle ear cavity.

The ossicles consist of compact bone formed by endochondral ossification which accounts for the cartilage **Ca** seen in this specimen from a kitten. Note also the tensor tympani muscle **Mu**.

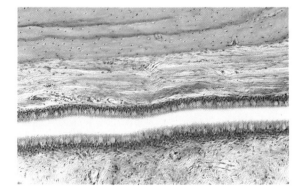

Fig. 21.23 Auditory (Eustachian) canal
H & E × 320

The auditory canal connects the cavity of the middle ear with the nasopharynx and allows for equalisation of air pressure between the middle ear and the external environment. From the middle ear, the tube first passes through bone, but towards the pharynx, the wall is supported on two sides by cartilage and on the remaining two sides by fibrous tissue.

The tube is lined by typical pseudostratified respiratory epithelium with numerous goblet cells particularly towards the pharyngeal end. The ***salpingo-pharyngeus, tensor palati*** and ***levator veli palati*** muscles are connected to the fibrocartilaginous part of the tube causing it to dilate during swallowing.

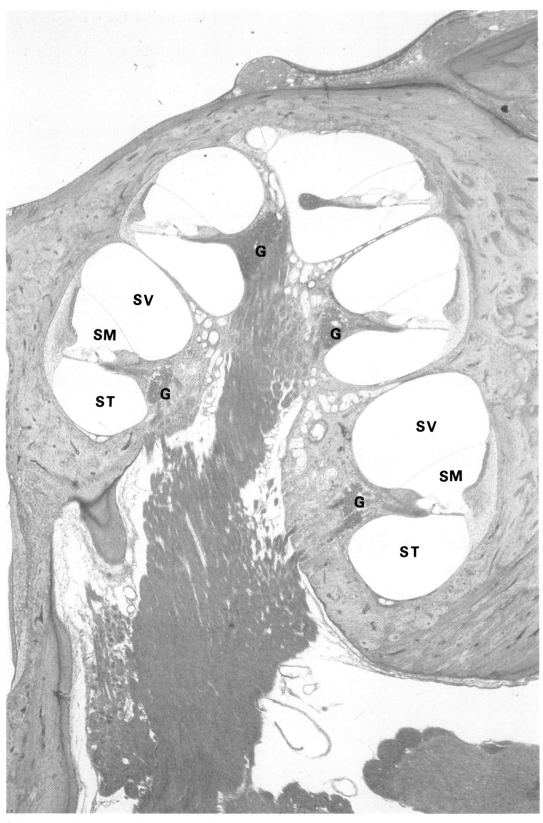

(a)

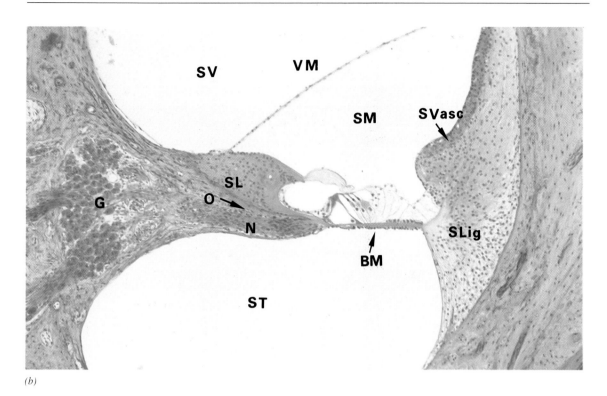

(b)

Fig. 21.24 **Cochlea** (a) H & E × 20 *(opposite)* (b) H & E × 96

The cochlea is the component of the internal ear which contains the auditory sense organ. The conical spiral-shaped form of the cochlea can be visualised in micrograph (a) which shows a cochlea cut in a plane of section which includes its long bony axis. Note that the cavity in the petrous temporal bone is reminiscent of the space inside a conical snail shell. The cochlea has two-and-a-half full turns and in this section, therefore, five separate cross-sections of the cochlea can be seen, each turn of the spiral being separated from the next by a thin plate of bone. A corkscrew-like bony structure, the *modiolus*, forms the central axis of the cochlea.

Each turn of the cochlear canal can be seen to be divided into three compartments, shown at higher magnification in micrograph (b). The central compartment, the *scala media* **SM**, is roughly triangular in cross-section, with the apex attached to a spicule of bone spiralling outwards from the modiolus and known as the *osseous spiral lamina* **O**. Above the free edge of the osseous spiral lamina is a thickened mass of tissue known as the *spiral limbus* **SL**. The base of the scala media is thickened and attached to the outer wall of the cochlea. The membrane making up the walls of the scala media represents that part of the membranous labyrinth extending up into the cochlea from the saccule, and the scala media is thus filled with endolymph.

Above the scala media is the *scala vestibuli* **SV** originating in the vestibule near the oval window and the base of the stapes; vibrations are conducted towards the apex of the cochlea in the perilymph of the scala vestibuli. Below the scala media is the perilymphatic space which spirals down from the apex to the secondary tympanic membrane, the *scala tympani* **ST**.

The membrane separating the scala media and the scala tympani, known as the *basilar membrane* **BM**, supports the *organ of Corti* which contains the auditory receptor cells; the organ of Corti is described in detail in Figure 21.25. The cells of the organ of Corti are derived from the simple epithelium lining the membranous labyrinth which embryologically is of ectodermal origin. The basilar membrane is composed of fibrous tissue. Axially, it is attached to the osseous spiral lamina and laterally to the *spiral ligament* **SLig** which consists of a marked thickening of the endosteum of the lateral wall of the cochlear canal. The thickened outer wall of the scala media is highly vascular and lined by a stratified epithelium; this area, known as the *stria vascularis* **SVasc**, is responsible for maintaining the correct ionic composition of endolymph.

The membrane between the scala media and scala vestibuli, the *vestibular (Reissner's) membrane* **VM**, is composed of extremely delicate fibrous tissue lined by simple squamous epithelium on both sides. The scala vestibuli and scala tympani are lined by a simple unspecialised squamous epithelium of mesodermal origin.

In micrograph (b) bundles of afferent nerve fibres **N** can be seen arising from the base of the organ of Corti and converging towards the *spiral ganglion* **G** in the modiolus at the base of the spiral lamina. These ganglion cells represent the cell bodies of bipolar sensory neurones, and their proximal axons form the auditory component of the eighth cranial nerve (see Fig. 21.26).

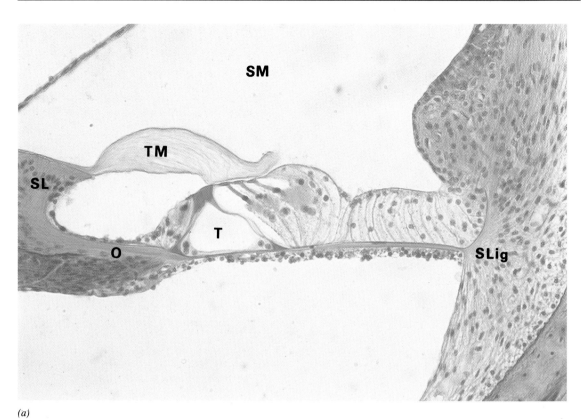

(a)

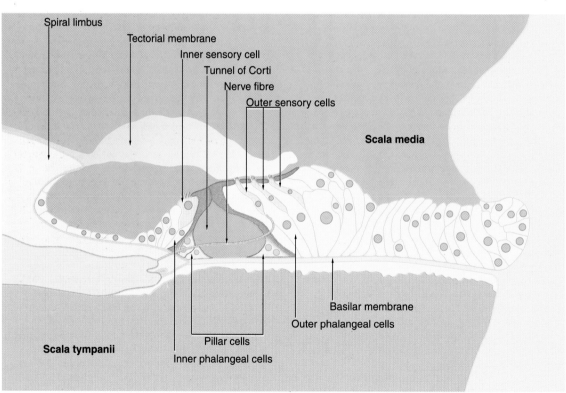

(b)

The organ of Corti is a highly specialised epithelial structure containing receptor cells which convert (transduce) mechanical energy in the form of vibrations into electrochemical energy, resulting in excitation of auditory sensory receptors.

The organ of Corti lies in the scala media **SM** supported on the basilar membrane. The basilar membrane consists of a thin sheet of fibrous tissue stretched between the osseous spiral lamina **O** of the modiolus and the spiral ligament **SLig** laterally; its undersurface, exposed to the scala tympani, is lined by a simple epithelium. The basilar membrane is thinnest at the base of the cochlea and becomes progressively thicker as it spirals towards the apex.

The organ of Corti consists of two basic types of cells, *sensory (hair) cells* and *support cells* of several different types, including among others the *inner* and *outer pillar cells* and *inner* and *outer phalangeal cells*. At the centre of the organ is a triangular-shaped canal, the *inner tunnel* or *tunnel of Corti* **T**, bounded on each side by a single row of tall columnar cells called *pillar cells*. Each pillar cell contains a dense bundle (pillar) of microtubules and the pillars on either side of the tunnel of Corti converge at the surface and then curve laterally to form a thin, hood-like structure containing small fenestrations. The cell bodies of the pillar cells lie in the acute angles formed by the pillars and the basilar membrane at the floor of the tunnel.

On the inner aspect of the inner row of pillar cells is a single row of flask-shaped cells, the inner phalangeal cells, which support a single row of *inner sensory (hair) cells*. The phalangeal cells contain microtubules, some of which support the base of the hair cells while others extend to the free surface around the hair cells. Beyond the outer row of pillar cells there are three to five rows of outer phalangeal cells which support the same number of rows of *outer sensory (hair) cells*. Cytoplasmic extensions of the phalangeal cells extend to the surface between and around the hair cells and their microtubules support the fenestrated hood-like structure formed by the pillar cells. Through the fenestrations project the free ends of the sensory cells. A variety of other specialised epithelial cells provides the remaining support for the organ of Corti.

The sensory cells are known as hair cells because numerous sterocilia, i.e. very long microvilli (see Fig. 5.17), project from their free ends. The sterocilia are embedded in the surface of the *tectorial membrane*. As previously described, the spiral ganglion of the cochlea contains bipolar cell bodies of first order sensory neurones. From here, axons pass towards the base of the rows of hair cells, those going to the outer hair cells traversing the tunnel of Corti as shown in the diagram (b). The end of

each fibre ramifies into a number of dendrites which make synaptic contact with several hair cells; each sensory cell may synapse with dendrites of several different sensory neurones. In addition, inhibitory neurones arising in the brain stem send fibres which also synapse with the sensory cells and exert a suppressive effect.

From the layer of *border cells* which cover the spiral limbus **SL**, there extends a flap-like mass of glycosaminoglycans called the *tectorial membrane* **TM** overlying the sensory cells and within which the tips of the stereocilia are embedded.

Function of the organ of Corti

Details of the exact physiological processes of the sense of hearing remain to be discovered. However, in brief, the mechanism is as follows. Sound waves are funnelled into the external auditory meatus and impinge on the tympanic membrane which vibrates at the appropriate frequency. These vibrations are transmitted to the stapes bone via the malleus and incus and, in the process, their amplitude is enhanced about 10-fold. The base of the stapes, which lies in the oval window, conducts the vibrations into the perilymph of the vestibule of the inner ear and pressure waves pass from here into the scala vestibuli of the cochlea. These pressure waves are probably conducted directly to the endolymph of the scala media across the delicate vestibular membrane from which vibrations are induced in the basilar membrane upon which rests the organ of Corti. From here, spent vibrations are transmitted into the perilymph of the scala tympani and dissipated at the secondary tympanic membrane over the round window.

The basilar membrane is thinnest at the base of the cochlea and thickest at the apex. It appears that, at every point on the spiral, the membrane is 'tuned' to vibrate to a particular frequency of sound waves reaching the ear; the overall range of frequencies encompassed is of the order of 11 octaves, with the highest frequencies (pitch) being sensed towards the base of the cochlea and progressively lower frequencies being sensed along the spiral towards the apex. For any given sound frequency, only one specific point of the basilar membrane and organ of Corti is thought to vibrate and thereby activate the appropriate hair cells to initiate afferent sensory impulses which then pass to the auditory cortex of the brain. Deformation of the stereocilia of the hair cells results in either depolarisation or hypopolarisation of the cell membrane, which in turn excites the sensory nerves which synapse with them.

The sensory input from the cochlea is integrated in the brain stem and auditory cortex from which efferent suppressor pathways can modulate receptor activity to enhance auditory acuity.

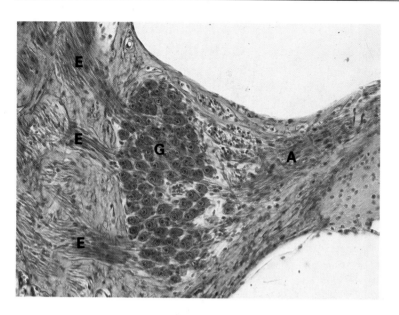

Fig. 21.26 Spiral ganglion
H & E × 320

The spiral ganglion is a spiral-shaped mass of nerve cell bodies lying in a canal at the extremity of the osseous spiral lamina of the modiolus.

As seen in this micrograph, the ganglion cells **G** have the typical appearance of somatic ganglion cells (see Fig. 7.17) and represent the cell bodies of bipolar sensory neurones, relaying information from the receptors of the organ of Corti to the brain.

Note the afferent fibres **A** entering the ganglion from the organ of Corti and numerous bundles of efferent fibres **E** which pass to the centre of the modiolus to form the *cochlear nerve*, the auditory component of the eighth cranial nerve; the cochlear nerve is readily seen in Figure 21.24(a).

Fig. 21.27 Receptor organs of the saccule and utricle *(illustrations opposite)*
(a) H & E × 480 (b) H & E × 600 (c) Scanning EM × 5000 (d) Schematic diagram

The saccule and utricle are two dilated regions of the membranous labyrinth lying within the vestibule of the inner ear and filled with endolymph. The walls of each are composed of a fibrous membrane which is bound down in places to the periosteum of the vestibule and, in other areas, is attached to the periosteum by fibrous strands, the intervening space being filled with perilymph. Internally, the saccule and utricle are lined by simple cuboidal epithelium but in each there is a small region of highly specialised epithelium called the *macula*, shown in micrographs (a) and (b), containing receptor cells which contribute part of the sensory input to that part of the brain responsible for maintaining balance and equilibrium. The macula of the utricle is oriented at right angles to that of the saccule.

The maculae are made up of two basic cell types, *sensory hair cells* and *support cells*. The support cells are tall and columnar with basally located nuclei and microvilli at their free surface. The hair cells lie between the support cells, with their larger nuclei placed more centrally. Each hair cell has a single eccentrically located cilium of typical conformation, often called the *kinocilium* (see Fig. 5.15), and many stereocilia (long microvilli) projecting from its surface; hence the name hair cells. The 'hairs' are embedded in a thick, gelatinous plaque of glycoprotein probably secreted by the supporting cells; this is lost during histological preparation. At the surface of the glycoprotein layer is a mass of crystals mainly composed of calcium carbonate and known as *otoliths*. These are shown in micrograph (c).

There are two different forms of hair cells. *Type I hair cells (goblet cells)* are bulbous in shape and stain poorly, their nuclei tending to lie at a lower level than those of

type II hair cells (*columnar cells*) which are more slender in shape. The type I hair cells are invested by a meshwork of dendritic processes of afferent sensory neurones, whereas the type II hair cells have only small dendritic processes at their bases. The hair cells also have synaptic connections with modulatory (inhibitory) neurones from the CNS.

Function of the maculae

The function of the maculae relates mainly to the maintenance of balance by providing sensory information about the static position of the head in space. This is of particular importance when the eyes are closed, or in the dark or under water, and the maculae are consequently more developed in animals other than humans.

When the head is moved from a position of equilibrium, the otolithic membrane tends to move with respect to the receptor cells, thus bending their stereocilia. When the stereocilia are bent in the direction of the cilium, the receptor cell undergoes excitation and, when the relative movement is in the opposite direction, excitation is inhibited. The orientation of the hair cells in different directions in the maculae causes different hair cells to be stimulated with different positions of the head. The pattern of hair cell stimulation allows the central nervous system to determine the position of the head very accurately with respect to gravity.

The neural pathways of the balance and equilibrium mechanism are extremely complex and the sensory input from the maculae is integrated with that of proprioceptors, muscle spindles etc. to elicit reflex responses directed towards the maintenance of postural equilibrium.

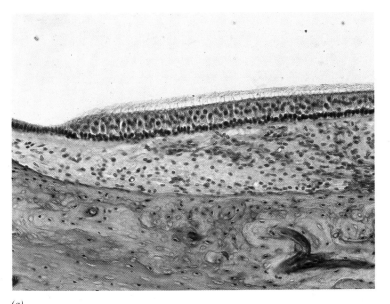

(a)

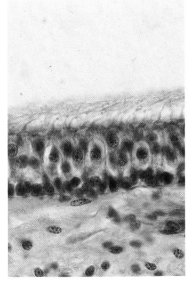

(b)

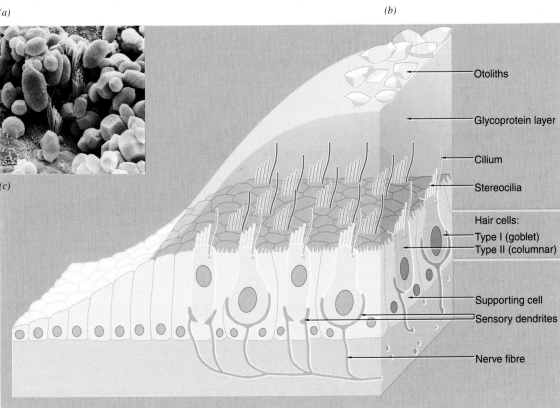

(c)

Otoliths

Glycoprotein layer

Cilium

Stereocilia

Hair cells:
Type I (goblet)
Type II (columnar)

Supporting cell

Sensory dendrites

Nerve fibre

(d)

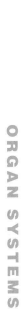

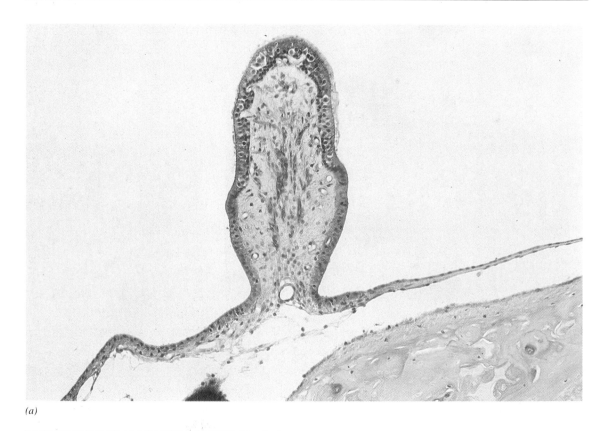

(a)

Fig. 21.28 **Receptor organs of the semicircular canals**
(a) Masson's trichrome × 200 (b) Schematic diagram *(opposite)*

Three semicircular canals arise from the vestibule of the inner ear, each containing a membranous semicircular duct which opens at both ends into the utricle. At one end of each duct is a dilated portion, the ampulla, which contains a receptor organ called the *crista ampullaris*.

Each crista ampullaris is an elongated epithelial structure situated on a ridge of supporting tissue arising from the membranous wall of the ampulla and oriented at right angles to the direction of flow of the endolymph in the semicircular canal. Structurally, the cristae ampullares bear many similarities to the maculae of the utricle and saccule (see Fig. 21.27). The hair cells are of the same two morphological forms, *type I* and *type II cells*, the former being invested by a basket of sensory dendrites and the latter having small dendritic endings at the base only. The hair cells are supported by a single layer of columnar cells which is continuous with the simple cuboidal epithelium lining the rest of the membranous labyrinth.

Like those of the maculae, the hair cells of the cristae have numerous stereocilia and a single kinocilium, the kinocilium being situated at the margin of the cell nearest to the utricle. The stereocilia and the kinocilia of the hair cells are embedded in a ridge of gelatinous glycoprotein which is tall and cone shaped in cross-section giving rise to the term *cupula*. In contrast to the macula, the cupula does not contain otolithic crystals. Traces of the cupola can be seen on the surface of the crista ampullaris in micrograph (a), although most of it has been lost during histological preparation of the specimen.

Function of the crista ampullaris

When the head is moved in the plane of a particular semicircular canal, the inertia of the endolymph acts so as to deflect the cupula in the opposite direction. The stereocilia of the sensory cells are then deflected towards or away from the cilia, resulting in excitation or inhibition, respectively.

In each ear there are three semicircular canals, two at right angles to each other in vertical planes and one in a near-horizontal plane. Each is paired with a semicircular canal in the other ear, the members of each pair being oriented in parallel. The sensory input from the cristae ampullares mainly concerns changes in the direction and rate of movement of the head. Afferent impulses pass via bipolar sensory neurones with cell bodies in the vestibular ganglion which lies at the base of the internal auditory meatus. Afferent fibres pass via the vestibular part of the eighth cranial nerve to the brain stem, cerebellum and cerebral cortex where sensory information from various other sources is integrated for the maintenance of balance, position sense and equilibrium.

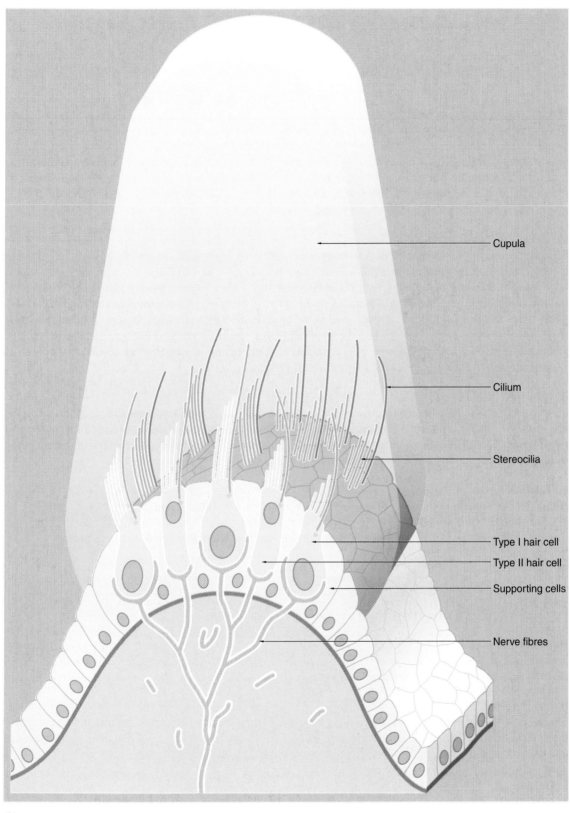

Cupula

Cilium

Stereocilia

Type I hair cell

Type II hair cell

Supporting cells

Nerve fibres

(b)

Notes on staining techniques

Haematoxylin and eosin (H & E)

This is the most commonly used technique in animal histology and routine pathology. The basic dye, haematoxylin, stains acidic structures a purplish blue. Nuclei, ribosomes and rough endoplasmic reticulum have a strong affinity for this dye owing to their high content of DNA and RNA, respectively. In contrast, eosin is an acidic dye which stains basic structures red or pink. Most cytoplasmic proteins are basic and hence cytoplasm usually stains pink or pinkish red. In general, when the H & E staining technique is applied to animal cells, nuclei stain blue and cytoplasm stains pink or red.

Periodic acid–Schiff reaction (PAS)

Staining techniques which specifically stain components of cells and tissues are called histochemical staining techniques. Such techniques are invaluable for the understanding of cell and tissue structure and function, and for making a diagnosis on diseased tissues. The PAS reaction stains complex carbohydrates a deep red colour, traditionally described as magenta. The mucin produced by goblet cells of the gastrointestinal and respiratory tracts stains magenta with this technique (and is therefore termed PAS-positive). Basement membranes and the brush borders of kidney tubules and the small and large intestines are also PAS-positive, as is cartilage and to some extent collagen. Glycogen, the intracellular storage form of carbohydrate found in cells such as hepatocytes and muscle cells, is also PAS-positive.

Masson's trichrome

This technique is a so-called connective tissue technique since it is used to demonstrate supporting tissue elements, principally collagen. As its name implies, the staining technique produces three colours: nuclei and other basophilic structures are stained blue; collagen is stained green or blue depending on which variant of the technique is used; and cytoplasm, muscle, erythrocytes and keratin are stained bright red.

Alcian blue

Alcian blue is a mucin stain which may be used in conjunction with other staining methods such as H & E or van Gieson (see below). Certain types of mucin, but not all, are stained blue by the Alcian blue method, as is cartilage. When the technique is combined with van Gieson, the Alcian blue colour becomes green.

van Gieson

This is another connective tissue method in which collagen is stained red, nuclei are blue and erythrocytes and cytoplasm yellow. When used in combination with an elastic stain, elastin is stained blue/black in addition to the results described above. This staining technique is particularly useful for blood vessels and skin.

Reticulin stain

This method demonstrates the reticulin fibres of supporting tissue which are stained blue/black by this technique. Nuclei may be counterstained blue with haematoxylin or red with the dye, neutral red.

Azan

This technique is traditionally classed as a connective tissue method but is excellent for demonstrating fine cytological detail, especially in epithelium. Nuclei are stained bright red; collagen, basement membrane and mucin are stained blue; muscle and red blood cells are stained orange to red.

Giemsa

This technique is a standard method for staining blood cells and other smears of cells, e.g. bone marrow. Nuclei are stained dark blue to violet, background cytoplasm pale blue and erythrocytes pale pink.

Toluidine blue

This is a basic stain which stains acidic components various shades of blue. It is commonly employed on very thin, resin embedded specimens. Some tissue components are able to turn the blue dye red, a phenomenon known as metachromasia.

Silver and gold methods

These methods were extremely popular at the end of the nineteenth century and are occasionally used today to demonstrate such fine structures as cell processes, e.g. in neurones, motor end-plates and intercellular junctions. Depending on the method used, the end product is either black, brown or golden.

Chrome alum/haematoxylin
This method is rarely used and is similar to the H & E method in principle, in that nuclei are stained blue and cytoplasm is stained red. Empirically this method demonstrates the glucagon-secreting cells of the pancreas pink and the insulin-secreting cells blue.

Isamine blue/eosin
This method is also similar to the H & E method but the blue component is rather more intense.

Nissl and methylene blue methods
These techniques use a basic dye to stain the rough endoplasmic reticulum found in neurones; when this is seen as clumps it is called Nissl substance.

Sudan black and osmium
These dyes stain lipid-containing structures such as myelin a brownish-black colour.

Immunohistological techniques
A variety of immunohistological techniques are now used routinely for diagnostic purposes as well as for research. Micrographs employing the immunoperoxidase technique are used in several chapters of this book to highlight specific histological features (see for example Figs 1.9e, 11.5, and 17.21a). For this reason the basic technique is described here in some detail.

Immunohistochemical techniques depend on the exquisite specificity of antibodies for their antigen. Thus any substance (antigen) can be specifically identified provided antibodies for it are available. To demonstrate a particular substance, such as insulin, in sections of tissue, antibodies must be produced. This is done by injecting human insulin into a laboratory animal which obligingly recognises the human peptide as foreign and produces antibodies to it. A virtually inexhaustible source of antibody can then be created using monoclonal technology. (In actual practice you order a vial of antibody from a recognised supplier.)

A section of tissue is placed on a glass slide (a) and a solution of antibody is laid over the tissue. The antibody binds to the antigen and excess antibody is washed away so that only cells containing the particular antigen have antibody bound to them. To demonstrate the position of antibody, the antibody is prelinked to an indicator substance. This may be a fluorescent substance such as fluorescein, in which case the technique is known as immunofluorescence and the position of antibody can be visualised using a fluorescence microscope. It is more useful to bind to the antibody an enzyme which is able to convert a colourless substrate to a coloured product. A solution of the substrate is laid over the tissue section (b) with the bound antibody. After a period of incubation, the coloured product can be seen on the section using an ordinary light microscope (c). An enzyme commonly used for this purpose is horseradish peroxidase and the technique is then called the immunoperoxidase technique. A further modification of this principle for electron microscopy uses antibodies linked to gold which, as gold is electron-dense, can be detected by electron microscopy (immunogold labelling). Many other variants of this technique are available.

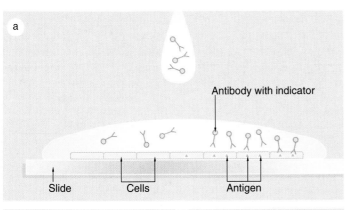

a

Antibody with indicator

Slide   Cells   Antigen

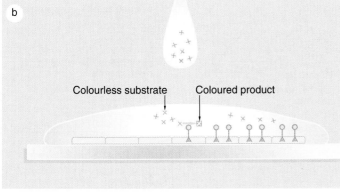

b

Colourless substrate   Coloured product

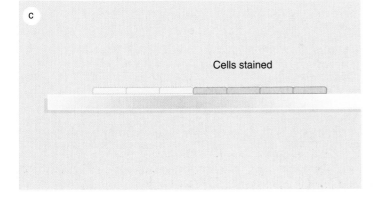

c

Cells stained

Index

Acetylcholinesterase, 128
Acid phosphatase, 20
Acidophilia, 11
Acidophils, pituitary, 312, 313
Acinar glands, 94
Acini
　liver, 274
　pancreas, 284
Acrosomal vesicle, Acrosomal head cap, 332
ACTH, 313
Actin, 27, 91, 103, 111
　salivary myoepithelial cells, 248
Action potentials, 116
Active transport, 8
Addressins, 211
Adenohypophysis (Anterior pituitary), 311, 312
Adhering junctions, 86, 87, 88
Adipocytes, 26, 73, 74
Adipose tissue, 26, 73–75
Adrenal gland, 319–323
Adrenaline, 323
Aerobic respiration, 22, 107
Airways, 222–223
Aldosterone, 321
Alkaline phosphatase
　intestinal, 266
　neutrophils, 50
Alpha cells, islets of Langerhans, 325
Alpha granules, platelets, 57
Alveoli, 222, 230–235
Ameloblasts, 241
Amnion, 367
Amphipathic phospholipids, 7
Ampulla of Vater, 282
Ampullae (semicircular canals), 394
Anaerobic respiration, 22, 51, 107
Anal canal, 271, 273
Anaphase, 36
Angiotensin, 303
Annulus fibrosus, 191
Antibodies, 195, 197, 200, 213, 407
Antidiuretic hormone, 304, 311
Antigen presenting cells, 79, 194, 197, 198, 204
Aorta, 148
Apocrine secretion, 93, 164, 170
Apoptosis, 42–44
Appendix, 216, 271, 273
APUD cells, 327
Aqueous humor, 382, 389
Arachnoid mater, 138
Areola (breast), 368
Argentaffin cells, 326
Argyrophil cells, 326
Arrector pili muscles, 164, 168
Arteries
　arterial system, 147
　arteriovenous shunts, 150
　coronary, 144
　elastic, 72, 147, 148
　muscular, 147, 148–149
　pulmonary, 223, 226, 229, 236
Arterioles, 147, 149

kidney, 289, 291, 293
Aryl sulphatase, eosinophils, 52
Astrocytes, 134, 135
Asymmetrical unit membrane, urinary epithelium, 309
ATP, 22
ATPase
　bile canaliculi, 279
　skeletal muscle, 107
Atrioventricular node, 146
Auerbach's (myenteric) plexus, 250, 252
Auricle, 394
Autonomic nervous system
　gastrointestinal tract, 250
　synapses, 127
Autophagy, 19
Axonemes, 90
　spermatozoa, 333
Axons, 29, 117, 121–125
　myelination, 121, 123–125, 137
Azurophilia, 46
Azurophilic granules, 50

B lymphocytes, 195, 197
　lymph nodes, 210, 211
　spleen, 221
　thymus, 204
Band forms (Stab cells), 61, 62
Barr bodies, 11, 50
Basal vacuolation, endometrium, 354
Basement membranes, 67–68, 86, 160
　glomerular, 294
Bases, DNA, 34
Basilar membrane, 401
Basket cells, cerebellum, 376
Basophilia, 46
Basophils, 54, 64, 78
　vs mast cells, 77
Basophils (pituitary), 312, 313
bcl-2 gene, 42
Bellini, ducts of, 289
Beta cells, islets of Langerhans, 325
Beta thromboglobulin, 57
Betz cells, 379
Bile acids, 260
Biliary system, 276, 279–282
Bipolar cells, retina, 387
Birbeck granules, 162
Bladder, 309
Blastocyst, 360
Blood, 46–64
Blood–brain barrier, 139
Blood pressure, juxtaglomerular apparatus on, 303
Blood–testis barrier, 334
Blood–thymus barrier, 203
Bone, 172, 175–188
　bone fluid, 179
　bone marrow, 46, 58–62
　bony endplates, 189
　cancellous bone, 175, 176, 182
　compact bone, 175-179
　cortical bone, 177,179
　development and growth, 183–188

histological preparation of, 178, 181
　lamellar bone, 176
　matrix, 187
　mineralisation, 182–183
　repair, 187
　woven bone, 176, 187, 188
Bone marrow, 46, 58–62
Bowman's capsules, 288–289
Bowman's glands, olfactory epithelium, 381
Bowman's membrane, 392
Brain, 372
Breast, 341, 368–371
Bronchi, 222, 227–228
Bronchial vascular system, 223
Bronchioles, 229, 230
Brown adipose tissue, 73, 75
Bruch's membrane, 384
Brunner's glands, 251, 260, 263
Brush borders, 82, 91
　small intestine, 266
　proximal convoluted tubules, 298
Bulbo-urethral glands of Cowper, 340
Bulk transport, 8

C cells, 316
Caecum, 249, 270
Cajal, horizontal cells of, 379
Calcitonin, 315, 316, 318
Calcium
　bone, 178, 181
　cardiac muscle, 112
　and connexons, 89
　parathyroid hormone on, 318
　pineal gland, 325
　smooth muscle, 111
Callus, 187
Calmodulin, 111
Calyces, kidney, 287
Canalicular membrane system, platelets, 57
Canalicular system, gastric parietal cells, 258
Canaliculi (bone), 177
Canaliculi (liver), 279, 280
Capillaries, 150–153
Capping proteins, 27
Capsules of organs, 71
Cardia (stomach), 254
Cardiac muscle, see Muscle, cardiac
Cartilage, 172–175
　articular, 189, 190
　elastic, 175
　fibrocartilage, 175, 189
　hyaline, 173
　joints, 189
Catalase, 21
Catecholamines, 319–320, 323
Caveolae, 110
CD system (lymphocyte surface markers), 195, 201
Cell cycle, 33–41
Cell death, 42, 89
Cell-mediated cytotoxicity, 197

Cell movement, 27–31
Cells, 4–32
Cellular respiration, 22
Cementum, 239, 243
Central nervous system, 134–139, 372–379
Central retinal artery, 388
Centrioles, 27, 28, 30
Centroacinar cells, pancreas, 284
Centromeres, 34
Centrosomes, 27, 28, 30, 31
Cerebellar peduncles, 375
Cerebellum, 376
Cerebral cortex, 379
Cerebrospinal fluid, 138
Ceruminous glands, 396
Cervix, 357–358
Chemotaxis, 51
Chiasma formation, 40, 41
Chief cells (parathyroid), 319
Chief cells (stomach), 255, 257
Cholecystokinin-pancreozymin, 260, 283
Cholesterol
    membranes, 7
    steroids from, 322
Chondroblasts, 172
Chondrocytes, 172, 173, 174
Chordae tendinae, 144, 147
Chorion, 360–363, 367
Choroid (eye), 382, 384
Choroid plexus, 138
Chromaffin cells, 323
Chromatids, 34
Chromatin, 11
Chromogranin A, 229
Chromophils, Chromophobes (pituitary), 312
Chromosomes, 34–35
Chylomicrons, 266, 269
Chymotrypsin, 260, 283
Cilia, 27, 30, 83, 86, 90
    basal bodies, 28, 30, 90
    olfactory receptors, 381
Ciliary body, eye, 382, 389
Circulatory system, 144–156
Circumvallate papillae, 244, 245
Clara cells, 229, 230
Clathrin, 19
Clear cells (C cells), 316
Cleavage furrow, cell division, 36
Coated pits, 19
Coated vesicles, 15, 19
Cochlea, 394, 399
Cochlear nerve, 402
Codons, 34
Collagens, 66, 69
    bone, 175, 179, 182
    cartilage, 173
Collecting system, kidney, 289, 304–305
Colon, 270–271, 273
Colostrum, 370
Columnar epithelia, 82, 83
Communicating junctions, 86, 89
Complement, 193
Cones, 386, 387
Conjunctiva, 392
Connective tissue, 65–79
Connexons, 89
Constrictor pupillae muscle, 390
Cornea, 382, 392
Corona radiata, ovarian follicle, 345

Corpora amylacea, prostate, 338
Corpora cavernosa, 339
Corpus albicans, 342, 347, 349
Corpus fibrosum, 348
Corpus luteum, 44, 342, 347, 348
Corpus spongiosum, 339
Corti, organ of, 394, 399, 401
Cortical sinuses, lymph nodes, 206
Corticotrophs, 313
Cortisol, 321
Counter-current multiplier system, 289, 300, 306
Crista ampullaris, 394, 404
Crystalloids, eosinophils, 52
Cuboidal epithelia, 82, 85
Cumulus oophorus, 345
Cupula, 404
Cutaneous plexus, 171
Cystic duct, 282
Cytokeratin, 27
Cytokinesis, 34, 36
Cytology, exfoliative cervical, 358
Cytoskeleton, 4, 27–31
    enterocytes, 269
    linkage with extracellular matrix, 67
    platelets, 57
Cytosol, 4
Cytotoxic T cells, 195
Cytotrophoblast, 360, 364, 365

Decidua, 363
Deciduous dentition, 239
Demarcation membrane system, megakaryocytes, 63
Dendrites, 117
Dendritic cells, 198
    lymph nodes, 210, 211
Dense-cored vesicles, 127
Dense granules, platelets, 57
Dense tubular system, platelets, 57
Dental pulp, 242
Dentine, 239, 242
Dermis, 157, 163
Descemet's membrane, 392
Desmin, 27
Desmosomes, 86, 87, 88
Diarthroses (Synovial joints), 189
Differentiation, cells, 32, 33
Diffuse neuroendocrine system, 327
Digestion, 249, 254, 262
Dilator pupillae muscle, 390
Diploidy, 34
Diplosomes (centrioles), 27, 28, 30
Discs (intervertebral), 191
Disse, space of, 277, 280
Distal convoluted tubules, 289, 301
DNA, 34
DOPA, Dopamine, 377
Ductuli efferentes, testis, 329, 335
Ductus (Vas) deferens, 336
Duodenum, 260, 263, 267, 273
Dura mater, 138
Dynein, 27, 90

Ear, 393–405
Eccrine secretion, 93, 164, 169
Efferent arterioles, kidney, 291, 293
Ejaculatory ducts, 336
Elastin, 66, 72–73
    in arteries, 147, 148
    in cartilage, 175

    in lung, 235
Electron microscopy, 2–3
Enamel, 239, 241
Endocardium, 144, 145
Endocervical glands, 358
Endochondral ossification, 183, 185, 186, 187
Endocrine system, 96, 310–327
    gastrointestinal tract, 326, 327
    respiratory tract, 326
Endocytosis, 8, 15, 19
    small intestine, 269
Endolymph, 394
Endomembrane system, smooth muscle, 110
Endometrium, 341, 351–356
Endomysium, 98
Endoneurium, 130
Endoplasmic reticulum, 4–5, 11, 13–14, 15
Endothelium, 76, 80, 81
    capillaries, 138–139, 150, 151–153
Energy production and storage, 22–26
Enkephalins, 323
Enterochromaffin cells, 324, 326
Enterocytes, 264, 269
Enterokinase, 260, 283
Enzyme histochemistry, 3, 407
Eosin, 11, 406
Eosinophilia, 46
Eosinophils, 52–53, 64, 78
Ependymal cells, 134, 137
Epicardium, 144, 145
Epidermis, 85, 157–162
Epididymis, 329, 336
Epimysium, 98
Epineurium, 130
Epiphyses, 185–186
Epithelia, 80–96
    basement membranes, 67, 80
Erectile tissue, 339–340
Erythroblastic islands, 61
Erythrocytes, 47–48, 64, 218
Erythropoiesis, 61, 62
Erythropoietin, 286
Euchromatin, 11
Eukaryotes, 4
Eustachian tube, 222, 394, 397
Exfoliative cytology, 358
Exocrine glands, 93–95
Exocytosis, 8, 15, 18
External auditory canal, 394, 396
External lamina, 67
Extracellular matrix, 65
Extraembryonic coelom, 361, 367
Eye, 382–392
Eyelid, 393

Facilitated diffusion, 8
Facultative dividers, 33
Fallopian tube, 83, 341, 349–350
Fascia adherens, 115
Fascia occludens, 88
Fast-twitch fibres, 105, 107
Female reproductive system, 341–371
Fertilisation, 360
Fibrillin, 66, 67
Fibroblasts, 65, 69–70
    bone marrow, 59
Fibronectin, 67
Filiform papillae, 244
Filtration, glomerular, 294

Fixation, *see* Histological techniques
Flagella, 30, 332, 333
Fluorescence microscopy
  immunohistochemistry, 407
  noradrenaline, 127
  nucleic acids, 11
Focal densities, smooth muscle, 111
Follicle stimulating hormone, 341
Follicles (lymphoid), 206, 208, 210,
    215, 221, 271
Follicles (ovary), 342, 344–346, 348
Follicles (thyroid gland), 96, 315–317
Fovea, 382, 387, 388
Freeze-etching, 12
Fungiform papillae, 244
Fusiform cells, cerebral cortex, 379
Fusiform vesicles, urinary epithelium,
    309

G cells, 259
Gall bladder, 282
Gametogenesis, 330
Ganglia, 133, 250
Gap junctions, 86, 89
Gastrin, 259, 283
Gastrin cells, 327
Gastro-oesophageal junction, 254
Gastrointestinal tract, 249–273
  endocrine system, 326, 327
Genital tract
  female, 349–359
  male, 328–340
Genome, 34
Germinal centres, lymph nodes, 210
Germinal epithelium, 342, 344
Gingiva, 238, 243
Glands, 80
  exocrine, 93–95
  endocrine, 310
Glassy membrane, 348
Glial cells, 134
Glial fibrillary acidic protein, 27, 135
Glomeruli, 288–289, 293–297
Glomus bodies, 171
Glucagon, 324
Glucocorticoids, 319, 321
Glycocalyx, 7, 265, 269
Glycogen, 22, 25
Glycolysis, 22
Glycoproteins, structural, 67
Glycosaminoglycans, 65–66
Goblet cells, 92, 263, 267
Gold immunohistochemistry, 407
Golgi apparatus, 4–5, 16–17, 25
Golgi cells, 376
Gonadotrophs, 313
Goormaghtigh cells, 303
Graafian follicle, 345
Granular cells, cerebellum, 376
Granule cells, cerebral cortex, 379
Granulocytes, 49, 61, 62, 78
Granulosa cells, 344, 347, 348
Grey matter, 134–135
Growth plates, 185–186
Gustatory cells, 380

Haemopoiesis, 58–63, 279
Hair cells, 401, 402, 404
Hairs, Hair follicles, 164, 166, 167, 168
Haploidy, 40, 330
Hassall's corpuscles, 204

Haversian systems, 177, 178
Hearing, 401
Heart, 144–147
Heister, spiral valve of, 282
Helicine arteries, 340
Helicotrema, 394
Helper T cells, 195
Hemidesmosomes, 86, 89
Henle, loop of, 289, 300, 305
Heparin, mast cells, 228
Hepatocytes, 277, 278, 280
Hering, canals of, 276, 279
Hertwig, epithelial sheath of, 241
Heterochromatin, 11
High endothelial venules, 205, 211
His, bundle of, 146
Histiocytes, 76, 78
Histological techniques
  enzyme histochemistry, 3, 24, 107,
    128, 266, 279
  fixation, 3
    chrome, 323
    osmium, 26, 131
  histochemistry, 3, 50 *see also*
    Staining methods
  immunochemistry, 3, *see also*
    Staining methods
  methods for bone, 178, 181
  methods for nerve tissue, 120–121,
    128, 135, 154, 155, 372
  methods for teeth, 239
Histone proteins, 11, 34
Holocrine secretion, 93, 168
Horizontal cells (retina), 387
Horizontal cells of Cajal, 379
Hormones, 309
Horseradish peroxidase, 16, 407
Howell–Jolly bodies, 62
Howship's lacunae, 181
Human chorionic gonadotrophin, 347
Hyaloid canal, 382
Hyaluronic acid, 66
Hyaluronidase, spermatozoa, 333
Hydrochloric acid secretion, 258
Hydrogen peroxide, 21
Hypoglossal nerve, central nuclei, 374
Hypophysis *see* Pituitary gland
Hypothalamus, hormone secretion and
    control, 311

Ileocaecal junction, 267
Ileum *see* Small intestine
Immune system, 193–221
  macrophages, 79
Immunoglobulins, 195, 200, 213
Immunohistochemistry, 3
Implantation, 360
Inflammation, 193
Infundibulum, Fallopian tube, 349
Inner cell mass, 360
Insulin, 324, 325
Integrins, 67, 89
Intercalated cells, renal collecting
    ducts, 304
Intercalated discs, cardiac muscle,
    112, 113, 115
Intercalated ducts, salivary glands,
    246, 247
Intermediate filaments, 27, 28, 29, 30
Interphase, 33
Intervertebral joints, 191
Intrafusal fibres, 142

Intramembranous ossification, 188
Intrinsic factor, 258
Introns, 13
Iodine, thyroid gland, 317
Iris, 382, 390
Islets of Langerhans, 324–325
Ito cells, 278

Jejunum *see* Small intestine
Joints, 172, 189–191
Junctional complexes, 86, 87
Junctions, cells, 86–89
Juxtaglomerular apparatus, 303

Karyolysis, Karyorrhexis, 43
Karyotyping, 34
Keratinising epithelia, 85, 158–161
Keratinocytes, 43, 158
Keratohyalin, 159
Kerkring, valves of (Plicae circulares),
    260, 261, 262
Kidney, 287–308
Kinesin, 27
Kinetochores, 34, 36
Kinocilia, 402, 404
Kulchitsky cells, 223, 229
Kupffer cells, 278

Labyrinth, 394, 402
Lacis cells, 303
Lacrimal gland, 392
Lactation, 370–371
Lacteals, 265
Lactiferous ducts and sinuses, 368
Lactotrophs, 313
Lamellar bodies, pneumocytes, 232, 235
Lamellar bone, 176
Lamina fibrosa, heart valve, 146, 147
Lamina propria, definition of, 250
Laminin, 67
Langerhans, islets of, 324–325
Langerhans cells, 162, 198
  see also Veiled cells
Late endosomes, 19
Lens, 382, 391
Leucocytes, 49–56, 78
Leydig cells, 331, 335
Lieberkühn, crypts of, 264
Ligaments, 172, 192
Light microscopy, 2
Limiting plates, liver, 276
Lingual tonsils, 245
Lip, 237, 238
Lipid laden interstitial cells, 300
Lipids, 26
  in adipocytes, 73
  lactation, 371
  small intestine, 266
Lipofuscin, 21, 321
Liver, 274–281
Long bones, 176
Loop of Henle, 289, 300, 305
Low-density lipoprotein receptors, 19
Luteinising hormone, 313, 341, 347
Lymph, 156, 213
Lymph nodes, 44, 205–212, 215
Lymphatic vessels, 144, 156, 236
Lymphocytes, 49, 55, 64, 78, 194–199
  clonal deletion, 42, 204
  formation, 61

in lymph nodes, 205, 208
MALT, 213–214
spleen, 221
surface markers, 201
see also B lymphocytes;
   T lymphocytes
Lysosomal enzymes, 20
Lysosomes, 15, 19, 20, 50

M cells, 215
Macrophages, 56, 78, 79
   alveolar, 231, 233
   lymph nodes, 209, 210
   tissue-fixed, 76, 78
Macula densa, juxtaglomerular
      apparatus, 303
Macula lutea, 382
Maculae (vestibule), 394, 402
Magnification, electron microscopy, 3
Major histocompatibility complex, 201
Malassez, epithelial rests of, 243
Male reproductive system, 328–340
Mammotrophs, 313
Martinotti, cells of, 379
Mast cells, 54, 76, 77, 228
Mastication, 237
Medial lemniscus, 375
Medulla oblongata, 374
Medullary cords, lymph nodes, 212
Medullary pyramids, kidney, 287
Medullary rays, kidney, 290
Megakaryocytes, 63
Meibomian glands, 393
Meiosis, 40–41, 330, 344
Meissner's corpuscles, 141
Meissner's plexus, 250, 252
Melanin, 21, 162, 166, 377
Melanocytes, 162, 166
Melatonin, 325
Membranes, 7–9
Meninges, 138–139
   optic nerve, 388
   spinal, 373
Menstrual cycle, 341, 351–355
Menstruation, 351, 355
Merkel cells, 140, 162
Merocrine secretion, 93, 164, 169
Mesangium, renal corpuscle, 292, 293,
      297, 303
Mesaxons, 122, 123
Mesenchyme, 69
Mesothelium, 80, 81, 236
Metachromasia, 54, 77
Metamyelocytes, 61, 62
Metaphase, 36
Metaphysis, 186
Metarterioles, 150
Microcirculation, 150–153
Microfibrils, 73
Microfilaments, 27, 28
Microglia, 134, 137
Microscopy, 2–3
Microtubule-associated proteins, 27
Microtubules, 27, 28, 29, 30, 31, 36
Microvilli, 7, 27, 82, 86, 87, 91, 269
Middle ear, 394
Milk, 371
Mineralocorticoids, 319, 321
Mitochondria, 4–5, 11, 22–24
Mitosis, 33, 34–39, 41
Mitotic index, 38
Moll, glands of, 393

Monocyte–macrophage system, 56
Monocytes, 49, 56, 61, 64
Morula, 360
Motor end plates (Neuromuscular
      junctions), 126, 128–129
Mouth, 237–248
Mucociliary escalators, 83
Mucosa, definition of, 250
   gastric, 254, 256
   gastrointestinal, 250, 251
   middle ear, 397
   nasal, 225
   neuroendocrine cells, 326
   oral, 237
   respiratory, 222
Mucosa-associated lymphoid tissue
      (MALT), 213–216, 223, 250
Mucous cells
   gastric glands, 255, 256
   salivary glands, 246
Mucus, Mucigens, 92, 247
Muller cells, 385
Multinucleate giant cells, 56
Multivesicular bodies, 19
Muscle, 97–115
   cardiac (myocardium), 23, 97,
      112–115, 144–145, 146
   skeletal, 24, 97–107
      fibre types, 107
      insertions into bone, 180
      neuromuscular spindles, 142
      tendinous insertion, 180
   smooth, 97, 108–111
      airways, 223
      gastrointestinal, 250
      uterus, 357
Muscular arteries, 147, 148–149
Muscularis mucosae, 252
Myelin, staining for, 372
Myelination, 121, 123–125, 137
Myelocytes, 61, 62
Myeloid cells (Granulocytes), 49, 61,
      62, 78
Myeloperoxidase, 50
Myenteric (Auerbach's) plexus, 250, 252
Myoblasts, Myotubes, 100
Myocardium, *see* Muscle, cardiac
Myoepithelial cells, 93, 97
   breast, 368
   iris, 390
   salivary glands, 248
Myofibrils, 101
Myofibroblasts, 97
Myointimal cells, 148
Myometrium, 357
Myosin, 27, 103, 111

Na⁺-K⁺ ATPase, 8, 9
   see also Sodium pump
Nails, 170
Natural killer cells (NK cells), 194
Necrosis, 42
Neocortex, 379
Nephrons, 286, 288–289
Nerve endings, 140–142
Nerve tissue, 11, 29, 116–142
   see also Central nervous system
Neurocrine action, 326
Neuroendocrine cells, 326, 327
   C cells, 316
   gastrointestinal, 255, 257, 259, 265,
      326, 327

respiratory, 326
Neurofilament proteins, 27
Neurofilaments, 30, 118
Neuroglia, 134
Neurohypophysis (Posterior pituitary),
      311, 314
Neuromuscular junctions, 126, 128–129
Neuromuscular spindles, 142
Neurones, 29, 117–129
   retina, 385–387
Neuropil, 134
Neurosecretion, 311
Neurotransmitters, 8, 116, 126
Neurovascular bundles, 155
Neutrophilia, 46
Neutrophils, 50–51, 64, 78
Nexus (Communicating) junctions,
      86, 89
Nissl substance, 118, 121
Noradrenaline, 127, 323
Normoblasts, 61, 62
Nose, 225
Nuclear envelopes, 4–5, 12, 16
Nuclear pores, 12
Nuclei, 4–5, 11–12, 25
Nucleoids, 21
Nucleoli, 11
Nucleoprotein, 11
Nucleus pulposus, 191
Nurse cells, 202

Occluding junctions, 86, 87, 88, 138
Oddi, sphincter of, 282
Odland bodies, 161
Odontoblasts, 241, 242
Oesophagus, 252, 253, 273
Oestrus cycle, 341
Olfactory mucosa, 225
Olfactory receptors, 381
Oligodendrocytes, 121, 123, 134, 137
Oocytes, 345
Oogonia, Ova, 40, 344, 346
Opsonisation, Opsonins, 51, 79, 193
Optic disc, 382, 388
Optic nerve, 388
Oral tissues, 237–248
Organs, 32
Ossicles, 394, 397
Ossification, 183–188
Osteoblasts, 175, 178, 180, 181
Osteoclasts, 175, 178, 181
Osteocytes, 175, 178, 179
Osteoid, 181
Otoliths, 402
Ova, 330, 345
Oval window, 394
Ovary, 341, 342–349
Ovulation, 345, 346
Oxidases, 21
Oxyntic cells, 255, 256, 257, 258
Oxyphil cells, parathyroid, 319
Oxytocin, 311
   lactation, 370

p53 gene, 42
Pacinian corpuscles, 141
Palate, 238
Palatine tonsils, 214
Pancreas, 95, 260, 283–285
   endocrine, 324–325
   exocrine, 18, 284

Paneth cells, 264, 265
Papillae (renal), 308
Papillae (tongue), 244–245
Papillary muscles, 144
Paracortex, lymph node, 208, 211
Paracrine hormones, 326
Parasympathetic ganglia, 133, 250, 252
Parathyroid gland, 318–319
Parathyroid hormone, 181, 318
Paraurethral glands, 340
Paraventricular nucleus, 311
Parenchyma, 32
Parietal (Oxyntic) cells, 255, 256, 257, 258
Parkinson's disease, 377
Parotid gland, 246
Pars intermedia, pituitary gland, 314
Parturition, 357
Passive diffusion, 8
Pelvicalyceal system, 287, 308
Penis, 339–340
Pepsin, Pepsinogen, 257
Peptic (Chief) cells, 255, 257
Periarteriolar lymphoid sheaths, spleen, 217, 218
Pericardium, 144, 145
Perichondrium, 172, 173
Pericytes, 151
Perilymph, 394
Perilymphoid zones, spleen, 218
Perimysium, 98, 99
Perineurium, 130
Periodontium, 238, 243
Periosteum, 179, 180
Peripheral nervous tissue, 130–133
Peristalsis, 108, 249
Peroxisomes, 21
Peyer's patches, 215
Phagocytosis, 19–20, 51, 294
    see also Macrophages
Phagolysosomes, 19, 20
Phagosomes, 51
Phospholipids, 7
Photoreceptors, 385–388
Physaliphorous cells, 191
Pia mater, 138
Pigmented cells, retina, 386
Pigments, 21
    iris, 390
Pillar cells, organ of Corti, 401
Pilosebaceous units, 168
Pineal gland, 325
Pinna, 394
Pinocytosis, 8, 19
Pituicytes, 314
Pituitary gland, 4–5, 309–314
Placenta, 359, 360, 362–366
Plasma cells, 11, 16, 78, 200
Plasma membranes, 4–5
Plasma, Plasma proteins, 46
Platelets, 57, 63, 64
Pleura, 236
Plicae circulares, 260, 261, 262
Pneumocytes, 231, 232, 235
Podocalyxin, 294
Podocytes, 288–289, 293, 294, 295
Polar trophoblast, 360
Polarity, 82
Polymorphs (Granulocytes), 49, 61, 62, 78
Polysomes, 13
Pons, 375
Portal tracts, liver, 276

Pregnancy
    breast, 370
    corpus luteum, 347
Preproinsulin, 325
Prickle cell layer, 158, 159
Principal cells (parathyroid), 319
Principal cells (renal collecting ducts), 304
Pro-opiomelanocortin, 313
Proerythroblasts, 61, 62
Progesterone, 347
Programmed cell death, 42
Proinsulin, 325
Prolactin, 311, 313
Prophase, 36
Prostate gland, 337–339
Proteins
    of membranes, 7
    synthesis, 12–13, 14
Proteoglycans, 54, 66, 172, 182
Proximal convoluted tubules, 9, 289, 298–299
Pseudopodia, 50, 51
Purkinje cells, 121, 376
Purkinje fibres (heart), 146
Pyknosis, 43
Pylorus, 259–260, 273
Pyramidal cells, cerebral cortex, 379

Ranvier, nodes of, 125
Rathke's pouch, 311
Receptor-mediated endocytosis, 19
Rectum, 271
Recycling endosomes, 19
Red pulp, 217, 218, 220
Reinke, crystals of, 335
Renal corpuscles, 287, 288–297
Renin, 286, 303
Reproductive system
    female, 341–371
    male, 328–340
Reserve cells, 33
Residual bodies, 19, 20
Respiration (cellular), 22
Respiration (mechanical), 222
Respiratory system, 222–236
    endocrine system, 326
    epithelia, 83, 223, 225, 226, 228, 231
Rete ridges, 157, 158
Rete testis, 329, 335
Reticular cells, 76
    bone marrow, 59
Reticulin, 66, 72
Reticulocytes, 48
Reticuloendothelial system, 56, 76
Retina, 382, 385–388
Rhodopsin, 386
Ribosomes, 13
Rods, 386, 387
Rough endoplasmic reticulum, 13–14
    neurones, 118, 121
Round window, 394
Ruffled borders, osteoclasts, 181

S phase, 33
Saccule, 394, 402
Saliva, 246
Salivary glands, 24, 95, 246–248
Saltatory conduction, 125
Sarcomeres, 103, 106, 114, 115

Sarcoplasmic reticulum, 15, 104
Satellite cells, skeletal muscle, 100
Scala media, 394, 399
Scala tympani, 394
Scala vestibuli, 394, 399
Scalp, 165, 393
Scanning EM, 2
    renal glomeruli, 295
Scars, 193
Schlemm, canal of, 382, 389, 390
Schmidt–Lanterman incisures, 125
Schwann cells, 29, 121–125, 128
Sclera, 382, 384
Sebum, Sebaceous glands, 95, 164, 168
Second messengers, 8
Secretin, 260, 283
Secretory IgA, 213
Secretory vesicles, 4–5
Self-tolerance, 194, 204
SEM see Scanning EM
Semen, 340
Semicircular canals, 394, 404–405
Seminal vesicles, 337
Seminiferous tubules, 329, 331
Sensory receptors, 140–142
Serotonin, platelets, 57
Sertoli cells, 331, 332, 334
Sharpey's fibres, 179, 180, 243
Sinoatrial node, 146
Sinusoids, liver, 274, 278
Skeletal tissues, 172–192
Skin, 157–171
    epithelium, 80, 85
    nerve endings, 140
Sliding filament theory, 102, 103
Small intestine, 260–269, 273
    absorption, 262
Smooth endoplasmic reticulum, 15
Sodium pump, 8
    proximal convoluted tubule, 298
Somatostatin, 324
Somatotrophs, 313
Sorting endosomes, 19
Spermatids, 331–332
Spermatogenesis, 330–333
Spermatogonia, 40, 331–333
Spermatozoa, 40, 331–333, 340
Spermiogenesis, 330–332
Spinal cord, 372, 373
Spindles, 27, 36
Spiral ganglion, 399, 402
Spiral valve of Heister, 282
Spleen, 216–221
Squamous epithelia, 81, 84–85
Stab cells, 61, 62
Staining methods
    electron microscopy, 3
    light microscopy, 2, 406–407
    particular methods
        acridine orange, 11
        alcian blue, 175, 186, 191, 225, 263, 270, 406
        azan, 11, 21, 71, 82, 83, 298, 302, 305, 308, 312, 320, 321, 344, 345, 350, 406
        Bielschowsky, 376
        chrome alum/haematoxylin, 407
        cresyl violet, 14
        elastin, 72, 66, 131, 146, 147, 148, 163, 165, 167, 175, 228, 229, 235, 406
        Giemsa, 17, 37, 47, 50, 52, 54, 55, 56, 57, 58, 62, 63, 406

gold methods, 28, 121, 406–407
Goldner's trichrome, 181
haematoxylin and eosin (H&E), 11, 406, and numerous examples throughout book
immunoperoxidase method, 17, 135, 202, 203, 210, 211, 216, 229, 245, 248, 259, 313, 339, 312, 314, 325, 339, 369, 407
iron haematoxylin, 17, 24, 108, 279
isamine blue/eosin, 96, 314, 407
lipid methods, 26, 407
Masson's trichrome, 71, 74, 99, 108, 109, 132, 141, 142, 144, 145, 159, 179, 253, 308, 309, 359, 388, 406
methylene blue, 379, 407
Nissl method, 121, 379, 407
Papanicolou method, 84, 358
PAS, 25, 68, 92, 256, 259, 263, 265, 278, 292, 298, 301, 406
Phloxine-tartrazine, 265
Reticulin, 72, 209, 212, 217, 220, 279, 406
Silver impregnation, 27, 68, 81, 120–121, 140, 141, 406
Supravital staining, 48
Toluidine blue, 54, 77, 90, 113, 159, 173, 211, 228, 231, 293, 406
Weigart-Pal, 373, 374, 375
Stapedius, 394
Starry sky appearance, 204
Stave cells, 220
Stellate cells
cerebellum, 376
cerebral cortex, 379
liver, 278
Stellate reticulum, 241
Stem cells, haemopoiesis, 58
Stereocilia, 86, 91, 336
hair cells, 401, 402
Steroid-secreting cells, 322, 345, 347
Steroids, adrenal, 319
Stomach, 254–260, 273
mucosa, 251
Stretch reflex, 142
Striated borders, 82, 91
Striated ducts, salivary glands, 246, 247, 248
Subarachnoid space, 138
Subcapsular sinus, lymph node, 206, 209
Sublingual gland, 246, 247
Submandibular gland, 246, 247
Submucosa, definition of, 252
Subpapillary plexus, 171
Substantia nigra, 377
Substantia propria, cornea, 392
Succinate dehydrogenase, 24
skeletal muscle, 107
Supporting tissues, 65–79
Suppressor T cells, 195
Supraoptic nucleus, 311
Surface immunoglobulins, 201
Surface markers, lymphocytes, 201
Surfactant, 235
Sustentacular cells
olfactory receptors, 381
taste buds, 380
Sutures, skull, 188
Sweat glands, 94, 164, 169, 170

Sympathetic nervous system
adrenal medulla, 323
ganglia, 133
Symphyses, 189
Synapses, 126–127
Synchondroses, 189
Syncytial knots, placenta, 366
Syncytiotrophoblast layer, 360, 364, 365
Syndesmoses, Synostoses, 189
Synovial joints, 189
Synovium, Synovial fluid, 190

T cell receptors, 201
T lymphocytes, 194–195
lymph nodes, 211
spleen, 221
thymus, 202, 204
T system, skeletal muscle, 104
Tamm–Horsfall protein, 300
Tarsus (eyelid), 393
Taste buds, 245, 380
Tectorial membrane, 401
Teeth, 238–243
mineralisation, 241
Telophase, 36
Tendons, 172, 192
Tensor tympani, 394
Terminal boutons, 126, 127, 128
Terminal bronchioles, 230
Terminal webs, 87, 88
Testis, 329–331, 334–336
Testosterone, 335
Thalamus, 377
Theca externa, 345, 348
Theca folliculi, 344
Theca interna, 345, 348
Theca lutein cells, 347, 348
Thymus, 202–204
Thyroglobulin, 316, 317
Thyroid gland, 96, 315–317
Thyrotrophs, 313
Thyroxine, 315, 317
Tight junctions, 86, 87, 88, 138
Tingible body macrophages, 210
Tissue-fixed macrophages, 76, 78
Tissues, 32
Tongue, 244–245
Tonofibrils, 159
Tonsils, 214
lingual, 245
Tooth, 238–243
Trachea, 226
Transcription, 13, 34
Transcytosis, 8
Transfer RNA, 13
Translation, 13
Transmembrane proteins, 7
Transmission EM, 2
Transport
across membranes, 8–9
intracellular, 15
Tri-iodothyronine, 315, 317
Trigeminal nerve, central nuclei, 374
Triglyceride, 22
Trophic hormones, 310, 311
Trophoblast, 360, 365
Tropocollagen, 66
Trypsin, 260, 283
Tubular myelin, pulmonary alveoli, 235
Tubules, kidney, 24, 289–300, 304–307

Tubulins, 27
Tubuloglomerular feedback mechanism, 303
Tubulovesicular system, gastric parietal cells, 258
Tunica albuginea, 329
Tunica vaginalis, 329
Tympanic cavity, 394
Tympanic membrane, 397

Umbilical cord, 367
Umbrella cells, 309
Upper respiratory tract, 222
Urate oxidase, 21
Ureter, 308
Urethra, 337, 340
Urinary tract, 286–309
Uterus, 351–358
Utricle, 394, 402
Uvea, 382

Vagina, 341, 359
Valves
heart, 146–147
lymphatic vessels, 156
veins, 154
Vas deferens, 336
Vasa recta, 289
Vasa vasorum, 144
Vasculature see Circulatory system
Vasopressin (ADH), 304, 311
Vater, ampulla of, 282
Veiled cells, 209, 211
Veins, 144, 154–155
Vellus hair, 166
Venules, 153, 154
Vermilion border, 237
Verumontanum, 338
Vestibule, 394
Villi (intestinal), 264, 265–266, 267
Villi (placental), 363, 366
Vimentin, 27
Vitamin D, 286
Vitello-intestinal duct, 367
Vitreous body, 382
Volkmann's canals, 177
Von Ebner's glands, 245, 380

Waldeyer's ring, 214, 245
Weibel–Palade bodies, 152
Weil, cell free zone of, 242
Wharton's jelly, 367
White adipose tissue, 73, 74
White matter, 134
White pulp, spleen, 217, 221
Wound healing, 70

Yolk sac, 367

Zeis, glands of, 393
Zona granulosa, 344, 345
Zona pellucida, 344
Zonula adherens, 86, 87, 88
Zonula occludens, 86, 87, 88, 138
Zymogen granules
pancreas, 284
peptic cells, 257
submandibular gland, 247